The BIG DOCTORS BOOK *of* HOME REMEDIES®

The BIG DOCTORS BOOK of HOME REMEDIES

QUICK FIXES, CLEVER TECHNIQUES, AND UNCOMMON CURES TO GET YOU FEELING BETTER FAST

BY THE EDITORS OF **Prevention**

RODALE

Rodale books may be purchased for business or promotional use or for special sales. For
information, please write to: Special Markets Department, Rodale Inc., 733 Third Avenue, New
York, NY 10017

Prevention is a registered trademark of Rodale Inc..
The Doctors Book of Home Remedies is a registered trademark of Rodale Inc.

Printed in the United States of America
Rodale Inc. makes every effort to use acid-free ∞, recycled paper ♻.

Icon art © iStock photo

Book design by Carol Angstadt

Library of Congress Cataloging-in-Publication Data

The big doctors book of home remedies : quick fixes, clever techniques, and uncommon
cures to get you feeling better fast / by the editors of Prevention.
      p.   cm.
Includes bibliographical references and index.
ISBN-13 978-1-60529-867-2 hardcover
ISBN-10 1-60529-867-0 hardcover
ISBN-13 978-1-60529-866-5 paperback
ISBN-10 1-60529-866-2 paperback
1. Medicine, Popular.   I. Prevention (Emmaus, Pa.)
RC81.B54   2009
616—dc22   2009015656

Distributed to the book trade by Macmillan

              10   9   hardcover
     4   6   8   10   9   7   5   3   paperback

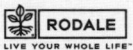

RODALE
LIVE YOUR WHOLE LIFE

We inspire and enable people to improve their lives and the world around them
For more of our products visit rodalestore.com or call 800-848-4735

Contents

C

D

E

Introduction

We can't pinpoint the exact moment in human history when home remedies came to be, but we imagine a scenario something like this: A crude hammer, fashioned from a stone, landed on an unfortunately placed finger. Throbbing pain ensued, perhaps accompanied by the muttering of a prehistoric blue streak. Our handyman ancestor may not have had access to a gel pack, but he would have instinctively sought relief in another way—by plunging his hand into a nearby cool stream, for example, or simply rubbing his finger until it felt better. Not very sophisticated, by today's standards, but it did the trick!

Whatever their origin, home remedies have stood the test of time. They grew from necessity, when formal medical care either didn't exist or wasn't widely available to everyone. Our forebears made do by using whatever they had on hand to treat their various ills, then sharing what worked through word of mouth.

The amazing thing about home remedies is that they have not just survived but thrived through the evolution of modern medicine. Despite all of the marvelous advances that have transformed how we treat illness and injury, home remedies tend to be our go-to choice for all but the most severe conditions.

It's easy to understand why: They're inexpensive (even free!), they're convenient, and most important, they work.

For this book, we've defined a home remedy as one that you can use on your own, with materials that you're likely to have at your disposal. You've got hundreds of tips and techniques to choose from, as you'll see in the pages that follow. The vast majority of the remedies come from interviews with M.D.s and other health professionals, all experts in their respective fields. They've helped us to separate the proverbial wheat from the chaff in creating the definitive home remedy resource for your bookshelf.

As our expert panelists would tell you, while certain remedies have been validated by clinical research, for many others the proof comes from the laboratory of real life. In other words, we don't know why they're effective; they just are. Indeed, a good number of them have found their way into our doctors' clinical practices.

The remedies presented here address a wide range of health concerns, from the mildly annoying to the more serious. Generally, any chronic condition—like asthma or diabetes, for example—requires proper medical care. In this case, home remedies can be helpful for easing symptoms and preventing flare-ups or complications, as long as your doctor okays them. Likewise, never stop taking a medication or otherwise change your treatment plan without consulting your doctor first.

Nearly all of the health concerns covered in this book are accompanied by a "When to Call a Doctor" box. Please read this information carefully and take it to heart. Sometimes professional medical attention is critical to getting a proper diagnosis and treatment. Time is of the essence, and spending it by trying one home remedy after another may not pay off in the long run.

Fortunately, such urgent situations are more the exception than the rule. You can use home remedies for the vast majority of common health concerns—and, in the process, continue the time-honored tradition of self-care that took root millennia ago. Let this book be your guide to your best health!

—*The Editors of Prevention*

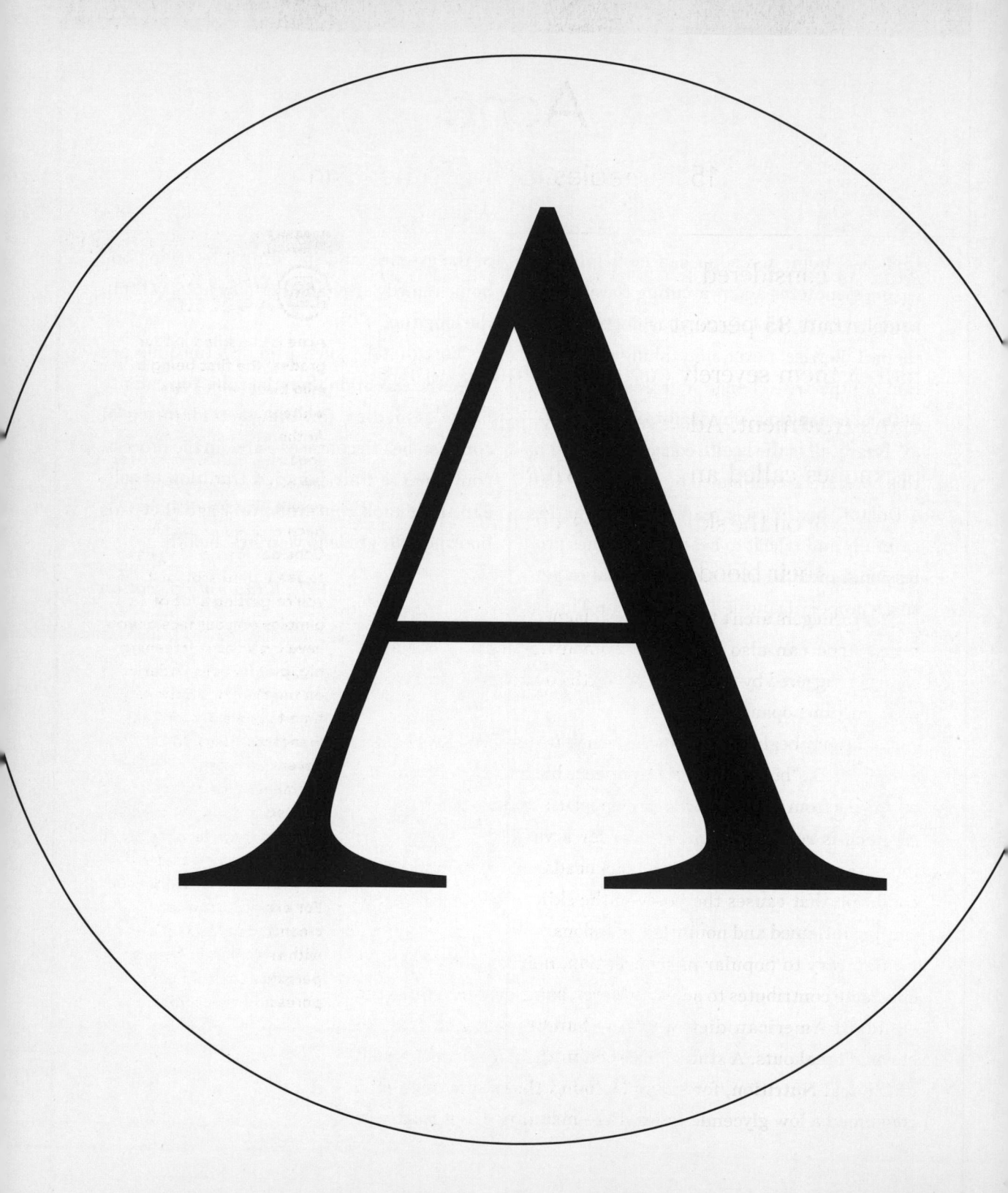

Acne

15 Remedies for Smoother Skin

Acne is considered a natural rite of passage. In fact, about 85 percent of teenagers have pimples, half of them severely enough to require a physician's treatment. Adolescents develop acne when hormones called androgens, which increase the amount of oil the skin produces, circulate at higher levels in their blood.

Yet teenagers aren't the only ones plagued by nasty skin eruptions. Acne can also beleaguer women undergoing hormone changes triggered by menstruation, birth control pills, pregnancy, even early menopause.

"Acne may begin and end in the teen years for men," says Laurie J. Polis, M.D., "but women can experience blemishes, pimples, and outbreaks from puberty through menopause and beyond."

Acne is really a catchall term for a variety of symptoms, including pimples, whiteheads, blackheads, and skin cysts. It's a condition that causes the pores of the skin to become clogged, causing inflamed and noninflamed lesions.

Contrary to popular misconception, neither dirty hair nor chocolate contributes to acne. However, some evidence links the standard American diet of greasy hamburgers and fries to chronic breakouts. A study published in the American Journal of Clinical Nutrition, for example, found that young men who consumed a low glycemic index diet—meaning a diet relatively

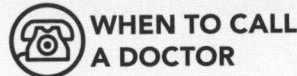
WHEN TO CALL A DOCTOR

Acne is classified in four grades, the first being a mild bout, with a few whiteheads and blackheads. At the other end of the spectrum, grade four cases are often accompanied by severe inflammation that becomes red or purple. Consider it a flashing light to see a dermatologist. "If you're getting a lot of pimples on your face or you have cystic acne (meaning big, painful boils under or on the skin), it's definitely time to see a doctor," says Francesca Fusco, M.D. Severe acne can result in permanent scarring if it isn't treated properly. A dermatologist can offer prescription medications that will help clear even severe acne. For example, topical creams, gels, and lotions with vitamin A or benzoyl peroxide can help unblock pores and reduce bacteria.

void of junk food—developed significantly fewer acne lesions than those who munched on high GI fare.

Nevertheless, experts agree that genetics is the major risk factor for chronic acne. So if both of your parents had acne as adults, there's a very good chance that you will, too. But being at risk for acne and actually experiencing it are two different things. Usually it takes some other factor to trigger a breakout, explains Francesca Fusco, M.D. That something can be hormonal fluctuations, stress, sun exposure, or seasonal changes. Certain types of makeup, as well as oral contraceptives, also can cause pimples to appear.

So what can you do to keep your skin smooth and clear? Start with these tips.

■ **CHANGE YOUR MAKEUP.** "Oil-based makeup is a big problem," says Dr. Fusco. "The pigments in foundation, rouge, cleansing cream, and night moisturizer aren't the problem, and neither is the water in the products. It's just the oil." The oil is usually a derivative of fatty acids, which are intended to keep skin soft and supple. In some people, though, they can cause breakouts.

"Use a non-oil-based makeup if you are prone to acne, and avoid layering mineral makeup throughout the day," says Dr. Fusco. "There's some preliminary evidence suggesting that mineral powder makeup contributes to inflammatory acne, which looks like little red bumps."

■ **READ THE LABELS.** The most important thing to look for on a label is the term "noncomedogenic," says Dr. Fusco. Beyond that, avoid cosmetic products that contain lanolins, isopropyl myristate, sodium lauryl sulfate, laureth-4, and D & C red dyes. Like oil, these ingredients are too rich for the skin.

■ **LATHER UP.** "Wash your makeup off thoroughly every night," says Dr. Fusco. Use a mild soap twice a day and wash away any soap film left behind. Rinsing well will help remove any debris, dead skin cells, and all traces of cleanser. Splashing the face five to ten times with fresh water should do it, says Dr. Fusco.

■ **BLAME IT ON THE PILL.** Research suggests that certain birth control pills, such as Ovral (norgestrel and ethinyl estradiol), Loestrin (norethindrone acetate and ethinyl estradiol), and Norinyl (norethindrone and ethinyl estradiol) can aggravate acne. If you're on the Pill and have an acne problem, discuss it with your doctor. She may be able to switch you to another brand or prescribe a different birth control method.

"Several brands of oral contraceptives can help reduce moderate acne and promote clearer, more healthful looking skin," says Dr. Polis. "Ask your dermatologist or ob-gyn for recommendations. Just remember that it might take a month or two before you'll see an improvement in your skin."

Other medications, including lithium (for mood disorders), steroids (such as prednisone),

How Hollywood Hides Blemishes

Don't celebrities ever break out? "You bet they do," says Hollywood makeup artist Maurice Stein. "The difference is, they can't let their pimples or any other blemish show."

Stein has been a makeup artist for more than 30 years, touching up famous faces in such movies as *M*A*S*H*, *Funny Girl*, and the original *Planet of the Apes* films.

Guerrilla warfare is the only way to fight the pimple that always sprouts at the wrong time. So here are two combat tips from the trenches in Hollywood. Stein says that he has used these on "some of the most expensive faces in the world."

Put makeup to the test. The right makeup will totally block out the discoloration, whether it's pink, red, or purple. While you can't really tell the pigment level of a product by looking at it, you can tell by sampling it. "Take a drop and rub it on your skin," suggests Stein. "If it's so solid in color that you can't see your own skin underneath, then you know it has a high pigment level and will cover your blemish well."

Try a layered look. "When I cover a pimple on an entertainer's face, I use two thin layers of foundation with a layer of loose translucent powder between each layer," Stein says. This helps set each layer.

and thyroid medications, also can contribute to acne, says Dr. Fusco. Talk to your doctor about potential outbreaks.

Otherwise, there isn't much you can do to a pimple to make it go away faster.

■ **ATTACK BLACKHEADS.** The black part of a blackhead is not dirt. In fact, dermatologists aren't sure what it is, but they do know that squeezing won't result in a pimple. "If you suffer from a lot of clogged pores or blackheads, try using topical treatments containing retinoic acid (retinol, Retin-A, Tazorac, and others)," says Dr. Polis. "Those medications loosen the sticky cells and facilitate removal." You should also have a properly trained aesthetician steam open the pores and clean them periodically, she says, or use pore-cleaning strips such as Biore.

■ **USE OTCS TO KNOCK OUT ACNE.** You can fight back an acne attack with over-the-counter products like salicylic acid, benzoyl peroxide, or sulfur. "My first choice is salicylic acid," says Dr. Fusco. "It unclogs already clogged pores and exfoliates the top layer of skin. Plus, not many people are allergic to salicylic acid." Her second choice is benzoyl peroxide. It unclogs the pores and it's also bacteriostatic, meaning it may reduce the amount and strength of bacteria on the skin so they're less likely to multiply in the pores.

Sulfur helps reduce redness of the skin and dries out the area.

OTC acne products come in various forms, such as gels, liquids, lotions, and creams. They come in a range of concentrations, too—and the stronger they are, the more likely they are to irritate the skin. Dry skin, in particular, can be sensitive to benzoyl peroxide.

No matter what sort of OTC acne product you choose, experts recommend starting with a lower-strength concentration and then increasing slowly. For benzoyl peroxide, a low strength would be about 2.5 percent; for salicylic acid and sulfur, more like 0.5 to 3 percent. "In cases of sensitivity, it's a good idea to spot-test a small patch of skin—on the side of the face, for example—for a few days before applying a new product all over," Dr. Polis advises.

"Be sure to clean your skin thoroughly before applying any over-the-counter acne medication," Dr. Fusco adds. "And if you have sensitive skin, wait a bit after cleansing before treatment."

You may notice some redness at first, which is normal. But if the redness doesn't clear or it develops into a rash, stop using the product altogether.

■ **GET A PEEL.** Both glycolic acid and salicylic peels (and products) can help combat acne, but salicylic acid components provide a more prolonged effect against pimples and clogged pores, says Dr. Polis.

■ **STAY OUT OF THE SUN.** Acne medications may cause adverse reactions after sun

exposure, so you should minimize time in sunlight and under infrared heat lamps until you know how you will react. Even more important, cautions Dr. Polis, is to know that sunlight aggravates acne. "Most people think it helps clear the skin, but this is a temporary reaction and sun exposure can actually cause a flare-up of acne 2 to 4 weeks after exposure," she says.

■ **USE ONE REMEDY AT A TIME.** Be careful not to mix treatments. If you use an OTC acne product, stop using it if you get prescription medication for your acne. Slowly introduce products so you can see how your skin reacts, says Dr. Fusco. Benzoyl peroxide, for example, is a close cousin to tretinoin (Retin-A) and other products containing vitamin A derivatives, so don't use both at the same time.

■ **TREAT IT WITH TEA.** Research shows that using a 2 percent tea lotion significantly reduces acne flare-ups. If a pimple is red or inflamed, soak a chamomile tea bag in cold water and then apply it to your skin for 30 seconds or so, suggests Dr. Polis. Chamomile is a

A

natural anti-inflammatory and will calm an angry pimple.

■ **DON'T TOUCH YOUR FACE.** "Frequently touching or rubbing your face, which we all do without thinking, can aggravate acne," says Dr. Polis. In fact, rubbing from a cell phone is a common culprit of acne along the jaw line or chin.

■ **LEAVE WELL ENOUGH ALONE.** Don't squeeze pimples or whiteheads. A pimple is an inflammation, and squeezing it could increase the redness and even cause an infection. Squeezing a whitehead could burst the wall of the skin pore and spill the contents onto the skin, ending in a pimple. The one exception is a pimple with a head of yellow pus. Gentle pressure will usually pop the head, and once the pus is out, the pimple will heal more quickly.

PANEL OF ADVISORS

FRANCESCA FUSCO, M.D., IS A CLINICAL ASSISTANT PROFESSOR OF DERMATOLOGY AT MOUNT SINAI MEDICAL CENTER IN NEW YORK CITY.

LAURIE J. POLIS, M.D., IS A BOARD-CERTIFIED COSMETIC DERMATOLOGIST AT SOHO SKIN AND LASER DERMATOLOGY IN NEW YORK CITY.

MAURICE STEIN IS A COSMETOLOGIST AND HOLLYWOOD MAKEUP ARTIST. HE IS THE OWNER OF CINEMA SECRETS, A FULL-SERVICE BEAUTY SUPPLIER FOR THE PUBLIC AND A THEATRICAL BEAUTY SUPPLIER FOR THE ENTERTAINMENT INDUSTRY IN BURBANK, CALIFORNIA.

Addiction

11 Ways to Conquer Unhealthy Behaviors

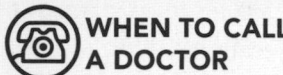

WHEN TO CALL A DOCTOR

Denial is one of the hallmarks of addiction. People with drug, alcohol, or other addictions often insist that their behavior is normal, even when the destruction is all around them.

Are friends, family members, or coworkers gently suggesting that you may have a problem? Listen to them. Look at your recent behavior. Ask yourself if they're seeing something that you don't.

"Try to solve the problems on your own," advises Tom Horvath, Ph.D. "Try cutting back or quitting entirely—and get the support of the people around you. If you've made one or several attempts that don't seem to be going far or fast enough, then it's time to get professional help."

Imagine a man who knocks back a few stiff drinks after work. Is he a "pleasure" drinker or an alcoholic? What about the woman who raids the refrigerator when she's tired or depressed, or the millions of Americans who spend hours sitting in front of the TV or surfing the Internet?

Harmless diversions—or addictions?

Most people have compulsive behaviors that they'd like to change. They find something they like that makes them feel good, and they use it again and again as a kind of coping mechanism, says Tom Horvath, Ph.D.

We tend to think of addictions in their most severe forms: the drug abuser who steals for the next fix, for example, or the compulsive gambler who empties the family bank account into slot machines. But many Americans have milder addictions. They crave substances or experiences that make them feel good temporarily, but that often have harmful long-term consequences.

If you suspect that you have an addiction—to alcohol, cigarettes, gambling, food, the Internet, or anything else—ask yourself this question: Has the behavior caused enough problems for you to consider stopping or cutting back? "In some cases, it's not clear whether a person's substance use reflects abuse or a more serious addiction," says Peter A. DeMaria Jr., M.D. The following techniques might help you determine whether your problem is a compulsive behavior that you can curb on your own, or a more serious addiction that requires professional help.

■ **START BY LISTING PROS AND CONS.** It's difficult for most people to recognize that they have an addiction. One way to find out is to list the pros and cons of the behavior that's troubling you.

First, write down all the things that you like about the substance or activity. If you drink, for example, the list might include things such as "It helps me unwind" or "I like the feeling of euphoria it gives me."

Second, write down the benefits of quitting: "I'd be more productive if I didn't drink" or "I'd have fewer Friday night fights with my spouse."

Now, compare the lists. Does it appear that the costs of your behavior outweigh the benefits? You've just recognized that you have some problems—the first step toward making the necessary changes, says Dr. Horvath.

Dr. DeMaria also suggests asking friends and family members how the substance or activity affects your life and if they see negative consequences to your behaviors. If they answer yes, you need to decide for yourself what steps you're willing to take to curb some of your behaviors. You're never cured of a true addiction, he adds, but you can bring your addictions under control.

■ **TAPER OFF—OR STOP COMPLETELY.** Some people wean themselves from addictions by initially smoking 10 fewer cigarettes each day, for example, or gambling once a week instead of every night. Others find it easier to stop the behavior cold turkey.

Both approaches can be effective. "With weaning, people are generally less scared, so they're more motivated," says Dr. Horvath. Going cold turkey is harder initially, but the process is faster. "You pay more up front, but it's easier to maintain because there is a shorter transition period," he explains.

■ **DISTANCE YOURSELF FROM CRAVINGS.** Anyone who curtails addictive substances or behaviors will go through a withdrawal period. The desire—for one more cigarette, one more drink, one more day at the track—can be unbearably intense.

"I advise people to keep their cravings at a distance," says Dr. Horvath. Distract yourself by calling a friend, walk around the block, washing the dishes. Do whatever you can to take your mind off the craving.

In other words, acknowledge how you're feeling. Admit to yourself your discomfort. But don't give in. "Just because you have an itch doesn't mean you have to scratch," Dr. Horvath adds. Be strong. Individual cravings will disappear in minutes or even seconds, and the entire urge will often leave in a month or two.

■ **STAY BUSY.** "A lot of people who make the commitment to quit an addiction find themselves sitting at home all the time," says Dr. DeMaria. If you don't keep busy—with exercise, hobbies, or other activities that keep your mind and body active—you'll find yourself focusing more and more on the addiction.

"Exercise can be especially helpful, because it's a way of reconnecting to things that are healthy," Dr. DeMaria adds.

■ **GET YOUR MIND RACING.** One way to distract yourself from cravings is to think about something—anything—at high speed. Count ceiling tiles as quickly as you can. Try reading book titles backward. Do repetitious math problems in your head—such as subtracting 7 from 1,000, 7 from 993, and so on.

"When you do these sorts of things quickly, they take up your entire mind, which will help you get past the desire," says Dr. Horvath.

■ **AVOID BEHAVIOR TRIGGERS.** If you've just quit smoking, the last thing you need is an evening at a smoke-filled party. If you've been obsessed with the Internet, it's probably a good idea to avoid shopping for Christmas gifts online.

Alcoholics Anonymous (AA), SMART Recovery, and other self-help programs teach members to steer clear of people, places, or things that are associated with their addictions. "Some people will alter their walking or driving routes to avoid parts of the city where they used to buy drugs or to stay away from people that were a bad influence," says Dr. DeMaria. "With smoking, talking on the phone may be a trigger. You have to recognize your triggers and figure out how to respond when you're confronted."

As time goes by, you'll find that addiction triggers will lose some of their pull.

■ **SUBSTITUTE GOOD BEHAVIORS FOR BAD ONES.** Avoidance is helpful in the early stages of fighting addictions, but no one can avoid all sources of temptation indefinitely. You can, however, develop substitute habits or ways to manage your cravings, says Dr. DeMaria. When you crave a cigarette, for example, chew gum. In some cases, the substitute may be temporary—you probably don't want to be eating celery for the rest of your life every time you feel hungry—but some substitutes may become healthful habits that you can sustain for life. After a while, your new habits will take the place of the old ones.

■ **MAKE IT HARDER TO INDULGE.** Addictions are grounded in habits, which means people sometimes indulge without thinking about what they're doing. Smokers, for example, may puff on a cigarette that they don't remember lighting. People with eating problems may raid the refrigerator and be unaware that they left the living room.

One way to break unconscious habits is to make them harder to practice. A smoker, for example, might put a pack of cigarettes inside a box and wrap the whole thing with rubber bands. You still may smoke, but at least you won't be doing it automatically.

The same approach works with other addictions. Turn off the computer when you sign off the Internet—and maybe crawl under the desk to pull the plug. Clear the house of alcohol, pornography, or other "forbidden" things. Putting obstacles between you and your addiction will force you to think about what you're doing, which in turn will make the addiction easier to overcome, says Dr. Horvath.

■ **FIND NEW WAYS TO BE FULFILLED.** It's not enough merely to give up unhealthy behaviors. If you're going to be successful, you need to replace addictions with something positive.

"In order to develop new habits, you need to gradually change the sources of satisfaction in your life," says Dr. Horvath. This could be as simple as creating a healthier lifestyle. Instead of spending the night in front of the television, for example, go to bed early and get more rest. You might focus more of your energy on eating healthful foods, exercising regularly, or even donating several hours a week to a charity. Spending time with friends is a good idea, too, because studies show that the more social support the less likelihood for relapse.

■ **JOIN A SUPPORT GROUP.** There are thousands of self-help groups for overcoming every sort of addiction—to alcohol, drugs, sex, overeating, and the Internet, to name a few. These groups are free, don't require insurance, and can be very effective, either by themselves or in combination with therapy, says Dr. DeMaria.

In a support group, you spend time with people in various stages of recovery, says Dr. DeMaria. "They've been through it all before, and they can act as role models and mentors."

Every group has a different mix of messages and personalities. If you find yourself in a gathering that doesn't feel right, don't give up on the idea. "I usually advise people to go to at least six different meetings in order to find one they like," he says.

Keep in mind, too, that different groups offer different approaches to recovery. Besides the traditional Alcoholics Anonymous (AA) model, options include SMART Recovery, Moderation Management, Women for Sobriety, LifeRing Secular Recovery, and Secular Organizations for Sobriety. Even if you can't find a meeting in your locality, most offer free online support in various formats.

■ **LEARN FROM SETBACKS.** Nearly everyone who struggles with addictions reverts on occasion. Expect it, says Dr. Horvath. Don't get discouraged, and don't give up.

"When slips happen, ask yourself why they happened. Then learn from them," says Dr. Horvath. "Persistence is the most important virtue. Everyone who keeps going will be successful. Eventually, you run out of ways to make mistakes and you will build a life that eliminates addiction problems and is also filled with satisfactions and pleasures that would not have been possible while you were engaged in an addictive behavior."

PANEL OF ADVISORS

PETER A. DEMARIA JR., M.D., IS A CLINICAL ASSOCIATE PROFESSOR OF PSYCHIATRY AND BEHAVIORAL SCIENCE AT TEMPLE UNIVERSITY SCHOOL OF MEDICINE IN PHILADELPHIA.

TOM HORVATH, PH.D., IS PRESIDENT OF PRACTICAL RECOVERY SERVICES, AN ADDICTION TREATMENT CENTER IN LA JOLLA, CALIFORNIA, AND PRESIDENT OF SMART RECOVERY, AN ABSTINENCE-ORIENTED SUPPORT GROUP FOR THOSE WITH ADDICTIVE BEHAVIORS.

Age Spots

9 Ways to Out the Spots

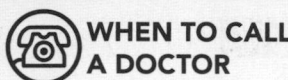
WHEN TO CALL A DOCTOR

If your age spots don't respond to home remedies, or if you have an age spot that bleeds, itches, tingles, or changes in size or color, it's time to see your doctor. Some skin cancers, such as melanoma, can look like age spots.

The term *age spots* is a misnomer. These flat, circular, brown areas that commonly appear on the backs of hands as well as on necks, faces, and shoulders are actually large, sun-induced freckles with no relation to age, says Audrey Kunin, M.D.

"The reason they're called age spots is because they usually occur from sun exposure over time—which means that for a lot of people they won't show up on their skin until they get a little older," she says.

While age spots are common during the fifth decade of life and beyond, they can appear on someone who's had significant sun exposure as early as the late twenties or thirties. Sunlight contains ultraviolet (UV) rays that cause suntans and sunburns. As time goes by, this sun damage causes excess pigment to deposit in the skin, which eventually leads to the flat, brown, skin freckles known as age spots, liver spots, or sun spots.

No matter what they're called, they're unsightly. And, if they change in size, they may indicate skin cancer, which is why it's a good idea to have a dermatologist examine your skin at least once a year.

Assuming they are indeed age spots, here are some tips on concealing and fading them (as well as preventing more).

■ **LIGHTEN UP.** If your age spots aren't too big or too dark, over-the-counter bleaching agents could help fade them, Dr. Kunin says. Look for products such as Porcelana and Palmer's Skin Success Cream, which contain 2 percent hydroquinone, the best-known active ingredient used in many types of bleaching agents. Hydroquinone lightens age spots until they become less noticeable or even disappear. It works best with a glycolic acid moisturizer, like Neutrogena Pore Refining Cream or Alpha Hydrox Enhanced Creme, which smooths the skin.

Apply the bleaching agent twice a day to your sun spots, carefully following the manufacturer's directions. Dab the cream directly onto

Prescription-Strength Help to Fade Spots

For especially stubborn age spots that have been given the all-clear by your dermatologist, a prescription-strength fade cream with 4 percent hydroquinone could be your first course of action. "Rub it on twice a day for 21 to 28 days, and you may see marked improvement," says C. Ralph Daniel III, M.D. For a stronger, quicker bleaching effect, some doctors prescribe vitamin A creams such as tretinoin (Retin-A and Renova) along with prescription-strength hydroquinone. Some studies involving laboratory animals have raised questions about the safety of hydroquinone—specifically, whether it might contribute to cancer. To date, no such link has been identified in humans, and doctors continue to prescribe hydroquinone to patients. Still, you should talk with your doctor about the benefits and risks, based on your own health history.

If creams fail to do the trick, your doctor has several treatment options at his disposal to make age spots disappear, says Dr. Daniel. For instance, your doctor can freeze them with liquid nitrogen. After a few weeks, the spots peel off. "This is a highly effective procedure for many benign age spots," he says.

A second treatment procedure is a chemical peel—done with trichloroacetic acid (TCA) or glycolic acid. These treatments can be quite effective for all body areas but may cause scarring and whitening of the skin if not done properly. The upper layer of affected skin takes 2 to 3 days to peel from your face or 5 to 7 days from your arms and chest.

A third, and much more expensive, procedure (average cost ranges between $2,000 and $6,000, depending on how large an area is treated) is laser resurfacing. During this procedure, the doctor uses pulses of laser light to fade the spots. The laser resurfacing procedure can take a half hour to an hour to perform and 2 to 6 weeks to heal.

"A much less expensive and quicker procedure than lasers is a relatively new technique known as Collagen Induction Therapy (CIT) or more simply microneedling," says Nelson Lee Novick, M.D. "The procedure takes only about 5 minutes to perform and has little or no downtime; most people return to work or social activities immediately afterward." Two to four treatments, spaced at 4 to 6 week intervals, are generally required for optimal lightening. Treatment costs may range between $350 and $450 per session, depending upon the number and location of the age spots.

the age spots with a cotton swab so that you don't bleach the pigment in unaffected areas.

"Be patient," says Dr. Kunin. "You won't see results overnight. These lightening agents often take 6 to 12 months to do the job." Stop the treatment when the age spots disappear, or the affected area may become lighter than your normal skin tone.

Want a more natural approach? Some plant extracts, such as aloe, flavonoids, licorice, yeast derivatives, and polyphenols can lighten the skin when applied topically.

■ **SLATHER ON THE SUNSCREEN BEFORE HEADING OUTDOORS.** Even if you already have age spots, sunscreen keeps existing ones from darkening and helps prevent more from popping up, says Dr. Kunin.

Buy a broad-spectrum sunblock (which protects you from both the UVA and UVB rays of the sun) with a sun protection factor (SPF) of at least 30. Apply it to exposed skin 10 to 15 minutes before you go outside, says C. Ralph Daniel III, M.D. Tests show that SPF 30 sunblock protects the skin against about 93 percent of the sun's UV rays, he says.

Cures from the Kitchen

 Cut a few lemon slices and place them directly onto your age spots for 10 to 15 minutes once a day, suggests Audrey Kunin, M.D. "The acid in the fresh lemon juice helps lighten the age spots in some cases." It won't happen overnight, though. Dr. Kunin says that you'll notice a difference in 6 to 12 weeks. Watch carefully. Overuse may cause the upper layer of skin to peel.

Be sure to use sunblock whenever you're planning to be outdoors for more than 10 to 15 minutes, whether you'll be on the golf course, tennis court, or ski slope. It's especially important if you spend a lot of time on a boat or at the beach, because the sun's rays reflect off the water.

Remember, too, to reapply sunscreen frequently, because perspiration and water can wash it off. Experts suggest using enough sunscreen to fill a shot glass every time you slather up. Dr. Daniel recommends Neutrogena #70. "It's water resistant and not greasy," he says.

■ **COVER YOUR HEAD.** Whether you're heading to the beach or spending extended time in the midday sun, wear a hat with at least a 4-inch-wide brim to keep the sun off your face and neck. Dr. Daniel's favorite: Tilley Hats (www.tilley.com).

Baseball caps, assuming they're worn with the bill in front, don't protect your ears, the back of your neck, or even most of your face from full sun, says Dr. Kunin. Straw hats don't usually offer much protection either. If the hats are unlined and loosely woven, the sun shines directly through them.

"Choose a hat with an extra-long bill and sun-protective cloth inside," says Dr. Kunin. "It will give you more protection and help limit your chances of developing age spots."

■ **PROTECT YOUR LIPS.** Most people don't think about their lips when it comes to sun protection. But age spots can show up there, too. Many women believe that their lipstick will protect them. The sun, however, can penetrate many lighter shades, and lipstick typi-

What the Doctor Does

There is a wart-remover product called Wart Stick that contains 40 percent salicylic acid, which is also the beta hydroxy acid that doctors use to treat wrinkles. "Because the stick allows you to concentrate on one specific spot or area to treat, I got the idea to use the Wart Stick for people who have brown spots, dark circles, and roughened areas of the skin," explains Nelson Lee Novick, M.D. "It's convenient, it doesn't run, and it works." He recommends applying it at bedtime. It may take 8 to 12 months to see results. Wart Stick is available at some drugstores, at mass merchandisers, and online.

cally wears off throughout the day, leaving the lips naked and unprotected.

Apply either a lip balm or lipstick with an SPF of 15 to 30 before you head outside. Dr. Kunin recommends DERMAdoctor Climate Control Lip Balm SPF 15 (available online) or Neutrogena Lip Moisturizer SPF 15 (available in drug stores). If you still want to wear your favorite non-SPF lipstick, apply it over a layer of the protective balm.

■ **SHUN THE SUN.** Since these brown blotches are caused by the sun's UV rays, limiting sun exposure is an important first step in the battle against age spots. "Avoid the sun as much as possible during peak hours (10:00 a.m. to 4:00 p.m. during spring, summer, and fall or 10:00 a.m. to 2:00 p.m. during winter), when the ultraviolet radiation is the strongest," says Dr. Kunin. If you have to do outdoor chores like gardening, perform them early in the morning or in the evening. And remember that sunblock is needed even during winter months and on cloudy days.

■ **TAKE A BREAK IN THE SHADE.** Excessive sun exposure causes age spots, so periodically retreat to a shady place on sunny days. At the beach or a backyard barbecue, park yourself under a big umbrella. "It sounds simple, but protecting yourself with sunblock and staying out of the sun are the two best ways to keep new age spots from forming," says Dr. Kunin. Also, whenever you're in the sun, wear tightly woven, light-colored clothing if it's not too hot outside. It helps keep UV rays from penetrating your skin. Dr. Daniel recommends a line of clothing called Sun Precaution. "It provides an SPF of 30 and keeps you relatively cool," he says.

■ **COVER UP THE SPOT.** If the other at-home remedies don't do the trick and you don't want to spend the money on a dermatologist-administered chemical peel or a laser resurfacing treatment, you can always reach into your cosmetics bag. "Brown age spots can be hidden by applying a cream-based or water-based concealer," says Dr. Kunin. Pick a lighter version of your skin tone to best hide age spots.

PANEL OF ADVISORS

C. RALPH DANIEL III, M.D., IS A CLINICAL PROFESSOR OF DERMATOLOGY AT THE UNIVERSITY OF MISSISSIPPI MEDICAL CENTER AND CLINICAL ASSOCIATE PROFESSOR OF DERMATOLOGY AT THE UNIVERSITY OF ALABAMA IN BIRMINGHAM.

AUDREY KUNIN, M.D., IS A COSMETIC DERMATOLOGIST IN KANSAS CITY, MISSOURI, THE FOUNDER OF THE DERMATOLOGY EDUCATIONAL WEB SITE WWW.DERMADOCTOR.COM, AND AUTHOR OF THE DERMADOCTOR SKINSTRUCTION MANUAL.

NELSON LEE NOVICK, M.D., IS A CLINICAL PROFESSOR OF DERMATOLOGY AT MOUNT SINAI SCHOOL OF MEDICINE IN NEW YORK CITY.

Allergies

15 Ways to Alleviate the Symptoms

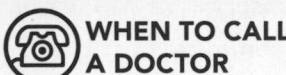 **WHEN TO CALL A DOCTOR**

If you have a known allergy and you notice any of the following symptoms, you should see your doctor.

■ Welts that spring up in response to exposure to an allergen, also known as hives. They may indicate the onset of anaphylactic shock, an allergic reaction severe enough to kill. Seek medical attention promptly.

■ Wheezing—a whistling sound when you breathe

■ Asthma—congestion of the chest severe enough to make breathing difficult, often accompanied by wheezing

■ An allergy attack that doesn't respond to over-the-counter medications within a week

"If your allergy symptoms are preventing you from doing the things you want to do, or you're missing work or school, you should see a doctor," says David Lang, M.D.

Allergies are the result of an immune system run amok. They develop when your immune system overreacts to a normally harmless substance, such as pollen, cat dander, or dust. About one in five Americans are plagued by sneezing, coughing, wheezing, chest tightness, difficulty breathing, itchy eyes, hives, and rashes, which are all hallmarks of allergy symptoms.

How can you tell the difference between a cold and an allergy? David Lang, M.D., offers this rule of thumb: If you have nasal symptoms and it feels like you have a cold but it's with more itching and sneezing, and it lasts for more than 2 weeks, you probably have an allergy.

Allergies come in almost infinite variety. But most triggers, called allergens, stimulate the immune system through four basic routes: ingestion (eating peanuts or shrimp, for example), injection (such as getting a penicillin shot), absorption through the skin (touching poison ivy), and inhalation (breathing in cat dander).

For food and drug allergies, avoidance is the only option. To prevent or treat contact allergies caused by poison plants, see Poison Plant Rashes on page 486 But when you want relief from inhalant allergies, the answer is probably right under your nose, because house dust, pollen, pet dander, and mold are the most common triggers.

"You find a bit of everything in house dust," says Thomas Platts-Mills, M.D. "Different people are allergic to different things—pieces of cockroach are pretty potent, actually—but the single biggest cause of problems is the dust mite."

The dust mite is an almost microscopic relative of ticks and spiders. But living mites are not the problem. People react, instead, to the fecal material that mites expel on carpets, bedding, and upholstered furniture. The bodies of dead mites also trigger allergies.

Dust mites have been isolated in dust samples from the five major continents of the world, and are frequently a big allergen for those with allergies and asthma. Because dust mites require heat and humidity to survive, and can live only below an altitude of 1500 meters, they are not found in areas of the United States such as Denver, Vail, Santa Fe, and Lake Tahoe.

The other common trigger, the cockroach, is pervasive. "Although most species of cockroaches live in the tropics, they are also found in North America, particularly in homes in large cities," says Dr. Lang. Not surprisingly, cockroach allergen is most abundant in kitchen areas where there is food debris.

Airborne allergens are hard to escape. Pollen fills the air in almost every region with seasonal regularity. Mold grows wherever it's dark and humid—under carpets, in dank basements, and in leaky garages and storage sheds. And with millions of dogs and cats in America,

it's not easy to escape pet dander. If you're sensitive to any of these allergens—most likely because you've inherited the tendency—contact with them will trigger a sneezing, wheezing, itchy reaction.

Fortunately, there's much you can do to help minimize the misery. The following doctor-tested and recommended tips will help plant you firmly on the wellness path to easy breathing and dry eyes.

■ **TREAT YOUR SYMPTOMS.** A certain amount of exposure to whatever bothers you is unavoidable. Allergy shots, available from your doctor, are a great way to make sure that your forays into the outside world are pleasant instead of painful. But you don't have to rely on them. Over-the-counter, nonsedating antihistamines, available from your local pharmacy, work wonders on drippy noses and red, itchy eyes, and are well tolerated. However, according to the Joint Council of Allergy, Asthma, and Immunology, the most effective medication for the treatment of nasal allergies is an intranasal steroid spray, which is available only by prescription.

■ **AIR-CONDITION YOUR HOUSE (AND CAR).** This is probably the single most important thing you can do to alleviate pollen problems, and it can help with two other chief inhalants: mold and dust mites.

The basic idea is to create an oasis of sorts," says Richard Podell, M.D. "You want your home to be a place of sanctuary, a place you can count on to provide escape."

Air conditioners help in two ways. They keep humidity low, which discourages mites and mold, and they can filter the air in the course of cooling it—if you also install an air cleaner. But it's the sealing of the house that provides the real benefit, Dr. Podell says. If you have the windows open, the inside of the house is essentially the same environment as the outside of the house—full of pollen.

If walking outside makes you start wheezing and sneezing, imagine what tearing through all those pollen clouds at 55 miles per hour is going to do. Be sensible and remember to use the air conditioner in your car, too.

■ **INSTALL AN AIR FILTER.** Keeping the air clean in your home can bring relief from pollen, mold, and pet dander. HEPA (high-energy particulate-arresting) filters are most efficient. When you use an air filter in your room, remember to keep the door closed to reduce the overall volume of air that the machine is trying to clean.

Air filters, however, aren't much use against dust mites. The dead mites float in the air for only a few minutes before falling, not long enough for the filter to draw them in.

■ **BUY A DEHUMIDIFIER.** Keeping the air in your home dry will help put a stop to dust mite problems.

Dust mites don't thrive in low humidity, below about 45 percent, says Dr. Platts-Mills. "Generally, the drier, the better."

Remember to empty the unit's water often and clean it regularly, according to the manu-facturer's instructions, to prevent mold. If your dehumidifier creates a problem for a child or someone else sensitive to dry air, try using a small room humidifier in the bedroom.

■ **KEEP IT CLEAN, BUT NOT TOO CLEAN.** People with allergies fare better when dust and grime are kept to a minimum. But your home will need more than a dusting with a dry cloth, which just propels allergens into the air. Instead, wipe down hard surfaces and floors with a slightly damp cloth. Try not to use aerosol sprays or products containing harsh chemicals or odors that may irritate airways.

In humid areas, use a bleach solution. Bleach kills mold, and, unlike some other exotic (and potentially dangerous) chemicals, you can get it at the grocery store. Wipe down surfaces in your bathroom as needed. The label on a bottle of bleach suggests that you clean floors, vinyl, tile, and your kitchen sink with a solution of ¾ cup of bleach per gallon of water. Let it stand for 5 minutes and then rinse. Use a regular fungicide for tough locations such as the basement. Of course, if you use bleach on fabrics they'll lose their color.

If you're allergic to house dust, pet dander, or another common household allergen, hire someone else to clean that carpet, such as a professional cleaning service or carpet cleaner. The cost of hiring a helper is a small price to pay to avoid an allergic reaction.

All of that said, some researchers believe that our excessively sanitized Western lifestyle keeps our immune systems confused, off bal-

How the Home Became a Dust Mite Haven

In the 1940s, American homeowners welcomed the vacuum cleaner with enthusiasm. Before long, no homemaker could live without one.

But the same technology that made our lives easier has indirectly contributed heavily to one common medical problem: allergies to dust mites.

"The vacuum cleaner made carpeting more attractive than throw rugs," says David Lang, M.D. With central heating, homes tended to stay warm year-round. Add well-insulated homes and cold-water washes to the mix (courtesy of the energy crisis), and you end up with a perfect environment for dust mites.

ance, and unable to distinguish friend from foe. In fact, increasing evidence shows that a baby's immature immune system can develop properly only if it's exposed to some bacteria.

■ **ISOLATE YOUR PETS.** The furry friends that occupy America's homes can worsen allergies. Cat dander usually causes the most problems, but dogs, birds, rabbits, horses, and other pets with hair or fur also stir up allergic reactions. "One walk a week through a room is all it takes for a pet to keep a dander allergy going," Dr. Podell says.

"Unfortunately, no secondary measure can rival the benefit that will occur with elimination of a pet from the home," says Dr. Lang. "If a cat or dog is removed from the home, however, clinically relevant levels of pet allergen may persist in 'reservoirs' like upholstered couches and chairs, wallpaper, and other areas for several months." So be patient.

If you can't bear to part with your pet (and most pet owners can't), make your bedroom a haven, sealed off from the rest of the house and absolutely forbidden territory for critters. There's evidence to suggest that washing a cat or dog frequently will reduce its level of allergens.

■ **WEAR A FACE MASK.** Don a mask when doing anything that's likely to expose you to a problem allergen. A simple chore like vacuuming can throw huge quantities of dust and contaminants into the air, where it will hang for several minutes, says Dr. Lang. Similarly, gardening can expose you to huge volumes of pollen. A small mask that covers your nose and mouth, known professionally as a dust and mist respirator, can keep the pollen from reaching your lungs. The 3M Company makes an effective, inexpensive version that can be found in most hardware stores.

■ **ENFORCE A NO-SMOKING POLICY.** Tobacco smoke is a significant irritant for not only the smoker but also anyone else nearby. Smoke can worsen allergies, so if you wish to breathe easier if you keep your home, office, and car smoke-free.

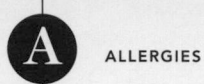
Don't Buy into the Allergen-Free Cat Claims

You may have heard the buzz about "allergen-free" cats. Most of these animals cost several thousand dollars, but the experts claim they offer more hype than hope. "I have yet to see any quantitative data to show that these animals lack Fel d 1, the main cat allergen," cautions Scott P. Commins, M.D., Ph.D. Before you buy one of these animals, he suggests waiting for some solid research indicating they are, indeed, allergen-free.

■ **MAKE YOUR BED A MITE-FREE ZONE.** Encase your pillows, mattress, and box spring in allergen-proof covers. These covers provide a barrier between you and any allergens found inside them. Look for a fabric weave of 10 microns, which is tight enough to keep out dust mite allergens. These products are available from companies such as American Allergy Supply, National Allergy Supply, Allergy Control Products, and at www.stopallergy.com.

■ **CHOOSE THE HOT CYCLE ON LAUNDRY DAY.** Linens should be washed in water that is at least 130°F to rid them of dust mites and their wastes. To test your water temperature, stop the washer once it's filled and dip a meat thermometer into the water. (This works only for top-loading machines, of course!) If you're worried about scalding people by setting your water heater that high, consider taking your bedding to a professional laundry service where you're assured that the bedding will be washed at a sufficiently high temperature.

■ **THROW OUT YOUR CARPETS.** Carpets may look nice, but they make an almost perfect home for dust mites and mold. Plus, tightly woven carpets very effectively attract and hold pollen and pet dander. Even steam cleaning may not help.

"It's not hot enough to kill the mites," says Dr. Platts-Mills. All steam cleaning really does is make it warmer and wetter underneath—an ideal climate for both mites and mold.

■ **BUY THROW RUGS.** Replace your carpets with throw rugs to achieve two major benefits. First, you'll eliminate your home's biggest collector of dust, pollen, pet dander, and mold. Second, you'll make keeping your home allergen-free much easier. Rugs *can* be washed at temperatures hot enough to kill dust mites. Also, the floors underneath—courtesy of a rug's loose weave—stay cooler and drier, conditions distinctly hostile to mold and mites.

"Mites can't survive on a dry, polished floor," Dr. Platts-Mills says. "That kind of floor dries in seconds versus days for a steam-cleaned carpet."

■ **BUY SYNTHETIC PILLOWS.** Dust mites like synthetic (Hollofil and Dacron) pillows just as much as those made from down and foam, however, synthetic pillows do have one major advantage: You can wash them in hot water and kill the dust mites.

■ **REDUCE CLUTTER.** Dried flowers, books, stuffed animals, and other homey touches collect dust and allergens. So keep knickknacks to a minimum, or get rid of them entirely.

■ **MAKE AT LEAST ONE ROOM A SANCTUARY.** If you can't afford central air and don't want to rip the wall-to-wall carpeting out of every room in your house, there's still hope. Make just *one* room a sanctuary.

"Most people spend the largest part of their time at home in the bedroom," Dr. Platts-Mills says. Making just that one room an allergen-free area can help a great deal to alleviate your allergy symptoms.

Do it by air-conditioning the room in summer, sealing it from the rest of the house (by keeping the door closed), replacing carpets with throw rugs, encasing linens in allergen-proof cases, and keeping it dust-free.

PANEL OF ADVISORS

Anal Fissures and Itching

17 Soothing Solutions

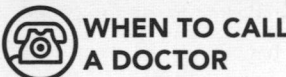 **WHEN TO CALL A DOCTOR**

Fissures don't require special medical attention, unless they persist.

The real caution with fissures is not to put them off forever—an ulcer that doesn't heal may be cancer.

If you have fissures that don't heal within 4 to 8 weeks, get them evaluated. A sore that will not heal is one of the seven classic warning signs of cancer. In addition, if you notice a mucus discharge from your anus, have it checked out by a doctor. The possibility of perirectal/perianal abscess formation should be considered if there's any persistent pain or discharge, says Judy Gerken, M.N., F.N.P.-B.C. Abscesses can be very serious in that area.

Even though the symptoms are comparable—pain, bleeding, and itching—the similarities between anal fissures and hemorrhoids are largely superficial. Hemorrhoids are generally swollen veins. In contrast, fissures are ulcers, or breaks in the skin, which just happen to occur in the same general area.

"Fissures are tears or ulcers in the lining of the anal canal most often caused by trauma, the most common being a hard bowel movement," says Edmund Leff, M.D.

New research points to anatomical problems that can contribute to chronic anal fissures, as opposed to isolated problems with the painful lesions. Increased pressure in the internal anal sphincter muscle and reduced blood flow to the area in which fissures occur may make you more prone to chronic problems.

If you have fissures, you know these little sores can make your life—at least your sitting life—miserable. Take comfort in the fact that about 60 percent of anal fissures heal within a few weeks. In severe, chronic cases, surgery may be required, but it carries considerable risks, including the possibility of fecal incontinence if the anal sphincter is injured. But according to Dr. Leff, some fissures will respond to Botox injections, eliminating the need for surgery. And a number of nonsurgical remedies exist to help fissures heal. Here's what our experts suggest.

■ **ELIMINATE HARD STOOLS WITH FIBER AND FLUID.** The anal opening was never meant to accommodate large, hard stools. Generally a by-product of a Western diet lacking in fiber, rock-hard stools tug and tear at the anal canal, which can result in anal fissures and hemorrhoids.

The solution? Adapt yourself to a diet high in fiber and fluids that produce soft bowel movements. Eating more fruit, vegetables, and whole grains, and drinking six to eight glasses of water a day are the best remedies and preventive measures you can use for anal fissures, says Dr. Leff. Once your stool is soft and pliable, your anal fissures should begin to heal on their own.

■ **TRY THE PETROLEUM SOLUTION.** Eating more fiber will soften your stool, but you can also protect your anal canal by lubricating it before each bowel movement. A dab of petroleum jelly inserted about a ½ inch into the rectum may help the stool pass without causing any further damage, says Dr. Leff.

■ **BUFF YOURSELF WITH BABY POWDER.** Following each shower or bowel movement, sprinkle on baby powder. This helps keep the area dry, which can help to reduce friction throughout the day. If the area is actively inflamed, skip this step, cautions Wal Baraza, M.B. CH.B., M.R.C.S., because it can worsen anal itching. And steer clear of the powders with perfumes, which may be irritating, adds Judy Gerken, M.N., F.N.P.-B.C. "People generally like to search for things that make them smell like a flower, but sometimes that can do more harm than good."

■ **WATCH THE WIPES.** Over-the-counter "wipes" are widely available, but many of them contain alcohol, which is the last thing you want to use if you have a fissure, says Gerken.

■ **AVOID DIARRHEA.** It may seem odd that not only can hard, constipated stools worsen anal fissures—but so can diarrhea. Watery stools can soften the tissues around them, and they also contain acid that can burn the raw anal area. "If you tend toward loose stools and have a fissure, taking fiber supplements with a minimum of water can firm up your stools," says Dr. Leff.

■ **DON'T SCRATCH.** Anal fissures may be itchy as well as painful, but using sharp fingernails on your tender anus can further abrade the skin and lead to a vicious cycle in terms of itching, says Dr. Baraza.

■ **SHED THOSE EXCESS POUNDS.** The more weight you carry, the more likely you are to sweat. Perspiration in your anal area irritates the skin and slows the healing of fissures, says Dr. Leff.

■ **MINIMIZE SWELLING WITH HYDROCORTISONE.** Nonprescription topical creams containing hydrocortisone can help reduce the inflammation that often comes with anal itching, says Dr. Baraza.

■ **TRY A VITAMIN SOLUTION.** Nonprescription ointments containing vitamins A and D, as well as aloe, may be particularly helpful for soothing pain and helping fissures heal.

■ **SOAK IN A HOT TUB.** Whether you fill your bathtub with hot water or slip into an outdoor hot tub, warm water helps relax the muscles of the anal sphincter, increases blood flow, and reduces much of the discomfort of fissures, says Dr. Leff.

■ **STEER CLEAR OF CERTAIN FOODS.** While no food directly causes fissures, some foods may irritate the tissues of the anal canal. "Hot, spicy foods, as well as caffeine, are irritating," says Dr. Leff. "Excess caffeine is probably the major cause of anal itching."

■ **AVOID ANAL ENTRY.** Anal intercourse can be a source of tears, says Gerken. The best treatment is prevention, so use adequate lubrication, she says.

■ **BUY YOURSELF A SPECIAL PILLOW.** Alleviate the pain associated with the anal area by sitting on a soft or gel-filled pillow. "But avoid doughnut-shaped pillows," cautions Gerken, "because they may restrict blood flow to the area."

■ **DON'T READ ON THE TOILET.** "People shouldn't be reading their morning paper or a novel while they're sitting on the toilet," says Gerken. "The seat has a constricting effect, and prolonged sitting causes engorgement of the blood vessels."

■ **WIPE GENTLY.** Rough toilet paper and overzealous wiping slows healing of your fissures. Use only white, unscented, top-quality toilet paper. Perfumes and dyes can irritate the anus. You can soften toilet paper by moistening it with water before wiping. Make sure you dab after a bath, don't wipe, says Dr. Baraza. Applying petroleum jelly after a bath can help soothe itching, too.

■ **SUBSTITUTE FACIAL TISSUE.** The very best toilet paper isn't a toilet paper at all. Facial tissues coated with moisturizing lotion offer the least amount of friction.

■ **USE A BIDET, IF YOU HAVE ONE.** There are portable bidets available, which divert water from your bathroom faucet to underneath your toilet seat. A narrow stream of water, aimed right where you need it most, does all your "wiping" for you. There's no need for toilet paper, except for one or two sheets to pat yourself dry. This is the best way to cleanse the area, says Dr. Leff.

PANEL OF ADVISORS

WAL BARAZA, M.B.CH.B., M.R.C.S., IS A SPECIALIST REGISTRAR IN GENERAL SURGERY AT SHEFFIELD TEACHING HOSPITALS IN SHEFFIELD, UK.

JUDY GERKEN, M.N., F.N.P.-B.C., IS A NURSE PRACTITIONER AND THE HIV PROGRAM COORDINATOR AT THE VA LONG BEACH HEALTH CARE SYSTEM IN LONG BEACH, CALIFORNIA.

EDMUND LEFF, M.D., IS A COLON AND RECTAL SURGEON IN PHOENIX AND SCOTTSDALE, ARIZONA.

Angina

10 Long-Life Strategies to Protect the Heart

More than a few people confuse the symptoms of angina with those of a heart attack. Angina isn't quite that serious, but it's close. Think of it as a warning sign that your heart needs some tender loving care.

Angina (the full name is angina pectoris) occurs when the heart gets insufficient blood and oxygen, which may result in temporary nausea, dizziness, or a burning or squeezing pain in the chest. Angina itself isn't a disease. It's a symptom of underlying problems, usually coronary artery disease.

"When you have chronic worsening angina (meaning your episodes become more frequent or occur with less activity), you're at a much higher risk of having a sudden 'cardiac event,' such as a heart attack or sudden cardiac arrest," says David M. Capuzzi, M.D., Ph.D. "Unfortunately, up to 50 percent of people who experience heart attack do not have prior angina as a warning."

Anything that increases the heart's demand for oxygen, such as exercise or emotional stress, can trigger bouts of angina. This is especially likely if the heart's supply of blood is decreased by a narrowing of one or more of the heart's blood vessels. The attacks normally last fewer than 5 minutes and are unlikely to cause permanent damage to the heart. The underlying problems, however, can be life-threatening.

The discomfort of angina can be relieved with nitroglycerine, beta-blockers, or other medications that dilate arteries or fulfill the heart's demand for oxygen. In addition, it's essential

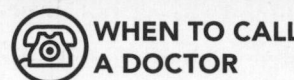

WHEN TO CALL A DOCTOR

Most people with angina have a form called chronic stable angina. This means that it occurs in predictable ways—during exercise, for example, or at times of emotional stress—with the pain lasting 5 minutes or less. Most chronic stable angina can easily be managed with medications and lifestyle changes.

Unstable angina, on the other hand, is much more serious. The discomfort can occur out of the blue and may last 20 minutes or more.

"If there's any change in your usual pattern of angina—if pain or shortness of breath get more intense—head to an emergency room right away," says David M. Capuzzi, M.D., Ph.D.

While you're en route, chew two aspirin tablets. "Aspirin thins the blood and can help dissolve blood clots that may be blocking circulation to the heart." says Dr. Capuzzi.

to make some lifestyle changes to reduce angina episodes and prevent the problem from getting worse.

■ **KEEP CHOLESTEROL AND TRIGLYCER-IDES UNDER CONTROL.** Along with other fatty substances in the blood, cholesterol slowly accumulates on the linings of arteries and restricts blood flow to the heart. If you're having episodes of angina, it probably means fatty buildups have reached dangerous levels, says Howard Weitz, M.D.

Keep your total cholesterol below 200. In addition, levels of low-density lipoproteins (LDL, or "bad" cholesterol) should ideally be below 100. "Apart from the use of medications, reducing the amount of saturated fat in your diet and increasing the fiber from whole grains are two of the most effective ways to control cholesterol," says Christine Gerbstadt, M.D., R.D.

Saturated fat is mainly found in fatty meats, whole-fat dairy (such as whole milk, cheeses, butter, cream, and ice cream), rich desserts, and snack foods. If you have high cholesterol, limit red meat to lean cuts no more than twice a week, and avoid snack foods that are made with butter or other fats, suggests Dr. Gerbstadt.

■ **INCREASE THE FIBER IN YOUR DIET.** Found in whole grains, legumes, fruits, and other plant foods, fiber helps prevent cholesterol from passing through the intestinal wall into the bloodstream. High-fiber foods are also filling, which means you'll naturally eat smaller amounts of other, fattier foods.

■ **LOAD UP ON FRUITS AND VEGETABLES.** A low-fat, meat-free diet isn't for everyone, but it's an ideal way for those with angina to partially control the underlying coronary artery disease. Most vegetarian diets tend to be lower in fat and also provide a bounty of antioxidants. These chemical compounds help prevent cholesterol from sticking to artery walls.

"Diet alone can lower cholesterol by up to 20 percent," says Dr. Weitz. "At the same time, it decreases your risk of heart attack by as much as 25 percent if you can lower LDL levels to 100 or less, which makes arterial plaques more stable and less likely to rupture and form clots. Patients frequently require both diet and cholesterol-lowering medication to help them achieve this goal.

■ **GET MOVING.** "Exercise is a major lifestyle component to prevent coronary disease, although we usually make sure people also take the appropriate medication," says Dr. Weitz. Strive to perform moderate to intense exercise such as brisk walking for 30 minutes a day, 7 days a week. If you haven't exercised in a while, start with as little as 5 minutes a day, suggests Dr. Gerbstadt, and build up from there.

If you've experienced angina, be sure to talk to your doctor before starting an exercise plan. You'll be advised to build up your fitness gradually—by starting with short walks or water-resistance walking (in a pool), for example, and increasing the exertion over a period of weeks or months. "Swimming may be added once a baseline test of a few months shows no signs of angina during the activity," says Dr. Gerbstadt.

■ **EXERCISE LATER IN THE DAY.** Morning can be a risky time for people with angina because fight-or-flight hormones, such as cortisol and norepinephrine, rise overnight and peak in the morning, says Dr. Gerbstadt. The levels stay elevated until about noon, and intensive morning exercise is probably not a good idea for most patients with angina.

"Don't sprint in the morning or do any heavy lifting or other stressful exercises," Dr. Gerbstadt says. "Ease into the morning and follow your doctor's advice. Some people with angina should never do heavy weight or strength training that requires bearing down, because this impedes blood return from the body to the heart, which can cause angina."

■ **AVOID EXERCISE FOLLOWING A MEAL.** Large meals, especially those containing saturated fats from fatty meats or fried foods, are a common angina trigger, because blood diverted to the intestine during digestion is not available to the heart, Dr. Weitz says.

■ **STAY AT A HEALTHFUL WEIGHT.** Those extra pounds that tend to accumulate over the years put an incredible load on the heart. For one, the heart has to work harder to supply blood to all that extra body tissue. What's more, being overweight can result in elevated levels of cholesterol, which makes it harder for blood to circulate.

■ **STAY AWAY FROM SMOKE.** Whether you smoke yourself or are exposed to second-

What the Doctor Does

For years author and cardiologist Ralph Felder, M.D., Ph.D., has been eating what he calls the seven bonus-years foods every day— red wine (5 ounces daily), dark chocolate (2 ounces daily), fruits and vegetables (4 cups daily), fish (three 5-ounce servings a week), garlic (one clove daily), and nuts (2 ounces daily). "Eat these seven foods every day in the recommended doses and you'll add an average of 5 to 6 years to your life," he says. In fact, a study published in the *British Medical Journal* suggests that people who eat these foods regularly can reduce their risk of heart disease by more than 75 percent. "The dark chocolate and fruits and vegetables lower your blood pressure. Garlic and nuts lower LDL (bad) cholesterol. Fish helps protect against cardiac arrhythmias, blood clotting, and inflammation," says Dr. Felder. "Together these foods help protect the endothelium (the Teflon-like coating around your blood vessels) and reduce the risk of heart disease."

hand smoke on a regular basis, now's the time to clear the air. Smoking even one cigarette temporarily reduces your heart's supply of oxygen, which can trigger painful angina.

■ **TAKE ASPIRIN.** If your stomach can handle it, experts generally agree that taking one 81-milligram aspirin daily is good protection. It won't stop the pain of angina, but it does reduce the risk of blood clots that can lead to heart attacks. In fact, taking an aspirin each day can reduce the risk of coronary heart disease by 28 percent. "Previously, doctors may have recommended higher doses (up to 325 milligrams), but with the higher dose there is generally an increased chance of

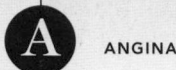

bleeding, says Ralph Felder, M.D., and it is probably not worth the risk.

■ **GET SOME CALM IN YOUR LIFE.** Emotional stress is an inevitable part of daily life, but when tension and anxiety soar, the body's demand for blood and oxygen increases, which can result in angina. Regular exercise is an excellent way to reduce stress. Some people meditate. Others practice yoga or deep breathing. Experiment to find what works best for you.

PANEL OF ADVISORS

DAVID M. CAPUZZI, M.D., PH.D., IS A PROFESSOR OF MEDICINE, BIOCHEMISTRY, AND MOLECULAR PHARMACOLOGY AND DIRECTOR OF THE CARDIOVASCULAR DISEASE PREVENTION CENTER AT THOMAS JEFFERSON UNIVERSITY HOSPITAL IN PHILADELPHIA.

RALPH FELDER, M.D., PH.D., IS A CARDIOLOGIST AND THE AUTHOR OF *THE BONUS YEARS DIET*.

CHRISTINE GERBSTADT, M.D., R.D., IS A NATIONAL SPOKESPERSON FOR THE AMERICAN DIETETIC ASSOCIATION AND PRESIDENT OF NUTRONICS HEALTH.

HOWARD WEITZ, M.D., IS DIRECTOR OF THE JEFFERSON HEART INSTITUTE OF THOMAS JEFFERSON UNIVERSITY HOSPITAL AND SENIOR VICE CHAIR OF THE DEPARTMENT OF MEDICINE AT JEFFERSON MEDICAL COLLEGE, BOTH IN PHILADELPHIA.

Anxiety

19 Ways to Control Excessive Worrying

Anxiety is a natural reaction to some of life's most challenging situations. In small, occasional doses, it can be a good thing—motivating you to meet a deadline, pass a test, or deliver a well-crafted presentation. As part of what's known as the fight-or-flight response, anxiety triggers the physiological changes that allow you to deal with stressors large and small. Your heart rate speeds up, you breathe faster, and your muscles tense, so you can take action if you need to.

A little bit of anxiety can be good. It helps motivate you to meet a deadline, pass a test, or deliver a well-crafted presentation at work. It also keeps you from meeting danger head-on. As part of the fight-or-flight response, anxiety causes your heart rate to increase and your muscles to tense should you need to act.

If your anxiety becomes so severe that it takes over your thinking and undermines your ability to function, then you may have an anxiety disorder. About 25 million Americans experience these disorders, which include panic attacks, generalized anxiety disorder, phobias, post-traumatic stress disorder, and obsessive-compulsive disorder. Anxiety disorders require medical attention and sometimes medication.

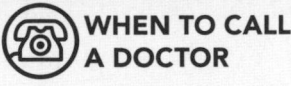 **WHEN TO CALL A DOCTOR**

The line between normal worrying and an anxiety disorder can be hard to discern. "If your life is restricted by anxiety, get medical attention," advises Bernard Vittone, M.D. Also see a doctor if you:

■ Experience more than one panic attack a month

■ Are nervous or anxious most of the time, particularly if your worry is attached to situations that would not make other people anxious

■ Have frequent insomnia, shakiness, poor concentration, tight muscles, or heart palpitations

■ Feel nervous in or avoid facing particular situations, such as crossing bridges or tunnels

■ Take refuge from fear or worry by using drugs, including alcohol, or overeating

■ Obsess or ruminate about the past or the future

■ Fear you might harm yourself or others

Millions of people fall somewhere in between these two extremes. They worry too much but don't have an actual disorder. Chronic worriers are able to function from day to day, but the anxiety eats away at their emotional and physical health. Edward M. Hallowell, M.D., calls this "persistent toxic worry."

"We virtually train ourselves to worry, which only reinforces the habit," Dr. Hallowell says. "Worriers often feel vulnerable if they're not worrying."

But they have good reason to stop. Excessive worry, or anxiety, is associated with increased risk for depression, heart disease, and other medical conditions.

Here are some tips for getting a handle on excessive worry.

■ **TAKE SLOW, DEEP BREATHS.** When you're anxious, you tend to hold your breath or breathe too rapidly or shallowly, and that makes you feel more anxious. "Regulating your breathing is a surprisingly effective antianxiety

measure," says Bernard Vittone, M.D. He recommends inhaling slowly through your nose holding one nostril, then holding your breath for about 10 seconds, and finally slowly exhaling through your mouth. Then repeat the process holding the other nostril. To make sure you're breathing correctly, place your hand on your diaphragm, just below your rib cage. Feel it rise with each inhalation and fall with each exhalation. Practice this technique regularly throughout the day for about a minute at a time, or any time you're feeling anxious.

■ **MAKE CONTACT.** The more isolated you feel, the more likely you are to worry, says Dr. Hallowell, who recommends daily doses of human contact. Go to a restaurant, a supermarket, or a library and start a conversation with someone. Call a friend or relative. Feeling connected reduces anxiety, Dr. Hallowell says.

■ **BE SURE TO MEDITATE.** Do some sort of meditative activity for at least 15 minutes, three or four times each day. Research shows that meditation can significantly lower anxiety. Find a quiet environment, clear your mind, and actively relax, says Dr. Vittone. "Focus on a mantra or make your mind a blank slate, whatever works for you."

■ **STAY IN THE PRESENT.** Pay attention to what's happening *now*, not to the past or the future. Take 1 day, 1 hour, or even 1 minute at a time, says Dr. Vittone.

■ **PASS UP PASSIVITY.** Don't be a passive victim, says Dr. Hallowell. If you're worried about your job, health, or finances, for

Cures from the Kitchen

To calm yourself before bedtime, reach for a glass of warm milk. "The old wives' tale of having warm milk really does help," says Bernard Vittone, M.D. Milk contains the amino acid tryptophan, which can cause a certain amount of relaxation. Chamomile tea is another folk remedy for anxiety—and there's evidence from test tube studies that the herb contains compounds that have a calming action. Experts recommend drinking one cup of tea at least three times a day.

How to Choose a Therapist

Edward M. Hallowell, M.D., offers these tips for choosing a mental-health professional, such as a licensed clinical social worker, psychologist, or psychiatrist. To start, consult two or three licensed professionals with good reputations in your community. Keep these questions in mind as you talk with each of them.

- Does she have a pleasant disposition and a sense of humor?

- Do you feel at ease with her?

- Is she sincere about trying to understand and help you?

- Does she treat you with dignity and respect?

- Is she honest, nondefensive, and kind?

- Is she willing to explain her approach, including strategies, goals, and length of treatment?

- Does she make you feel accepted?

- Can she understand your background and cultural heritage, if relevant?

- Does she treat you like an equal—or as though you are flawed or defective?

- Do you leave the sessions feeling more hopeful and empowered most of the time?

- Do you feel that she understands your pain?

- Do you feel safe disclosing your innermost feelings and that they are held in confidence?

- Does she give you homework assignments between sessions?

As you talk with potential therapists, keep in mind that research shows that the therapist's personal style, such as empathy, is more important in determining therapeutic success than is a therapist's theoretical persuasion or choice of techniques, says Dr. Hallowell.

These tips also apply if you're seeking help for depression, the symptoms of which are often intertwined with those of anxiety or other serious mental disorders. (For more information on depression, see page 173.)

example, create a plan to solve potential problems. Start a savings account or schedule a work evaluation with your boss. Taking action reduces anxiety.

■ **GET REAL.** Or, at least, get the facts, says Dr. Hallowell. Exaggerated worry often stems from a lack of information. If your CEO snubs you in the hall, you may worry that you're not doing a good job. But the CEO may have been pondering a personal matter, not even aware of your presence.

■ **STOP THE STIMULUS.** People who are too anxious need to decrease stimulation, says Dr. Vittone. Eliminate some of the racket vying for your attention. Turn off the car radio, don't answer the telephone at home, take a lunch break away from your office—and away from your cell phone.

■ **TAKE A "NEWS FAST."** Turn off the TV. Leave the morning paper on the porch. Taking a break from the news for a few days may decrease feelings of anxiety and lessen personal worries.

■ **ENVISION THE WORST.** Ask yourself, "What's the worst that could happen?" "How bad would it be?" "What's the likelihood of it happening?"

The worst thing that can happen usually isn't that bad, Dr. Vittone says. What's more, it seldom happens. Later, you may even wonder why you worried at all.

■ **WRITE IT DOWN.** Journaling or writing your worries down can help to put them in perspective and free you to think of solutions, says Dr. Vittone.

■ **PREPARE TO SLEEP.** At night, that is. "Give yourself time to unwind and relax," says Dr. Vittone. Take 30 to 50 minutes to do something quiet and nonstressful before bed. Read a light novel, watch a TV comedy, or take a warm bath. Avoid active tasks such as housework.

■ **LAUGH AT YOURSELF.** Take another

view of your worries. Ask yourself: "What's funny about this situation?" "When I think about this 2 years from now, will I laugh?"

If we can find humor in a situation, we immediately defuse the danger, Dr. Vittone says.

■ **SHARE YOUR WORRY.** Never worry alone. "When we talk about our worries, the toxicity dissipates," says Dr. Hallowell. Talking it through helps us find solutions and realize that our concerns aren't so overwhelming.

■ **LET IT GO.** Chronic worriers have a tough time letting go. You may hold on to worry as though it will fix the problem, Dr. Hallowell says. It won't. So train yourself to let go. He suggests meditation or visualization using your own technique. One patient "sees" worries in the palm of her hand and blows them away. Another takes a shower and "watches" worries go down

What the Doctor Does

Bernard Vittone, M.D., who considers himself "more anxious than the average individual," banishes worry by exercising for 30 to 40 minutes every day after work. He also tries to view his anxiety as energy to help him perform his job better and more efficiently—and he takes short breaks to meditate and clear his mind.

If you experience anxiety, he suggests exercising for at least a half hour each day. Try running, cycling, walking, or swimming laps. The repetitive action of these activities produces the same calming effect as meditation. Of course, yoga and stretching are good choices, too. The more vigorous the exercise, the more anxiety you'll eliminate from your system.

ANXIETY

Put a Cap on Caffeine

Nothing is worse for anxiety than caffeine, says Bernard Vittone, M.D. Found in beverages such as coffee, tea, and cola, and medications like Excedrin, caffeine affects neurotransmitters in the brain, which causes anxiety. Research shows that people who are predisposed to anxiety and those with panic disorders are especially sensitive to caffeine's effects.

Caffeine is deceptive, says Dr. Vittone. When you drink a cup of coffee, for example, you're likely to feel more vivacious for up to an hour afterward. Two to 12 hours after that, caffeine's anxiety-producing effects kick in. Because of this delayed reaction, people rarely connect anxiety to their morning java.

If you consume a lot of caffeine, try this test: Abstain from coffee and other caffeine-containing foods for 2 weeks. Then, drink three cups in one sitting and see how you feel. You're likely to notice a tightening of muscles, worry, nervousness, or apprehension several hours later.

"I really advocate trying to cut out caffeine completely," Dr. Vittone says. If that's asking too much, then limit coffee, tea, or cola to one cup a day.

the drain. "Don't feel like a failure if you can't do it at first," he says. Keep practicing.

■ **HANDLE WITH LESS CARE.** Stop treating yourself as fragile. If you believe that you're fragile, it becomes a self-fulfilling prophecy. Instead, learn to make anxiety a stimulus, not a hindrance. If you're about to give a speech, for example, imagine it as a thrill instead of a threat.

■ **FIND YOUR CHALLENGE.** Anxiety often arises when people are juggling too many responsibilities. Instead of viewing your busyness as negative, think of life as action-filled, rich, or challenging. If you're raising a family, for example, consider how one day you will miss your children's presence at home. The way you interpret things makes all the difference in the world, Dr. Vittone says.

■ **AVOID ALCOHOL.** Beer, wine, and other alcoholic beverages can exacerbate anxiety. "Alcohol reduces the anxiety when you first take it in," says Dr. Vittone. "But when it wears off, it has the opposite effect." People are often more anxious the day after a night of heavy drinking, he says. Avoid alcohol, or limit consumption to one or two drinks a day.

PANEL OF ADVISORS

EDWARD M. HALLOWELL, M.D., IS A PSYCHIATRIST AND FOUNDER OF THE HALLOWELL CENTER FOR COGNITIVE AND EMOTIONAL HEALTH IN SUDBURY, MASSACHUSETTS, AND NEW YORK CITY. HE IS THE AUTHOR OF *WORRY: HOPE AND HELP FOR A COMMON CONDITION AND CONNECT: 12 VITAL TIES THAT OPEN YOUR HEART, LENGTHEN YOUR LIFE, AND DEEPEN YOUR SOUL.*

BERNARD VITTONE, M.D., IS A PSYCHIATRIST AND FOUNDER OF THE NATIONAL CENTER FOR THE TREATMENT OF PHOBIAS, ANXIETY, AND DEPRESSION IN WASHINGTON, D.C.

Asthma

29 Steps to Better Breathing

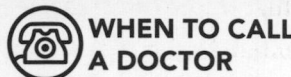 **WHEN TO CALL A DOCTOR**

The symptoms of asthma are often subtle at first, but they can get much worse in a hurry. Report any changes in your usual breathing patterns to your doctor.

You also should see a doctor if your wheeze, cough, or shortness of breath worsens after you take your rescue medication. It means the asthma isn't well controlled, and you have a higher risk for a flare-up, which may be serious.

You may think of asthma as a childhood illness, not one that's much of a problem for adults. Yet of the 22 million Americans who have asthma, only 9 million are children. Every day in America, 5,000 people visit the emergency room, 1,000 are admitted to the hospital, and 11 die due to asthma.

Of course, asthma doesn't always require hospitalization. It may cause only occasional and short-lived symptoms, such as breathlessness, coughing, or wheezing. But unless your asthma is well controlled, it may subtly interfere with normal activity and get out of hand quickly. In fact, a person with "mild asthma" can have a fatal attack.

Asthma occurs when the main air passages in the lungs, called bronchioles, become inflamed and overly sensitive to "triggers." During attacks, the lungs produce extra mucus and the bronchiole walls narrow, making breathing difficult.

No cure exists yet, but nearly everyone can dramatically reduce—and maybe even eliminate—symptoms. Even if you currently use medications to treat your asthma, you may be able to reduce the dose or frequency by more than 50 percent if you practice good lifestyle control, says Thomas F. Plaut, M.D.

Here are some doctor-recommended approaches.

■ **LOOK INTO ALLERGIES.** More than 70 percent of adults with asthma have allergies that set off or worsen symptoms. "Everyone who takes medications daily for asthma needs to find out if they have allergies," says Dr. Plaut. Think about when your symptoms occur and what you are doing at the time. Any patterns may help indicate if you have an allergy. You might want to keep an asthma journal. A board certified allergist can identify your allergens by taking a careful history and performing skin testing for inhalant allergens, including pollen (tree, grass, weed), mold, dust mites, cockroaches, and pet dander, says David Lang, M.D.

■ **WATCH THE SULFITES.** Food allergies are commonly suspected as relevant for asthma, but rarely confirmed, says Dr. Lang. Generally allergies influencing your asthma symptoms are those that are inhaled. That said, an estimated 5 to 10 percent of asthmatics suffer from a sensitivity to sulfites, which are often added to wine, beer, dried fruit, and frozen food.

■ **AVOID PLANT POLLEN.** It's a main asthma trigger. Plants pollinate at specific times of the year, so once you know those that are your triggers, take steps to avoid them. Stay indoors between 5:00 a.m. and 10:00 a.m. and on dry, hot, windy days, when pollen counts tend to be highest. During the warm months, keep your windows closed and air-condition your house. Doing these two things can cut down on the indoor pollen count by 90 percent or more, says Dr. Lang. Air conditioning also eliminates the high indoor humidity that promotes mold and dust mites.

Ragweed is the most common pollen allergen for Americans. This plant's season runs from August to November, usually peaking in early to mid-September. Check your local TV or newspaper for daily pollen counts to determine when it's best to stay inside.

■ **SWITCH ON THE BATHROOM FAN.** Mold is a common asthma trigger, and it thrives in bathrooms and other high-moisture areas, so good ventilation is essential. Use the bathroom fan every time you bathe or shower to reduce the moisture that mold needs to thrive.

Using a squeegee to wipe water off the bathroom tiles is a terrific strategy for preventing mold—and takes only about 30 seconds, says Dr. Plaut.

■ **WASH YOUR PETS WEEKLY.** Dogs and cats are loaded with dander—a combination of skin cells and allergy-causing proteins that can provoke asthma attacks. Some pet owners with asthma may find they are allergic to dander, and the only solution is remove animals from the home. At the very least, wash your pets weekly—with or without shampoo—to reduce dander. And keep your bedroom pet-free, says Dr. Lang.

■ **OPEN WINDOWS WHEN YOU COOK.** Strong food odors—from a smoking frying pan, for example, or the pungent oils in onions and garlic—can irritate airways and trigger asthma attacks. Open the windows during low-pollen months or use an exhaust fan when you cook to help vent the odors outside.

■ **FREQUENTLY CHANGE FURNACE FILTERS.** During the cold months, central heating systems circulate dust all over the house.

Installing electronic air cleaners in place of the standard furnace filters is one of the best ways to control this spread, Dr. Plaut says. These devices, available from heating contractors, act almost like dust magnets.

■ **REDUCE EXPOSURE TO DUST MITES.** Despite the name, these microscopic creatures live on the dead skin cells in your home. When they die, their bodies dry up and are ground into dust. They're a potent asthma trigger—and because people shed millions of skin cells every day, dust mites are hard to eliminate. They can, however, be reduced.

Wash sheets, pillowcases, and bathroom towels at least once a week in water 130°F or hotter to kill adult mites as well as the eggs, says Dr. Plaut.

"It's also important to encase pillows, mattresses, and box springs in covers made specifically to act as a barrier against dust mites. These covers are available at allergy supply stores," he adds. These products are available from companies such as American Allergy Supply, National Allergy Supply, and Allergy Control Products.

■ **INVEST IN A GOOD AIR FILTER.** A good air purifier, ideally with a HEPA filter, can really help clear indoor air of allergens, says Elson Haas, M.D.

■ **KEEP YOUR HOUSE PEST-FREE.** Studies have shown that cockroaches—which thrive in the same areas as humans—can trigger asthma. Like dust mites, their dry, dead bodies and feces turn into dust and can trigger an asthma episode, says Dr. Plaut.

Cockroaches are difficult to get rid of, even if your house is always squeaky-clean. One of the safest ways to control roaches is to sprinkle boric acid in areas where they congregate—around drainpipes, for example, or along kitchen and bathroom baseboards.

"Don't have an exterminator spray the house if you can help it," says Dr. Plaut. The fumes can irritate the airways for days, making asthma symptoms much worse. Many asthmatics are very sensitive to chemical exposures at home and work, adds Dr. Haas.

■ **MAKE YOUR HOUSE A SMOKE-FREE ZONE.** Cigarette smoke is extremely irritating. It not only triggers asthma attacks but also can increase the risk of asthma in children. If you smoke, take advantage of nicotine patches, prescription medications, or smoking-cessation programs. Let others know that smoking in the house is *verboten*.

■ **LOAD YOUR DIET WITH FLAVONOIDS.** Fight the inflammation that accompanies asthma by eating foods loaded with flavonoids—tiny crystals found in onions, apples, blueberries, and grapes that give them their blue, yellow, or reddish hues. Flavonoids not only strengthen the capillary walls, but they are also antioxidants, and so they help protect the membranes in the airways from being damaged by pollution. Eat a couple of servings of flavonoid-rich foods every day.

■ **TAKE FISH OIL.** Preliminary research shows that diets containing the fatty acids gamma linolenic acid (GLA) and eicosapentaenoic acid (EPA)—found in such fatty fish as salmon, sardines, tuna, and mackerel—may improve the quality of life in people with asthma and decrease their reliance on rescue medication. Plus, studies show that fish oil partially reduces reactions to allergens that can trigger attacks in some asthmatics. Other studies suggest fish oil supplements may prevent exercise-induced asthma attacks. "The best natural sources of omega-3s are fish, particularly salmon or other cold-water fish," says Dr. Plaut. Fish oil capsules are a good alternative, but they can cause "fish burps." "This can usually be avoided if the capsules are taken frozen right before a meal," he adds.

■ **TAKE MAGNESIUM.** Magnesium levels are frequently low in asthmatics. Research shows that taking a supplement may improve lung function and reduce reaction of the bronchial passages. Extra magnesium may help to decrease muscle tension and airway spasms,

Cures from the Kitchen

If you or anyone in your family has asthma, put fish on the menu at least twice a week. Fatty fish such as tuna, salmon, and mackerel contain beneficial fats called omega-3 fatty acids. Asthma is an inflammatory disease, and the omega-3s help to damp down many of the body's processes that create inflammation.

explains Kendall Gerdes, M.D. But high doses of magnesium (350 milligrams or more) can cause cramps, gas, or diarrhea for some people, so take what your gut will allow. Dr. Gerdes suggests starting with 100 milligrams twice a day and increasing it gradually until you experience some of these side effects. Then cut back the dosage a level at a time until problems subside, and then hold that dose. Make sure you're taking a form of magnesium that can be easily absorbed by the body, says Dr. Gerdes. Magnesium citrate, magnesium chloride, and magnesium glycinate are all good options.

Note: If you have heart or kidney problems, be sure to talk to your doctor before taking supplemental magnesium.

■ **SUPPLEMENT WITH QUERCETIN.** This flavonoid is extracted from certain fruits and vegetables, such as apples, onions, and the white rinds of citrus, and helps reduce the histamine reactions that can lead to asthma. Quercetin can also be taken as a supplement, says Dr. Haas, who recommends 250 to 300 milligrams twice or three times a day along with 500 to 1,000 milligrams of vitamin C. At higher intakes, vitamin C has a mild antihistamine, antiallergy effect. Because asthma is a serious, individualized condition, it's a good idea to talk with your doctor before making any changes to your treatment plan, he adds.

■ **STAY ACTIVE.** An active lifestyle can help control asthma much better than a sedentary one. Physical activity helps improve lung capacity and may enable people to use lower doses of medications or to use them less often. All asthma patients should discuss a fitness program with their physicians. It is important to first warm up by either stretching, jogging, or sprinting for 20 to 30 minutes before exercising.

■ **AVOID EXERCISING IN COLD AIR.** Cold air may irritate the airways and trigger an asthma episode. It is important, however, to exercise throughout the year. If you enjoy skiing or skating, make sure you wear a mask to create a reservoir of warm air, advises Dr. Plaut. If you notice that you're having more asthma episodes during the cold months, consider shifting to warm-weather activities. Swimming is especially good because the moist air soothes the airways and reduces the risk of attacks.

■ **CHANGE YOUR BREATHING STYLE.** Most people breathe using only their chest muscles. This makes it difficult to empty air from the lungs completely. For those with asthma, it's important to use the diaphragm as well. This large muscle between the chest and abdomen adds power to your breathing and helps remove "used" air from the lungs, which can reduce feelings of breathlessness, explains Dr. Plaut.

It takes practice to develop the habit of diaphragmatic breathing (also called abdominal, or belly, breathing). Several times a day, lie on your back with one hand on your belly and the other on your chest. As you breathe in, the hand on your belly should rise slightly, while the hand on your chest should barely move.

■ **TAKE UP A WIND INSTRUMENT.** Playing a reed instrument, like the oboe, saxophone, or trumpet, requires diaphragmatic breathing, Dr. Plaut says. Even if you aren't especially musical, playing the instrument is great practice for your breathing muscles.

■ **PRACTICE STRESS CONTROL.** Yoga, self-hypnosis, deep breathing, and other techniques for reducing stress are good techniques for dealing with asthma because they help the airways open more fully, says Dr. Plaut.

■ **WASH YOUR HANDS OFTEN.** Asthma episodes surge in the autumn and winter, when colds are more common. Even a mild case of the sniffles can make asthma harder to control. A viral infection is a common trigger of an asthma attack.

Cold viruses can survive for hours on doorknobs, handrails, and even money. Washing your hands often—at least every few hours—will flush away the viruses before they have a chance to take hold. Some people have infectious asthma, meaning they wheeze only when they have a cold or flu, says Dr. Haas.

■ **THINK TWICE ABOUT ASPIRIN.** Close to 5 percent of those with asthma are sensitive to aspirin, ibuprofen, and related pain relievers, known as nonsteroidal anti-inflammatory drugs (NSAIDs). For those who are sensitive, an asthma attack or other respiratory problems can begin within 3 hours of taking the drugs. If you have asthma and chronic sinusitis with nasal polyps, your chances of developing a sensitivity to aspirin (known as "aspirin exacerbated respiratory disease") is about one in three, says Dr. Lang.

If you need long-term pain relief—from arthritis, for example—your doctor may advise you to switch to acetaminophen or other analgesics that are less likely to trigger asthma attacks. Because acetaminophen may also "cross-react" in those sensitive to aspirin, you should take regular rather than extra-strength acetaminophen, and always avoid not only aspirin but also medications otherwise known as NSAIDs, including ibuprofen, naproxen, and others, says Dr. Lang. If you have aspirin sensitivity, the reaction to it and these other drugs can be serious or even life-threatening.

■ **DON'T PUT UP WITH HEARTBURN.** The upward surge of stomach acids that cause the telltale pain of heartburn can also trigger asthma attacks. One of the best ways to prevent heartburn is to eat four or more small meals daily, instead of two or three large meals, says Dr. Plaut. Also, don't eat 2 hours before bedtime. To help prevent stomach acid from going "upstream," create an incline by raising the head of your bed 4 to 6 inches by putting blocks under the top legs.

You can also treat heartburn with over-the-counter antacids or acid-suppressing drugs, such as cimetidine (Tagamet) and ranitidine (Zantac), or proton pump inhibitors (Prilosec).

■ **FLUSH YOUR SINUSES.** Millions of Americans get sinus infections every year, and the inflammation and mucus drainage can make asthma worse. Sinusitis often requires treatment with antibiotics, but you may be able to prevent infections by flushing your sinuses at home, says Dr. Plaut.

Mix $\frac{1}{2}$ teaspoon of salt in 1 cup of warm water. Put the solution into a plastic squeeze bottle (available at drugstores), a neti pot, or a measuring cup. Use the solution to rinse out one nostril, then repeat with the other nostril. People susceptible to sinus infections should repeat the treatment at least once daily. If you get infections less often, flush the sinuses only at the first sign of a cold or when your allergies are worse than usual.

■ **ACT QUICKLY IF ASTHMA STRIKES.** Don't ignore early signs of asthma attacks, even if the symptoms—wheezing, coughing, or faster breathing—seem mild at first. Use your rescue medication promptly. It will help reverse airway narrowing before the attack gets more serious, says Dr. Plaut.

■ **KEEP TRACK OF INHALER "PUFFS."** Many inhalers have a built-in dose counter. If you use medication to control asthma, the worst thing is to discover that your inhaler is empty right when you need it. To prevent this, put a piece of masking tape on the inhaler and make a mark on the tape every time you use it. If you take a medicine on a regular basis—for example, two puffs a day—you can calculate the date you will run out simply by dividing the total number of doses in the inhaler by the number of puffs you take in a day.

■ **OR USE THE DOSER.** Available at allergy supply stores and catalogs, the Doser attaches to metered inhalers and automatically keeps track of how many doses you have left.

■ **USE A PEAK-FLOW METER.** A peak-flow meter is a device that measures the speed at which air leaves the lungs. It's available in drugstores and is an invaluable way to detect the airway narrowing that occurs prior to asthma attacks. A reading between 80 to 100 percent indicates that your breathing is healthy, says Dr. Plaut. Lower scores may indicate that you need higher doses of medication or your asthma isn't adequately controlled. Keep a daily diary that lists the following: peak-flow levels, frequency and severity of symptoms, number of medicine usages, and exposure to possible triggers. By consulting the diary regularly, you'll be able to detect factors that cause your asthma to get worse—and those that cause it to improve, Dr. Plaut says.

PANEL OF ADVISORS

KENDALL GERDES, M.D., IS DIRECTOR OF ENVIRONMENTAL MEDICINE ASSOCIATES IN DENVER.

ELSON HAAS, M.D., IS DIRECTOR OF THE PREVENTIVE MEDICAL CENTER OF MARIN, AN INTEGRATED HEALTHCARE FACILITY IN SAN RAFAEL, CALIFORNIA, AND AUTHOR OF SEVEN BOOKS ON HEALTH AND NUTRITION, INCLUDING *THE FALSE FAT DIET, STAYING HEALTHY WITH NUTRITION,* AND *THE NEW DETOX DIET.*

DAVID LANG, M.D., IS HEAD OF ALLERGY AND IMMUNOLOGY IN THE RESPIRATORY INSTITUTE AT CLEVELAND CLINIC IN OHIO.

THOMAS F. PLAUT, M.D., IS AUTHOR OF *DR. TOM PLAUT'S ASTHMA GUIDE FOR PEOPLE OF ALL AGES* AND *ONE-MINUTE ASTHMA: WHAT YOU NEED TO KNOW.*

Athlete's Foot

18 Ways to Get Rid of It

You don't have to be an athlete to catch athlete's foot. You can pick up the fungal infection, which is caused by organisms that live on the skin and breed best in warm, moist conditions, by letting your bare feet touch wet areas in locker rooms, pools, and bathrooms. And even though these humid climates encourage the growth of the fungus, sweaty footwear (including thermal socks, insulated boots, and stinky sneakers) is the more usual culprit.

Athlete's foot is the most common form of tinea, a fungal infection of the nails, skin, hair, or body. The fungus triggers redness, swelling, cracking, burning, scaling, and intense itching between your toes, and your skin may also appear puckered.

Once you have the fungus, it takes at least 4 weeks to make headway against a savage case. Worse, it will return unless you stamp out the conditions that caused it in the first place. So here are some tips on dealing with an active infection and some ways to guard against an encore.

■ **TAKE IT EASY AT FIRST.** Athlete's foot can come on suddenly and be accompanied by oozing blisters and intermittent burning, says Frederick Hass, M.D. When you're going through this acute stage, baby your foot. Keep it uncovered and at constant rest.

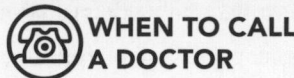

WHEN TO CALL A DOCTOR

How do you know if that red, itching splotch between your toes is a true case of athlete's foot? And when should tinea between your toes send you scrambling to see a doctor? If the condition hasn't improved and you're in a lot of pain, it's time to see your doctor, says Suzanne M. Levine, D.P.M., P.C. And be wary of infection. You can't assume that athlete's foot will go away on its own, says Dr. Levine. An unchecked fungal infection can lead to cracks in the skin and invite a nasty bacterial infection. Consult your physician if:

■ Your foot is swollen and warm to the touch, especially if there are red streaks

■ The inflammation proves incapacitating

■ You have diabetes and develop athlete's foot

■ Pus appears in the blisters or the cracked skin

Although the inflammation itself is not dangerous, it can lead to a bacterial infection if you're not careful.

■ **SOOTHE THE SORES.** Use compresses to cool the inflammation, ease the pain, lessen the itching, and dry the sores, says Dr. Hass. Dissolve one packet of Domeboro powder or 2 tablespoons of Burow's solution (both available without a prescription at drugstores) in 1 pint of cold water. Soak an untreated white cotton cloth in the liquid and apply three or four times daily for 15 to 20 minutes.

■ **USE A SALTY SOLUTION.** Soak your foot in a mixture of 2 teaspoons of salt per pint of warm water, says Suzanne M. Levine, D.P.M., P.C. Do this for 5 to 10 minutes at a time, and repeat until the problem clears up. The saline solution provides an unappealing atmosphere for the fungus and lessens excess perspiration. What's more, it softens the affected skin so that antifungal medications can penetrate deeper and be more effective.

■ **MEDICATE YOUR FOOT.** An over-the-counter antifungal medication may contain miconazole nitrate (found in Micatin products, for example), tolnaftate (Aftate or Tinactin), or fatty acids (Desenex). Dr. Levine recommends using antifungal gels instead of creams or lotions, since the gels contain a drying agent. Lightly apply the medication to the area involved and rub in gently. Continue two or three times a day for 4 weeks (or for 2 weeks after the problem seems to have cleared up).

■ **AVOID ALUMINUM CHLORIDE.** It used to be the popular treatment for athlete's foot, but experts claim all aluminum chloride does is remove heat and moisture from the fungus's habitat. It doesn't kill the fungus, says Neal Kramer, D.P.M.

■ **RUB IN BAKING SODA.** For fungus on your feet, especially between the toes, apply a baking soda paste, suggests Dr. Levine. Add a little lukewarm water to 1 tablespoon of baking soda. Rub the paste on the fungus, then rinse and dry thoroughly. Finish the treatment by dusting on cornstarch or powder.

■ **SCRUB AWAY DEAD SKIN.** When the acute phase of the attack has settled down, remove any dead skin, advises Dr. Hass. "It houses living fungi that can reinfect you. At bath time, work the entire foot lightly but vigorously with a bristle scrub brush. Pay extra attention to spaces between toes—use a small bottle brush or test-tube brush there." If you scrub your feet in the bathtub, shower afterward to wash away any bits of skin that could attach themselves to other parts of the body and start another infection.

■ **KEEP APPLYING MEDICATION.** Once your infection has cleared, help guard against its return by continuing to use (less often) the antifungal medication that cured your problem, says Dr. Levine. This is especially prudent during warm weather. You should continue using the cream for 50 percent longer than it took to clear up the problem. Once the condition is gone, if it took a month to knock out the fungus, for example, use the medication faithfully for an additional 2 weeks to get the last of it.

■ **CHOOSE PROPER SHOES AND SOCKS.** Avoid plastic shoes and footwear that has been treated to be waterproof, says Dr. Levine. They trap perspiration and create a warm, moist spot for the fungus to grow. Natural materials such as cotton and leather provide the best environment for feet, while rubber and even wool may induce sweating and hold moisture.

■ **CHANGE THEM OFTEN.** Don't wear the same shoes 2 days in a row, says podiatrist Dean S. Stern, D.P.M. It takes at least 24 hours for shoes to dry out thoroughly. If your feet perspire heavily, change shoes twice a day.

■ **AIR THEM OUT.** Dr. Hass recommends giving your shoes a little time in the sun to air out. Remove the laces, open each shoe, and prop it in the sun. You should even leave sandals outdoors to dry between wearings. And wipe the undersides of their straps clean after every wearing to remove any fungi-carrying dead skin. The idea is to reduce even the slightest possibility of reinfection.

■ **KEEP THEM DRY—AND CLEAN.** Dust the insides of your shoes frequently with antifungal powder or spray. Another good idea, says Dr. Kramer, is to spray some disinfectant (such as Lysol) on a rag and use it to wipe the insides of your shoes every time you take them off. This kills any fungus spores.

■ **SOCK THE INFECTION.** If your feet perspire heavily, says Dr. Hass, change your socks three or four times a day. And wear only clean cotton socks, not those made with synthetic yarns. Be sure to rinse them thoroughly during laundering, because detergent residue can aggravate your skin problem. To help kill fungus spores, says Dr. Kramer, wash your socks twice in hot water.

■ **POWDER YOUR TOES.** To further keep your feet dry, allow them to air for 5 to 10 minutes after a shower before putting on your socks and shoes. If you eliminate anything that's hot, dark, and moist, you're better off, says Dr. Kramer. To speed drying, hold a hair dryer about 6 inches from each foot, wiggle your toes, and dry between them. Then apply powder. To avoid a powder mess, place it in a plastic or paper bag, then put your foot into the bag and shake it well.

■ **COVER UP IN PUBLIC PLACES.** You can decrease your exposure to the fungus by wearing slippers or shower shoes in areas in which other people go barefoot, says Dr. Levine. This includes gyms, spas, health clubs, locker rooms, and even around swimming pools. If you're prone to fungal infections, you can pick them up almost any place that is damp—so be prudent.

PANEL OF ADVISORS

FREDERICK HASS, M.D., IS A GENERAL PRACTITIONER IN SAN RAFAEL, CALIFORNIA.

NEAL KRAMER, D.P.M., IS A PODIATRIST IN BETHLEHEM, PENNSYLVANIA.

SUZANNE M. LEVINE, D.P.M., P.C., IS A PODIATRIC SURGEON AND CLINICAL PODIATRIST AT NEW YORK HOSPITAL-CORNELL MEDICAL CENTER. SHE IS THE AUTHOR OF *YOUR FEET DON'T HAVE TO HURT.*

DEAN S. STERN, D.P.M., IS A PODIATRIST AT RUSH–PRESBYTERIAN–ST. LUKE'S MEDICAL CENTER IN CHICAGO.

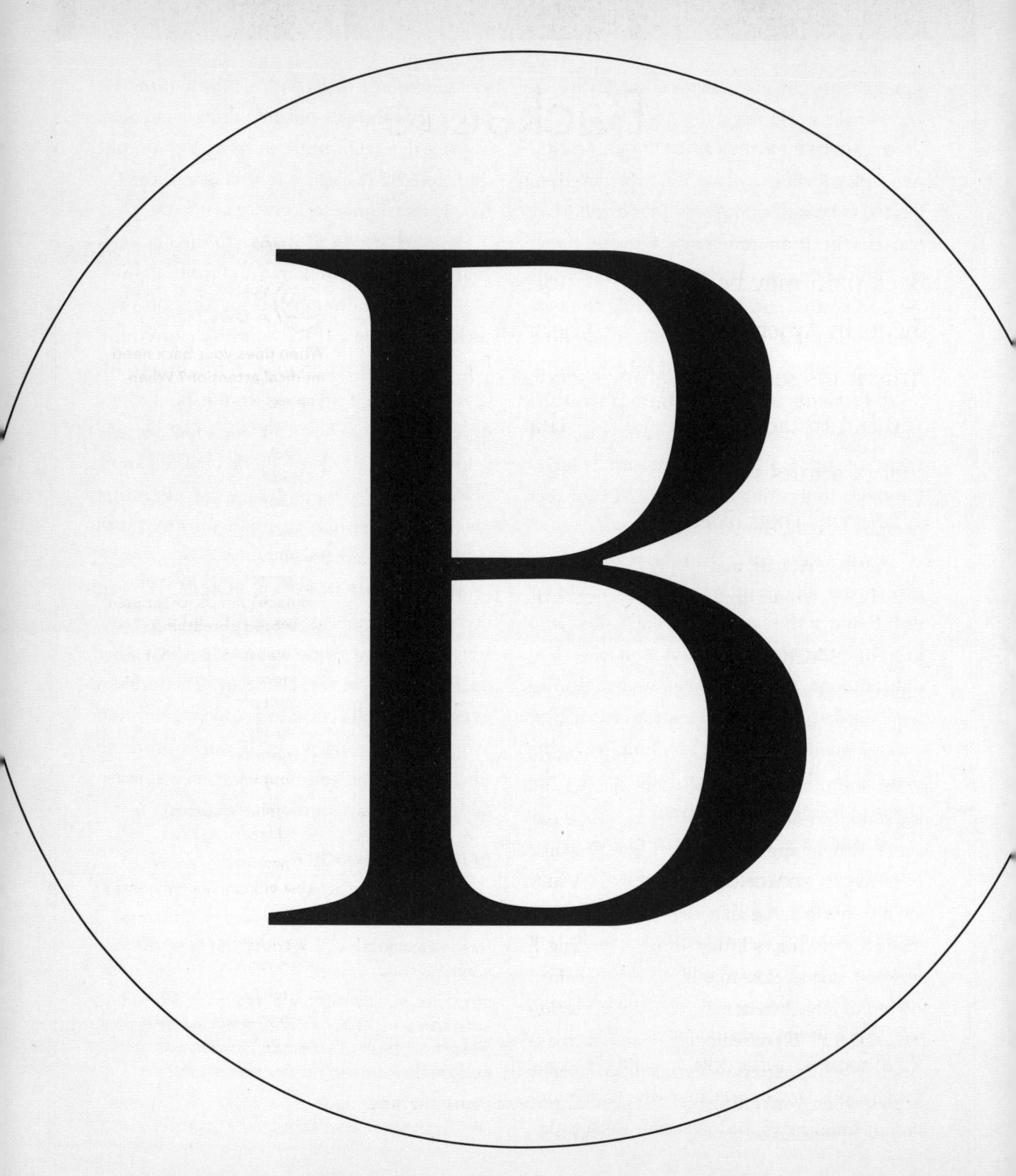

Backache

22 Pain-Free Ideas

Back pain may be one of the most pervasive ailments in America. It's the number two reason that Americans see their doctors—second only to colds and flu. In fact, research shows that up to 90 percent of adults suffer from back pain at some time or other in their lives.

Lower-back pain may be acute (short-term), lasting less than 1 month, or chronic (ongoing), lasting more than 3 months.

ACUTE BACK PAIN

Acute pain comes on suddenly and intensely. It's the kind you might experience from doing something that you shouldn't be doing or from doing it the wrong way. The pain can come from sprains, strains, or muscle pulls in your back. It may hurt like crazy for several days, but doctors say that you can be pain free within 4 to 6 weeks without any lasting effects by following these self-help tips.

■ **AVOID PROLONGED STOOPING OR BENDING POSTURES.** If you'll be performing an activity that requires prolonged stooping, bending, twisting, or lifting (think gardening, filing, or cleaning out drawers), stay as close to your work as comfortably possible and try to keep your back in its natural upright position, says Gregory Snow, D.C., C.C.S.P. "If you're unable to maintain a neutral posture, treat the activity like exercise—warm up, do the activity, take breaks, and stretch when you're finished." A neutral position puts the least amount of tension on bones, joints, and muscles.

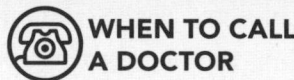

WHEN TO CALL A DOCTOR

When does your back need medical attention? When you experience any of the following:

■ Back pain that comes on suddenly and for no apparent reason

■ Back pain that is accompanied by other symptoms, such as fever, stomach cramps, chest pain, or difficulty breathing

■ An acute attack that lasts for more than a week or so without any pain relief

■ Chronic pain that lasts for more than 2 weeks without relief

■ Burning with urination or blood in your urine

■ Uncontrollable loss of urine or stool (incontinence)

■ Weakness or numbness in your buttocks, leg, or pelvis region

■ Back pain that radiates down your leg to your knee or foot

■ **STAY ACTIVE.** Forget the old adage about plenty of bed rest. In a study at the Texas Tech University Health Sciences Center School of Nursing, researchers found that patients who exercised returned to work more quickly than those who didn't. After a day or two of rest, begin light cardio training such as walking, riding a stationary bicycle, or swimming. Aerobic activities can help blood flow to your back and promote healing. They also help strengthen muscles in your stomach and your back. "Return to as much of your usual routine as possible, as long as there's no severe pain," says Dennis C. Turk, Ph.D. "But do it gradually. If you experience pain, just cut back and increase your activity over time."

■ **IF YOU MUST GO TO BED, KEEP IT SHORT.** Most people believe that a week of bed rest will cure the pain. But that's not so. For every week of bed rest, it takes 2 weeks to rehabilitate.

A study at the University of Texas Health Sciences Center bears this out. Researchers there tracked 203 patients who came into a walk-in clinic complaining of acute back pain. Some were told to rest for 2 days, others for 7 days. There was no difference in the length of time it took the pain to diminish in either group, reports Richard A. Deyo, M.D., one of the researchers. But those who got out of bed after only 2 days returned to work sooner.

■ **PUT YOUR PAIN ON ICE.** The best way to cool down an acute flare-up is to ice the area within the first hour or two, says Dr. Turk. This helps reduce inflammation. You might also want to try ice massage. "But place the ice in a towel, not directly on the skin," Dr. Turk advises. Apply the ice for 15 minutes, then repeat every hour.

■ **TRY SOME HEAT RELIEF.** After the first day or two of ice, switch to heat, says Dr. Turk. Take a soft towel and put it in a basin of very warm water. Wring it well and flatten it so that there are no creases. Put a layer of plastic wrap over the towel, and then a heating pad set on medium on the plastic. Lie on your stomach, with pillows under your hips and ankles, and lay the towel sandwich across the painful part of your back. If possible, place something, such as a phone book, on top to create a little pressure. You can also take hot baths or showers to relax the muscles, says Dr. Turk. Once you get past the inflammation, heat helps relax the muscles. In fact, in one study of 30 patients with lower-back pain published in the *Clinical Journal of Pain*, those who used a heat wrap along with oral pain relievers reported significantly less lower-back pain than those who took just the pain relievers.

■ **USE HEAT *AND* COLD.** For those of you who can't make up your mind which feels better, it's okay to use both methods, says Edward Abraham, M.D. Do 30 minutes of ice, then 30 minutes of heat, and keep repeating the cycle, ending with the ice.

■ **STRETCH TO SMOOTH A SPASM.** Stretching a sore back will actually enhance the healing process. "It's also helpful for preventing another flare-up," says Dr. Turk. He recom-

Exercise Your Pain Away

Exercise may be the last thing on your mind when your back is hurting, but you should get up and moving as soon as you're able. Experts agree that a little gentle physical activity is the best Rx for back pain, especially the chronic kind that tends to vary in intensity over the course of your day. Be sure to check with your doctor before beginning any sort of exercise program. Once you've got the ok, try these expert-approved moves.

Do pressups. Pressups are something like half of a pushup. Lie on the floor on your stomach. Keep your pelvis flat on the floor and push up with your hands, arching your back as you lift your shoulders off the floor.

This helps strengthen your lower back. Do it once in the morning and once in the afternoon.

Move into a crunch. While you're on the floor, turn onto your back and do what's called a crunch situp. Lie flat with both feet on the floor and your knees bent. Cross your arms and rest your hands on your shoulders. Raise your head and shoulders off the floor as high as you can while keeping your lower back on the floor. Hold for 1 second, then repeat.

Swim on dry land. You don't need a pool—you can swim on your floor. Lie on your stomach and raise your left arm and your right leg. Hold for 1 second, then alternate with your left leg and right arm as if you were swimming. This will extend and strengthen your lower back.

Get into the pool. A good exercise for acute lower-back pain is a swim in a warm pool. "Swimming can be very beneficial because the water is so therapeutic," says Dennis C. Turk, Ph.D. "Make sure you don't do too much too fast." Try using a snorkel and a mask while you're swimming so you don't have to worry about breathing and turning your neck, says Edward Abraham, M.D.

Take an indoor spin. Ride a stationary bike with a mirror set up so that you can see yourself. Be sure to sit up straight without slouching. If you have to, raise the handlebar so that you're not bent too far forward.

Listen to your body. Be careful and know your limits with these and any other exercises. If the activity you're doing hurts or aggravates your condition, don't do it anymore. If you feel fine a day or two after you exercise, then it's safe to continue exercising. "Back exercise doesn't seem to help for acute pain," says Richard A. Deyo, M.D. "It's better to wait until it has improved, at which point exercise may help to prevent recurrences."

mends the following stretch for lower-back pain: Lie on your back and gently bring your knees up to your chest. Once there, put a little pressure on your knees. Stretch, then relax. Repeat. You can also try gently stretching your body side to side and then forward and back. "The most important thing is to take any stretching exercises slowly and gently," he adds.

■ **ROLL OUT OF BED.** Each morning, when you're ready to get out of bed, slowly and carefully roll onto your side with your knees bent, says Dr. Snow. Push yourself up with your arms or elbows into a seated position. Place your feet flat on the floor before you start to stand up, suggests Dr. Turk. And move slowly, keeping your back as rigid as possible.

CHRONIC BACK PAIN

For some people, back pain is chronic, a part of everyday life. The pain lingers for what can seem like an eternity. Other people experience recurring pain, which can happen unpredictably. The following tips are particularly helpful for those with chronic pain, although people with acute pain can benefit from them as well.

■ **FIRM UP YOUR MATTRESS.** Lumber under the mattress will help the lumbar on top. The object is to have a bed that doesn't sag in the middle when you sleep on it. "If you don't have a firm mattress, put a ¾-inch piece of plywood between the mattress and the box spring to end the sagging problem," says Dr. Turk.

■ **BECOME A "LAZY S" SLEEPER.** A bad back can't stomach lying facedown. "The best position for someone resting in bed is what we call the lazy S position," says Dr. Abraham. "Put a pillow under your head and upper neck, keep your back relatively flat on the bed, then put a pillow under your knees."

When you straighten your legs, your hamstring muscles pull and put pressure on your lower back, he explains. Keeping your knees bent puts slack into the hamstrings and takes the pressure off your back.

■ **DEVELOP FETAL ATTRACTION.** You'll sleep like a baby if you sleep on your side in the fetal position. "It's a good idea to stick a pillow between your knees when you sleep on your side," adds Dr. Turk. The pillow stops your leg from sliding forward and rotating your hips, which puts added pressure on your back.

■ **TAKE AN ASPIRIN.** Aspirin helps reduce inflammation, says Dr. Turk. "Take it with a full 8-ounce glass of water and follow the dose instructions on the bottle. If you aren't experiencing any benefit after 3 or 4 days, stop taking the aspirin and talk to your doctor. Acetaminophen may be effective for the pain, but it is not an anti-inflammatory drug."

■ **VISUALIZE YOURSELF PAIN-FREE.** The middle of the night can be the worst time for pain. Pain wakes you up, and it keeps you up. "Using visualization is a particularly good thing to do at times like this," says Dr. Turk.

"Close your eyes and imagine something pleasant," suggests Dr. Turk. "Think of yourself on a ski slope, for example, if that's something you enjoy. The idea is to bring as much detail to the image as possible so you can actually smell the trees and feel the mountain air. The more involved you are in the image, the more you are engaged with it, and the quicker you will become distracted from the pain," he says.

Protect Your Back When You Sit

Does your back drive you crazy every time you buckle up? It could be that the seat is your problem. While there are many causes for back pain, most people have what is called mechanical back pain, or pain related to sitting, standing, lifting, or bending. Riding in the car or sitting at a desk can be a real source of pain for people in this category, says Dennis C. Turk, Ph.D.

Take a new car for a "test sit." Next time you're in the market for a car, check for cushion comfort, too. The back of the seat should push against your lower back around your waist. "Better cars have built-in lumbar support," says Dr. Turk. A smart thing to do is rent the same make and model for a weekend and take a long drive to see how comfortable the seat is. For a less-expensive solution than buying a new car—or a different seat in the one you own—Dr. Turk suggests placing a pillow or towel behind the small of your back while you're driving to make you more comfortable.

Use a pillow for support. If you're working at your desk, or lounging on soft, mushy home furniture, a small pillow offers a quick fix for mechanical back pain, says Dr. Turk. Place the pillow in the curve of your lower back, which will put the spine into "neutral" and prevent slouching. Blow-up cushions are also available in health catalogs and online.

■ **TRY TAI CHI TO UNTIE MUSCLE KNOTS.**
Tai chi is an ancient Chinese discipline of slow, fluid movements. "It's a great relaxation method that helps the muscles in your back," says Dr. Abraham, who uses the method himself. "There are a lot of breathing exercises and stretching activities that foster a harmony within the body."

Tai chi takes time and self-discipline to learn, but Dr. Abraham says that it's worth it. Yoga is another good form of exercise to try. In fact, evidence supports the use of a type of yoga called viniyoga for easing back pain, says Dr. Deyo.

PANEL OF ADVISORS

EDWARD ABRAHAM, M.D., IS A CLINICAL ASSISTANT PROFESSOR OF ORTHOPEDICS AT THE UNIVERSITY OF CALIFORNIA, IRVINE, COLLEGE OF MEDICINE, AND HAS A PRACTICE IN SANTA ANA. HE ORIGINATED THE CONCEPT FOR OUTPATIENT BACK THERAPY IN THE UNITED STATES.

RICHARD A. DEYO, M.D., IS A PROFESSOR OF FAMILY MEDICINE AND INTERNAL MEDICINE AT OREGON HEALTH SCIENCE UNIVERSITY IN PORTLAND.

GREGORY SNOW, D.C., C.C.S.P., IS DEAN OF CLINICS AT PALMER COLLEGE OF CHIROPRACTIC, WEST CAMPUS IN SAN JOSE, CALIFORNIA.

DENNIS C. TURK, PH.D., IS THE JOHN AND EMMA BONICA PROFESSOR OF ANESTHESIOLOGY AND PAIN RESEARCH AT THE UNIVERSITY OF WASHINGTON IN SEATTLE.

Bad Breath

15 Ways to Overcome It

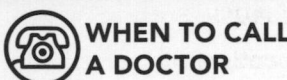 **WHEN TO CALL A DOCTOR**

If your halitosis hangs on for more than 24 hours without an obvious cause, call your dentist or doctor. "When you have bad breath, it's usually a sign of an imbalance in the system," says John C. Moon, D.D.S. It can be a sign of gum disease, diabetes, abscess, or bacterial or fungi overgrowth. "Bad breath often stems from some form of inflammation," says Dr. Moon. It can also be a sign of dehydration or zinc deficiency, or it can be caused by drugs, including penicillamine and lithium.

In Roman times, people used sticks for toothbrushes and tooth powder so abrasive that it ground away the surface of the teeth, exposing the pulp. When their teeth hurt, they applied olive oil in which earthworms had been boiled. After all of that, it's safe to say, they had bad breath.

Today, dental hygiene is big business, and the space allocated to it in the average grocery store rivals that of the produce section. Still, people worry about their breath. The good news is that for the most part—with proper dental care—bad breath, also called halitosis, can be avoided for good. Here's how.

■ **GO EASY ON THE GARLIC.** Highly spiced foods like to linger long after the party's over. Certain tastes and smells linger in the form of the essential oils that they leave in your mouth. Depending on how much you eat, the odor can remain up to 24 hours, no matter how often you brush your teeth. Some foods to avoid include onions, hot peppers, and garlic.

■ **DELAY THE DELI RUN.** Spicy deli meats such as pastrami, salami, and pepperoni also leave their oils behind long after you've swallowed that sandwich. You breathe. They breathe. "Since these are acidic foods, they promote bacteria colonization and dry mouth, which causes bad breath," says John C. Moon, D.D.S. If an occasion calls for sweet-smelling breath, avoid these meats for 24 hours beforehand to keep them from talking for you.

■ **SAY, "PLEASE, NO CHEESE."** Camembert, Roquefort, and blue cheese are called strong for good reason—they get a hold on your breath and don't let go. Some other dairy products may have the same effect.

■ **WELCOME YOGURT.** Preliminary research shows that the live bacteria in yogurt can suppress levels of bad-breath-causing bacteria. Researchers think yogurt reduces the smell-inducing bacteria coating the tongue. The theory: Good bugs in yogurt may crowd out the stink-causing bacteria or create an unhealthy environment for it. Yogurt promotes good bacteria, says Dr. Moon.

■ **LIMIT FISH.** Some fish, like the anchovies on your pizza or the tuna you tuck into your brown-bag lunch, can leave a lasting impression.

Cures from the Kitchen

EAT YOUR VEGETABLES. "Vegetables help decrease acidity," says John C. Moon, D.D.S. "That not only promotes good breath, but also good overall health." If all else fails, eat your garnish. Parsley contains chlorophyll, a known breath deodorizer. Toss a few handfuls (even add some watercress to the mix) in a juicer. Sip the juice anytime you need to refresh your breath.

THINK "SPICE IS NICE." Other herbs and spices in your kitchen are natural breath enhancers. Carry a tiny plastic bag of cloves, fennel, or anise seeds to chew after odorous meals.

TRY A GARGLE SPECIAL. Mix extracts of sage, calendula, and myrrh gum (all available at health food stores) in equal proportions and gargle with the mixture four times a day. Keep the mouthwash in a tightly sealed jar at room temperature.

■ **WATCH WHAT YOU DRINK.** Coffee, beer, wine, and whiskey are at the top of the list of liquid offenders. Each leaves a residue that can attach to the plaque in your mouth and infiltrate your digestive system. Each breath you take spews traces back into the air.

■ **CARRY A TOOTHBRUSH.** Some odors can be eliminated—permanently or temporarily—if you brush immediately after a meal. The main culprit in bad breath is a soft, sticky film of living and dead bacteria that clings to your teeth and gums, says Dr. Moon. This film is called plaque. At any time, there are 50 trillion of these microscopic organisms loitering in your mouth. They sit in every dark corner, eating each morsel of food that passes your lips, collecting little smells, and producing little odors of their own. As you exhale, the bacteria exhale. So brush away the plaque after each meal and get rid of some of the breath problem.

■ **SIP ON WATER.** Even when you can't brush, you can rinse. Take a sip of water after meals, swish it around, and wash the smell of food from your mouth, says Jerry F. Taintor, D.D.S. In fact, experts claim that drinking at least eight 8-ounce glasses of water daily keeps your mouth moist and helps wash away the food debris on which bacteria thrive. "Dry mouth is a serious problem for people who take certain medications such as antihistamines, and for our growing elderly population who are on multiple medications," says Dr. Taintor. In fact, dry mouth is one of the main culprits behind bad breath.

How to Test Your Breath

How horrible is your halitosis? If you don't have a friend to tell you the truth, there are a couple of ways you can test your breath.

Cup your hands. Breathe into them with a great, deep "ha-a-a-a." Sniff. If it smells rank to you, then it's deadly to those around you. "Most people who have bad breath, know it," says John C. Moon D.D.S. "People who have bad breath also have a taste indifference, so that's another indication that something is going on."

Floss. Pull the floss gently between your teeth and then sniff some of the gunk you unearth. It will have an odor no matter what, but if it smells bad, you smell bad.

■ **GARGLE A MINTY MOUTHWASH.** If you need 20 minutes of freedom from bad breath, gargling with a mouthwash is a great idea. But like Cinderella's coach-turned-pumpkin, when your time is up, the magic will be gone, and you'll be talking from behind your hand again. Want extra protection? Dip your toothbrush in a mouth rinse with 0.12 percent chlorhexidine gluconate (such as Peridex, an over-the-counter mouth rinse made by Procter & Gamble) and brush your tongue, too.

■ **CHOOSE YOUR MOUTHWASH BY INGREDIENTS.** Medicine-flavored mouthwashes contain essential oils such as thyme, eucalyptus, peppermint, and wintergreen, as well as sodium benzoate or benzoic acid. Herbs and essential oils help neutralize the odor-producing waste products of your mouth bacteria, says Dr. Moon. He recommends Biotene, Crest ProHealth, or The Natural Dentist mouthwashes. "They taste very refreshing and there's no alcohol in them," he says. No matter which mouthwash you choose, avoid products containing alcohol, which causes dry mouth.

■ **CHEW A MINT OR SOME GUM.** Like mouthwash, a breath mint or minty gum is just a cover-up, good for a short interview, a short ride in a compact car, or a very short date. But avoid gum containing sugar, cautions Dr. Moon. "Sugar can breed bacteria and promote bad breath. Instead, chew on sugarless gum or Biotene gum." Biotene has a complete line of products, including rinse, gum, and spray. Dr. Moon recommends all three. Just keep gum chewing to a minimum, because it wears down teeth.

■ **BRUSH YOUR TONGUE.** "Most people overlook their tongues," says Dr. Moon. Your tongue is covered with little hairlike projections, which under a microscope look like a forest of mushrooms. Beneath the caps of the "mushrooms," there's room for plaque and some of the things we eat to get lodged. This stuff causes bad breath.

What the Doctor Does

Jerry F. Taintor, D.D.S., chews sugarless, minty gum with sips of water. It moves the minty flavor throughout the mouth and makes your breath smell better. What about the bacteria? Good question. Dr. Taintor uses mouthwash before brushing and after brushing. "This helps reduce the amount of oral bacteria," he says. Less bacteria equals better breath and less dental decay.

His advice? When you brush your teeth, gently go over your tongue, too. This will help clear away the food and bacteria that lead to bad breath. If you want, you can buy a tongue scraper just for this purpose; they're sold in many drugstores and discount department stores.

Dr. Moon also recommends a product called Breath Rx, which loosens debris on the tongue and helps kill odor-causing bacteria.

PANEL OF ADVISORS

JOHN C. MOON, D.D.S., IS A COSMETIC AND GENERAL DENTIST IN HALF MOON BAY, CALIFORNIA.

JERRY F. TAINTOR, D.D.S., IS FORMER CHAIR OF ENDODONTICS AT THE UNIVERSITY OF TENNESSEE COLLEGE OF DENTISTRY IN MEMPHIS AND UCLA SCHOOL OF DENTISTRY. HE IS AUTHOR OF *THE COMPLETE GUIDE TO BETTER DENTAL CARE*.

Bed-Wetting

6 Options for Sleep-Through Nights

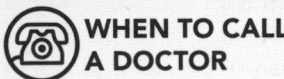

WHEN TO CALL A DOCTOR

"If your child has been previously dry at night but then starts wetting, it can be a sign of diabetes or a urinary tract infection," says Tanya Remer Altmann, M.D. "If you go to the doctor and get a simple urine test, at least you can rule out more serious issues." Chances are, reverting to nighttime wetting is an emotional issue caused by a new baby in the family or another significant transition.

Bed-wetting, also called enuresis, is such a common childhood challenge that millions of boys and girls regularly wake up to sopping sheets and pajamas. Roughly 15 percent of all 5-year-olds, 5 percent of 10-year-olds, and 1 percent of 15-year-olds wet the bed. The problem is more common among boys.

The causes are varied. Sometimes the bladder is too small to handle all the urine, says Jennifer Shu, M.D. Other reasons point to slow physical development and an inability to recognize a full bladder during sleep. After the age of 4, anxiety may play a role. Finally, genetics may be to blame: In the 1990s, Danish scientists found a sign that human chromosome 13 may be at least partly responsible for bed-wetting.

The good news? Almost all kids outgrow bed-wetting. In the meantime, try these remedies.

■ **BE REALISTIC.** "It's completely normal for children not to be dry at night up to age 6 or 7," says Tanya Remer Altmann, M.D. "Potty training really refers to daytime use of the toilet, so even if your child is wetting the bed at night, he may still be potty trained." It's also a good idea to let kids know that they're not alone and that some of their friends probably wet the bed, too. "If you have a school of 100 fifth graders, for example, about five of them still wet the bed," says Dr. Shu. "Putting this into perspective can sometimes make kids feel less embarrassed about the condition."

■ **STOP THE FLUIDS.** Decrease the amount of fluids children drink before bed; make up the difference earlier in the day, recommends Dr. Altmann.

■ **SCHEDULE A MIDNIGHT WAKE-UP CALL.** If you're up late, take your sleeping child to the bathroom before you go to bed. "That helps prevent nighttime accidents," says Dr. Shu. "Or, if you wake up to urinate, wake up your child at that time so she can go, too."

■ **BUY ABSORBENT BRIEFS FOR BEDTIME.** To help minimize psychological stress, Dr. Altmann recommends using nighttime pull-ups or absorbent underwear. "They make little boxers in pink or blue, so even girls can wear them with a T-shirt and look like they're wearing shorts," she says. "It's much easier now than when we were kids, because you can buy absorbent bed pads and after your child has an accident, you just change the pad and the bottom sheet."

■ **SET THE ALARM.** "Bed-wetting alarms can work," says Bryan P. Shumaker, M.D. "But you'd better have patience. The alarm is loud, and chances are good it will wake up everybody in the house when it goes off."

Bed-wetting alarms emit a buzzing or ringing sound when the child is wet. The theory is that the sound will condition him to awaken when he needs to urinate. Eventually, wetting will ease, and a full bladder will signal the child to awaken.

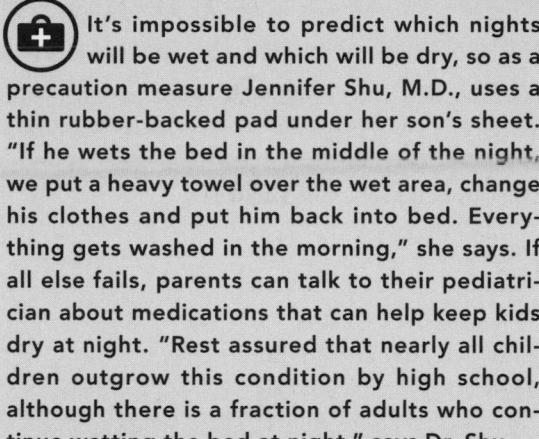

What the Doctor Does

It's impossible to predict which nights will be wet and which will be dry, so as a precaution measure Jennifer Shu, M.D., uses a thin rubber-backed pad under her son's sheet. "If he wets the bed in the middle of the night, we put a heavy towel over the wet area, change his clothes and put him back into bed. Everything gets washed in the morning," she says. If all else fails, parents can talk to their pediatrician about medications that can help keep kids dry at night. "Rest assured that nearly all children outgrow this condition by high school, although there is a fraction of adults who continue wetting the bed at night," says Dr. Shu.

The newer alarms, which are much smaller and more sensitive to wetness than the bulky, complicated mats and pads of yesterday, run on hearing-aid batteries and have moisture sensors that attach directly to underwear. Best of all, the relapse rates with new alarms is only 10 to 20 percent, compared with the 50 percent relapse rate with older models. A second round of alarm use is usually enough for lasting success.

Most children respond to this conditioning strategy within 60 days, says Dr. Shumaker. Bed-wetting is considered cured when the child remains dry for 21 consecutive nights.

■ **PRACTICE PATIENCE AND LOVE.** "Understand that all kids outgrow bed-wetting at a rate of 15 percent a year," says Dr. Shumaker. "Which means by the time they go through puberty, less than 1 or 2 percent will still wet the bed. So be patient and supportive. No kid wants to wet himself; it's unpleasant, uncomfortable, and cold. "It's embarrassing, too. So help your child, but don't badger him. Time is on your side."

PANEL OF ADVISORS

TANYA REMER ALTMANN, M.D., IS A PEDIATRICIAN IN WESTLAKE VILLAGE, CALIFORNIA AND AUTHOR OF *MOMMY CALLS*.

JENNIFER SHU, M.D., IS A PEDIATRICIAN AND PARENTING BOOK AUTHOR IN ATLANTA.

BRYAN P. SHUMAKER, M.D., IS A UROLOGIST AT MICHIGAN INSTITUTE OF UROLOGY IN ST. CLAIRE SHORES.

Belching

11 Steps to Banish the Burps

Everyone belches on occasion, but when it happens often or interferes with your normal activities, it's called aerophagia, a medical term for swallowing air. The purpose of belching is to release air from the stomach. Every time you swallow, you gulp air, fluid, or food. As the air builds up in the stomach, pressure also builds, causing the stomach to stretch. When the lower esophageal sphincter muscle relaxes, it lets the gas out—causing a belch.

Drinking lots of soft drinks and beer is guaranteed to cause problems, but your saliva also contains tiny air bubbles that travel to your stomach with every swallow.

Some people naturally swallow excessive air when they eat or drink, and patients who have gastroesophageal reflux disease (GERD) tend to belch more frequently because they swallow often to drive stomach acid out of the throat, says William J. Snape Jr., M.D. But belching is a problem that is controllable. Most of us can, with practice, reduce the amount of air we swallow. Here's how.

■ **BECOME AWARE OF AIR.** "You can swallow up to 5 ounces of air each time you swallow," says André Dubois, M.D. People who are feeling anxious or nervous will do this quite frequently.

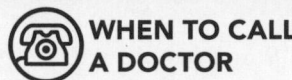

WHEN TO CALL A DOCTOR

Some individuals may have a mild medical condition called functional dyspepsia, says Douglas A. Drossman, M.D. They often fill up after eating and feel discomfort in their stomachs, which is relieved by belching. On rare occasions, belching can relate to an underlying medical problem such as gallbladder disease or a bowel obstruction. In these cases, a doctor can identify any medical condition and offer specific treatments to help relieve the excessive belching.

Many physicians see no physiological need to stifle belching. They view it as a natural body function. "If you swallow too much air, it's actually good for you," says André Dubois, M.D. In fact, in other countries, it's perfectly normal to belch in public.

Some people are compulsive swallowers and create a problem by habitually swallowing too much saliva. "You can learn to control your swallowing reflexes simply by becoming aware of it," he says. "Ask your friends or relatives to tell you if they notice you swallowing a lot. You probably won't notice it in yourself."

Once you're aware of a swallowing habit, it's easier to curb it, says Dr. Dubois. There are also some personal habits you can change to help you take in less air.

- Avoid carbonated beverages.

- Eat slowly and chew your food completely before swallowing.

- Always eat with your mouth closed.

- Don't chew gum.

- Don't drink out of cans or bottles, or through a straw.

- Avoid foods high in air content such as beer, ice cream, soufflés, omelets, and whipped cream.

■ **EAT SMALL MEALS.** Large meals means you're swallowing more (and swallowing more air) in one sitting. You may be able to avoid discomfort by eating smaller meals five or six times a day rather than two or three large meals, Dr. Snape says.

■ **NIX A NERVOUS BELCHING HABIT.** Chronic air swallowers can belch forever—belching begets more belching—but even chronic swallowers can be helped. When all else fails, see a psychologist or counselor for relaxation exercises that may help reduce nervous swallowing, says Douglas A. Drossman, M.D.

■ **SAY GOOD-BYE TO GASSY GOODIES.** On occasion, we all eat a little too much just a little too quickly, and we belch. Take small bites and chew carefully, says Dr. Dubois. You don't want to eat big chunks of meat because big air comes with them.

For people with upper-digestive-system gas, it may be useful to eat fewer foods that produce the problem. Those foods include fats and oils such as salad oil, margarine, and sour cream.

■ **SMASH BUBBLES WITH SOOTHING SIMETHICONE.** To help alleviate a problem that already exists, digestive experts sometimes recommend over-the-counter antacids containing simethicone, such as Di-Gel, Mylanta, Mylanta Supreme, and Maalox Max, says Dr. Snape.

Simethicone breaks large bubbles into small bubbles in the stomach, which may decrease belching. The caveat: It does not reduce the amount of gas, says Dr. Dubois.

PANEL OF ADVISORS

DOUGLAS A. DROSSMAN, M.D., IS A PROFESSOR OF MEDICINE AND PSYCHIATRY, AND CODIRECTOR OF THE UNIVERSITY OF NORTH CAROLINA CENTER FOR FUNCTIONAL GI AND MOTILITY DISORDERS AT CHAPEL HILL.

ANDRÉ DUBOIS, M.D., IS A GASTROENTEROLOGIST IN BETHESDA, MARYLAND.

WILLIAM J. SNAPE JR., M.D., IS DIRECTOR OF NEUROGASTROENTEROLOGY AND MOTILITY AT CALIFORNIA PACIFIC MEDICAL CENTER IN SAN FRANCISCO.

Bites, Scratches, and Stings

28 Hints to Relieve the Pain

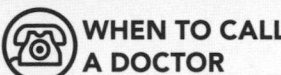 **WHEN TO CALL
A DOCTOR**

Any bite could develop
complications. Stay alert for
these potential problems.

■ **ALLERGIC REACTION.** A bee
sting can cause someone
who's allergic to go into
anaphylactic shock.
Pay attention for chest
tightness, hives, nausea,
vomiting, wheezing,
hoarseness, dizziness,
swollen tongue or face, or
fainting. These are signs of
a medical emergency and
require immediate medical
attention.

■ **RABIES.** All warm-blooded
animals can carry rabies. If
you're bitten by a dog or
cat, contact the animal's
owner to determine
whether its rabies shots are
up to date. Any bite from a
wild animal should be
evaluated by a doctor.

■ **LYME DISEASE.** The
characteristic symptom of
this tick-borne illness is a
bull's-eye rash, often
accompanied by a fever.

Most insect bites and stings are minor annoyances that itch like crazy and produce ugly, little welts that last a few days. Even love nips from Fifi and Fido are often more insult than real injury. But on those occasions when the bite is a little worse than the bark (or the buzz), doctors suggest the following.

FLIES AND MOSQUITOES

A bite from one of these insects can be pretty uncomfortable. Here's what to do for relief.

■ **DISINFECT THE BITE.** Wash the bite area thoroughly with soap and water. Then apply an antiseptic.

■ **STOP THE ITCHING.** Fly and mosquito bites may produce swelling and intense itching that can last for 3 to 4 days. Try the following to control these symptoms.

- An oral antihistamine (Choose an over-the-counter nonsedating antihistamine such as Claritin or Zytec.)

- Calamine lotion

- Ice packs

- Baking soda (Dissolve 1 teaspoon in a glass of water, dip a cloth into the solution, and place it on the bite for 15 to 20 minutes.)

■ **PRACTICE PREVENTION.** The hotter the weather, the more active are flies and mosquitoes. Mosquitoes, in particular, will likely plague you in places with standing water, such as swamps and marshes, where female mosquitoes lay their eggs. "They're attracted to a human's warmth 'scent,' carbon dioxide, and dark clothing," says Mark S. Fradin, M.D. Three ways to avoid mosquito bites is to stay clear of wet breeding areas, wear protective clothing, and apply an insect repellent, he says.

TICKS

Because ticks transmit Lyme disease, which untreated can cause long-term cardiac and neurological problems, they present a big threat to humans. Named in 1977 after doctors discovered arthritis in a cluster of children in and near Lyme, Connecticut, the disease can trigger a rash, fever, fatigue, headache, muscle aches, and painful joints.

Here's what you need to know so you're prepared.

■ **DON'T BE A TARGET.** You can reduce your chances of getting bitten, or contracting Lyme, in three simple steps.

■ Leave as little skin exposed as possible, says Richard Hansen, M.D. Wear long pants, high socks, and long sleeves. Tuck your shirt into your pants, your pants into your socks, and wear boots, not sandals.

■ Spray your pant legs, socks, and boots with a permethrin spray (available at sporting goods stores) before heading out. Permethrin binds tightly to fabric and can be effective for up to 2 weeks, killing any ticks that try to crawl past it, says Dr. Fradin.

■ Inspect your body for any free-loading ticks after being outdoors. Certain species are quite small, and you might otherwise overlook them.

■ **EASE IT OUT.** Ticks pose a special problem because they burrow into your skin and hold on for dear life. "If you get them early, you can pull them off with your fingers," says Dr. Hansen. Trying to brush away a tick as you would a fly has no effect. And forcefully plucking it out may leave its mouthparts embedded, setting the stage for infection. So use a gentler approach: Dr. Fradin recommends taking a pair of fine-tipped tweezers and grabbing the tick as close to the attachment site as possible. Then very slowly pull the tick out in the direction its back end is pointing. Ease the tick off. Don't jerk it out, he says. And do not squeeze the tick's body, because it can regurgitate into your skin.

■ **CLEAN UP.** Once you've removed the tick, wash the bite area with soap and water and apply iodine or another antiseptic to guard against infection.

DOGS AND CATS

When it comes to animal bites, anyone can become a victim. Between a half million to 1 million people seek medical attention for dog bites each year, and countless other bites go unreported and untreated, according to the American Veterinary Medical Association. Here's what to do if you are bitten.

■ **ASSESS THE DAMAGE.** Seek medical help for all but the most minor wounds, say doctors.

■ **THOROUGHLY WASH THE BITE.** Animal bites—especially from cats—may transmit infections, so pour some hydrogen peroxide or alcohol on the wound. Then cleanse it thoroughly with soap and water to remove saliva and any other contamination. Wash for at least 5 minutes.

■ **CONTROL BLEEDING.** If there is bleeding, apply direct pressure and cover the entire wound with thick sterile gauze or a clean cloth pad, says Dr. Hansen. He recommends gauze that will breathe rather than plastic, to allow air to get to the wound. If you don't have an appropriate bandage, thoroughly cleanse your hand and press it firmly against the wound. You may also put some ice against the pad (not directly on the skin) and raise the wound above heart level to help stop bleeding.

■ **BANDAGE THE AREA.** When the bleeding stops, cover the bite with a new sterile gauze bandage or clean cloth. Tie or tape it loosely in place.

■ **REDUCE PAIN.** Use aspirin or acetaminophen to ease pain. This is appropriate even if the bite did not break the skin. Elevate the wound and ice it if there is any swelling.

■ **GET A TETANUS SHOT.** Anyone bitten by an animal should have a tetanus booster, says Dr. Fradin. If you haven't had a booster shot in the past 5 to 8 years, get one now.

■ **TREAT THE WOUND.** Apply antibiotic ointment to the wound and cover with an adhesive bandage two times a day until it heals, says Dr. Hansen.

INSECT STINGS

Compared with insects, we're far outnumbered. Bees, wasps, and their ilk inject venom into our skin when they attack us, and their sting ends in pain, redness, and swelling. Discomfort can last from several hours to a day, depending on what stings and how many times. If you happen to make contact with an angry stinging insect, these tips can minimize the damage.

■ **IDENTIFY YOUR ATTACKER.** Knowing which insect did the damage can provide a clue to treatment—and help you avoid more stings. A honeybee, which has a fuzzy, golden-brown body, can sting only once. That's because its barbed stinger remains embedded in your skin. Without the stinger, the bee dies.

Bumblebees, wasps, hornets, and yellow jackets, on the other hand, have smooth stingers that can zap you repeatedly. So be prepared to flee. They sting harder and more vigorously, says Dr. Hansen. There is one type of yellow jacket, though, that does leave the

When the Itsy Bitsy Spider Turns Nasty

Certain kinds of spiders, like the black widow and brown recluse, have reputations for inflicting especially nasty bites. The fact is, all spiders are poisonous. It's just that most aren't big or strong enough to penetrate the skin and do much harm.

The general advice for treating a spider bite is pretty much the same as for any bite:

- Wash the wound, then disinfect it with an antiseptic.

- Apply an ice pack to slow the absorption of venom.

- Neutralize the poison by moistening the bite with water and running an aspirin tablet over it. (Skip this if you're alleric to aspirin.)

If you do happen to encounter one of the more notorious spider species, a trip to the doctor may be necessary to treat or prevent a serious reaction. Here's what you need to know.

Black widow. This black spider with the distinctive red hourglass shape on its abdomen is not aggressive and will bite only when disturbed, says Mark S. Fradin, M.D. That said, its venom is a potent neurotoxin that can cause serious symptoms such as muscle pain and cramping, abdominal pain, and headache. Definitely see your doctor if you've been bitten; he may pre-scribe pain relievers, muscle relaxants, or calcium gluconate injections. A more severe reaction may require antivenom, says Dr. Fradin.

Brown recluse. A bite from the brown recluse may be painless at first, but within 3 days or so, the skin tissue at the bite site can begin to blister and die off. The resulting ulceration can be very painful and cause scarring, Dr. Fradin says. Your doctor can help minimize the tissue damage, provided you see him as soon as possible after you're bitten.

stinger in the skin more than 25 percent of the time, says David Golden, M.D., so you can't assume that if the stinger is left in the skin it's an absolute sign of a honeybee sting.

Yellow jackets pose an additional problem. Smashing one of them can lead to a full-scale attack by its nest mates. That's because breaking its venom sac releases a chemical that incites other yellow jackets to attack.

■ **ACT FAST.** The key to effective treatment is quick action. The faster you apply some sort of first-aid treatment, the better your chances of controlling pain and swelling.

■ **REMOVE THE STINGER.** If a honeybee got you, remove the stinger as soon as possible. Otherwise, the venom sac attached to it will continue to pump for 20 to 30 seconds, driving the stinger and its poison deeper into your skin. But be careful not to squeeze the stinger or the sac—doing so will release more poison into your wound.

To remove it before the damage worsens, flick it out with your fingernails or use the flat edge of a knife blade, suggests Dr. Hansen. Scraping the stinger out is the best approach. Use your fingernail, a nail file, or even the edge of a credit card to gently scrape under the stinger and flip it out.

■ **RELIEVE THE PAIN.** At this point, your wound is still throbbing, so you want to deaden the pain *fast*. The following treatments are effective—but for them to work, you must act quickly after being stung.

- **Ice.** An ice pack, or even an ice cube, placed over the sting can cut down on swelling and keep the venom from spreading, says Dr. Golden. It can also reduce the pain.

- **Baking Soda.** A paste of baking soda and water may be mildly effective. The alkali in the baking soda tends to neutralize the toxin, says Dr. Hansen.

- **Meat Tenderizer.** "An enzyme-based meat tenderizer, such as Adolph's or McCormick's, breaks down the proteins that make up insect venom," says Dr. Golden. You have to use it right away, however, for it to be effective.

- **Activated Charcoal.** "A paste of powdered activated charcoal will draw the

poison out very quickly, so the sting won't swell or hurt," according to Dr. Hansen. Carefully open a few charcoal capsules and remove the powder. Moisten it with water and apply it to the sting. The charcoal works best if it stays moist, so cover it with gauze or plastic wrap.

■ **TAKE AN ANTIHISTAMINE.** An over-the-counter oral antihistamine may help relieve pain, says Dr. Hansen. Parents can give their children a cough syrup containing an antihistamine, such as Benylin. The antihistamine helps sedate the child a little and also lessens the swelling, throbbing, and redness caused by the insect venom. Some children have reverse reactions to antihistamines and become hyper rather than sedated, says Dr. Fradin. So be prepared for both.

■ **DON'T GET STUNG IN THE FIRST PLACE.** A bit of prevention can save you a lot of anguish later. Here's how to minimize your chances of getting stung.

- Stinging insects prefer dark colors. That's why beekeepers generally wear khaki, white, or other light colors. Plus, dark colors retain heat, which draws mosquitoes in because they have an odd affinity for sweat compounds. The hotter, stinkier, and sweatier you are, the more likely you'll be attacked.

- Avoid perfume, aftershave, or any other fragrance that will lead a bee to confuse you with a nectar-bearing flower. Bees are attracted to fragrances and perfumes, says Dr. Hansen. When a bee finds out you're not a flower, it'll get mad.

- If you're being pursued by a buzzing horde, run indoors, jump into water, or head for the woods. Stinging insects have trouble following their prey through a thicket or woods, say researchers at the Cornell University Cooperative Extension Service.

PANEL OF ADVISORS

MARK S. FRADIN, M.D., IS A CLINICAL ASSOCIATE PROFESSOR OF DERMATOLOGY AT THE UNIVERSITY OF NORTH CAROLINA IN CHAPEL HILL.

DAVID GOLDEN, M.D., IS AN ASSOCIATE PROFESSOR OF MEDICINE AT JOHNS HOPKINS UNIVERSITY IN BALTIMORE.

RICHARD HANSEN, M.D., IS MEDICAL DIRECTOR OF EMERALD VALLEY WELLNESS CENTER IN CRESWELL, OREGON, AND AUTHOR OF *GET WELL AT HOME*.

Black Eye

10 Ways to Clear Up the Bruise

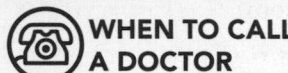

WHEN TO CALL A DOCTOR

Black eyes shouldn't be taken lightly, since they can involve serious internal eye injuries, including retinal detachment and internal hemorrhages that may not be evident at first.

If you have difficulty seeing, you need medical attention immediately. And if you have pain in the eye, sensitivity to light, blurred or double vision, or the sensation of objects floating through your field of vision, you should also be seen.

"I think every patient with a black eye should be examined at an emergency room or by an ophthalmologist," says Anne Sumers, M.D. "Many times, serious complications will have no symptoms."

"Black eye" is somewhat of a misnomer. "Very dark blue eye" or "rainbow-of-color eye" would be better. Whether you ran into a door frame or got punched, blood instantly filled this plentiful space under your eye. Since the skin is so thin, the pooled blood beneath is readily seen as a very dark blue, says Audrey Kunin, M.D. During the week most black eyes take to heal, the blood is slowly reabsorbed into the body, evolving into a kaleidoscope of colors that actually signifies healing.

Throughout the centuries, there have been a host of wild and sundry treatments for black eyes, ranging from leeches to liver to raw-steak compresses. They all share the same goal: to reduce swelling. But, it turns out, there are plenty of efficient ways to achieve that objective in a more pleasant manner. Here are some to try.

■ **PACK IT IN ICE . . . THEN HEAT.** A cold pack keeps the swelling down and, by constricting the blood vessels, helps decrease the internal bleeding. Apply ice on and off for the first 48 hours, says Randy Wexler, M.D. Or, if you don't have an ice pack handy, use a bag of frozen vegetables. Then switch to warm compresses.

■ **FADE THE BLACK WITH BROMELAIN.** "I used to tell my patients with black eyes to eat fresh pineapple," says Jay Zimmerman, M.D. "But now they can buy supplements that contain bromelain, the active ingredient in pineapple. The supplements are even more effective than applying bromelain topically."

Bromelain is sold in different amounts, but Dr. Zimmerman recommends taking 1 to 2 grams of it with water before meals.

■ **GO FOR GREEN ICE.** Parsley is a very old folk remedy for bruising; it has anti-inflammatory and anesthetic properties. Combine it with ice, because cold causes blood vessels to constrict, which reduces swelling. To make this remedy, combine a cup of fresh parsley with about 2 tablespoons of water, whisk it into a fine slurry in the blender, and freeze the mixture in an ice cube tray. Wrap the cubes in a soft cloth before holding them under your eye for 15 to 20 minutes.

■ **BOOST VITAMIN K.** Increasing your intake of vitamin-K-rich foods like alfalfa sprouts will help slow the spread of black eye bruising. "Vitamin K is an old Chinese remedy for black eye. It helps the blood clot so it doesn't spread so far across your face," says Georgianna Donadio, Ph.D. You can increase your intake of vitamin K by eating alfalfa sprouts or taking a few hundred milligrams of vitamin K per day in the form of an alfalfa tablet, she says. Don't use vitamin K if you are pregnant or taking a blood thinner such as Coumadin.

■ **TURN TO A BOTANICAL.** Herbal experts recommend both creams and gels made from the bright flowers of the arnica plant as remedies for bruises. You can find these products in health food stores.

■ **SPICE IT UP.** A few days into the black eye, Dr. Donadio recommends applying a Chinese remedy of 1 part cayenne pepper to 4 to 6 parts petroleum jelly. "Heat up the petroleum jelly, mix in the cayenne, and apply the concoction around the black eye once a day," she says. "It will help flush out the stagnant blood."

■ **DE-COLORIZE WITH C.** Vitamin C will help prevent the wild discoloration that sometimes accompanies a black eye, Dr. Donadio says. When it comes to vitamin C, you can't have too much. So drink lots of fortified orange juice, eat oranges, and load up on green, leafy vegetables—any food that has lots of vitamin C in it, she says.

■ **REDUCE SWELLING WITH TEA.** "You can minimize some of the swelling of a black eye by using a black tea bag as a topical compress," Dr. Kunin explains. "The chemical epigallocatechin gallate (EGCG) in the tea acts as an anti-inflammatory, and the caffeine is a natural diuretic, so it will help reduce the swelling," she says.

■ **BE PATIENT.** Once the eye bruises, there's not much you can do except control the swelling. Even makeup can't disguise it totally, although a good foundation will help once any cuts heal, says Anne Sumers, M.D.

■ **AVOID ASPIRIN.** It's simply bad news for black eyes. As an anticoagulant, aspirin prevents blood from clotting and helps it spread more easily. Depending on exactly why you take aspirin (if it's for a heart-related condition, talk to your doctor first), you may want to stop for a few days to keep the bruising from spreading, says Dr. Kunin.

PANEL OF ADVISORS

GEORGIANNA DONADIO, PH.D., IS DIRECTOR OF THE NATIONAL INSTITUTE OF WHOLE HEALTH, A HOLISTIC CERTIFICATION PROGRAM FOR MEDICAL PROFESSIONALS.

AUDREY KUNIN, M.D., IS A COSMETIC DERMATOLOGIST IN KANSAS CITY, MISSOURI, THE FOUNDER OF THE DERMATOLOGY EDUCATIONAL WEB SITE WWW.DERMADOCTOR. COM, AND AUTHOR OF *THE DERMADOCTOR SKINSTRUCTION MANUAL.*

ANNE SUMERS, M.D., IS TEAM OPHTHALMOLOGIST FOR THE NEW YORK GIANTS AND THE NEW JERSEY NETS, AND HAS A PRACTICE IN RIDGEWOOD, NEW JERSEY. SHE SERVES AS A SPOKESPERSON FOR THE AMERICAN ACADEMY OF OPHTHALMOLOGY.

RANDY WEXLER, M.D., IS AN ASSISTANT PROFESSOR IN THE DEPARTMENT OF FAMILY MEDICINE AT OHIO STATE UNIVERSITY MEDICAL CENTER IN COLUMBUS.

JAY ZIMMERMAN, M.D., IS A BOARD-CERTIFIED DERMATOLOGIST AND CLINICAL INSTRUCTOR IN THE DEPARTMENT OF DERMATOLOGY AT UCLA.

Blisters

20 Hints to Stop the Hurt

Blisters are your body's way of saying it's had enough. Be it too much friction or too much ambition, a blister—much like a muscle cramp or a side stitch—is designed to slow you down and make you better prepared for physical activity. "A blister forms because you've ruptured cell tissue and released plasma (the fluid in the blister), and the outside skin is your body's way of trying to prevent infection," says Georgianna Donadio, Ph.D.

Though most of these remedies are for blisters on the feet, many can be applied to friction blisters on the hands or any place where your body has said "slow down."

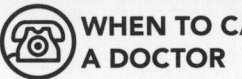

WHEN TO CALL A DOCTOR

Head to the doctor if your blister is very large (more than 2 inches across) or possibly infected. Symptoms of infection include persistent pain, fever, yellow crusting, oozing pus, and redness that extends beyond the edge of the blister. If you have a condition that causes blisters, such as eczema, chicken pox, or impetigo, a trip to the doctor is also in order.

BLISTER TREATMENT

Here's how experts recommend you handle the discomfort of blisters.

■ **MAKE A DECISION.** Once you develop a blister, you either have to protect it and leave it alone, or pop it and drain the fluid.

"I think it depends on the size of the blister," says Suzanne Tanner, M.D. "A purist will probably tell you not to prick it, because then you don't run any risk of infection. But for most people that's just not very practical."

While purists do indeed exist, most experts agree that it's best to drain large, painful blisters and any likely to break on

Two Socks Are Better Than One

If you're prone to blisters, you may want to double up on your socks for extra protection. In preparation for a long walk or hike, put on two pairs of socks to reduce the chance of any friction. The inner pair should be made from a thinner, wicking material like acrylic or silk, and the outer socks should be made of cotton.

their own. If you pop them yourself, you decide how and when. Leave smaller, painless blisters intact.

■ **MAKE A MOLESKIN DOUGHNUT.** If you decide not to drain the blister, one way to protect it is to cut a moleskin pad into a doughnut shape and place it over the blister. "The blister can sit in the open center," says Dr. Tanner. The surrounding moleskin will absorb most of the shock and friction of everyday activity. As long as the skin is clean and dry, the sticky moleskin will adhere.

■ **BE WISE AND STERILIZE.** If you choose to drain a blister, first clean it and the surrounding skin, and sterilize the needle you'll use to puncture it. "Sterilize the needle by heating with a match for a few seconds (let it cool) or washing it with antiseptic lotion," Dr. Donadio says. "Then pierce the blister and allow the plasma to release," she says. Wash the blister several times a day with antiseptic lotion, and press a piece of folded gauze on the spot where the plasma emerged, she says.

■ **KEEP THE ROOF ON.** Leave the skin on the blister—the part that's worn loose. Think of the top of a blister as nature's bandage, says Audrey Kunin, M.D.

■ **OR EVEN ADD ON AN ARTIFICIAL ROOF.** Randy Wexler, M.D., enthusiastically recommends over-the-counter blister covers. "They actually work quite well," he says.

■ **DRESS A BROKEN BLISTER.** If a blister pops by accident, wash it with soap and water and apply a triple antibiotic ointment such as Neosporin.

Keep the dressing simple. After you've treated the blister, keep it covered and protected while it heals. You might reach for gauze pads and special bandages, but there's a much simpler approach. "My first choice is an adhesive bandage," says Richard M. Cowin, D.P.M.

Gauze pads, however, are recommended for blisters that are just too big to cover with an adhesive bandage. Keep them in place with waterproof adhesive tape. Whatever bandage you choose, change it once a day.

■ **USE SECOND SKIN FOR A SECOND WIND.** If you've treated and covered your blister and want to get back to your active lifestyle, try Spenco Second Skin dressing, a spongy material that absorbs pressure and reduces friction against blisters and surrounding skin.

■ **GIVE IT SOME AIR.** Remove the dressing at bedtime to let the blister air. "Air and water are very good for healing," says Dr. Cowin, "so soaking it in water and keeping it open to the air at night is helpful."

■ **CHANGE WET DRESSINGS.** If a dressing becomes wet, it should be replaced. Change it often if your feet perspire heavily or if an activity leads to a sweaty or damp dressing.

■ **TREAT IT WITH PREPARATION.** If your blister is itching and burning, use a little of the hemorrhoid-relieving cream Preparation H. The cream will not only ease the discomfort of a blister but also add a protective coating.

■ **USE A SEA SALT SOLUTION.** To mimic the healing properties of ocean water, Janet Maccaro, Ph.D., C.N.C., suggests the following compress for blisters: Combine ⅛ cup ice water with ¼ cup sea salt. "Apply the mixture to a damp washcloth and wrap it around the blister for 1 hour," she says.

■ **SMEAR IT WITH ALOE.** Turns out aloe vera gel is as good for blisters as it is for burns. Apply some pure aloe gel directly from the plant onto your blister and cover it with an adhesive bandage or gauze pad. Stay away from commercial aloe products, however— some of them contain alcohol, which can have a drying effect.

■ **DRY IT WITH MOUTHWASH.** The classic breath freshener Listerine also does a number on blisters. Moisten a cotton ball with Listerine and dab it on your blister three times a day until the area "dries out" and no longer hurts, Dr. Maccaro says.

■ **PREVENT INFECTION.** If your blister is raw and oozing pus, cover it with an antibiotic ointment such as Neosporin a few times a day to prevent infection, says Dr. Kunin.

BLISTER PREVENTION

Prevention is always the best option, so here's how to keep blisters from developing.

■ **TRY A HEEL LIFT.** Blisters form on the back of the foot when your shoe's heel counter hits in the wrong place, says Dr. Cowin. The fix is quite simple. "All you usually have to do is add a heel lift," he says.

■ **KEEP YOUR SOCKS ON.** As a general rule, avoid sock-free fashions. "The people who don't wear socks suffer blisters on the back of their heel all the time," says Dr. Cowin. He recommends that those who want to flash some ankle without suffering the consequences invest in "low-cut socks that only go around the foot area."

■ **DEODORIZE YOUR FEET.** Dry feet are less likely to develop blisters than moist ones. One way to keep feet dry is to rub on antiperspirant once a day.

■ **SHOP FOR SHOES IN THE P.M.** Your feet swell during the course of a day, so if you buy shoes in the morning, they may be too small. To make sure your new shoes are roomy enough, shop after lunch. And make sure you have plenty of toe space; when you're standing up, you should have a thumb-width of space between the end of the shoe and your longest toe.

■ **TREAT YOUR FEET TO TREATED INSOLES.** Chemically treated insoles can prevent blisters on the bottom of the foot. Spenco makes a version that is highly recommended. The best insoles have "bubbled-in nitrogen," add some cushioning, and help the foot glide over the bottom of the shoe to prevent sticking, a cause of blisters, says Dr. Cowin.

■ **BEWARE TUBE SOCKS.** While tube socks, those unformed heelless wonders you can slip into without thinking, can be tempting to wear, it's best to avoid them. "I personally don't believe in tube socks," says Dr. Cowin. "I don't think they ever fit properly. You need a regular, fitted sock to help prevent blisters."

Body Odor

12 Ways to Feel Fresh and Clean

Some scientists believe that body odor is a vestige of our evolution. That is, the smells we give off from certain areas of our bodies, primarily our armpits and groin, may have once served to advertise our sexuality.

However, in modern society, this form of advertisement is far from desirable. Many of us go to great lengths to avoid offending those around us with unpleasant smells.

Easier said than done? Actually, there are quite a few ways to take on body odor and come up smelling like a rose.

■ **SCRUB-A-DUB-DUB.** The most basic way to avoid body odor is to scrub with soap and water, particularly in those areas of the body most likely to smell, such as the armpits and groin, says Randy Wexler, M.D.

Body odor is most often caused by a combination of perspiration and bacteria. Scrubbing with soap and water washes both away.

The best type of soap for a body odor problem is an antibacterial version because it hinders the formation of bacteria. How often you need to wash depends on your individual body chemistry, your activities, your mood, and the time of year. If you're not sure if you're clean enough, ask a trusted friend. Remember that sweat glands and bacteria work night as well as day shifts, which could mean you need to shower both morning and evening.

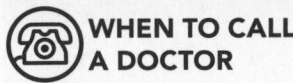

WHEN TO CALL A DOCTOR

Frequent, heavy sweating can be more than embarrassing. It can be a sign that you have an overactive thyroid or low blood sugar. You may also have an abnormality in the part of the nervous system that controls sweating. In any case, check with your doctor.

You should also see your doctor if after you've tried all the suggested remedies, your body odor persists. "Body odor can be caused by some pretty serious diseases," says Georgianna Donadio, Ph.D. "You could have anything from a zinc deficiency that is causing your pancreas to malfunction to diabetes that is causing you to give off an acetone smell," she says. So it is important to get checked.

■ **WASH MORE THAN YOUR BODY.** You can wash till your skin shrivels like a prune, but you'll still smell bad if your clothes aren't clean. How often do you need to change into a fresh shirt? It depends on you as an individual. A daily change should suffice for most. On hot summer days, more than once a day might be in order.

■ **CHOOSE NATURAL FABRICS.** Natural fabrics such as cotton absorb perspiration better than synthetic materials. The absorbed sweat is then free to evaporate from the fabric.

■ **REALIZE YOU'RE A SPONGE FOR ODOR.** "If you've been surrounded by cooking foods, such as garlic, onions, and strong spices, or smoke or fuel, these odors can cling to your clothing and hair," Lenise Banse, M.D. says. "Until your clothing and hair are washed, these odors will be carried with you," she says.

■ **STOP PERSPIRATION BEFORE IT STARTS.** Commercial deodorants leave chemicals on the skin that kill odor-causing bacteria, making them effective at masking underarm odor in most people. Deodorants, however, don't control perspiration. So if you sweat heavily, you may need an antiperspirant.

Cures from the Kitchen

To keep yourself smelling sweet, try the following concoction: Mix ½ cup honey with 2 cups of uncooked oatmeal. Apply the mixture to your body with a loofah, a dry washcloth, or your hands, and then shower off.

"People who perspire excessively can use an underarm antiperspirant daily to stop the sweating," says Terry Spilken, D.P.M. "Most antiperspirants contain aluminum chlorhydrate, a very good drying agent," he says.

■ **CLEAR THE AIR WITH CHLOROPHYLL.** "In some cases, body odor is from putrefaction—an incomplete elimination of organic matter," says Georgianna Donadio, Ph.D. "The most successful thing you can do to fight this is to start eating lots of chlorophyll-rich plants, because chlorophyll is a natural detoxifier," she says. You can take liquid chlorophyll, but Dr. Donadio cautions that dizziness and diarrhea can be side effects. "You get chlorophyll by eating green plants such as spinach and kale." The greener the plant, the more chlorophyll, she says.

■ **APPLY SOME APPLE CIDER VINEGAR.** "Apple cider vinegar is a great natural underarm deodorant," Dr. Donadio says. Apply it directly to your armpit with a washcloth, and it will kill body odor, she says.

■ **WATCH WHAT YOU EAT.** Extracts of proteins and oils from certain foods and spices remain in your body's excretions and secretions long after eating them, and they can impart an odor. "A vegetarian diet, low in meat and fat, will alkalinize the body and decrease odor," says Ellen Kamhi, Ph.D., R.N.

■ **BENEFIT FROM GOOD BACTERIA.** For a natural deodorant that fights odor from the inside out, Dr. Kamhi recommends taking a daily acidophilus supplement. Acidophilus is a probiotic bacteria that helps aid digestion.

■ **LET YOUR FEET BREATHE.** If the source of your body odor is your feet, make sure they see the light of day. Bacteria grow in warm, dark, moist places, like inside your shoes. If you have foot odor, take your shoes off as often as possible, wear socks, and choose canvas instead of leather sneakers.

■ **CLEANSE YOUR SOLES.** Dogs release toxins through the soles of their feet, and people do this too, Dr. Donadio says. If your feet stink, help draw out the odor-causing toxins out by using raw sliced potatoes. "Tape the sliced potatoes to the bottom of your feet or put them in your socks," she says. "When you take them off a few hours later, you will find that they have turned black—there are chemicals in the potatoes that help draw the toxins out through your soles," she says.

PANEL OF ADVISORS

LENISE BANSE, M.D., IS A DERMATOLOGIST IN CLINTON TOWNSHIP, MICHIGAN, WHERE SHE IS DIRECTOR OF THE NORTHEAST FAMILY DERMATOLOGY CENTER. SHE HAS SPECIAL EXPERTISE IN CUTANEOUS ONCOLOGY AS WELL AS COSMETIC DERMATOLOGY.

GEORGIANNA DONADIO, PH.D., IS DIRECTOR OF THE NATIONAL INSTITUTE OF WHOLE HEALTH, A HOLISTIC CERTIFICATION PROGRAM FOR MEDICAL PROFESSIONALS.

ELLEN KAMHI, PH.D., R.N., IS THE NATURAL NURSE, CLINICAL INSTRUCTOR IN THE DEPARTMENT OF FAMILY MEDICINE AT STONY BROOK UNIVERSITY IN NEW YORK, AND AUTHOR OF *THE NATURAL MEDICINE CHEST, ARTHRITIS: THE ALTERNATIVE MEDICINE DEFINITIVE GUIDE,* AND *CYCLES OF LIFE: HERBS FOR WOMEN.*

TERRY SPILKEN, D.P.M., IS A FORMER DEAN AND CURRENT ADJUNCT ASSOCIATE PROFESSOR AT THE NEW YORK COLLEGE OF PODIATRIC MEDICINE IN NEW YORK CITY.

RANDY WEXLER, M.D., IS AN ASSISTANT PROFESSOR IN THE DEPARTMENT OF FAMILY MEDICINE AT OHIO STATE UNIVERSITY MEDICAL CENTER IN COLUMBUS.

Boils

14 Tips to Stop an Infection

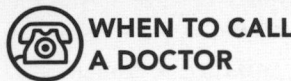

WHEN TO CALL A DOCTOR

Some boils warrant medical care. See your doctor if:

■ The boil is near your eye, on your nose or lips, or in your armpit or groin

■ The boil is on your breast and you're nursing

■ The boil is more than ¼ inch in diameter

■ The boil appears to be extremely tender

■ You notice red lines radiating from the boil

■ Your boil is accompanied by fever, chills, or swelling of the lymph nodes

■ You get boils frequently

In general, if the person with the boil is very young, elderly, or ill, he or she should be treated by a doctor, advises Rodney Basler, M.D.

A boil, also called an abscess, is an infection deep inside the skin that produces redness, pain, swelling, and pus.

Boils generally develop when *Staphylococcus* bacteria invade the body through a break in the skin, a blocked sweat gland, or an ingrown hair. The body's immune system sends in white blood cells, which collect as pus, to fight the bacteria. A pus-filled abscess begins to grow beneath the skin surface, rising up red and painful. Sometimes the body reabsorbs the boil; other times the boil swells and erupts before it drains and subsides.

Boils are uncomfortable and unsightly. Sometimes they leave scars. Occasionally, they can be dangerous. But for the most part, you can treat them safely at home. Here's how.

■ **APPLY HEAT.** "Applying a warm compress is the very best thing you can do for a boil," says Rodney Basler, M.D. The heat will cause the boil to form a head, drain, and heal a lot faster.

At the first sign of a boil, place a warm, moist washcloth over it for 20 to 30 minutes three or four times a day. Change the cloth a few times during each session to keep it warm. It's not uncommon for a boil to take 5 to 7 days to break on its own, he says.

■ **PREVENT A RECURRENCE.** It's important to continue the warm compresses for 3 days after the boil breaks, Dr. Basler says. All of the pus must drain from the tissues, and it is important that the area kept clean. Covering the open boil is one way to do that, but it's not critical. "A bandage is mainly to keep the drainage off your clothes," he adds.

■ **LANCE THE LESION.** When the boil comes to a pus-filled head, if it's small and there are no signs of spreading infection, you may want to break it. Do this when and where it's convenient. Letting the boil break on its own can be messy if it should happen, for example, while you're sleeping. To lance the boil, sterilize a needle with a flame, nick the head, and squeeze gently.

Some doctors worry that squeezing a boil can drive the infection deeper into the skin, and possibly into the lymph system. This rarely happens, says Dr. Basler. "In the office, we just squeeze the dickens out of them."

■ **CLEAN IT.** Audrey Kunin, M.D., recommends keeping a boil clean to guard against spreading the infection. Wipe it with hydrogen peroxide or apply an over-the-counter antibiotic ointment such as Polysporin or Neosporin as insurance.

■ **KEEP IT LOCALIZED.** When a boil is draining, keep the skin around it clean. Take

Cures from the Kitchen

Folklore has it that home remedies for boils are as close as your vegetable bin. All the following are variations of the warm-washcloth compress. They should be wrapped in a thin cloth and changed every few hours.

■ A heated tomato slice
■ A raw onion slice
■ A mashed garlic clove
■ An outer cabbage leaf
■ A tea bag of black tea

showers instead of baths to reduce the rare chance of spreading the infection to other parts of the body. After treating a boil, wash your hands well and especially before preparing food because staph bacteria can cause food poisoning.

■ **APPLY A SWEET HEALING PASTE.** Once the boil pops, apply a mixture of honey and iodine, which should help treat the infection, says Jacob Teitelbaum, M.D. "It makes an excellent antibacterial mix. The honey works on an osmotic basis, sucking liquid right out of the bacteria and killing them," he says.

■ **TACKLE IT WITH TEA TREE OIL.** After a boil has opened and drained, put a little tea tree oil on a cotton ball and dab it onto the area a few times a day until it is no longer painful. "Tea tree oil is a natural antiseptic," says Georgianna Donadio, Ph.D.

■ **QUIET A BOIL BY USING SOME CLAY.** "Bentonite clay is an effective treatment for boils," says Carolyn Dean, M.D., N.D. You can purchase the powdered clay in a health food store or online. Using a blender, mix purified or boiled water with just enough clay to make a thick paste. Then apply the paste to the boil, which should draw out the pain, heat, and inflammation, Dr. Dean says.

■ **SET THE STAGE FOR PREVENTION.** If you're prone to boils, you may be able to reduce their frequency by cleaning your skin with an antiseptic cleanser like Betadine to keep the staph population down.

PANEL OF ADVISORS

RODNEY BASLER, M.D., IS A DERMATOLOGIST AND ASSOCIATE PROFESSOR OF INTERNAL MEDICINE AT THE UNIVERSITY OF NEBRASKA COLLEGE OF MEDICINE IN LINCOLN.

CAROLYN DEAN, M.D., N.D., IS MEDICAL DIRECTOR OF VIDACOSTA SPA EL PUENTE, A MEDICAL SPA IN COSTA RICA, OPENING IN 2010. SHE IS AUTHOR OF *THE MAGNE-SIUM MIRACLE.*

GEORGIANNA DONADIO, PH.D., IS DIRECTOR OF THE NATIONAL INSTITUTE OF WHOLE HEALTH, A HOLISTIC CERTIFICATION PROGRAM FOR MEDICAL PROFESSIONALS.

AUDREY KUNIN, M.D., IS A COSMETIC DERMATOLOGIST IN KANSAS CITY, MISSOURI, THE FOUNDER OF THE DERMATOLOGY EDUCATIONAL WEB SITE WWW. DERMADOCTOR.COM, AND AUTHOR OF *THE DERMA-DOCTOR SKINSTRUCTION MANUAL.*

JACOB TEITELBAUM, M.D., IS A BOARD-CERTIFIED INTER-NIST AND MEDICAL DIRECTOR OF THE FIBROMYALGIA AND FATIGUE CENTERS, WITH LOCATIONS THROUGHOUT THE COUNTRY.

RANDY WEXLER, M.D., IS AN ASSISTANT PROFESSOR IN THE DEPARTMENT OF FAMILY MEDICINE AT OHIO STATE UNIVERSITY MEDICAL CENTER IN COLUMBUS.

Breast Discomfort

19 Ways to Reduce Soreness

Benign breast changes may be as bewildering as they are uncomfortable, but they are not unusual. The majority of women experience breast discomfort at some point in their lives, often during pregnancy and before menstruation.

This tenderness occurs because of the natural cycles of the reproductive hormones, estrogen and progesterone. These hormones trigger cell growth in the milk-producing glands, which requires nourishment from blood and other fluids that fill the surrounding areas. These fluid-logged tissues can stretch nerve fibers, causing pain and tenderness.

Another cause of breast pain is fibrocystic changes, which include lumps and cysts. These changes usually affect the non-working areas of your breasts: the fat cells, fibrous tissues, and other parts not involved in the making or transporting of milk.

In either case, the following strategies provide relief and promote healing.

■ **SWITCH YOUR DIET.** "Eat a diet high in whole grains, vegetables, and beans, and low in animal fat, especially a week to 10 days before your period," says Carolyn Dean, M.D., N.D. Such a diet can help ease breast tenderness, she says. A study at Tufts University School of Medicine in Boston found that women who maintained this kind of diet metabolized estrogen differently. The

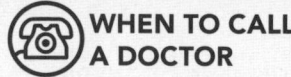
WHEN TO CALL A DOCTOR

Whenever you find a lump during your monthly self-examination, consult your physician—whether or not a previous lump was diagnosed as benign. Your doctor may order a biopsy of the lump or use a needle to aspirate a fluid-filled cyst.

The best time to do a self-exam is 1 week after your menstrual period begins. That's because lumps that sometimes surface just prior to menstruation can disappear just as quickly when your period ends.

increase in fiber helps your body excrete estrogen, Dr. Dean says.

■ **STAY SLIM.** Keep your weight within the proper range for your height. For seriously overweight women, losing weight can help relieve breast pain and lumpiness. "Estrogen dominance can stimulate fibrocystic breasts, and overweight women have too much estrogen," says Dr. Dean.

■ **EASE THE PAIN WITH IODINE.** "Breast pain and tenderness are sometimes caused by an iodine deficiency," says Jacob Teitelbaum, M.D. "so taking iodine tabs (follow label directions) or eating kelp (seaweed is very high in iodine) over a 6-week period can help," he says.

Cures from the Kitchen

To get relief from breast inflammation, try this castor oil compress recommended by Ellen Kamhi, Ph.D., R.N. She says it helps heal minor breast infections, too.

You'll need cold-pressed castor oil, a wool flannel cloth, a piece of plastic, and a heating pad.

Fold the cloth into a square and saturate it with the oil, but make sure it's not so wet that it will drip on the breast. Put the cloth on the breast, cover with plastic, and then apply the heating pad. Turn the setting on the pad up to moderate heat, then to hot if you can stand it, says Dr. Kamhi. Leave it on for an hour.

Cold-pressed castor oil contains a substance that increases lymphocyte function, says Dr. Kamhi. Lymphocytes are white blood cells that help speed healing of infection.

You may need to use the compress for 3 to 7 days to really be able to see results. "This can often be extremely beneficial for taking away pain," she says.

■ **GET YOUR VITAMINS.** Be sure to eat plenty of foods rich in vitamin C, calcium, magnesium, and B vitamins, says Christiane Northrup, M.D. These vitamins and minerals help regulate the production of prostaglandin E, which in turn reins in prolactin, a hormone that activates breast tissue. In addition, Dr. Dean recommends taking 400 IUs of vitamin E as mixed tocopherols and tocotrienols a day to prevent breast tenderness.

■ **PASS ON THE MARGARINE AND OTHER HYDROGENATED FATS.** Hydrogenated fats interfere with your body's ability to convert essential fatty acids from the diet into gamma linoleic acid, says Dr. Northrup. This acid contributes to the production of prostaglandin E, which is essential to help keep prolactin, a breast tissue activator, in line.

■ **KEEP CALM.** Epinephrine, a substance produced by the adrenal glands during stress, also interferes with gamma linoleic acid conversion, says Dr. Northrup.

■ **CUT OUT ALL CAFFEINE.** Caffeine's role in contributing to breast discomfort is not proven. Some studies say it does; other studies are inconclusive. Some experts think that caffeine triggers an adrenal immune response that causes your lymphatic glands not to work as well. As a result, the lymphatic tissue doesn't drain properly and the breasts then become engorged. But no matter the exact link, Dr. Teitelbaum strongly recommends cutting out caffeine.

And just cutting the java isn't enough.

Pine Relief

Native Americans used poultices made with pine to relieve pain and inflammation. If you wish to try a modern version of this time-honored remedy, wash your breasts with pine tar soap, suggests Ellen Kamhi, Ph.D., R.N.

You can buy pine tar soap at some drugstores or your local health food store.

You really have to cut out all caffeine. This means forgoing soft drinks, chocolate, ice cream products, tea, and over-the-counter pain relievers that contain caffeine, such as diet aids and Excedrin.

■ **SKIP THE PEPPERONI PIZZA.** Highly salted foods bloat you, says Yvonne S. Thornton, M.D. Restrict your salt for 7 to 10 days before your menstrual period, before the monthly hormonal changes occur.

■ **STAY AWAY FROM DIURETICS.** It's true that diuretics can help flush fluid from your system. And that can help reduce the swelling in your breasts. But the immediate relief will cost you, says Dr. Thornton. Overuse of diuretics can cause an imbalance in your electrolyte system and lead to dehydration and muscle weakness.

■ **TAKE THE PRIMROSE PATH.** Evening primrose oil is an anti-inflammatory that can soothe pain and shrink lumps. Take one or two 1,000-milligram capsules of evening primrose oil with food three times a day for several months.

■ **FIND A GOOD BRA.** A sturdy sports bra can help support nerve fibers in the breast already stretched by engorged tissue. Some women find that wearing the bra to bed helps, says Gregory J. Radio, M.D., FACOG. When you shop for a new bra, try it on to see if it gives enough lift without pinching, and toss old bras that are misshapen or stretched out.

■ **COOL THEM DOWN.** When your breasts feel swollen and painful, wrap a towel around a bag of ice or a bag of frozen vegetables and put it on each breast for 10 minutes or so for quick relief.

■ **CONSIDER RECONSIDERING THE PILL.** "Women on a birth control pill can be affected by the daily estrogen stimulation," says Dr. Dean. If you're on the Pill and suffer from breast discomfort, consider another form of birth control, she says.

■ **COVER IT WITH CABBAGE.** To temporarily relieve breast discomfort, place a cabbage leaf against your breast in your bra, suggests Ralph Boling, D.O.

■ **CREATE A COMPRESS.** Dr. Kamhi suggests a breast compress, made by mixing nettles (3 tablespoons of the dried leaf or 30 drops of tincture), ginger (1 tablespoon of grated root), lavender (2 tablespoons of flower tops or 5 drops of essential oil), and fenugreek (1 teaspoon of ground seeds) in 1 quart of water. "Heat the water just below a full boil," she says. Allow the water to cool until comfortable to the touch. "Soak a clean washcloth in the solution and cover your breast with the cloth, focusing on the affected area," she says. Repeat several times until you feel some relief.

■ **TRY SELF-MASSAGE.** Georgianna Donadio, Ph.D., says a gentle breast self-massage helps move built-up breast fluid into the lymph passageways, providing pain relief. "Massage your breasts in a clockwise motion," she says. "It's best to do this around the time of ovulation, when breasts are least sore," she says. "It's great for breast discomfort and overall breast health."

■ **DISCOVER THE EMOTIONAL AND PHYSICAL TIE.** "This is absolutely the first thing I consider," says Dr. Northrup. "When I ask my patients 'what's going on in your life around the issue of nurturing or being nurtured?' I often see tears."

"Breasts as the symbol of nurturance are highly charged for women," she adds. "You know that tingling feeling that accompanies the letdown of milk? Some women who have gone through menopause still feel that when they hear a baby cry. That's how closely linked breasts are to the emotions."

Breastfeeding

22 Problem-Free Nursing Ideas

Breastfeeding is a wonderful way for mother and child to bond, and breast milk is nature's nearly perfect food. It not only contains all the nutrients that your baby needs, but it also helps protect your infant against infections.

Some studies show that breastfeeding significantly reduces the risk of diarrhea and pneumonia during a child's first year, as well as allergies, ear infections, and other illnesses well beyond the first year.

Less than an hour after birth, a full-term baby is physically able to nurse. "Many hospitals place the baby skin-to-skin on Mom's chest at delivery and watch the baby find the nipple and start breastfeeding all on his own. He knows what to do!" says Kittie Frantz, R.N., C.P.N.P., "Ask the staff to do this when you deliver—you will be amazed."

The beauty of breastfeeding is, there are no bottles to prepare or wash and no formula to buy. Plus, you have a ready supply of milk all the time.

Here's how to make breastfeeding trouble-free.

■ **DO A LITTLE PREPARATION.** "You're less likely to get sore, cracked nipples if you prepare in advance by rubbing your nipples daily with a terry cloth to 'toughen' them," says Ellen Kamhi, Ph.D., R.N.

■ **SET YOUR MILK SUPPLY.** Get your baby used to nursing and establish your milk supply by breastfeeding exclusively for the first

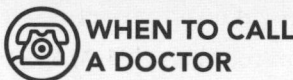

WHEN TO CALL A DOCTOR

If your breast feels inflamed, you're running a fever, or you have flulike symptoms, call your doctor. You could have mastitis, a breast infection.

Mastitis is usually treated with 10 days of antibiotics. If that's what your doctor prescribes, be sure to finish all the medication even if symptoms have already disappeared. This helps prevent recurrent infections.

Meanwhile, you can help speed healing on your own by going to bed, drinking lots of clear fluids, and nursing more frequently, says Carolyn Rawlins, M.D. Don't stop nursing. The milk isn't infected, and if you stop nursing while you have mastitis, it could trigger a breast abscess.

6 weeks. Hold off on bottles, and don't give your baby a pacifier unless you are sure he has nursed well beforehand. "This is the secret to a bountiful milk supply," Frantz says.

■ **PRACTICE GOOD NUTRITION.** Although you're no longer "eating for two," some of what you eat does make it into your breast milk, and into your baby. "Plus, proper nutrition is essential to milk production," adds Dr. Kamhi. She recommends eating plenty of protein, vitamins, minerals, and essential fatty acids. "Oats, sea vegetables, and green foods can help provide the extra nutrients needed at this cycle of life," she says. "And this is a time to pay particular attention to organic food sources, because pesticides and herbicides come through the milk."

■ **CHECK YOUR BABY POSITION.** Be sure your baby's mouth is open wide before putting him to your breast; he should latch onto the areola (the darker area around your nipple), says Frantz. You should see more areola above his top lip than below his bottom lip. "Sit reclined in a comfortable chair or couch, place the baby clad only in a diaper to your bare chest—this skin-to-skin triggers his search for the breast," Frantz says. "He will scoot down and move to one side to try to get under the breast. Then, when his chin touches the breast, he will open his mouth wide, reach up, and attach himself. It really is wondrous to see babies do this," she says. Once your baby does this at the hospital or at home, all you need to do is put him near your breast and he will take over. "This makes it easy when you are away

from home—just put a shawl over your shoulder and the baby to cover up," she says.

■ **SWITCH IT UP.** Leave the baby on your breast as long as he is swallowing every suck or two. If you see him drifting off to sleep or he lets go of the breast, burp him, and switch sides. Let him nurse on the second breast as long as he wants until he falls asleep or lets go again. In general, feeding time is a minimum of 20 to 30 minutes during the newborn period, and even longer is normal, Frantz says.

■ **DON'T SHOW FAVORITISM.** If either breast hurts from milk engorgement, make sure the baby nurses equally from both. "Usually, a baby will drink from one breast (say the right breast), drain that breast, and move to the other one," says Donna Hallas, Ph.D., C.P.N.P. "But the baby may get full halfway through the left breast and leave milk behind. To avoid milk buildup, start with the breast you ended with the time before, she says.

As an easy reminder, put a safety pin on the side of the bra where you need to start the next feeding.

■ **NURSE OFTEN.** "New mothers are often shocked at how often a baby wants to nurse. Well-meaning family and friends may offer advice more appropriate for bottle-feeding," says Frantz. You'll probably find yourself nursing 8 to 12 times each 24 hours in the early weeks.

■ **TURN INTO A NIGHT OWL.** "Babies are night people in the first 3 weeks—you will find that your newborn nurses more at night than in the morning," Frantz says. You will also find she will be more awake and smile more at night. This is a normal rhythm for a newborn. "So nurse her a lot at night, nap or sleep later in the morning, and know that it will get better in a few weeks," she says.

■ **GET COMFORTABLE.** A horseshoe-shaped nursing pillow will make you and your baby more comfortable during nursing sessions. This cushion fits around your midriff and provides a convenient armrest. Two popular brands of nursing pillows are Boppy and My Brest Friend.

■ **DON'T GET TOO COMFORTABLE.** If your baby nods off at the breast but cries when you put him down, "you may have made him too cozy," Frantz says. "Infants wrapped in blankets or swaddled in too many clothes often fall asleep before they are finished nursing—they feel like they are back in the womb," she says. And be mindful that a baby warm to the point of sweating is more prone to sudden infant death syndrome (SIDS), Frantz says.

■ **FORGET THE SOAP.** When you lather up, skip your nipples—soap dries them out. The little bumps around the areola are glands that produce an antiseptic oil, so there's no need to wash, too. "We now know that this oil also helps your baby smell the nipple and he can find it faster," Frantz says.

■ **BE SURE TO AIR-DRY.** Before you cover up after nursing make sure your nipples are dry, says Dr. Hallas. And don't use breast pads that hold in moisture, particularly those made with plastic.

■ **FIND THE RIGHT POSITION.** Most of the time nipple soreness comes when the baby attaches and sucks from the wrong angle, says Dr. Hallas. "If you hear a clicking or popping sound as your baby sucks, he's not latched on properly," she says. "Gently put your finger in the baby's mouth and take him away, then adjust him so his mouth is on the nipple properly." Rawness stops after you correct the position, though you may take a day or two to heal. To speed healing, air-dry your nipples when you finish a feeding, express a little milk, and rub it on your sore nipple. Milk left at the end of the feeding is high in lubricants and contains a natural antibiotic, she says.

Can't pump milk successfully? You can also rub vitamin E, avocado, or almond oil on sore nipples for a soothing effect, adds Dr. Kamhi.

■ **WEAR THE RIGHT NURSING BRA.** "For comfort and body tone, a good supportive nursing bra is important," Dr. Hallas says. Resist the urge to overbuy bras in the beginning, because your breasts will change, she says. Instead, wait until a few days after your milk has come in. "To find a nursing bra, I recommend going to someone who really knows how to measure women," she adds.

Here are tips for selecting a good nursing bra.

■ Choose all-cotton versus nylon.

■ Make sure the cup opening is big enough and doesn't compress the breasts, which could lead to clogged milk ducts.

- Check for ease in opening and closing the bra with one hand. This will help you be discreet.

- Be sure straps are comfortable and the bra isn't tight across the chest.

■ **STAY ALERT FOR PLUGGED DUCTS.** Binding clothes, your own anatomy, fatigue, or prolonged periods without nursing can cause clogged milk ducts. "This can cause areas of the breast to get hot, red, and sometimes hard or swollen," Dr. Kamhi says. A plugged duct can lead to an infection if ignored. "In most cases, you can treat this problem by applying hot compresses to the reddened area, and by expressing milk manually and allowing the baby to nurse," she says.

■ **TRY WARM COMPRESSES TO HELP WITH OVERPRODUCTION.** If you have more milk than your baby can drink and your breasts are full and painful, apply warm, wet compresses, says Frantz. This opens the ducts so milk flows more freely. Nurse the baby more often and longer, and take in enough fluids so that you urinate more often.

■ **CONTROL LEAKING.** To stop leaking, press the heel of your hand down on the nipple into the chest. Or buy reusable breast pads that you can launder. All-cotton pads work well.

■ **FILL UP ON FENUGREEK.** Much like oxytocin, a naturally occurring hormone, fenugreek seeds help stimulate milk production in nursing mothers. The recommended dosage is $\frac{1}{2}$ to $1\frac{1}{2}$ teaspoons of seeds a day, or capsules of 600 to 700 milligrams a day. Start with a low dose and slowly increase it if necessary. "Fenugreek may give the urine a maple syrup aroma, and in rare cases, this may lead to a misdiagnosis of maple urine disease in an infant," adds Dr. Kamhi.

■ **INCREASE FLOW WITH GALACTAGOGUES.** "These herbs have traditionally been used to increase the flow of milk," Dr. Kamhi says. In addition to fenugreek, galactagogues include blessed thistle, chaste berry, fennel seed, dill, black cohosh, milk thistle, nettles, and hops. "You can start any one of these in small amounts (1 cup of tea or 10 drops of tincture a day) and then increase them once it is determined that neither mother nor baby experiences any ill effects," she says.

PANEL OF ADVISORS

Bronchitis

10 Tips to Stop the Cough

Murphy's Law being what it is, you can count on bronchitis to trigger a stubborn cough when it is least welcome: in the middle of a long sermon, during a big presentation at work, in the wee hours of the morning when the entire household is trying to sleep.

Bronchitis is an infection and inflammation of the lining of the bronchial passages, the airways that connect the windpipe to the lungs. It is often triggered by an upper respiratory infection, and if it doesn't improve, bronchitis can lead to pneumonia.

In many ways, bronchitis is a lot like a cold. It's usually caused by a virus, says Randy Wexler, M.D., and antibiotics won't do much good. Sometimes, though, bronchitis is caused by bacteria, and in this case antibiotics may clear it up.

Acute bronchitis most often goes away by itself in a week or two. But people with chronic bronchitis can cough and wheeze for months. Although you have to let bronchitis take its course, there are things that you can do to breathe easier while you have it.

■ **STOP SMOKING.** It's the most important thing to do, especially if you're a chronic sufferer. Quit smoking, and your chances of ridding yourself of bronchitis go up dramatically.

■ **GET ACTIVE ABOUT PASSIVE SMOKING.** Avoid those who smoke, and if your spouse smokes, your coughing might be incentive to kick the habit. Other people's smoking could be causing *your*

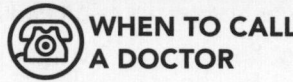

WHEN TO CALL A DOCTOR

Bronchitis requires a doctor's attention when:

■ You find your cough is getting worse, not better, after a week.

■ You have a fever or are coughing up blood.

■ You are older and get a hacking cough on top of another illness.

■ You are short of breath and also have a very profuse cough.

■ You are elderly.

■ You also have heart or lung disease.

Why Antibiotics Generally Aren't the Answer

At the first sign of a nasty cough, fatigue, wheezing, sore throat, chest discomfort, and low-grade fever that characterize bronchitis, many people ask their doctors for antibiotics. Generally, though, antibiotics are a waste of time, because up to 95 percent of all cases are caused by viruses, which antibiotics won't touch. Bacteria trigger only a small portion of acute bronchitis infections.

Doctors are often reluctant to prescribe antibiotics because there's scant evidence that they shorten the course of the illness or ease symptoms. There is some evidence, however, that bronchodilators—asthma drugs that open the airways—can relieve symptoms. Patients who use bronchodilators are more likely to stop coughing within a week of starting the medicines compared with those who took a placebo. The patients who used bronchodilators also returned to work sooner than patients taking a sugar pill. Doctors caution, however, that bronchodilators are most likely to work in patients whose bronchial passages are inflamed. Bronchodilators such as albuterol (Ventolin) usually come in the form of inhalers.

bronchitis. Exposure to secondhand smoke (called passive smoking) can result in bronchitis.

■ **BOOST IMMUNITY WITH CALCIUM.** "Bronchitis is the 'low-calcium-level disease,'" says Georgianna Donadio, Ph.D. "It results when your immune function is lowered, and low calcium levels do suppress your immune system," she says. Just make sure you get plenty of both calcium and vitamin D, particularly in the winter time, she says. "I recommend taking 800-milligram capsules of vitamin D daily, and at least 500 milligrams of a combination calcium and magnesium powder per day—powder is much more effective than tablets," she says.

■ **BREATHE IN WARM, MOIST AIR.** Warm, moist air helps vaporize mucus. If you have mucus that is thick or difficult to cough up, a vaporizer will help to loosen the secretions. You could also close the door and run a hot shower in your bathroom, breathing in the warm steam.

Running a humidifier in your home is particularly important in the winter, when indoor heating systems dry the air—and your mucus membranes. When your mucus membranes dry out, it is harder for your immune system to move germs out of your body effectively, and you become more susceptible to illnesses like bronchitis.

■ **VAPORIZE FROM THE OUTSIDE IN.** To help suppress the cough associated with bronchitis, rub on a topical cough suppressant ointment such as Vicks VapoRub, suggests Rachel Schreiber, M.D. VapoRub contains camphor, a cough suppressant and topical analgesic from the camphor tree; eucalyptol, a cough suppressant and herbal extract; menthol, a cough suppressant and topical analgesic from mint oils; as well as cedar leaf oil, nutmeg oil, thymol, and turpentine oil. All of these ingredients are used for cough suppression in the traditional Indian practice of Ayurvedic medicine. Dr. Schreiber recommends applying VapoRub to the chest right before sleep.

■ **ELIMINATE MUCUS-CAUSING FOODS.** "One of the best ways to address any condition that involves the lungs is to stop eating foods that create mucus," says Ellen Kamhi, Ph.D., R. N. "This can vary due to individual sensitivities, but wheat and dairy products are the biggest culprits for most people," she says. Dr. Kamhi suggests people with bronchitis eat mostly homemade vegetable soup and drink hot tea.

■ **TRY AN AFRICAN REMEDY.** One of the best remedies for bronchitis is an African herb called pelargonium sidoides (you can find it as a glycerin extract in most health food stores), says Judith Stanton, M.D. "Take 1 dropperful every 2 hours," she says. Other helpful natural treatments include astragalus root, echinacea, garlic, licorice root, and vitamin C. Of course, getting plenty of sleep, drinking lots of fluids, and avoiding alcohol are all important as well, she says.

■ **FOCUS ON PREVENTION.** Infants, young children, smokers, people with heart or lung disease, and the elderly are more likely to develop bronchitis. They are also more likely to have a case of bronchitis balloon into pneumonia. Those who are vulnerable should curtail strenuous outdoor work and exercise on days when air pollution is high.

What the Doctor Does

"I recently had bronchitis, and this remedy cleared it up in 36 hours," says Georgianna Donadio, Ph.D. She recommends making a homemade antiviral poultice out of garlic and onions. "Mash up some fresh garlic and onions—both are natural virus fighters—and put them in an old sock. Then place a little cloth on your chest, put the garlic and onion sock on top of that, and put a hot-water bottle on top of the sock," she says. "The vapors will go right into your chest—it's fabulous for bronchitis," she says.

PANEL OF ADVISORS

GEORGIANNA DONADIO, PH.D., IS DIRECTOR OF THE NATIONAL INSTITUTE OF WHOLE HEALTH, A HOLISTIC CERTIFICATION PROGRAM FOR MEDICAL PROFESSIONALS.

ELLEN KAMHI, PH.D., R.N., IS THE NATURAL NURSE, CLINICAL INSTRUCTOR IN THE DEPARTMENT OF FAMILY MEDICINE AT STONY BROOK UNIVERSITY IN NEW YORK, AND AUTHOR OF *THE NATURAL MEDICINE CHEST, ARTHRITIS: THE ALTERNATIVE MEDICINE DEFINITIVE GUIDE,* AND *CYCLES OF LIFE: HERBS FOR WOMEN.*

RACHEL SCHREIBER, M.D., IS A BOARD-CERTIFIED PHYSICIAN IN ALLERGY/IMMUNOLOGY AND INTERNAL MEDICINE, AND WAS RECENTLY SUGGESTED AS ONE OF AMERICA'S TOP PHYSICIANS BY THE CONSUMER'S RESEARCH COUNCIL OF AMERICA.

JUDITH STANTON, M.D., IS A CLINICAL INSTRUCTOR AT UC BERKELEY-UCSF AND AN ATTENDING PHYSICIAN AT ALTA BATES HOSPITAL IN BERKELEY, CALIFORNIA.

RANDY WEXLER, M.D., IS AN ASSISTANT PROFESSOR IN THE DEPARTMENT OF FAMILY MEDICINE AT OHIO STATE UNIVERSITY MEDICAL CENTER IN COLUMBUS.

Cures from the Kitchen

At the first sign of bronchitis, try what Georgianna Donadio, Ph.D., calls "the bronchitis diet." "Drink orange juice and water for 2 or 3 days, followed by a few days of all fruits and vegetables—it will really clean out your respiratory system," she says.

Bruises

10 Healing Ideas

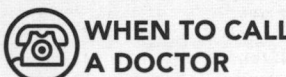

WHEN TO CALL A DOCTOR

Sometimes a bruise can be a sign of an underlying illness. A blood disorder can cause unexplained bruising, for example, while bruising that occurs along with nosebleeds could indicate a clotting disorder. So if you're prone to bruises and you don't know for sure what's behind them, talk with your doctor.

Also contact your doctor if any bruise is accompanied by extreme pain or broken skin with areas of redness, heat, or tenderness. These could be signs of an infection, says Monica Halem, M.D. "If you have bruising in your extremities combined with numbness, you could have a condition known as compartment syndrome," she says.

Unless you encase yourself in bubble wrap, you'll never be bruise-proof. But you can lessen the likelihood of a small bruise turning into a large one and help the black-and-blue fade quickly. Here's how.

■ **PUT THE CHILL ON BRUISES.** If the skin isn't broken, put ice on any injury that might bruise, advises Monica Halem, M.D. "Ice constricts the blood vessels and prevents more blood from seeping into the skin," she says. A cold pack also minimizes the swelling, numbs the area, and reduces pain. Wrap the ice pack in a thin cloth to protect your skin, put it on the bruise as quickly as possible, and keep it there for 15 minutes. If you suspect the bump will blossom into a severe bruise, continue this ice treatment every couple of hours for the first 24 hours. Allow your skin to warm naturally and don't apply heat between ice packs.

■ **FOLLOW ICE WITH HEAT.** After 24 hours, use heat to dilate the blood vessels and improve circulation in the area. "Warm compresses will help speed up the body's natural mechanisms for removing the blood in the bruise," says Randy Wexler, M.D.

■ **KEEP IT CLOSED AND CLEAN.** Leave the skin covering a bruise intact, says Dr. Halem. "If the skin is already broken, clean it with soap and water, and then apply an over-the-counter antibiotic ointment or petroleum jelly," she says. Then cover it with an adhesive bandage.

■ **PROP YOUR FEET UP.** Bruises are little reservoirs of blood. Blood, like any liquid, runs downhill. If you do a lot of standing, blood that has collected in a bruise will seep down through your soft tissues and find other places to puddle. "Elevation will also help ease any swelling," Dr. Halem says.

■ **ADD VITAMIN C TO YOUR DAILY DIET.** If you do bruise easily, there's a possibility you could be deficient in vitamin C.

Vitamin C is instrumental in helping build protective collagen tissue around blood vessels in the skin, says Sheldon V. Pollack, M.D. Your face, hands, and feet contain less collagen than, say, your thighs, so bruises in these areas are often darker.

If you bruise easily, Dr. Pollack suggests 500 milligrams of vitamin C three times a day to help build your collagen. Or you can boost

Cures from the Kitchen

Keep some apple cider vinegar on hand for instant bruise relief. Apple cider vinegar is an excellent natural anti-inflammatory. Put a little on a cotton ball and dab it directly on the bruise. Or make a paste out of apple cider vinegar and an egg white or petroleum jelly, and smear it on the bruised area.

your intake by eating foods rich in vitamin C such as citrus fruits, green leafy vegetables, and bell peppers.

■ **CONTROL A BRUISE WITH K.** Vitamin K decreases bruising—both inside and out—by helping blood to clot. Rub some vitamin-K cream (available in your local drugstore and online) on a bruise a few times a day to clear it up faster, Dr. Halem says. You can also minimize bruising or ease the severity of a bruise by boosting your intake of vitamin-K-rich foods. "Green leafy vegetables, alfalfa, broccoli, and seaweed are good dietary sources of vitamin K," she says.

■ **WATCH THOSE MEDICATIONS.** People who take aspirin to protect against heart disease or those on blood thinners will find that a bump easily turns into a bruise. Drugs such as anti-inflammatories, antidepressants, and asthma medicines can inhibit clotting under the skin and cause larger bruises. Alcoholics and drug abusers tend to bruise easily, too. If you're taking medicine that makes you prone to bruising, talk to your doctor about it.

■ **DE-BRUISE WITH BROMELAIN.** To help a bruise heal faster, take bromelain, a pineapple extract available in most health food stores. It "digests" proteins that cause inflammation and pain, says Jay Zimmerman, M.D. "Take 1 or 2 grams with water before meals."

PANEL OF ADVISORS

MONICA HALEM, M.D., IS A CLINICAL ASSISTANT PROFESSOR OF DERMATOLOGIC SURGERY AT NEW YORK–PRESBYTERIAN HOSPITAL/COLUMBIA IN NEW YORK CITY.

SHELDON V. POLLACK, M.D., IS AN ASSOCIATE PROFESSOR OF MEDICINE IN THE DEPARTMENT OF DERMATOLOGY AT THE UNIVERSITY OF TORONTO SCHOOL OF MEDICINE, AND DIRECTOR OF THE TORONTO COSMETIC SKIN SURGERY CENTRE INC.

RANDY WEXLER, M.D., IS AN ASSISTANT PROFESSOR IN THE DEPARTMENT OF FAMILY MEDICINE AT OHIO STATE UNIVERSITY MEDICAL CENTER IN COLUMBUS.

JAY ZIMMERMAN, M.D., IS A BOARD-CERTIFIED DERMATOLOGIST AND CLINICAL INSTRUCTOR IN THE DEPARTMENT OF DERMATOLOGY AT UCLA.

Burnout

25 Paths to Renewal

Stress is an inevitable, unavoidable fact of life. You do what you can to cope. Sometimes, though, it becomes so persistent and overwhelming that it just drains you, physically and emotionally. Experts refer to this state of complete exhaustion as burnout—and not surprisingly, it's more pervasive than ever.

Burnout seems to go hand-in-hand with job stress, but it isn't always work-related. The slide into burnout is gradual; loved ones and colleagues may be the first to notice that something isn't quite right.

A feeling of excessive responsibility or a sense of a lack of control contributes to burnout, which in turn can lead to serious medical problems, including high blood pressure, gastrointestinal problems, coronary artery disease, and sleep problems, says Peter S. Moskowitz, M.D.

The emotional signs often start first. "You may feel irritable, finding that you have less ability to deal with minor problems at home and at work," he notes. People under stress may begin to squabble with coworkers, experience road rage, or have an extra cocktail before dinner. They may show signs of depression—struggling to get out of bed in the morning—or symptoms of anxiety—lying awake at night.

Later, physical signs appear, such as headache, abdominal pain, backache, chronic fatigue, and a general I've-just-been-run-over-by-a-truck feeling.

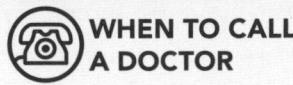 **WHEN TO CALL A DOCTOR**

If burnout goes unchecked, it can have serious repercussions on your physical and emotional health.

Clues that you need professional help may be external, such as a poor job evaluation, heavy absenteeism, or a major fight at home. Or the clues may be internal, such as anxiety or depression.

If your anxiety or depression interferes with your daily life or persists despite your self-help efforts, consult a doctor.

"Burnout is a serious situation," says Ellen Kamhi, Ph.D., R.N. "Feelings of high stress negatively impact all aspects of health."

Physically, burnout means that your adrenal glands have become exhausted—you have asked them to do too much for too long. "During acute stress, your body produces increased amounts of corticosteroids, which are anti-inflammatory," explains Georgianna Donadio, Ph.D. "When you are first under acute stress, you are okay, but after you've been stressed for weeks, your body runs out of steroids, especially if you are undernourished." At this point, you become completely exhausted and depleted—in other words, burned out.

Who's at greatest risk for burnout? Surprisingly, workers who burn out are often the most highly motivated, dedicated people on the job. "You can't burn out unless there's been a fire in the first place," explains Dr. Moskowitz. Some people may experience burnout as disillusionment with a job that no longer seems as challenging.

Other people at risk for burnout are those who tend to worry excessively or put work before self or family. "These people don't manage stress well, and they don't have a well-thought-out plan for taking care of themselves and balancing their lives," says Dr. Moskowitz. "They don't realize that lifestyle balance is the most potent form of stress management available."

Fortunately, burnout isn't inevitable. You can take steps to revitalize your outlook on your job, relationships, and life in general.

Here are a few strategies from our experts.

■ **DISCOVER WHAT IS ACTUALLY BURNING YOU OUT.** "It's so important to find the source of the burnout—it could be work, family, marriage, or keeping a clean house," says life-balance coach Wendy Kaufman, M.A. "There is no one right answer or source for everyone, but once you've narrowed it down, you can work on treating the things that give you the most stress," she says.

■ **STEP BACK FROM YOUR SITUATION.** If burnout is acute, meaning it's linked to only current circumstances, a brief time-out may be enough. "Take a vacation, go to a health spa, get a massage, learn yoga, or engage in another stress-reducing technique," Dr. Kamhi advises. Chronic burnout, on the other hand, may require more drastic measures. "The ultimate remedy may involve moving, switching jobs, leaving a toxic relationship, or making other major life changes," Dr. Kamhi says.

■ **REFRAME YOUR THOUGHTS.** You can't always control what happens around you, but you can control how you respond to those events, says Jack N. Singer, Ph.D. If layoffs in your company have led to a heavy workload for you, remind yourself that you were valuable enough to remain employed. Give yourself credit for being able to handle the extra work. Feel good about doing the best job you can. "To remind yourself of what a good job you do, keep a folder of your best work—this can be very motivating when you look back on it," Kaufman says.

■ **ASSERT YOURSELF.** Burnout can result from resentment caused by lack of recognition or by being taken for granted by your boss, coworkers, family members, and others, says Kate Muller, Psy.D. So don't be afraid to strongly express your heart-felt needs and feelings. "Assertiveness can be incredibly helpful and freeing," she says. "When you express yourself in a calm yet firm way, it can really strengthen and build relationships."

■ **PUT YOURSELF FIRST.** One of the most important things you can do to prevent burnout is to think about you. "Give yourself permission to take care of you first. It's like the oxygen mask on the plane theory: You can't help others properly until you've helped yourself," Kaufman says. "This may mean taking a day off from work and doing things just for you. It may be hard to do, but ultimately it will benefit those around you."

Cures from the Kitchen

During periods of burnout, certain vitamins and minerals, such as vitamins B and C, zinc, and magnesium, are important for immune health, says Janet Maccaro, Ph.D., C.N.C. To keep your body well nourished during times of stress, she recommends eating more foods rich in those crucial nutrients. Some of these foods include brown rice, grains, sunflower seeds, brewers' yeast, bran, eggs, leafy dark green vegetables, almonds, avocado, carrots, and citrus fruits.

■ **DEVELOP SELF-AWARENESS.** For those who want to take care of themselves, Dr. Moskowitz recommends some form of calm reflection daily. Relaxation techniques that foster health, healing, and self-awareness include prayer, meditation, yoga, tai chi, breathing exercises, journaling, and self-hypnosis. Psychotherapy and career coaching are additional pathways to greater self-awareness.

■ **ESCAPE.** Take a little time away from the thing that is burning you out, says Randy Wexler, M.D. Rent a movie, go to dinner, and turn off your cell phone.

Try different approaches until you find the best relaxation program for your needs, interests, and abilities. "Taking time to meditate, or just a few minutes to take some deep breaths, can really be helpful," says Machelle Seibel, M.D. Some, such as tai chi, involve both physical and mental exercises, while others, like meditation, chiefly are a mental discipline.

■ **SEE THE GLASS AS HALF FULL.** They say "perception is reality," and in many cases, this is true. If you train your mind to look for the positives in negative situations, you will develop a much more positive outlook overall, says Susan Mikolic, R.N.

■ **DE-CLUTTER.** By becoming better organized, you will improve your efficiency, Kaufman says. "This means organizing everything in your life—your closet, files, e-mail inbox, office supplies, drawers, and more," she says. "Getting rid of old stuff makes a difference psychologically," she says.

■ **DIG INTO YOUR WORK.** "Don't sit there fretting about how much there is to do, procrastinating out of fear that you'll never get it done," Dr. Singer says. Get organized and set goals at the beginning of each day, doing the toughest tasks first and crossing them off a list as you complete them. Build small rewards into your day, such as enjoying a cup of tea or a walk around the building, as you accomplish what you set out to do.

■ **MAKE YOUR WORK SPACE A PLACE YOU LIKE.** Hang cartoons that make you laugh, display pictures of people you love, or tack up photos of places you enjoy.

■ **LAUGH.** Humor and laughter lower blood pressure and boost immunity, says Dr. Singer. "Every time you laugh, it's like exercising your internal organs."

He recommends putting a "fun quotient" into every office. For example, keep a funny book next to your phone to flip through when you're on hold. Dr. Singer recommends *Chicken Poop in My Bowl* by John M. Irvin.

■ **HAVE AN ANNUAL CHECKUP.** Burnout takes a physical toll, so if you live a stressful life, make sure that your body is in good shape. Your doctor can help you develop a program of self-care designed to make you feel better by exercising, eating right, and getting the sleep you need. Knowing that you're taking care of your own body also helps you feel more in control of your life.

■ **EXERCISE OFTEN.** Regular exercise combats burnout by reducing stress. It also boosts your resistance to disease, lowers your blood pressure, improves your cholesterol profile, helps control weight, and may lift depression. Exercising at least 3 days a week for 30 to 60 minutes is especially important for people who feel frazzled and burned out, so make this a priority, recommends Dr. Moskowitz.

Exercise is particularly beneficial if you do it outside. "Exercise in a natural setting among trees, water, and other vegetation," Mikolic says. Trees and vegetation covert carbon dioxide into oxygen, which energizes your entire body, and natural sunlight will enrich your body with immunity-boosting vitamin D. "Plus, fresh air and moving water contain higher concentrations of negative ions (low concentrations of negative ions have been shown to create agitation and hostility)."

■ **EAT WELL.** You don't have control over all of the stressors making you feel burned out, but you do have control over what you eat. Eat a low-fat, high-fiber diet. "And stop eating junk food, which aggravates burnout by slowing down body systems and inducing inflammation," says Mikolic. You'll gain a sense of satisfaction knowing that you're doing right by your body, and you may even lose some weight to boot.

■ **PUT BACK IN WHAT YOU'VE BURNED OUT.** "Researcher and medical doctor Dr. Hans Seyle spent 55 years of his life identifying what the body needs to recover from burnout," Dr. Donadio says. "And he found that you need to boost your intake of protein, vitamins A, C, B, and E, essential fatty acids, minerals, cholesterol, and calcium," she says. "Why these substances? Because those are the things your body uses to make steroids, and steroids are what your body makes when it is under stress. Essentially, these are the raw materials of stress hormones," she says.

■ **BANISH BURNOUT WITH BANANAS AND OTHER FOODS RICH IN POTASSIUM.** "Potassium is lost when adrenal health is compromised," says Janet Maccaro, Ph.D., C.N.C. "Bananas, kiwis, potatoes, fish, and other foods high in potassium can help recharge your adrenal glands and give you more energy," she says.

■ **GET RESTFUL SLEEP.** Let go of the day's worries and unfinished business. Tell yourself that you will make decisions tomorrow, after a good night's rest. Visualize one of your favorite vacations or a serene scene from a movie. Imagine yourself in that place as you drift off to sleep. Avoid alcohol, tobacco, and exercise for at least 1 hour prior to sleep. "Invest in a firm, comfortable mattress," says Dr. Moskowitz.

■ **SLEEP AT THE RIGHT TIME.** Dr. Maccaro recommends going to bed by 10:00 p.m. and sleeping until 9:00 a.m. whenever possible. "These are the hours that help restore adrenal health and, therefore, help alleviate burnout and speed recovery," she says.

■ **DEEPEN YOUR RELATIONSHIPS.** People who feel burned out often take out their frustration on those who love them most. That's like shooting yourself in the foot, because time devoted to enriching relationships with family and friends will help to ease feelings of burnout, says Dr. Moskowitz.

■ **GET A LIFE AND A COMMUNITY.** Seek out a community of like-minded people to share your life, whether it's pursuing a hobby, finding a place of worship, or doing community service. "Connecting with people will give you a wonderful source of support and encouragement and make you more resilient to stress," Dr. Moskowitz notes.

■ **ACCEPT WHAT YOU CAN'T CHANGE.** The more you struggle against a situation, the more you suffer. "Recent research in the area of stress management suggests that learning to 'radically accept' situations you are not feeling good about can help you better cope with them," Dr. Muller says. "If you can let go of the struggle and live with some unchangeable factors, you will feel less frustrated," she says. For example, take a coworker who continuously comes in late, forcing you to cover for her. After asking, pleading, and demanding that she come in on time, nothing has changed. "Instead of looking at her empty chair and fuming, if you change your attitude about the situation and accept that this is how it will be, you will lower your frustration level significantly," Dr. Muller says.

■ **BE BRAVE—TAKE RISKS AND MOVE ON.** If you've determined that your unhappiness is coming from your job and you can't change or delegate the tasks that trouble you most, have the courage to find another job that better suits you. "It's scary, and it requires risk, but your risk will be rewarded tenfold," promises Dr. Moskowitz. "Nothing changes without some pain. With risk comes personal growth and renewal."

PANEL OF ADVISORS

GEORGIANNA DONADIO, PH.D., IS DIRECTOR OF THE NATIONAL INSTITUTE OF WHOLE HEALTH, A HOLISTIC CERTIFICATION PROGRAM FOR MEDICAL PROFESSIONALS.

ELLEN KAMHI, PH.D., R.N., IS THE NATURAL NURSE, CLINICAL INSTRUCTOR IN THE DEPARTMENT OF FAMILY MEDICINE AT STONY BROOK UNIVERSITY IN NEW YORK, AND AUTHOR OF *THE NATURAL MEDICINE CHEST, ARTHRITIS: THE ALTERNATIVE MEDICINE DEFINITIVE GUIDE,* AND *CYCLES OF LIFE: HERBS FOR WOMEN.*

WENDY KAUFMAN, M.A., IS A LIFE-BALANCE SPECIALIST AND THE FOUNDER AND PRESIDENT OF BALANCING LIFE'S ISSUES INC., A NATIONAL EXECUTIVE TRAINING COMPANY IN WEST CHESTER, NEW YORK.

JANET MACCARO, PH.D., C.N.C., IS A HOLISTIC NUTRITIONIST AND CERTIFIED NUTRITION CONSULTANT IN SCOTTSDALE, ARIZONA, PRESIDENT OF DR. JANET'S BALANCED BY NATURE PRODUCTS, AND AUTHOR OF *NATURAL HEALTH REMEDIES.*

SUSAN MIKOLIC, R.N., IS THE PRESIDENT OF STEPPING STONES MENTAL HEALTH EDUCATIONAL CONSULTING IN EASTLAKE, OHIO.

PETER S. MOSKOWITZ, M.D., IS DIRECTOR OF THE CENTER FOR PROFESSIONAL AND PERSONAL RENEWAL IN PALO ALTO, CALIFORNIA. HE CONDUCTS WORKSHOPS AND LECTURES AND PROVIDES CAREER/LIFE COACHING FOR PHYSICIANS AND OTHER PROFESSIONALS ON STRESS MANAGEMENT AND RELATED LIFE-BALANCE ISSUES.

KATE MULLER, PSY.D., IS DIRECTOR OF PSYCHOLOGICAL TRAINING AND THE COGNITIVE BEHAVIOR THERAPY PROGRAM AND ASSISTANT PROFESSOR OF PSYCHIATRY AND BEHAVIORAL SCIENCES AT THE ALBERT EINSTEIN COLLEGE OF MEDICINE IN BRONX, NEW YORK.

MACHELLE SEIBEL, M.D., IS A PROFESSOR AT THE UNIVERSITY OF MASSACHUSETTS SCHOOL OF MEDICINE AND AUTHOR OF *A WOMAN'S BOOK OF YOGA.*

JACK N. SINGER, PH.D., IS A CLINICAL PSYCHOLOGIST IN ORANGE COUNTY, CALIFORNIA, AND PRESIDENT OF WWW.ASKDRJACK.COM.

RANDY WEXLER, M.D., IS AN ASSISTANT PROFESSOR IN THE DEPARTMENT OF FAMILY MEDICINE AT OHIO STATE UNIVERSITY MEDICAL CENTER IN COLUMBUS.

Burns

15 Treatments for Minor Accidents

When you accidentally brush your hand on the burner, splash battery acid on your chest, or take a face full of steam when you lift the lid on a pot, you need to put the fire out—*fast!* Here's how.

■ **DOUSE THAT FLAME.** The first and most important thing is to stop the burning process. Flush your burns with lots and lots of tepid (not cold) water until the burning stops, says Rebecca Coffey, R.N., C.N.P. But *don't* use ice or ice water—they can make your burn worse, she adds.

"If it's a contact burn, and it covers more than 10 percent of your body or is on the hands, feet, face, perineum, or joints, cover it with a clean, dry dressing and seek medical attention right away," Coffey says. If it's hot grease or splattered hot material like battery acid, soup, or water, first remove any saturated clothing, wash the grease off your skin, then soak the burn in tepid water, she says. If the clothing sticks to the burn, rinse over the clothing, then go to the doctor. Do not attempt to pull the clothing off your skin.

Once you've put the fire out, you're halfway to healing. The coolness stops the burning from spreading through your tissue and works as a temporary painkiller.

■ **LEAVE THE BUTTER FOR BREAD.** This is one case the old wives got wrong—you shouldn't soothe a burn with butter, says Coffey. After all, you wouldn't try to smother a fire with a giant pat of butter, would you? The same goes for a burn. In fact, butter can actually make it worse by holding the heat in your tissue and possibly causing an infection.

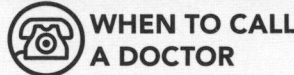

WHEN TO CALL A DOCTOR

For any third-degree burns, call 911 immediately. While you wait for help, elevate the burned area above the heart and cover it with a clean sheet to reduce heat loss.

Also seek immediate medical attention for the following:

■ A burn that you can't positively identify as first- or second-degree

■ Any burn on the face, hands, feet, pelvic or pubic area, or the eyes

■ Chemical or electrical burns. (For an electrical burn, don't touch the victim until the power is off.)

■ A burn that shows signs of infection, such as a blister filled with greenish or brownish fluid, or a burn that becomes hot again

■ Any burn that doesn't heal in 10 days to 2 weeks

Note: If you need to see a doctor about a burn, don't apply any ointments, antiseptics, or sprays. You may wrap the affected area in a dry, sterile dressing.

Know the Three Degrees

You can usually self-treat first- and second-degree burns smaller than a silver dollar. Third-degree burns are metaphorically too hot to handle on your own and need medical attention. Here's how to tell the difference between first-, second-, and third-degree burns.

■ First-degree burns, like most sunburns and scalds, are red and painful.

■ Second-degree burns, including severe sunburns or burns caused by brief direct contact with hot surfaces such as stove coils or an iron, tend to blister and ooze, and are painful.

■ Third-degree burns are charred and white or creamy colored. They can be caused by chemicals, electricity, or prolonged contact with hot surfaces. Usually, they are not painful because nerve endings have been destroyed, but they always require a doctor's care.

■ **REACH FOR WATER.** If you burn your mouth sipping a scalding cup of coffee or other hot food or drink, rinse your mouth and gargle with cool water for 5 to 10 minutes. Avoid hot foods and drinks for several days.

■ **COVER THE BURN.** After you cool and clean the burn, gently wrap the injury in a clean, dry cloth, such as a thick gauze pad.

■ **THEN DO NOTHING.** At least for the first 24 hours, leave the burn alone. Burns

Cures from the Kitchen

If you burn yourself while cooking, Janet Maccaro, Ph.D., C.N.C., suggests applying any of the following for instant relief:

■ The inside of a banana peel

■ Honey

■ A piece of raw potato

■ Baking soda or apple cider vinegar in warm water

should be allowed to begin the healing process on their own.

■ **BABY THE BLISTERS.** If the burn raised blisters and covers just a small area, resist the urge to pop the blisters. "Blisters are a great natural dressing for the burn—the best thing you can do is leave them alone and cover them with a dry dressing," says Coffey. "If the blisters break on their own or the burned skin is moist, use an over-the-counter antibiotic ointment such as Neosporin, following label directions," she says.

■ **SOOTHE WITH ALOE.** Two to 3 days after you burn, snip off a fresh piece of aloe and use the plant's natural healing moisture, or apply an over-the-counter aloe cream. Both have an analgesic action that will make your wound feel better. Or get to the core of the burn by drinking 8 ounces of unsweetened aloe juice, suggests Jacob Teitelbaum, M.D. "Available at Wal-Mart or Safeway, unsweetened aloe juice will dramatically speed burn healing," he says.

■ **MAKE SOOTHING SOLUTIONS.** When your burn starts to heal, cut open a capsule of vitamin E and rub the liquid onto your sore skin. It feels good and may prevent scarring. Or reach for an over-the-counter remedy such as the sunburn-cooler Solarcaine.

■ **COOL IT DOWN WITH A MINTY MIX-TURE.** For instant burn relief, Janet Mac-caro, Ph.D., C.N.C., suggests combining 10 drops of peppermint essential oil with ⅛ cup honey and generally applying it to the burn to ease pain, as needed.

■ **DAB ON AN ANTIMICROBIAL CREAM.** An over-the-counter antibiotic ointment containing the active ingredients polymyxin B sulfate or bacitracin zinc discourages infection and speeds healing. (For a list comparing the effectiveness of various over-the-counter ointments, see page 161.)

■ **PREVENT SCALDS.** Scalds account for one-third of admissions to burn centers, Coffey says. To protect yourself, make sure your hot water tank is set no higher than 120°F.

PANEL OF ADVISORS

REBECCA COFFEY, R.N., C.N.P., IS A NURSE PRACTITIONER AT THE BURN CENTER AT OHIO STATE UNIVERSITY MEDICAL CENTER IN COLUMBUS.

GEORGIANNA DONADIO, PH.D., IS DIRECTOR OF THE NATIONAL INSTITUTE OF WHOLE HEALTH, A HOLISTIC CERTIFICATION PROGRAM FOR MEDICAL PROFESSIONALS.

JANET MACCARO, PH.D., C.N.C., IS A HOLISTIC NUTRITIONIST AND CERTIFIED NUTRITION CONSULTANT IN SCOTTSDALE, ARIZONA, PRESIDENT OF DR. JANET'S BALANCED BY NATURE PRODUCTS, AND AUTHOR OF *NATURAL HEALTH REMEDIES*.

JACOB TEITELBAUM, M.D., IS A BOARD-CERTIFIED INTERNIST AND MEDICAL DIRECTOR OF THE FIBROMYALGIA AND FATIGUE CENTERS, WITH LOCATIONS THROUGHOUT THE COUNTRY.

Bursitis

15 Ways to Ease Your Pain

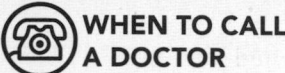

WHEN TO CALL A DOCTOR

Painful bursitis may subside with just a little TLC. But if it's caused by an infection or gout, you need to see a doctor. How can you tell? If the joint is tender, warm, and red, that's a definite sign. But sometimes these signs won't be present even if you have an infection, so it's best to get a doctor's advice when you have a flare-up of bursitis.

Bursitis is an inflammation of the fluid-filled sacs in the joints, called bursae, that ensure the body's movements are smooth and friction-free. You have more than 150 of them nestled in your shoulders, knees, and other joints. Bursitis pain flares whenever repeated movement stresses a specific joint, such as a long day of tennis or golf causing intense shoulder pain. The most frequent site of bursitis is the shoulder, followed by the elbow and the knee.

Bursitis strikes, it retreats, it strikes again. The acutely painful stage of bursitis lasts 4 to 5 days, sometimes even longer. The on-again, off-again nature of acute bursitis is aggravating for people with the condition and frustrating for those trying to determine what type of treatments actually work.

Right now, there is no "cure" for bursitis. Until medicine comes up with one, here are some tried-and-true remedies that may bring temporary relief from this painful condition.

■ **USE R.I.C.E.** This acronym stands for a treatment method used frequently to help ease inflammatory conditions like bursitis, says Carolyn Dean, M.D., N.D. It stands for the following:

R: Rest the joint in the initial stages of bursitis. If the bursitis is in your shoulder or elbow, wear a sling to take the pressure off of the joint.

I: Ice the area 10 minutes on, 10 minutes off. "Don't put the ice directly on the skin—wrap it in a cloth instead," Dr. Dean says.

C: Use compression. If the joint is swollen, a mild pressure bandage will keep fluid from building, Dr. Dean says.

E: Elevate your leg if the bursitis is in your knee or ankle.

■ **THEN HEAT IT UP.** After you've passed the acute phase of inflammation, apply warm compresses to the affected area to speed healing, says Janet Maccaro, Ph.D., C.N.C.

■ **OIL THE PAIN.** Tea tree oil is great for calming the inflammatory process, says Georgianna Donadio, Ph.D. Dab a little tea tree oil on a cotton ball and apply it directly to the painful joint as needed, she says.

■ **ADD SOME SPICE.** Mix up a natural warming solution by combining 1 part cayenne pepper to 4 to 6 parts petroleum jelly, suggests Dr. Donadio. Then apply it directly to the painful area. This is a Chinese remedy that works well, she says.

■ **PUT SOME SALT ON IT.** Epsom salt, that is. Dr. Maccaro recommends taking an Epsom salt bath once a week to ease bursitis, while also adding several drops of rosemary essential oil to the bathwater.

■ **AVOID ACID.** Decreasing the amount of acid in your body will help douse the burn of bursitis and encourage speedy healing. So Dr. Maccaro suggests steering clear of acid-forming foods like salt, caffeinated beverages, red meat, refined sugar, processed foods, and nightshade plants like tomatoes, potatoes, and eggplant.

■ **DECREASE INFLAMMATION NATURALLY.** Before you go on medication, try to treat bursitis with natural anti-inflammatories, Dr. Dean says. "The most effective is a combination of magnesium, vitamin C (food-based, organic), and pancreatic enzymes," she says. "Take one dose of angstrom-size magnesium, 1,000 milligrams of vitamin C, and two pancreatic enzyme tablets, three times a day." Look for a magnesium product that says "angstrom" on the label.

■ **CALM THE PAIN WITH CASTOR OIL.** When the pain is no longer acute, Alan Tomson, D.C., recommends a castor oil pack, which is as simple to make as it is effective. Spread castor oil over the afflicted joint. Put cotton or wool flannel over that and then apply a heating pad.

■ **APPLY SOOTHING BALM.** Alternative remedies can speed relief when used with standard treatments. One remedy worth trying is Tiger Balm, a Chinese massage cream containing menthol, which may ease bursitis pain when used one or two times a day. If you can't find Tiger Balm in your local health food store, you can make a homemade balm by mixing water and turmeric powder (a spice used in curry recipes) into a paste.

■ **GENTLY MOVE THE JOINT.** Once the pain is no longer acute, gentle exercises are in order. If elbow or shoulder pain is the problem, doctors recommend swinging the arm freely to relieve the ache. Exercise for only a couple of minutes at first, but do it often during the day.

"You want to maintain range of motion," says Edward Resnick, M.D. "You don't want to get a stiff shoulder, but you don't want to over-stretch it either."

Dr. Resnick recommends bending forward from a standing position, while supporting yourself with your good arm and placing your hand on a chair seat. Allow the painful arm to hang, then swing the arm back and forth, side to side, and finally in circles both clock-wise and counterclockwise.

Some experts recommend performing soothing exercises in a hot tub, bathtub, whirl-pool, or swimming pool. Float your limb on the surface of the water, then move it gently, without pushing it along.

■ **STRETCH.** The importance of exercise following a bursitis attack can't be over-emphasized. A common recommendation is to perform stretching techniques to return full, normal movement to the joint.

One effective primary stretching motion for stiff shoulder joints is called the cat stretch. Get down on your hands and knees. Put your hands slightly forward of your head, then keep your elbows stiff as you stretch backward and come down onto your heels.

Another stretching motion is to stand facing a corner and walk your fingers up the wall in the corner, Dr. Resnick says. "The object is to try and get your armpit in the corner. That way you know you're getting effective exercise."

■ **GIVE THE JOINT SOME FLAVOR.** Garlic is fabulous for any inflammatory process, bur-sitis included, Dr. Donadio says. She suggests making a paste of mashed garlic and placing it inside a piece of cheesecloth. To prevent any skin irritation from the garlic oils, fold the cheesecloth six to eight times, so it's nice and thick. Then lay the cheesecloth over the joint and top with a hot water bottle or compress. Leave it in place for 10 to 15 minutes, and repeat twice a day. "The garlic vapors will go directly into the joint and decrease inflamma-tion," Dr. Donadio says.

■ **FIGHT INFLAMMATION WITH FLAX-SEED.** Flaxseed oil, which contains omega-3 fatty acids known to reduce inflammation, is sometimes recommended for people with recurrent bursitis. Add 1 to 2 tablespoons to your salad dressing.

■ **START THE DAY PAIN-FREE.** When bur-sitis strikes, Dr. Maccaro recommends drinking a concoction of 2 tablespoons of vinegar and 2 tablespoons of honey in water. Repeat twice a day for 2 weeks.

■ **BE PATIENT.** Bursitis generally takes about 10 days to heal—sometimes more, sometimes less. If all else fails, say doctors, time will heal the pain.

PANEL OF ADVISORS

CAROLYN DEAN, M.D., N.D., IS MEDICAL DIRECTOR OF VIDACOSTA SPA EL PUENTE, A MEDICAL SPA IN COSTA RICA, OPENING IN 2010. SHE IS AUTHOR OF *THE MAGNESIUM MIRACLE.*

GEORGIANNA DONADIO, PH.D., IS DIRECTOR OF THE NATIONAL INSTITUTE OF WHOLE HEALTH, A HOLISTIC CERTIFICATION PROGRAM FOR MEDICAL PROFESSIONALS.

JANET MACCARO, PH.D., C.N.C., IS A HOLISTIC NUTRITIONIST AND CERTIFIED NUTRITION CONSULTANT IN SCOTTSDALE, ARIZONA; PRESIDENT OF DR. JANET'S BALANCED BY NATURE PRODUCTS, AND AUTHOR OF *NATURAL HEALTH REMEDIES.*

EDWARD RESNICK, M.D., IS AN ORTHOPEDIC SURGEON AT TEMPLE UNIVERSITY HOSPITAL IN PHILADELPHIA.

ALLAN TOMSON, D.C., IS A CHIROPRACTOR AT NECK, BACK, & BEYOND, AN INTEGRATED HEALING CENTER IN FAIRFAX, VIRGINIA.

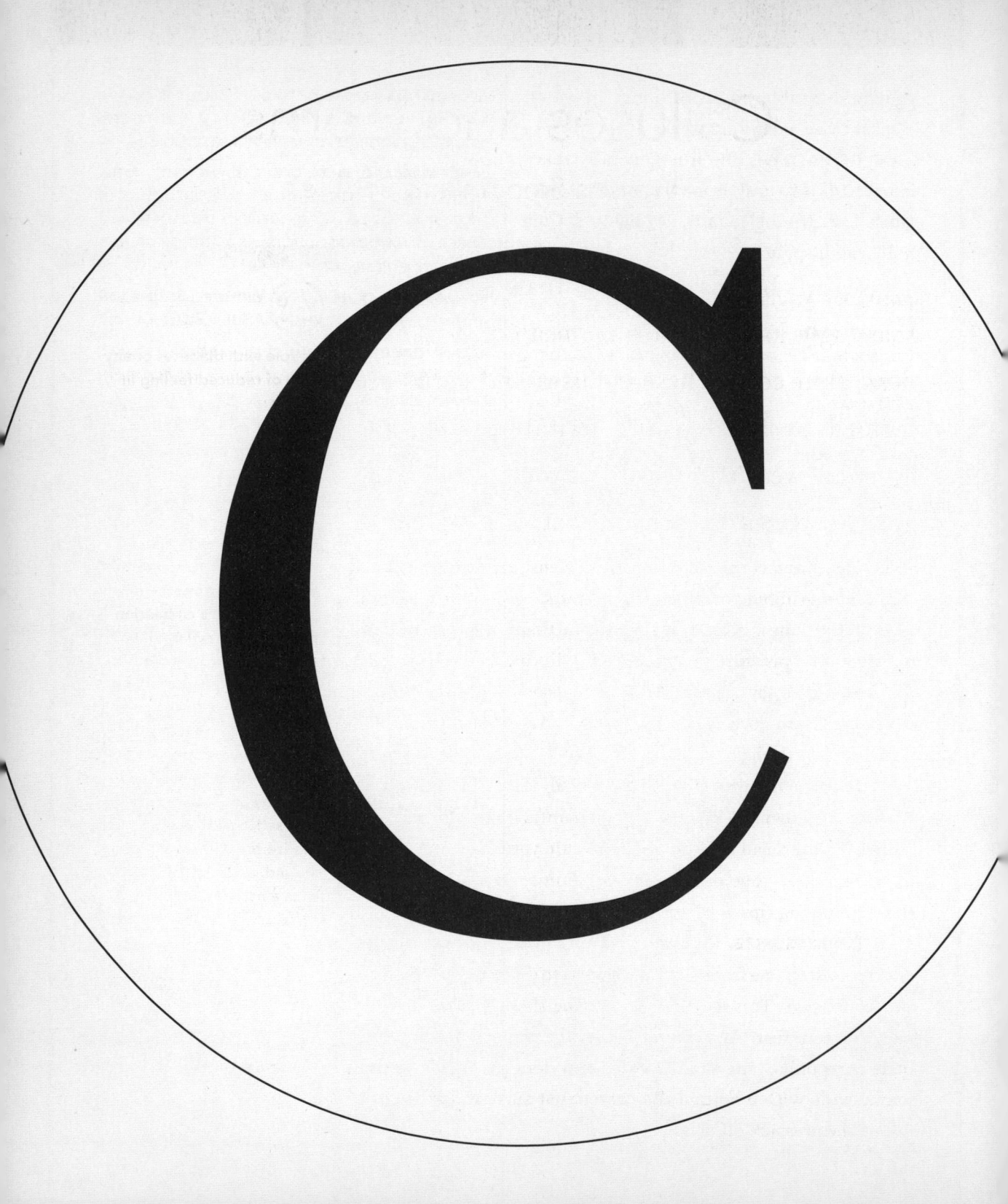

Calluses and Corns

17 Ways to Smooth and Soothe

Those little bumps and lumps that give your feet that "ugly look" are a trash heap of discarded dead skin cells. These calluses and corns are formed by friction and irritation from the everyday wear and tear from your shoes or the adjacent bones on the same foot.

"Calluses and corns are your body's defense mechanism to protect against rubbing over little bone spurs," says Audrey Kunin, M.D. "If the bone is not totally smooth and there's a spot that sticks out right on a pressure point, the skin will thicken up to protect that bone," she says. As pressure builds, so will the callus. If it develops a hard core, it becomes a corn. And not only are both unsightly, but they also can be painful.

"People can live with calluses more easily than with corns," says Richard M. Cowin, D.P.M. "If you get painful corns on your toes, it's like having a bad toothache—it can ruin your day."

So, to *start* your day—every day—on the right foot, heed these following tips.

■ **DEPRESSURIZE.** The best thing you can do to prevent a callus or corn, or stop one from getting worse, is to disperse the pressure, Dr. Kunin says. This may involve retiring shoes that rub certain places on your feet. "And you can relieve the pressure of corns with little corn pads," she says. "I call them doughnut pads—small foamy pads with a hole in the center that surrounds the corn, taking the pressure off of it."

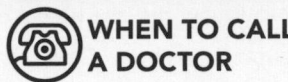 **WHEN TO CALL A DOCTOR**

People with diabetes or any kind of reduced feeling in their feet should never treat themselves. Diabetes affects tiny blood vessels throughout the body, including those in the feet. This leads to decreased circulation, which reduces the ability of wounds to heal and resist infection.

If you have a circulation disorder, you will be okay if your skin remains intact. But if you get any kind of abrasion or opening in the skin, it becomes very dangerous. If you can't feel pressure or pain very well, you may not know you cut yourself, or you may not realize the full severity of a wound, and could wind up with a nasty infection.

■ **STAY AWAY FROM SHARP INSTRUMENTS.** Resist the urge to play surgeon. Do not pare down calluses and corns with razor blades, scissors, or other sharp instruments, says Dr. Kunin.

■ **BE A LITTLE ABRASIVE.** "The secret to removing calluses and corns is to thin the skin in that area," Dr. Kunin says. A callus file or pumice stone will lightly abrade the area and rub off the top layers of skin. Finish with some hand cream. If you have particularly bad calluses, make this part of your daily routine directly after showering or bathing.

■ **TAKE FIVE.** Here's another way to soften stubborn calluses. Crush five or six aspirin tablets into a powder. Mix into a paste with $\frac{1}{2}$ teaspoon each of water and lemon juice. Smooth it on the hard-skin spots on your foot, then put your foot into a plastic bag and wrap a warm towel around everything. The combination of the plastic and the warmth will help the paste penetrate the hard skin. Sit still for at least 10 minutes. Then unwrap your foot and scrub the area with a pumice stone. All that dead, hard, callused skin should come loose and flake away easily. Because of the remote chance of a reaction, if you're allergic or sensitive to aspirin, don't use it on your skin.

■ **HEAL CALLUSES AND CORNS WITH LICORICE.** "Licorice contains estrogen-like substances that literally soften the hard skin of calluses and corns," says Georgianna Donadio, Ph.D. So she suggests making a homemade licorice paste. "Grind up a few licorice sticks, mix them with $\frac{1}{2}$ teaspoon of petroleum jelly, and rub the mixture into your calluses and corns," she says.

■ **AVOID MEDICATED PADS.** Over-the-counter corn plasters or medications for corns and calluses are nothing more than acid, which doesn't know the difference between corns and calluses and normal skin. So although they may get rid of your corn or callus, they may also eat away normal skin.

If you *must* use corn plasters or other over-the-counter salicylic acid products, which come in liquid, salve, and pad form, follow the advice of Suzanne M. Levine, D.P.M., P.C.: Apply *only* to the problem area, not surrounding skin. If treating a corn, first put a doughnut-shaped nonmedicated pad around the corn to shield adjacent skin. Never use this type of product more than twice a week, and see a doctor if there's no sign of improvement after 2 weeks.

■ **ENJOY A GOOD SOAK.** "Your corn pain may be coming from a bursa, a fluid-filled sac

Cures from the Kitchen

If you have a lot of callused tissue, Suzanne M. Levine, D.P.M., P.C., recommends soaking your feet in very diluted chamomile tea. The tea will both soothe and soften hard skin. The brew will stain your feet, but it comes off easily with soap and water.

that becomes inflamed and enlarged at the site between the bone and the corn," says Dr. Levine. "For temporary relief of the pain, soak your feet in a solution of Epsom salts and warm water. This will diminish the size of the bursa sac and take some pressure off the nearby nerves. But be aware that if you put your feet back into tight shoes, the bursa will soon swell again to its painful size."

■ **MAKE CORNS PUCKER.** Soak your feet in warm water for a few minutes, then apply a lemon compress, says Janet Maccaro, Ph.D., C.N.C. To make the compress, soak a washcloth in warm lemon juice. "Then dab some tea tree oil on a cotton ball and apply it to your corn two or three times a day," she says.

■ **CAP A CALLUS WITH ALOE.** Remove a callus by splitting an aloe leaf and taping the gel side down on the callus, says Carolyn Dean, M.D., N.D. "Wear this to bed, and in the morning rub off the callus with a dry washcloth or pumice stone," she says.

■ **FIX CALLUSES WITH FLAX.** To soften a tough callus, Dr. Maccaro suggests you soak your feet in warm water, then apply a flaxseed oil pack. To make the pack, soak a flannel cloth in warm flaxseed oil. Then apply the pack to the callus or corn and wrap the area in plastic wrap overnight.

■ **MIX OIL AND VINEGAR.** "An excellent foot soak consists of equal parts white vinegar and castor oil heated in an old pot," Dr. Dean says. "It's a very messy mixture, but it works

wonders," she says. "After soaking, preferably near a tub, wash off the oil and use a pumice stone to smooth away dead skin." Keep the solution in the pot and reheat it as needed.

■ **RUB AWAY WITH CALENDULA.** Apply calendula oil to calluses and corns each day to soften them, Dr. Maccaro says.

■ **GIVE SOFT CORNS SPACE.** Soft corns— the ones that form between two toes—require a different kind of care than regular corns. Soft corns are caused by bones from two adjacent toes rubbing together, says Dr. Cowin, "so you need to put something soft there to separate the toes. You can buy toe separators or toe spacers, which are simply little pieces of foam that you place between the toes."

■ **BECOME A SOFTY.** If your skin is dry and cracked and you tend to form calluses and corns, you may be deficient in essential fatty acids, Dr. Dean says. So soften your skin from the inside out by getting omega-3 fatty acids from fish oil or flax oil. Take 3 grams of either one each day, she says.

■ **MIX UP A NATURAL EXFOLIANT.** Combine 1 part olive oil with 1 part table salt. "Apply the mixture to your calluses and corns when you're showering to exfoliate, then wash away the salt with water, leaving smooth skin," says Jay Zimmerman, M.D.

To avoid problems, says Dr. Cowin, wear proper-fitting shoes that don't have exceptionally high heels. "For special occasions, high heels won't hurt," he says, "but for everyday situations, lower heels are better."

"If you must wear high heels," adds Dr. Levine, "look for a brand with extra cushioning in the forefoot area, or have your shoemaker add foam cushioning there. And if you have bad calluses on the backs of your heels, avoid open-backed shoes until the area heals."

■ **GET A PROPER FIT.** "The most important thing when buying a shoe is fit," says Terry L. Spilken, D.P.M. "Whether a shoe costs $20 or $200, if it doesn't fit correctly, it's going to give you problems. Make sure it's the proper length; you want a thumb's width from the end of your longest toe to the tip of your shoe. (And your longest toe isn't necessarily the big toe.) You should have enough width across the ball of the foot and enough room in the toebox so that there's no pressure across the toes."

"Look for natural materials, like leather, that breathe. And remember that it's just as harmful for the foot to be in a shoe that's too big as one that's too small," he says. "If the shoe's too big, the foot will slide, which causes friction. And the friction of the skin rubbing can cause a callus or corn just as easily as a tight shoe that pinches."

PANEL OF ADVISORS

Canker Sores

17 Ways to Ease the Sting

If you've ever had a canker sore, surely you've been amazed by how something so small can cause a sting so big. No one knows for sure why some people get canker sores and others don't. For most people, a hot pizza burn heals in 2 to 3 days with little or no pain, but for others it can lead to a lesion that won't heal for 2 weeks. Some experts think canker sores result from a body chemistry imbalance that can result after an illness, fever, or other body stress, leading to reduced immunity. Heredity, certain foods, overly aggressive toothbrushing, ill-fitting dentures, chewing on the inside of your mouth, and emotional stress are all thought to contribute to painful, craterlike canker sores.

Whatever the cause, medicating a canker sore is a difficult task. Nothing sticks well to the skin in your mouth, and it's one of the most bacteria-laden places in the body. Remedies have a double-barreled aim: Protect the sore to minimize pain and kill the organisms.

The good news is that canker sores tend to be more prevalent

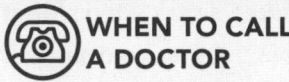

WHEN TO CALL A DOCTOR

A canker sore should heal within 2 weeks. If the sores last longer than that, or they are keeping you from eating or drinking, call your dentist. You should also contact your dentist if you have more than four sores at a time or you are getting sores frequently, says Chris Kammer, D.D.S.

in young people, becoming much less frequent with age. But meanwhile, a mouthful of sores can make you miserable. Here are a few escape routes.

■ **RINSE IT AWAY.** There are rinses that help normalize the pH in the mouth to fight canker sores, says Janet Maccaro, Ph.D., C.N.C. She suggests rinsing with salt water, echinacea tea, or aloe vera juice.

■ **READ LABELS.** Look for over-the-counter canker sore medications that contain benzocaine, menthol, camphor, eucalyptol, or alcohol in a liquid or gel. They often sting at first, and most need repeated application because they don't stick, but they're effective.

■ **APPLY A PASTE COATING.** Some over-the-counter pastes form a protective "bandage" over the sore. To get pastes like Orabase to work, dry the sore with one end of a cotton swab, then immediately dab on the paste with the other end. It works only on beginning sores.

■ **HAVE SOME TEA.** Several experts, among them dermatologist Jerome Z. Litt, M.D., recommend applying a wet, black tea bag to the ulcer. Black tea contains tannin, an astringent that "may pleasantly surprise you" with its pain-relieving ability, he says. There are over-the-counter medications available that contain tannin, such as Tanac.

■ **PUT A LID ON IT.** "There's a product out there called a 'canker cover' that offers immediate relief for canker sores," says Chris Kammer, D.D.S. The adhesive, dissolvable patch covers the sore and releases a numbing and healing gel. "One patch stays on securely for 12 hours and fully treats most canker sores in 24 hours," he says.

■ **DROWN IT IN APPLE CIDER VINEGAR.** Mix a teaspoon of apple cider vinegar in 6 to 8 ounces of warm water, and add a heaping teaspoon of a calcium-magnesium powder, says Georgianna Donadio, Ph.D. "Fill the rest of the glass with cool water and sip it—your canker sores will soon be gone," she says.

■ **SOOTHE IT WITH ALOE.** The ubiquitous "first-aid" plant aloe offers relief for canker sores, too. "Squeeze a bit of gel from an aloe vera leaf," says Dr. Kammer. "Dry the sore with a cotton swab, then dab on the gel, repeating as often as necessary," he says.

■ **AVOID FOOD IRRITANTS.** Coffee, spices, citrus fruits, nuts high in the amino acid arginine (especially walnuts), chocolate, and strawberries irritate canker sores and can even cause them in some people.

■ **PICKLE IT.** "You can treat a small, isolated canker sore by applying alum, a spice used in pickling," says James B. Towry, D.O. Alum is the active ingredient in a styptic pencil, an old-fashioned medicine cabinet standby for cuts and shaving nicks. "It's an antiseptic and pain reliever that can prevent the infection from getting worse," Dr. Towry says. You can find alum in the spice section of most grocery stores. Apply the alum powder directly to the sore. Be warned that it will cause stinging in the area and a general puckering sensation in your mouth. "If a person has multiple or large canker sores, however, this treatment shouldn't be used," Dr. Towry says.

■ **NEUTRALIZE IT.** The pain of a canker sore is usually caused by acids and digestive enzymes eating away at it. To neutralize these acids and speed healing, munch a chewable Pepto-Bismol, Tums, or Rolaids tablet, or apply it directly to the sore and allow it to dissolve, says Dr. Kammer.

■ **LEAVE IT TO MOM.** As an alternative to an antacid, you can use a small amount of milk of magnesia as a makeshift mouth rinse. "Or apply it to the canker sore three or four times a day," Dr. Kammer says.

■ **BRUSH CAREFULLY.** It is important to keep your mouth and teeth clean while a canker sore heals, but you must be cautious. You don't want to jab a healing sore with a toothbrush or toothpick and reinjure yourself. Also, read toothpaste labels if

Cures from the Kitchen

Eating 4 tablespoons of unflavored yogurt a day may help prevent canker sores by sending in helpful bacteria to counter the "bad" bacteria in your mouth, says Jerome Z. Litt, M.D. Look for yogurt that contains active cultures of *Lactobacillus acidophilus*.

you're someone who is prone to canker sores. Sodium lauryl sulfate, used as a detergent in some toothpaste, may trigger canker sores in some people. Other toothpastes contain triclosan, an antimicrobial ingredient that may help canker sores heal.

■ **FIGHT IT WITH LYSINE.** L-lysine is one of the essential amino acids, and it seems to have some power against canker sores. To prevent canker sore recurrence, take 1,000 milligrams of L-lysine daily on an empty stomach, says Craig M. Wax, D.O.

■ **COAT IT WITH A BALM.** Lemon balm, that is. Although lemon juice may be the last thing you want to dab onto a painful canker sore, lemon balm can be soothing. Jacob Teitelbaum, M.D., recommends applying lemon balm cream as needed to ease canker sore pain.

■ **RELY ON VITAMINS.** Craig Zunka, D.D.S., recommends squeezing vitamin E oil from a capsule directly onto your canker sore. Repeat this several times a day to keep the tissue well oiled. Also, at the first tingle of a canker sore, take 1,000 milligrams of vitamin C with bioflavonoids and then take 500 milligrams three times a day for the next 3 days. It's very important that you use vitamin C with bioflavonoids, he says, because vitamin C by itself doesn't work for canker sores. For those who chronically get canker sores, the homeopathic remedy Borax 12X may also help.

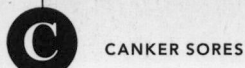

PANEL OF ADVISORS

GEORGIANNA DONADIO, PH.D., IS DIRECTOR OF THE NATIONAL INSTITUTE OF WHOLE HEALTH, A HOLISTIC CERTIFICATION PROGRAM FOR MEDICAL PROFESSIONALS.

CHRIS KAMMER, D.D.S., IS A DENTIST AT THE CENTER FOR COSMETIC DENTISTRY IN MIDDLETON, WISCONSIN.

JEROME Z. LITT, M.D., IS A DERMATOLOGIST AND CLINICAL ASSISTANT PROFESSOR OF DERMATOLOGY AT CASE WESTERN RESERVE UNIVERSITY SCHOOL OF MEDICINE IN CLEVELAND, AND AUTHOR OF *YOUR SKIN: FROM ACNE TO ZITS* AND *CURIOUS, ODD, RARE AND ABNORMAL REACTIONS TO MEDICATIONS.*

JANET MACCARO, PH.D., C.N.C., IS A HOLISTIC NUTRITIONIST AND CERTIFIED NUTRITION CONSULTANT IN SCOTTSDALE, ARIZONA, PRESIDENT OF DR. JANET'S BALANCED BY NATURE PRODUCTS, AND AUTHOR OF *NATURAL HEALTH REMEDIES.*

JACOB TEITELBAUM, M.D., IS A BOARD-CERTIFIED INTERNIST AND MEDICAL DIRECTOR OF THE FIBROMYALGIA AND FATIGUE CENTERS, WITH LOCATIONS THROUGHOUT THE COUNTRY.

JAMES B. TOWRY, D.O., IS AN AMERICAN OSTEOPATHIC ASSOCIATION BOARD-CERTIFIED DERMATOLOGIST IN JONESBORO, ARKANSAS.

CRAIG M. WAX, D.O., IS AN AMERICAN OSTEOPATHIC ASSOCIATION BOARD-CERTIFIED FAMILY PHYSICIAN IN MULLICA HILL, NEW JERSEY.

CRAIG ZUNKA, D.D.S., IS A DENTIST IN FRONT ROYAL, VIRGINIA, AND IS PAST PRESIDENT AND ADVISOR TO THE BOARD OF THE HOLISTIC DENTAL ASSOCIATION. HE ALSO IS A DIPLOMATE OF THE BOARD OF DENTAL HOMEOPATHY.

Carpal Tunnel Syndrome

17 Coping Techniques

Once the bane primarily of restaurant servers, carpenters, and journalists who used typewriters, carpal tunnel syndrome is now one of the most common ailments of the computer and cell phone age. It's a painful reminder of how much many of us depend on our hands to communicate and earn a living. At first, symptoms include numbness, tingling, loss of strength or flexibility, and pain. Yet carpal tunnel can progress over time, with a very small percentage of patients developing permanent injury. That's why it's best to address symptoms head- (or hands-) on.

The good news is that most people with carpal tunnel syndrome recover completely and avoid injury again by changing the way they work. What's more, those with carpal tunnel can make other changes that ease the pain.

Carpal tunnel syndrome isn't something that happens overnight. It's a cumulative trauma disorder that develops over time when your hands and wrists perform repetitive movements.

Think of New York City's Holland Tunnel. Imagine what a pain it is to try to get through it during rush hour as multiple lanes of traffic fight to squeeze into two-lane tubes. Your wrist, known as the

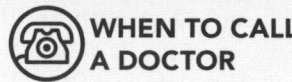

WHEN TO CALL A DOCTOR

Wrist and hand pain is not always the result of carpal tunnel syndrome and could actually be the sign of a more serious illness, cautions physical therapist Susan Isernhagen. "If you get a crackly or crunchy feeling in your wrist when you exercise it, that's not a sign of carpal tunnel syndrome," she says. "It may be a symptom of osteoarthritis." Ask your doctor to check it out.

The Vitamin B$_6$ Debate

Doctors first recommended vitamin B$_6$ supplements for carpal tunnel syndrome 30 years ago. Yet as the years passed, the debate over the vitamin's usefulness intensified.

Several books recommend taking 100 to 200 milligrams of vitamin B$_6$ every day to ease symptoms, with some studies suggesting that low levels of vitamin B$_6$ may increase the risk of carpal tunnel syndrome.

Critics say that large doses of vitamin B$_6$ are not only useless in the treatment of carpal tunnel syndrome, but can also be dangerous. Vitamin B$_6$ can be toxic at high levels, and it should be used only as a supplement under the supervision of a physician, because an excess can lead to nerve damage. The Daily Value is 2 milligrams.

Forego the supplements and boost your intake of B$_6$ by eating foods rich in the vitamin, including bananas, beef, brown rice, chicken, peanuts, and walnuts.

---

carpal tunnel, is a lot like the tunnel under the Hudson River during rush hour. When you use your hand in repeated motions—like writing, typing, or hammering—the tendons, which run like lanes through your wrist, swell and compress the median nerve that runs to your hand.

Sometimes the affected hand will feel numb or tingle, or feel like it's "fallen asleep."

When the feeling comes, it's time to look for relief. Here's how.

■ **CIRCLE AROUND THE PROBLEM.** "When symptoms such as tingling begin, correcting postures through exercise helps," says physical therapist Susan Isernhagen. Getting the "bend" out of the neck, wrist, and fingers through gentle circling exercises will restore circulation and oxygen flow, Isernhagen says. "Exercise also eliminates waste products and restores normal motion. Muscles, nerves, and joints all get relief," she says.

One of these is a simple circle exercise that rotates the wrist. Move your hands around in gentle circles for about 2 minutes. "This exercises all the muscles of the wrist, restores circulation, and gets your wrist out of the bent position that normally brings on the symptoms of carpal tunnel syndrome," Isernhagen says.

■ **REACH FOR THE SKY.** Get those hands off the keyboard and up into the air. "Stretch your hands up and try to touch the ceiling," Isernhagen says. "Fully straighten your neck, shoulders, and elbows. Hold each sky reach for 5 seconds, followed by gentle circling of each joint. You will feel the stress and tension disappear," she says.

■ **TAKE SOME ASPIRIN.** "To reduce pain and inflammation, take a nonsteroidal anti-inflammatory medication like aspirin or ibuprofen," says Stephen Cash, M.D. Don't take acetaminophen, though. "Acetaminophen reduces pain," he says, "but it doesn't do anything for inflammation."

■ **BOOST B₆.** There is some evidence that the swelling and inelasticity of the sheath surrounding a nerve in the wrist may be caused by a lack of vitamin B_6. Other research shows that B_6 helps interrupt the irritated nerve's ability to transmit pain signals. So boost your intake by eating more B_6-rich foods, such as avocados, bananas, beef, brown rice, chicken, eggs, oats, peanuts, soybeans, walnuts, and whole wheat, says Janet Maccaro, Ph.D., C.N.C.

■ **UNKNOT YOUR NECK.** To reduce carpal tunnel syndrome, Isernhagen recommends working from the neck down. "First, let your neck relax and hang your head forward. Then circle to the left, back, and right, making full circles. Go slowly, and repeat five times," she says. Clasp your hands and put them behind your neck, keeping your wrists straight. "Then move your elbows forward and backward to gently stretch your wrists, fingers, and shoulders."

■ **RELAX AT WORK.** "Take advantage of a good chair backrest," Isernhagen says. "Recline slightly backward and keep your neck upright. This position is the most relaxed for your neck and back, and it will let the chair support your weight, instead of your muscles," she says.

■ **DON'T BE A HUNCHBACK.** Whether it is from rushing to complete work or general tension, we tend to hunch our shoulders, which can lead to pinched nerves and arteries. "To combat this, consciously relax your shoulders," Isernhagen says. "With your arms at your sides, move your shoulders downward and away from your ears—it will give those tensed muscles a break," she says.

■ **FIGHT CARPAL TUNNEL WITH CASTOR OIL.** Make and apply a warm castor oil pack to your wrist every other night, says Dr. Maccaro. Here's how to make the castor oil pack: You'll need cold-pressed castor oil, a wool flannel cloth, a piece of plastic, and a heating pad. Fold the cloth into a square and saturate it with the castor oil. Wrap the cloth around your wrist, cover it with the plastic, and then apply the heating pad, set on the medium or hot setting. You may need to use the compress for 3 to 7 days to really see results. But once it starts working, the pack may be very effective.

■ **PERFORM A PLIÉ WITH YOUR HANDS.** This classic ballet move also helps prevent carpal tunnel syndrome. "Gently place your palms and fingers together as if you are praying," Isernhagen says. "Then raise your elbows and feel the gentle stretch in your wrists and fingers," she says. "Hold the stretch for 5 seconds."

■ **BE STRAIGHT AS AN ARROW.** Continuous bending of your neck puts pressure on the nerves in your wrist and other joints, Isernhagen says. "So at home, at work, and even when you are sleeping, hold your neck straight on your shoulders, relax your shoulders and elbows, and keep your wrist and fingers straight."

■ **WEAR A SPLINT.** To relieve symptoms of carpal tunnel syndrome, use a wrist splint to keep your wrist straight. "The splints help take pressure off the nerve," says Dr. Cash. He recommends a splint that has a metal insert and Velcro fasteners. It gives support without being totally rigid.

"The ones made out of plastic usually are hard, hot, and sticky," cautions Isernhagen. "Whatever kind of splint you get, it should fit into the palm of your hand, leaving the thumb and fingers free."

You may want to consider having the splint tailor-made. "You should really have a professional, such as a physical therapist or an occupational therapist, fit you to make sure it fits your hand exactly," says Isernhagen.

■ **DON'T GO TOO TIGHT.** You don't want to completely tie up traffic in your wrist. Don't wrap your wrist with an elastic bandage, because you could wrap it too tight and cut off the circulation, says Isernhagen.

■ **USE THE RIGHT GRIP.** If you have to carry anything with a handle, make sure the grip fits your hand. If the grip is too small around, build it up with tape or rubberized tubing. If it's too large, get another handle, says Isernhagen.

■ **HANDLE WITH CARE.** "Don't concentrate pressure at the base of the wrist when working with hand tools. Use your elbow and shoulder as much as possible," says Isernhagen.

■ **REMOVE ACID.** Some research shows that high acid levels in the body can contribute to pain and inflammation. To combat the discomfort associated with carpal tunnel syndrome, Dr. Maccaro suggests lowering your acid levels by avoiding acid-forming foods, such as soft drinks, caffeine, and hard liquor. In addition, she recommends drinking a glass of lemon juice and water each day to help keep your body alkaline. (Lemon juice is acidic, but it becomes alkaline once it's metabolized in the body.)

PANEL OF ADVISORS

STEPHEN CASH, M.D., IS AN ORTHOPEDIC SURGEON AT MAIN LINE HAND SURGERY, P.C. IN WYNNEWOOD, PENNSYLVANIA.

SUSAN ISERNHAGEN IS A PHYSICAL THERAPIST AND PRESIDENT OF DSI WORK SYSTEMS IN DULUTH, MINNESOTA. SHE ACTS AS A CONSULTANT TO INDUSTRIES TO HELP REDUCE WORK INJURIES AND REHABILITATE INJURED WORKERS.

JANET MACCARO, PH.D., C.N.C., IS A HOLISTIC NUTRITIONIST AND CERTIFIED NUTRITION CONSULTANT IN SCOTTSDALE, ARIZONA, PRESIDENT OF DR. JANET'S BALANCED BY NATURE PRODUCTS, AND AUTHOR OF *NATURAL HEALTH REMEDIES*.

Chafing

12 Ways to Rub It Out

What starts off innocently as your skin rubs on something else—be it more skin, jogging shorts, or the underside of a bra—can quickly become more sinister. Take the example of a marathon runner who, as he crosses the finish line, is more pained by his raw nipples against his T-shirt than by his tired joints. With just a few rubs—or in the case of the runner, 26 miles' worth—a little friction can make skin red, hot, inflamed, and in severe cases, even bleed. So when something rubs you the wrong way—and leaves a rash—find alternatives. Try these strategies.

■ **CHOOSE NATURAL FIBERS.** No matter what your sport, synthetic uniforms may be more durable, but when it comes to chafing, cotton is the fabric of choice.

■ **WASH BEFORE YOU WEAR.** Wash any new exercise clothes before you wear them. Washing sometimes softens the fabric enough to lessen abrasion.

■ **WRAP IT UP.** People who are overweight or who have big thighs, which makes chafing more likely, may find relief by wrapping elastic bandages around the portions of their legs that rub, says Tom Barringer, M.D. These bandages will shield the skin when your thighs rub together, and instead of skin against skin, the rubbing will be fabric against fabric. But be sure that the elastic bandages are secure so that they don't move across the skin.

■ **WEAR TIGHTS.** A pair of athletic tights or Lycra cycling shorts are snug, yet they stretch and cause no friction against the skin, says Dr. Barringer.

■ **GREASE YOUR BODY.** If you're experiencing chafing from clothing, Audrey Kunin, M.D., recommends trying a silicone or cyclomethicone gel. You can apply it between your thighs, under your arms, or beneath a sports bra—wherever clothing rubs, she says.

■ **ROLL ON RELIEF.** Most running stores carry sticks of roll-on lubricant that you can rub on before an activity that may lead to raw skin. "These work quite well," says Randy Wexler, M.D.

■ **KEEP YOUR SKIN DRY.** If excess moisture is the source of the irritation you are experiencing, try to keep the area as dry as possible, Dr. Kunin says. "Dry the area that is chafing, be it skin folds or your breasts, with a hair dryer on the cool setting to circulate some air there whenever possible," she says.

■ **SMOOTH THINGS OUT.** Cornstarch gives a double whammy to chafing—it keeps skin dry and helps heal the irritated area, says Georgianna Donadio, Ph.D. So sprinkle on the cornstarch to prevent and treat chafing. For extra lubrication and protection, Dr. Donadio suggests smearing a little petroleum jelly over the cornstarch.

■ **FIND POWDER POWER.** Your mother may have used this remedy when you were a child. An old tried-and-true treatment for chafing, baby powder works as a lubricant, just the way petroleum jelly does. It helps the skin slip past other skin without the friction that can lead to a rash, says Dr. Kunin.

If you don't like powdery floors, sprinkle the powder into the middle of a large, soft, white handkerchief, and tie the corners. Then, use the sack of powder like a powder puff. It will leave powder on you, and most importantly, not on the floor.

■ **BLOCK IT WITH A BANDAGE.** Simply block the rub with an adhesive bandage. Runners, for example, use bandages over nipples to prevent rubbing.

■ **FIGHT THE YEAST BEAST.** "If there is a lot of rubbing under the breasts or along the thighs, there could be a yeast infection going on, which can cause the skin to break down," Dr. Kunin says. "Try an over-the-counter anti-yeast medicated powder to see if it clears it up," she says.

■ **LOSE WEIGHT.** Overweight people may find chafing a regular problem until they lose a little girth, says Dr. Kunin. "This type of chafing usually happens when heavy skin folds rub on each other," she says.

PANEL OF ADVISORS

TOM BARRINGER, M.D., IS A FAMILY PHYSICIAN IN CHARLOTTE, NORTH CAROLINA.

GEORGIANNA DONADIO, PH.D., IS DIRECTOR OF THE NATIONAL INSTITUTE OF WHOLE HEALTH, A HOLISTIC CERTIFICATION PROGRAM FOR MEDICAL PROFESSIONALS.

AUDREY KUNIN, M.D., IS A COSMETIC DERMATOLOGIST IN KANSAS CITY, MISSOURI, THE FOUNDER OF THE DERMATOLOGY EDUCATIONAL WEB SITE WWW.DERMADOCTOR.COM, AND AUTHOR OF *THE DERMADOCTOR SKINSTRUCTION MANUAL.*

RANDY WEXLER, M.D., IS AN ASSISTANT PROFESSOR IN THE DEPARTMENT OF FAMILY MEDICINE AT OHIO STATE UNIVERSITY MEDICAL CENTER IN COLUMBUS.

Chapped Hands

23 Soothing Tips

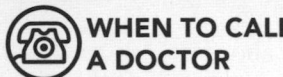

WHEN TO CALL A DOCTOR

If your chapped hands persist despite the use of creams and lotions, you could have a more serious condition, like psoriasis or allergic contact dermatitis, says Monica Halem, M.D. Also consult your doctor if you have cracked or fissured skin on your hands—"it could become infected," she says.

Sometimes it seems there's nothing more painful—or unattractive—than chapped hands. Blame it on aging and the weather. As you age, your body produces less of the oil you need to keep skin smooth and supple. Add in the low humidity of fall and winter, and you have a mess of dry and irritated skin. Fortunately, there are many soothing solutions for turning rough, dry hands into something soft enough to hold.

Here's what the experts recommend.

■ **KEEP THEM WARM.** It may sound simple, but wearing gloves religiously in cold weather will do wonders for preventing chapped hands, says Janet Maccaro, Ph.D., C.N.C.

■ **BOLSTER YOUR BARRIER.** The skin on the hands acts like a barrier to keep moisture in, says Monica Halem, M.D. If this barrier is disrupted by extreme weather conditions, sun exposure, dry air, or certain disease processes, the result can be very dry, itchy, red, cracked, and sore hands. To combat this, reestablish the skin barrier on your hands. "The skin barrier is made of three key elements—ceramide, cholesterol, and triglyceride," Dr. Halem says. There are several creams and lotions on the market that contain all three ingredients; check the label to make sure all three are listed. "And keep in mind that a cream (oil-water mix) is much richer than a lotion (water-oil mix), and better to use for dry hands," she says.

Cures from the Kitchen

To remove the top layer of dead skin cells from chapped hands, skin-care specialist Lia Schorr recommends a weekly sloughing treatment. "Process 1 cup of uncooked, old-fashioned (not instant) rolled oats in a blender until you have a very fine powder. Place it in a large bowl, then rub your hands in the powder, gently removing dry skin. Rinse with cool water, pat dry, and lavish on hand cream. Wait 2 minutes and apply more cream."

■ **DON'T GO NEAR THE WATER.** Although you were probably taught to wash your hands often throughout the day, if you have chapped hands, water is not your friend. In fact, water is *the worst* influence for chapped hands. Repeated hand washing strips the hands' natural oil layer and allows the skin's moisture to evaporate and escape. So always think twice about washing your hands unnecessarily. "If you have to wash your hands frequently because of your occupation, be sure to apply a hand cream after each wash," Dr. Halem says.

■ **BATHE WISELY.** To prevent chapped hands, Dr. Halem recommends you shower or bathe in warm—not hot—water, limit your bathing time, and keep your exposure to drying soaps to a minimum.

■ **SEAL IN MOISTURE.** Most people usually apply hand lotion to dry hands, but it's best to rub it in when your hands are still wet after you wash them. "If you add creams when your palms are dry, it will add some moisture and make your hands feel better for a few minutes,

but it will do little to help in the long run," says Jacob Teitelbaum, M.D. "Instead, put lotion on your hands immediately after washing them to trap moisture," he says.

■ **BE COMPULSIVE WITH CREAM.** If you have chapped hands, you simply can't apply hand cream too often, says Audrey Kunin, M.D. "So be obsessive about it—rub on hand cream throughout the day," she says. Dr. Kunin recommends you look for a hand cream that contains cyclomethicone, a silicone oil. "And try to stay away from creams and lotions that contain lanolin, because people prone to eczema are often allergic to it," she says.

■ **WEAR GLOVES TO BED.** "There are hydrating gloves available that you can put on at night. They have a thick gelatinous layer inside them," Dr. Kunin says. "They're great— it's like putting your hands into a humidifier."

■ **LET CREAM PENETRATE OVERNIGHT.** Randy Wexler, M.D., recommends applying a greasy hand cream, such as Eucerin, to your hands and covering them with gloves before you go to bed for an extra-soothing treatment. Leave the gloves on overnight. Your hands remain bandaged, in a sense, and can heal. "This can help chapped hands a lot," he says.

■ **REPLACE YOUR SOAP.** "Instead of using soap, clean your hands with an oil-free skin cleanser such as Cetaphil," says Joseph Bark, M.D. "Rub it on the skin, work it into a lather, then wipe it off with a tissue. It's a wonderful way to wash skin with no irritation whatsoever."

CHAPPED HANDS

■ TRY THE BATH OIL TREATMENT. Taking the no-soap concept one step further, Rodney Basler, M.D., recommends washing your hands with bath oil. "They may not *feel* really clean like they might with soap, but they won't get dried out either."

■ DON'T THROW IN THE TOWEL. If your workplace bathroom has a hot-air blower instead of hand towels, you should bring in a towel from home. Hot-air blowers are hard on hands. If you must use one, keep your hands at least 6 inches from the nozzle and dry them thoroughly.

■ GO SOAK YOUR HANDS. Although in general you should keep your hands out of water, sometimes a therapeutic soak is in order.

Favorite Fixes

WHAT IT IS: Heel Rescue Superior Moisturizing Foot Cream. It's a nongreasy intensive moisturizing treatment for the relief of dry, scaly, cracked feet, says Amy Fry of New York City.

WHY IT WORKS: This intensive foot cream is designed to penetrate, moisturize, and repair tough skin on the feet, so it is extra-effective for healing chapped skin on the hands.

HOW I USE IT: "I keep a tub of PROFOOT's Heel Rescue Superior Foot Cream on my desk for my hands," Fry says. Although it is made for feet, it works amazingly well for hands. There is no peppermint smell like typical foot creams, and its nongreasy texture helps it last, even after you wash your hands. It's great during the winter cold season, when washing hands is essential.

"For an inexpensive way to achieve the same moisturizing effects produced by skin creams, simply soak your hands in warm water for a few minutes. Then pat dry and smooth vegetable or mineral oil on your damp hands to seal in moisture," says Howard Donsky, M.D.

In the same vein, Dr. Basler recommends soaking in a water-and-oil solution. "Use 4 capfuls of a bath oil that disperses well (Alpha Keri is the best) in 1 pint of water. At the end of the day, soak for 20 minutes to get oil back into the skin. That alone will help chapped hands."

■ DOUBLE UP. "When applying any type of lotion or cream, use what I call Bark's double-layer application technique," says Dr. Bark. "Put on a very thin layer and let it soak in for a few minutes. Then apply another thin layer. Two thin ones work much better than one heavy one."

■ TRY LEMON OIL. "To smooth and soothe irritated hands, mix a few drops of glycerin with a few drops of lemon essential oil (both are available at drugstores or health food stores). Massage this into your hands at bedtime," says skin-care specialist Lia Schorr.

■ MIX RUBBER AND COTTON. "For wet work, it's extremely important to use cotton gloves under vinyl ones," says Nelson Lee Novick, M.D. Perspiration, lotions, and medications on your hands accumulate inside the gloves and may become irritating rather quickly. If the cotton gloves get wet, change them immediately. Otherwise, every 20 min-

Prevention Is Your Best Solution

Chapped hands are always easier to prevent than to treat. Here are some ways to do that.

Stay out of hot water. Avoid hot water, detergents, and strong household solvents.

Avoid soaping. Chapped hands occur when oil is washed from the skin, so you should not use a harsh or alkaline soap. Instead, use a mild soap, preferably with a little cold cream in it. "I often recommend Dove because it's virtually the mildest soap there is," says Joseph Bark, M.D.

Put moisture in the air. "Skin moisturizes itself from the inside out," says Rodney Basler, M.D. "If there's moisture in the air, not as much will be drawn out through the skin, so it's a good idea to use a home humidifier."

Pamper your hands. When you apply moisturizer to your face in the morning, apply some to your hands, too. At night do the same. This will help keep hands supple and resistant to chapping.

utes replace them with a fresh pair. "I don't recommend rubber gloves with built-in cotton linings, because it's very difficult to launder them," he says. "But you can launder separate cotton gloves in a mild detergent such as Ivory Snow or Ivory Flakes."

■ **TREAT YOUR HANDS LIKE YOUR FACE.** To keep hands soft, supple, and free of chapping, Dr. Maccaro recommends washing them with a soap that contains cold cream.

■ **CALL ON HYDROCORTISONE.** Over-the-counter (OTC) hydrocortisone creams and ointments are of value in treating chapped hands, particularly if you have painful fissures or splits around your fingers. Use an OTC 1 percent cortisone cream, Dr. Kunin says. Or ask your doctor for a prescription cortisone cream if the chapping is really out of control, she says.

■ **SATURATE WITH UNSATURATED FATTY ACIDS.** "Chapping can be caused by a lack of unsaturated fatty acid in the epithelial layer of the skin," says Georgianna Donadio, Ph.D. To combat this, she recommends rubbing an oil high in unsaturated fatty acids into your hands. "You can use borage oil, almond oil, or olive oil," she says. "Or find a hand cream that is very high in moisture and fatty acids."

PANEL OF ADVISORS

JOSEPH BARK, M.D., IS A DERMATOLOGIST IN LEXINGTON, KENTUCKY, AND DIRECTOR OF SKIN SECRETS, A COMPREHENSIVE SKIN-CARE FACILITY.

RODNEY BASLER, M.D., IS A DERMATOLOGIST AND ASSOCIATE PROFESSOR OF INTERNAL MEDICINE AT THE UNIVERSITY OF NEBRASKA COLLEGE OF MEDICINE IN LINCOLN.

GEORGIANNA DONADIO, PH.D., IS DIRECTOR OF THE NATIONAL INSTITUTE OF WHOLE HEALTH, A

123

Cures from the Kitchen

"If you want the cheapest home remedy going, use Crisco," says Joseph Bark, M.D. "It's a wonderful moisturizer that covers the skin and keeps water locked in. The key is to use very little and rub it in well so that your hands don't feel greasy. Your skin needs only two molecules' worth of barrier thickness to protect it from water loss. They used to call Crisco 'Cream C' at Duke University, where doctors dispensed it freely. It really works."

"You don't have to purchase expensive creams to get good results," agrees Howard Donsky, M.D. "Inexpensive substitutes for people with dry and normal skin include cocoa butter, lanolin, petroleum jelly, and light mineral oil."

HOLISTIC CERTIFICATION PROGRAM FOR MEDICAL PROFESSIONALS.

HOWARD DONSKY, M.D., IS A CLINICAL INSTRUCTOR OF DERMATOLOGY AT THE UNIVERSITY OF ROCHESTER SCHOOL OF MEDICINE AND DENTISTRY. HE IS A DERMATOLOGIST AT THE DERMATOLOGY AND COSMETIC CENTER OF ROCHESTER IN NEW YORK AND AUTHOR OF BEAUTY IS SKIN DEEP.

MONICA HALEM, M.D., IS A CLINICAL ASSISTANT PROFESSOR OF DERMATOLOGIC SURGERY AT NEW YORK–PRESBYTERIAN HOSPITAL/COLUMBIA IN NEW YORK CITY.

AUDREY KUNIN, M.D., IS A COSMETIC DERMATOLOGIST IN KANSAS CITY, MISSOURI, THE FOUNDER OF THE DERMATOLOGY EDUCATIONAL WEB SITE WWW.DERMADOCTOR.COM, AND AUTHOR OF THE DERMADOCTOR SKINSTRUCTION MANUAL.

JANET MACCARO, PH.D., C.N.C., IS A HOLISTIC NUTRITIONIST AND CERTIFIED NUTRITION CONSULTANT IN SCOTTSDALE, ARIZONA, PRESIDENT OF DR. JANET'S BALANCED BY NATURE PRODUCTS, AND AUTHOR OF NATURAL HEALTH REMEDIES.

NELSON LEE NOVICK, M.D., IS A CLINICAL PROFESSOR OF DERMATOLOGY AT MOUNT SINAI SCHOOL OF MEDICINE IN NEW YORK CITY.

LIA SCHORR IS A SKIN-CARE SPECIALIST AND DIRECTOR OF LIA SCHORR INSTITUTE OF COSMETICS SKIN-CARE TRAINING IN NEW YORK CITY.

JACOB TEITELBAUM, M.D., IS A BOARD-CERTIFIED INTERNIST AND MEDICAL DIRECTOR OF THE FIBROMYALGIA AND FATIGUE CENTERS, WITH LOCATIONS THROUGHOUT THE COUNTRY.

RANDY WEXLER, M.D., IS AN ASSISTANT PROFESSOR IN THE DEPARTMENT OF FAMILY MEDICINE AT OHIO STATE UNIVERSITY MEDICAL CENTER IN COLUMBUS.

Chapped Lips

14 Tips to Stop the Dryness

Chapped lips give new meaning to the expression "crack a smile." "Chapped lips can be caused by a range of problems—everything from medication to ingredients in your toothpaste to different disease disorders, says Audrey Kunin, M.D. "But in most cases, chapped lips are caused by dry, cold weather," she says. "The skin on the lips is very thin, so there is nothing to protect them from the elements."

■ **TRY THE PALM OR BALM SOLUTION.** "The best way to deal with chapped lips is to avoid the dry, cold weather that can cause them in the first place," says Joseph Bark, M.D. "But since heading for the tropics is not too practical for most people, you can head for the drugstore instead."

■ **PICK UP SOME LIP BALM.** Then, before you go outside—and several times while you're out—coat your lips with it. Lips don't hold anything on them very well, so reapply balm every time you eat or drink anything or wipe your mouth.

■ **USE A SUNSCREEN.** Remember, too, that the sun fries lips—any time of the year. So you're well advised to use a balm with built-in sunscreen, even in the wintertime, says Monica Halem, M.D. Or you can apply a lotion sunscreen directly on your lips to prevent sunburn and help treat any sun damage, she says.

■ **KEEP 'EM MOIST.** When it comes to treating chapped lips, moisture is key, Dr. Halem says. "It is important to protect the

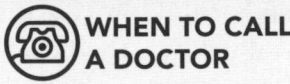 **WHEN TO CALL A DOCTOR**

If your chapped lips don't improve with any of the suggested remedies, you should see your dermatologist. "Persistent chapped lips can be a sign of acitinic chelitis, a pre-malignant condition that results from years of sun exposure," says Monica Halem, M.D. "You could also have contact dermatitis in response to something you've applied to your lips, such as lip balm or lipstick," she says.

mucosal barrier of the lips by applying an oil-based lip balm throughout the day and night." She notes that night is a particularly good time to apply lip balm because this is when skin repairs itself.

■ **USE THE RIGHT MOISTURIZER.** "A lot of people think putting a waxy lip balm on already chapped lips is going to be helpful and heal the skin, but that's a myth," Dr. Kunin says. "If your lips aren't chapped, applying a waxy lip balm can be preventative, but it won't impart the moisture required to get into the crevices of the lips," she says. "To soften lips and help the healing process from the deeper tissues outward, you really need to use a product that is more viscous, such as petroleum jelly or something of a similar texture," she says.

■ **HYDRATE YOUR ENVIRONMENT.** To fight chapped lips and dry skin in general, Dr. Kunin recommends running a humidifier in your bedroom in the winter. "Ideally, it's great to have a humidifier on your furnace, but that's not practical for everyone," she says. To keep lips and skin moist, a bedroom humidifier is the next best thing.

■ **SATURATE YOUR LIPS.** "Lip chapping can be caused by a lack of unsaturated fatty acids in the epithelial tissue," says Georgianna Donadio, Ph.D. "If you have a deficiency, cold weather will wreak havoc—the lack of fatty acids in the tissue will cause your lips to dry out." To keep lips hydrated, Dr. Donadio suggests boosting your intake of foods rich in omega-3 fatty acids, such as salmon, almonds, and walnuts.

■ **ARM YOUR LIPS AGAINST INFECTION.** If your lips are chapped to the point of cracking, Janet Maccaro, Ph.D., C.N.C., suggests putting some Polysporin antibiotic ointment on them to prevent infection.

■ **BE WISE.** "Nutritional deficiencies—such as those of B-complex vitamins and iron—can play a part in scaling of the lips. So make sure you're okay on that front with a multivitamin supplement," says Nelson Lee Novick, M.D.

■ **MIND YOUR OWN BEESWAX.** "To my mind, the single best product for chapped lips is Carmex," says Rodney Basler, M.D. "It's an old-fashioned product that comes in a white jar and contains, among other things, beeswax and phenol. No prescription medication is better than that."

■ **STOP LICKING.** "Chapped lips are a dehydration problem," according to Dr. Basler. "When you lick them, you momentarily apply moisture, which then evaporates and leaves your lips feeling drier than before. Besides, saliva contains digestive enzymes. Granted they're not very strong, but they don't do your sore lips any good."

"Licking chapped lips can lead to something called lip-licker's dermatitis," cautions Dr. Bark. "It's usually seen in kids but can occur in adults, too." What happens when you lick your lips is that you scrape off any oil that might be on them from surrounding areas.

(The lips themselves don't have any oil glands.) Pretty soon, you're licking not just the lips but also the area around them. Eventually, you end up with a red ring of dermatitis around the mouth. The moral: Don't lick in the first place.

If you *are* tempted to lick your lips, remember what Dr. Basler laughingly calls the old Nebraska treatment: chicken manure applied to the lips. "It doesn't make your lips better, but it sure keeps you from licking them," he says.

■ **THINK ZINC.** "Some people have a tendency to drool in their sleep, which can dry out lips or aggravate them if they're already chapped," says Dr. Novick. If that's a problem, apply zinc oxide ointment every night before bed. It acts as a barrier to protect lips.

■ **LAY A FINGER ALONGSIDE YOUR NOSE.** "Here's what I tell farmers, who may be working outside and may not have anything else handy," says Dr. Bark. "Put your finger on the side of your nose. Then rub your finger on your lips. Your finger picks up a little of the oil that's naturally there. It's the kind of oil the lips are looking for anyway, and they usually get it from contact with adjacent skin. You couldn't get any more of a home remedy than that."

PANEL OF ADVISORS

JOSEPH BARK, M.D., IS A DERMATOLOGIST IN LEXINGTON, KENTUCKY, AND DIRECTOR OF SKIN SECRETS, A COMPREHENSIVE SKIN-CARE FACILITY.

RODNEY BASLER, M.D., IS A DERMATOLOGIST AND ASSOCIATE PROFESSOR OF INTERNAL MEDICINE AT THE UNIVERSITY OF NEBRASKA COLLEGE OF MEDICINE IN LINCOLN.

GEORGIANNA DONADIO, PH.D., IS DIRECTOR OF THE NATIONAL INSTITUTE OF WHOLE HEALTH, A HOLISTIC CERTIFICATION PROGRAM FOR MEDICAL PROFESSIONALS.

MONICA HALEM, M.D., IS A CLINICAL ASSISTANT PROFESSOR OF DERMATOLOGIC SURGERY AT NEW YORK–PRESBYTERIAN HOSPITAL/COLUMBIA IN NEW YORK CITY.

AUDREY KUNIN, M.D., IS A COSMETIC DERMATOLOGIST IN KANSAS CITY, MISSOURI, THE FOUNDER OF THE DERMATOLOGY EDUCATIONAL WEB SITE WWW.DERMADOCTOR.COM, AND AUTHOR OF *THE DERMADOCTOR SKINSTRUCTION MANUAL.*

JANET MACCARO, PH.D., C.N.C., IS A HOLISTIC NUTRITIONIST AND CERTIFIED NUTRITION CONSULTANT IN SCOTTSDALE, ARIZONA, PRESIDENT OF DR. JANET'S BALANCED BY NATURE PRODUCTS, AND AUTHOR OF *NATURAL HEALTH REMEDIES.*

NELSON LEE NOVICK, M.D., IS A CLINICAL PROFESSOR OF DERMATOLOGY AT MOUNT SINAI SCHOOL OF MEDICINE IN NEW YORK CITY.

Colds

32 Remedies to Win the Battle

WHEN TO CALL A DOCTOR

If your cold is accompanied by one or more of the following symptoms, see your doctor. Your problem may be more serious than the common cold.

■ A fever that remains above 101°F for more than 3 days, or any fever above 103°F

■ Any hot, extreme pain, such as earache, swollen tonsils, sinus pain, or aching lungs or chest

■ Excessive amounts of sputum, or sputum that is greenish or bloody

■ Extreme difficulty swallowing

■ Excessive loss of appetite

■ Wheezing

■ Shortness of breath

If colds are so common, why isn't there a cure? The answer has to do with simple mathematics. More than 200 viruses are responsible for the 1 billion colds that Americans get each year, stymieing most scientists' ability to concoct a "cure" that will work against them all.

It's clear that antibiotics, highly effective at knocking out bacterial infections, are useless against colds, which are caused by viruses. So most people live with the sniffles and aches, maybe take an over-the-counter remedy or two, and hope the symptoms will disappear in the customary week or so.

But there's much more you can do to ease your way through a cold more comfortably, doctors say. Some remedies may even help you overcome a cold more quickly. Here's how.

■ **SEE IF VITAMIN C WORKS FOR YOU.** "Vitamin C works in the body as a scavenger, picking up all sorts of trash—including virus trash," says Keith W. Sehnert, M.D.

Vitamin C may also cut back on coughing, sneezing, and other symptoms, although scientific studies produce mixed results when the vitamin is put to the test. One summary of 30 studies, published in 2000, found "a consistently beneficial but generally modest therapeutic effect on duration of cold symptoms." On average, vitamin C reduced the number of days people experienced cold symptoms by 8 to 9 percent.

If you're going to take vitamin C, experts recommend that you take 100 to 500 milligrams a day. To help maintain levels of vitamin C throughout the day, take half of the recommended dose in the morning and half at night.

■ **ZAP IT WITH ZINC.** Sucking on zinc lozenges can cut colds short, from an average of 8 days to an average of 4, report researchers at the Cleveland Clinic. Study subjects sucked on four to eight lozenges a day, each containing 13.3 milligrams of zinc. Zinc can also dramatically reduce symptoms such as a dry, irritated throat, says Elson Haas, M.D. "It doesn't work for everyone, but when it works, it works," he says.

The downside is that zinc has an unpleasant taste. Fortunately, there are many brands of zinc lozenges available that come in a variety of flavors. But before choosing a brand, remember to check the label. Some lozenges have more zinc content than others. Always follow the directions on the package, and don't take more than the amount recommended. Also, don't take vitamin C and zinc at the same time, since the two bind together, making zinc less effective. Either take the vitamin first or wait half an hour after your zinc lozenge has disappeared to take it.

Taking more than 40 milligrams a day can cause nausea, dizziness, or vomiting. High doses over an extended period of time can hinder your ability to absorb copper, another vital mineral.

■ **TRY SOME NATURAL HEALING.** In the early stages of a cold, try this recipe from Brian Berman, M.D.: Place a whole unpeeled grapefruit, sectioned into four pieces, in a pot and cover with water; heat to just under a boil. Stir and add a tablespoon of honey, then drink the liquid as you would a tea. "The simmering releases immune boosters from the grapefruit into the water—vitamin C and flavonoids hidden between the rind and the fruit," he says. "The concoction packs more punch than store-bought grapefruit juice, plus the warmth eases a sore throat."

To beef up your body's healing response, Dr. Berman swears by liquid olive leaf extract, available at health food stores. Studies suggest that its antiviral qualities can help treat colds. "You end up getting rid of mucus sooner, and it helps your immune system fight back as well."

■ **EAT YOUR WHEATIES.** Really, any well-rounded breakfast may go a long way in helping to keep colds at bay, according to a current study in the United Kingdom. Researchers there found that people who regularly eat breakfast report having the fewest number of colds and illnesses, perhaps because breakfast is an indicator of healthy lifestyles.

■ **BE POSITIVE.** A positive attitude about your body's ability to heal itself can actually mobilize immune-system forces, says Martin Rossman, M.D. He teaches this theory by getting his patients to practice imagery techniques to combat colds. After bringing yourself into a deeply relaxed state, "imagine a white tornado decongesting your stuffed-up sinuses," he suggests, "or an army of

The Cold Truth

So you have a cold that won't let go, and you want to know who to blame. Elliot Dick, Ph.D., who conducted research for more than 30 years on how colds are transmitted, says a lot of suspects take a bum rap. They include:

- Sharing food or beverages with someone who has a cold
- Kissing someone who has a cold
- Stepping outside with a wet head

The *real* culprit, of course, is a virus transmitted through the air, says Dr. Dick. You can catch it, he says, when someone with a cold coughs, sneezes, or does a sloppy job of blowing his nose, sending the virus floating into your path.

---

microscopic maids cleaning up germs with buckets of disinfectant."

■ **REST AND RELAX.** Extra rest enables you to put all your energy into getting well. It can also help you avoid complications like bronchitis and pneumonia, says Samuel Caughron, M.D.

Take a day or two off from work if you're feeling really bad, he advises. At the very least, skip some of your everyday activities and reschedule your time. "Trying to keep up with your regular routine can be draining, because when you're not feeling well, your concentration is down, and you'll probably need to double the amount of time it takes you to do things," Dr. Caughron says.

■ **BE A HOMEBODY.** When you're sick, parties and other good times can wear you out physically, compromising your immune system

and causing your cold to linger, says Timothy Van Ert, M.D. Stay home and snuggle up.

■ **WARM UP.** Bundle up against the cold, advises Dr. Sehnert. This keeps your immune system focused on fighting your cold infection instead of displacing energy to protect you from the cold.

■ **TAKE A WALK.** Mild exercise improves your circulation, helping your immune system circulate infection-fighting antibodies, says Dr. Sehnert. Do gentle exercises indoors or take a brisk half-hour walk, he suggests. But refrain from strenuous exercise, he warns, which could wear you out.

■ **GO AHEAD, GO OUTSIDE.** Despite its name, getting a cold has nothing to do with temperature. (It's caused by a viral infection, period.) In fact, a classic 1968 study published in the *New England Journal of Medicine* showed that colds were no more frequent or severe in people who were chilled than in those who weren't chilled.

■ **FEED A COLD—LIGHTLY.** The very fact that you have a cold may indicate that your diet is putting a strain on your immune system, says Dr. Haas. Counteract the problem, he advises, by eating fewer fatty foods, meat, and milk products, and more fresh fruit and vegetables.

What you feed your immune system may also matter. A study conducted by Simin N. Meydani, M.V.M., Ph.D., looked into the effect of taking extra vitamin E (found in almonds, hazelnuts, peanuts, and wheat germ) for colds. Although popping a daily supplement of 200 IU of vitamin E didn't significantly shorten the duration of colds in the study, the participants who took the supplement had significantly fewer colds than those who didn't take vitamin E.

■ **LOAD UP ON LIQUIDS.** Drinking six to eight glasses of water, juice, tea, and other mostly clear liquids daily helps replace important fluids lost during a cold and helps flush out impurities that may be preying on your system. "Remember: Dilution is the solution to pollution," says Dr. Haas.

■ **STOP SMOKING.** Smoking aggravates a throat that may already feel irritated from a cold, says Dr. Caughron. It also interferes with the infection-fighting activity of cilia, the microscopic "fingers" that sweep bacteria out of your lungs and throat. So if you can't kick the habit for good, at least do it while you have a cold.

■ **EASE A SORE THROAT.** Gargle morning, noon, and night—or whenever it hurts most—with salt water, Dr. Van Ert says. Fill an 8-ounce glass with warm water and mix in 1 teaspoon of salt. The salt water will help soothes your sore throat.

Paul S. Anderson, N.D., says to mix a clove bud, which is antiseptic and fights infection, with ¼ teaspoon powered ginger (or 1 teaspoon grated fresh ginger) and ⅛ teaspoon cinnamon—the latter two because of their anti-inflammatory properties. Infuse the tea in 2 cups boiling water, and for every cup, stir in 2 teaspoons raw honey. Sip throughout the day until your throat settles down.

■ **TAKE GOLDENSEAL AND ECHINACEA.** Goldenseal stimulates your liver, whose job includes clearing up infections. It also strengthens the ailing mucous membranes in your nose, mouth, and throat. Echinacea cleans your blood and lymph glands, which help circulate infection-fighting antibodies and remove toxic substances. You can buy these herbs separately or in combination capsules. "I recommend these herbs at the early onset of a cold," says Dr. Haas. Whichever you choose, take them following the directions on the bottle for up to 2 weeks.

■ **SIP A HOT TODDY.** Clear your stuffed-up nose and help yourself to a good night's sleep by drinking a "hot toddy"—a hot drink consisting of a liquor, such as rum, water, sugar, and spices—or half a glass of wine before bedtime, suggests Dr. Caughron. Don't consume any more than that, however, because too much can stress your system, making recovery more difficult.

■ **DRINK TEA AT BEDTIME.** For a good night's sleep, brew a cup of hops, valerian herb tea, or Celestial Seasonings Sleepytime herbal tea, all of which have a natural tranquilizing effect. For even better results, Dr. Van Ert suggests adding a teaspoon of honey, a simple carbohydrate that has a sedative effect.

■ **SOOTHE YOUR THROAT WITH LICORICE ROOT.** Licorice root tea has an anesthetizing effect that soothes irritated throats and relieves coughs, says Dr. Van Ert. Although licorice root is available in tea bags, he prefers making his own. Just put the root in a nonmetallic tea ball and steep in hot water for the desired amount of time. Drink it daily.

■ **BREATHE STEAM.** Taking a steamy shower can help clear congestion, says Kenneth Peters, M.D. Or heat a teakettle or pot of water to boiling; turn off the flame; stand above the kettle and drape a towel over your head, creating a tent; and inhale the steam until it subsides. This also relieves your cough by moistening your dry throat, he says.

Woodson Merrell, M.D., suggests boiling a pot of water, letting it cool for about 1 minute, and then mixing in a teaspoon of medicated VapoRub. Lean over it with your head about a foot from the steam. Again, make a tent over your head with a towel, and inhale for 5 minutes.

Another idea: Put a few drops of eucalyptus oil in a hot, running shower and inhale the steam as it accumulates, says Benjamin Kligler, M.D., M.P.H. (Note: The room may be too hot for children.)

You may also find comfort using a humidifier close to your bed at night, adds Dr. Van Ert.

■ **RINSE OUT YOUR NOSE.** Your nasal congestion may also respond to saltier measures: Dr. Merrell rinses his sinuses with a store-bought nasal saline solution (or, in a pinch, dissolve a teaspoon of salt in a cup of water) to wash out pollen and thin mucus.

Dr. Kligler as well suggests irrigating your nose using contact lens saline solution and a neti pot.

Cures from the Kitchen

A longtime folk remedy is now a proven fact. A cup of hot chicken soup can help unclog your nasal passages. Researchers at Mount Sinai Medical Center in Miami Beach, found that chicken soup increases the flow of nasal mucus. Nasal secretions serve as a first line of defense in removing germs from your system, the scientists say.

It's also known that garlic and onions have antiviral properties, and adding some spice in the form of cayenne or chile peppers can help unclog nasal passages, too.

Andy Spooner, M.D., says his two children willingly "hose their nose" when they're sick by squirting the solution up each nostril with a bulb syringe. "Buy saline by the case, and start your kids early. It provides instant relief of congestion without side effects," he adds. "It won't shorten your cold, but being able to breathe through your nose makes the wait more pleasant."

■ **USE PETROLEUM JELLY ON A SORE NOSE.** Relieve a nose raw from blowing by using a cotton swab to dab on a lubricating layer of petroleum jelly around and slightly inside your nostrils, suggests Dr. Peters.

■ **MEDICATE AT NIGHT.** Don't let your cold symptoms keep you from getting a healing night's sleep. Numerous medications for colds are available without a prescription. Some treat specific symptoms. Others, like NyQuil and Contac, contain a combination of drugs—plus alcohol, in some cases—aimed at treating a wide range of symptoms. These combination drugs, however, can have many uncomfortable side effects, such as nausea and drowsiness, says Dr. Van Ert. "I recommend taking these at night, since you won't feel the side effects while you're sleeping."

If you need to be on medications during the day, he suggests using those that treat just the symptoms you're experiencing. Be sure to follow the instructions carefully, he advises. Here's what to reach for.

■ For relief of body aches or fever, take *aspirin* or *acetaminophen*.

■ To stop sneezing and dry up your runny nose and watery eyes, take an *antihistamine,* which blocks your body's release of histamine, a chemical that causes these symptoms. Look for products, like Chlor-Trimeton, that are available over-the-counter, advises Diane Casdorph, B.S., Pharm.D., Warning: Antihistamines frequently cause drowsiness, so save these for bedtime or for when you won't be driving or doing anything that requires quick reactions. If drowsiness is a problem, talk with your doctor about nondrowsy antihistamines, which are available by prescription.

■ To unstuff your nose, take a *decongestant.* First, check your medicine cabinet and make sure you aren't taking an old product that contains phenylpropanolamine, which was voluntarily withdrawn by manufacturers when the FDA warned that it was associated with an increased risk of stroke, especially in women. Products currently on the market that do not contain phenylpropanolamine include Sudafed, Actifed, Dristan, and Contac. Before taking a nonprescription antihistamine or decongestant, contact your doctor or pharmacist.

What's Behind the Ahchoo?

Sometimes it's hard to tell if your stuffy nose and frequent sneezing herald a cold or an allergy. Colds and allergies share some symptoms, but not all. Here's how to tell what you've got:

SYMPTOM	COLD	ALLERGY
Itchy eyes	Rarely	Often
Fever	Sometimes	Never
Aches and pains	Sometimes	Never
Duration	7 to 10 days	As long as allergen is present

■ *Nasal sprays and drops*, such as Afrin and Neo-Synephrine, are also effective decongestants. But they shouldn't be used for longer than 3 days, says Dr. Peters. Overuse can result in a "rebound effect," meaning your nose becomes more congested than ever, requiring more medication.

■ To relieve a cough, try *cough drops and syrups*. Look for a product that contains cough-suppressing antitussives such as dextromethorphan, says Dr. Casdorph. These include Vicks cough drops and Robitussin DM cough syrup, which also contains an expectorant to loosen phlegm.

■ *Lozenges* can also combat coughs. Many of them contain topical anesthetics that slightly numb your sore throat, says Dr. Van Ert, which relieves your need to cough. Sucrets, Cepacol, and Cepastat sore throat decongestant lozenges are among them.

■ *Menthol or camphor rubs* have a soothing, cooling effect and may relieve congestion and help you breathe more easily, especially at bedtime. Apply Vicks VapoRub or a similar product to your bare chest, cover up, and get a good night's sleep, recommends Dr. Van Ert.

■ **DON'T SPREAD YOUR GERMS.** When you need to cough, go ahead and cough. When you need to blow your nose, go ahead and blow. But cough and sneeze into disposable tissues instead of setting germs free in the environment, Dr. Van Ert advises, then promptly throw the tissue away and wash your hands. Your healthy friends and family who want to stay that way will appreciate it.

PANEL OF ADVISORS

PAUL S. ANDERSON, N.D., IS AN ASSOCIATE PROFESSOR OF NATUROPATHIC MEDICINE AT BASTYR UNIVERSITY IN SEATTLE.

BRIAN BERMAN, M.D., IS A PROFESSOR OF FAMILY MEDICINE AND FOUNDER AND DIRECTOR OF THE CENTER FOR INTEGRATIVE MEDICINE AT THE UNIVERSITY OF MARYLAND SCHOOL OF MEDICINE IN BALTIMORE.

DIANE CASDORPH, B.S., PHARM.D., IS A CLINICAL ASSISTANT PROFESSOR IN THE DEPARTMENT OF CLINICAL PHARMACY AT WEST VIRGINIA UNIVERSITY SCHOOL OF PHARMACY IN MORGANTOWN.

SAMUEL CAUGHRON, M.D., IS A FORMER CLINICAL ASSISTANT PROFESSOR IN FAMILY MEDICINE AT THE UNIVERSITY OF VIRGINIA, AND IS A FELLOW IN THE AMERICAN COLLEGE OF OCCUPATIONAL AND ENVIRONMENTAL MEDICINE AND THE AMERICAN COLLEGE OF PREVENTIVE MEDICINE. HE IS A FAMILY PHYSICIAN IN CHARLOTTESVILLE.

ELLIOT DICK, PH.D., WAS A VIROLOGIST AND PROFESSOR OF PREVENTIVE MEDICINE AT THE UNIVERSITY OF WISCONSIN–MADISON. HE CONDUCTED RESEARCH ON THE COMMON COLD FOR MORE THAN 30 YEARS.

ELSON HAAS, M.D., IS DIRECTOR OF THE PREVENTIVE MEDICAL CENTER OF MARIN, AN INTEGRATED HEALTHCARE FACILITY IN SAN RAFAEL, CALIFORNIA, AND AUTHOR OF SEVEN BOOKS ON HEALTH AND NUTRITION, INCLUDING *THE NEW DETOX DIET* AND *STAYING HEALTHY WITH NUTRITION*.

BENJAMIN KLIGLER, M.D., M.P.H., IS RESEARCH DIRECTOR AT THE CONTINUUM CENTER FOR HEALTH AND HEALING AND VICE CHAIR OF THE DEPARTMENT OF INTEGRATIVE MEDICINE AT BETH ISRAEL MEDICAL CENTER, BOTH IN NEW YORK CITY.

WOODSON MERRELL, M.D., IS EXECUTIVE DIRECTOR OF INTEGRATIVE MEDICINE AT THE CONTINUUM CENTER FOR HEALTH AND HEALING AND A CLINICAL ASSISTANT PROFESSOR OF MEDICINE AT COLUMBIA UNIVERSITY COLLEGE OF PHYSICIANS AND SURGEONS, BOTH IN NEW YORK CITY, AND AUTHOR OF *THE SOURCE*.

SIMIN N. MEYDANI, M.V.M., PH.D., IS ASSOCIATE DIRECTOR OF THE JEAN MAYER USDA HUMAN NUTRITION RESEARCH CENTER ON AGING AT TUFTS UNIVERSITY IN MEDFORD, MASSACHUSETTS.

KENNETH PETERS, M.D., IS MEDICAL DIRECTOR OF THE NORTHERN CALIFORNIA HEADACHE CLINIC AND PRACTICES GENERAL INTERNAL MEDICINE AT EL CAMINO HOSPITAL, BOTH IN MOUNTAIN VIEW. HE HAS PUBLISHED NUMEROUS ARTICLES ON EFFECTIVE HEADACHE MANAGEMENT AND HAS DONE EXTENSIVE CLINICAL RESEARCH IN THE AREA OF NEW HEADACHE MEDICATIONS.

MARTIN ROSSMAN, M.D., IS FOUNDER AND DIRECTOR OF THE COLLABORATIVE MEDICINE CENTER IN GREENBRAE, CALIFORNIA, AND CODIRECTOR OF THE ACADEMY FOR GUIDED IMAGERY IN MALIBU. HE IS A CLINICAL ASSOCIATE IN THE DEPARTMENT OF MEDICINE AT THE UNIVERSITY OF CALIFORNIA MEDICAL CENTER IN SAN FRANCISCO AND AUTHOR OF *FIGHTING CANCER FROM WITHIN* AND *GUIDED IMAGERY FOR SELF-HEALING*.

KEITH W. SEHNERT, M.D., WAS A PHYSICIAN WITH TRINITY HEALTH CARE IN MINNEAPOLIS AND IS AUTHOR OF SEVERAL BOOKS, INCLUDING *THE GARDEN WITHIN* AND *HOW TO BE YOUR OWN DOCTOR (SOMETIMES)*.

ANDY SPOONER, M.D., IS DIRECTOR OF THE DIVISION OF GENERAL PEDIATRICS IN THE COLLEGE OF MEDICINE AT THE UNIVERSITY OF TENNESSEE HEALTH SCIENCE CENTER IN MEMPHIS AND A FELLOW OF THE AMERICAN ACADEMY OF PEDIATRICS.

TIMOTHY VAN ERT, M.D., IS MEDICAL DIRECTOR OF THE STUDENT HEALTH AND COUNSELING CENTER AT WESTERN OREGON UNIVERSITY IN MONMOUTH, WHERE HE SPECIALIZES IN SELF-CARE AND PREVENTIVE MEDICINE.

Cold Sores

20 Tips to Halt Herpes Simplex

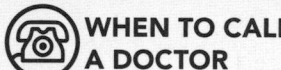 **WHEN TO CALL A DOCTOR**

Left alone, a cold sore will normally last 10 to 14 days, says Lenore S. Kakita, M.D. But if you're bothered by frequent, severe cold sores, it makes sense to see your doctor. Even if the cold sore develops, most people find that the outbreak will be milder, less painful, and shorter if they're taking medication. Prescription medications such as acyclovir (Zovirax) are available to fight the herpes simplex virus 1 responsible for cold sores, and they can stop a cold sore in its tracks, says Dr. Kakita.

If a cold sore develops pus, seek medical attention, advises James F. Rooney, M.D. You probably have a bacterial infection, which can benefit from antibiotic treatment.

Many people get an unsightly cold sore at least once during their lives. Generally, they were exposed during childhood to the highly contagious virus that causes cold sores, called herpes simplex virus 1, a different strain of herpes virus from the one that causes genital herpes.

The first cold sore you experience is probably the worst, says Lenore S. Kakita, M.D. Afterward, the virus lies dormant in nerve cells, but occasionally it becomes reactivated. When that happens, you may experience a telltale sensation of numbness, tingling, burning, or itching on your lip or the skin around your mouth before a cold sore appears. You might even feel a bit feverish, as though you have a touch of the flu.

The good news, says Dr. Kakita, is that most people develop a slight immunity to cold sores over the years, making outbreaks fewer and farther between. And fortunately, there are a number of steps you can take to minimize the pain of a cold sore and speed its healing.

■ **LET IT BE.** "If the cold sore isn't really bothersome, just leave it alone," says James F. Rooney, M.D. "Make sure to keep the sore clean and dry."

■ **KEEP YOUR HANDS OFF.** People don't realize how highly contagious cold sores are, says Geraldine Morrow, D.M.D. "If you have a cold sore on your lip, don't pull it, don't stretch it, don't touch it." You could get "very, very painful" cold sores on your hands, especially if the fluids from the blister get under a hangnail, Dr. Morrow says.

■ **REPLACE YOUR TOOTHBRUSH.** Your toothbrush can harbor the herpes virus for days, reinfecting you after a cold sore heals.

Researchers at the University of Oklahoma exposed a sterile toothbrush to the virus for 10 minutes. Seven days later, half of the disease-producing viruses remained, says Richard T. Glass, D.D.S., Ph.D.

Dr. Glass recommends that you throw away your toothbrush when you notice you're just beginning to get a cold sore. If you still develop a sore, get a new toothbrush after the blister develops and breaks. This can prevent you from developing multiple sores. And once the sore has healed completely, replace your toothbrush again. He says that patients who tried this method found it significantly reduced the number of cold sores they typically experienced in a year.

■ **DON'T STORE YOUR TOOTHBRUSH IN THE BATHROOM.** A damp toothbrush in a moist environment like your bathroom is a perfect environment for herpes simplex virus. That moisture helps prolong the life of the herpes virus on your toothbrush. That's why Dr. Glass recommends storing your toothbrush in a dry spot, preferably on a window ledge where the UV rays of sunlight can penetrate into the bristles, because UV light kills the virus.

■ **USE SMALL TUBES OF TOOTHPASTE.** Toothpaste can transmit disease, too, says Dr.

Glass. Buy small tubes so that you replace them regularly.

■ **PROTECT WITH PETROLEUM JELLY.** You can protect your cold sore by covering it with medicated petroleum jelly, says Dr. Glass. This will help keep the sore moist and prevent cracking. Be sure not to dip back into the jelly with the same finger you used to touch your sore. Better yet, use a cotton swab each time.

■ **ZAP IT WITH ZINC.** Many studies show that a water-based zinc solution, applied the minute you feel that tingling, will speed healing.

In a Boston study of 200 patients who were followed over a 6-year period, a 0.025 percent solution of zinc sulfate in camphorated water was found very effective. Sores healed in an average of 5.3 days. The solution was applied every 30 to 60 minutes during the onset of the cold sore.

Researchers in Israel also found a 2 percent water-based zinc solution, applied several times a day, was very helpful, says Milos Chvapil, M.D., Ph.D.

How does zinc help? The zinc ions crosslink with the DNA molecule of the herpes virus and prevent the DNA from replicating, reducing the number of viruses produced, he says.

Zinc gluconate is kinder to the skin than zinc sulfate, says Dr. Chvapil. The mineral is available at health food stores.

■ **IDENTIFY THE PATTERN.** What was going on in your life just before you got your

Cures from the Kitchen

 Fighting cold sores may involve your daily diet. Try these tips.

RELY ON LYSINE. Mark A. McCune, M.D., advises patients who have more than three cold sores a year to supplement their daily diets with 2,000 to 3,000 milligrams of the amino acid lysine. He also recommends that they double up on the dosage when they feel the itching and tingling that signals the start of another cold sore. However, don't take amino acids without your doctor's guidance. The supplement may not be safe for those with high cholesterol, heart disease, or high triglycerides.

Not all studies have found lysine helpful for people with cold sores. But in one study of 41 patients, Dr. McCune and his colleagues found that a daily dose of 1,248 milligrams of lysine helped subjects reduce the number of cold sores they have in a year.

Good food sources of lysine include dairy products, potatoes, and brewer's yeast.

AVOID ARGININE-RICH FOODS. The herpes virus needs arginine as an essential amino acid for its metabolism. So cut out arginine-rich foods such as chocolate, cola, peas, grain cereals, peanuts, gelatin, cashews, and beer.

APPLY LEMON BALM TEA. Also known as melissa, lemon balm is "a first-choice herbal treatment" for cold sores, according to botanist James Duke, Ph.D., author of *The Green Pharmacy*. Lemon balm has antiviral properties that work to tame herpes outbreaks. Prepare lemon balm tea by brewing 2 to 4 teaspoons of the herb per cup of boiling water. Let it cool, then apply it with a cotton ball to the cold sore several times a day.

last cold sore? What about the cold sore prior to that? If you do some sleuthing, you may figure out what triggers a cold sore for you. If you can find a trigger, take additional lysine

when you're most prone to cold sores, says Mark A. McCune, M.D. Common triggers include stress and a variety of foods.

■ **GRAB AN ICE CUBE.** Applying ice directly to a cold sore can reduce the swelling and provide temporary relief, says Dr. Morrow.

■ **FORM A BARRIER.** Abreva, an over-the-counter medication containing docosanol, works by protecting healthy cells from the infected cells. Applying it may make the cold sore infection less likely to penetrate the healthy cells.

Use the cream five times a day, beginning when you experience the first symptoms, says David H. Emmert, M.D. This can help your cold sore heal 1 to 2 days quicker.

■ **NUMB IT.** Most over-the-counter products contain an emollient to reduce cracking and soften scabs, and a numbing agent such as phenol or camphor.

Phenol may have some antiviral properties, says Dr. Rooney. "Theoretically, it is possible that phenol is capable of killing the virus."

■ **BLOCK SUN AND WIND.** Protecting your lips from trauma like sunburn or wind exposure was cited by all our experts as a key to preventing cold sores.

■ **PERFECT YOUR COPING SKILLS.** Studies have shown that stress can trigger recurrences of the herpes simplex virus. High levels of stress are not necessarily the culprit, says Cal Vanderplate, Ph.D. "How you cope with the stress—how you perceive it—is what's important."

His number one stress deflator is maintaining a loving social support system. "A sense of control is also very important. If you take a positive attitude toward your health, you'll be better able to influence your symptoms."

■ **RELAX.** "By the time symptoms appear, it's too late to intervene in stress reduction," says Dr. Vanderplate. "But you may be able to reduce the severity by doing some relaxation exercises." He favors deep muscle relaxation techniques, biofeedback, visualization, and meditation.

■ **EXERCISE.** "There is some evidence that exercise actually helps bolster the immune system," says Dr. Vanderplate. The stronger your immune system, the better able it is to defend you against viruses. Exercise is also a super way to relax, he says.

■ **SLEEP UPRIGHT.** If you have a cold sore, prop a few pillows behind your head at bedtime to let gravity help the blisters drain, says Dr. Kakita. Otherwise, fluid may settle in your lip during the night.

■ **CORRECT YOUR PERCEPTION.** No one likes getting a cold sore. But if you have one, focusing on it and worrying about how you look can make it worse. "Minimize any negative perceptions you have about it," says Dr. Vanderplate. "Tell yourself that it is just like a pimple and it won't interfere in your life in any way."

PANEL OF ADVISORS

MILOS CHVAPIL, M.D., PH.D., IS A PROFESSOR EMERITUS OF SURGERY IN THE SURGICAL BIOLOGY SECTION OF THE UNIVERSITY OF ARIZONA COLLEGE OF MEDICINE IN TUCSON.

JAMES DUKE, PH.D., HELD SEVERAL POSTS IN HIS MORE THAN THREE DECADES WITH THE USDA, INCLUDING CHIEF OF THE MEDICINAL PLANT RESOURCES LABORATORY. HE IS AUTHOR OF *THE GREEN PHARMACY.*

DAVID H. EMMERT, M.D., IS A FAMILY PHYSICIAN IN MILLERSVILLE, PENNSYLVANIA, WHO HAS SUMMARIZED COLD SORE TREATMENTS FOR THE MEDICAL JOURNAL *AMERICAN FAMILY PHYSICIAN.*

RICHARD T. GLASS, D.D.S., PH.D., IS A PROFESSOR OF FORENSIC SCIENCES, PATHOLOGY, AND DENTAL MEDICINE AT OKLAHOMA STATE UNIVERSITY CENTER FOR HEALTH SCIENCES IN TULSA, OKLAHOMA. HE IS A PROFESSOR EMERITUS AND FORMER CHAIR OF THE DEPARTMENT OF ORAL AND MAXILLOFACIAL PATHOLOGY AT THE UNIVERSITY OF OKLAHOMA, COLLEGES OF DENTISTRY, GRADUATE, AND MEDICINE, AND PROFESSOR OF PATHOLOGY.

LENORE S. KAKITA, M.D., IS A CLINICAL ASSOCIATE PROFESSOR OF DERMATOLOGY AT THE UNIVERSITY OF CALIFORNIA IN LOS ANGELES AND AN ADVISOR TO THE AMERICAN ACADEMY OF DERMATOLOGY.

MARK A. MCCUNE, M.D., IS A DERMATOLOGIST IN OVERLAND PARK, KANSAS. HE IS PRESIDENT OF KANSAS CITY DERMATOLOGY, P.A. AND PAST CHAIR OF THE DEPARTMENT OF DERMATOLOGY AT HUMANA HOSPITAL IN OVERLAND PARK.

GERALDINE MORROW, D.M.D., IS PAST PRESIDENT OF THE AMERICAN DENTAL ASSOCIATION, A MEMBER OF THE AMERICAN ASSOCIATION OF WOMEN DENTISTS, AND A DENTIST IN ANCHORAGE, ALASKA.

JAMES F. ROONEY, M.D., IS A FORMER SPECIAL EXPERT IN THE LABORATORY OF ORAL MEDICINE AT THE NATIONAL INSTITUTES OF HEALTH IN BETHESDA, MARYLAND.

CAL VANDERPLATE, PH.D., IS A CLINICAL FACULTY MEMBER AT EMORY UNIVERSITY SCHOOL OF MEDICINE IN ATLANTA AND A CLINICAL PSYCHOLOGIST SPECIALIZING IN STRESS-RELATED DISORDERS.

Colic

12 Ideas to Quiet the Cries

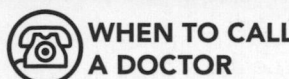
When writer Thomas Paine penned his famous line, "These are the times that try men's souls," he was referring to America's struggle for independence. Yet any parent who tries to soothe an inconsolable infant at the witching hour just before dinner will tell you the truly trying times come when a baby careens into incessant screams caused by colic.

Ancient scholars first described infantile colic in the 6th century. Modern parents have no trouble describing it today. The baby sobs, pulls her knees up to her abdomen, and appears to be in great pain. She may become gassy, then quiet, then scream again.

Nothing much seems to have changed over the centuries, and nothing much seems to help. Colicky babies cannot generally be quieted with feeding or a change of diaper, and episodes may last for several hours. Colic tends to be most severe at 4 to 6 weeks of age and gradually subsides by 3 to 4 months.

Though none of the remedies offered below will cure colic, most have brought some relief to suffering parents and their babies, so you may want to give them a try. And remember that this, too, shall pass. Colic disappears as mysteriously as it begins.

■ **TRY THE COLIC CARRY.** "I'm a big believer in the colic carry," says nanny industry expert Sharon Graff-Radell. Extend

2 Videos to Buy, Not Rent

Pediatric nurse Helen F. Neville, R.N., recommends two "groundbreaking" visual resources for parents struggling with a colicky baby:

The Happiest Baby on the Block. Pediatrician Harvey Karp, M.D., concludes that human babies are normally born three months early in order for their large heads to pass through the birth canal, and that colic is their demand to return to a womblike environment. He recommends "The 5 S's": swaddling, swinging, shooshing sound, sucking, and side or stomach position (while baby is falling asleep, that is. For safety, always turn baby on her back once asleep.) Dr. Karp's video is available at www.thehappiestbaby.com.

Dunstan Baby Language: Understand the Meaning of Your Baby's Cry. Priscilla Dunstan has translated babies' cries. Learn what to listen for to know if your baby is tired, hungry, or needs to burp or pass gas. Dunstan's video is available at www.dunstanbaby.com.

your forearm with your palm up, then place the baby on your arm chest down, with her head in your hand and her legs on each side of your elbow. Support the baby with your other hand and walk around the house with her in this position.

Another type of carry that works combines a tight swaddling with an over-the-shoulder carry. "This relieves gas, provides motion, and the tight swaddle helps baby feel secure," Graff-Radell says.

■ **BURP THAT BABE.** "My experience is that at least some colicky babies do have more abdominal gas than the norm and may be more difficult to burp," says pediatric nurse practitioner Linda Jonides, B.S., R.N., C.P.N.P. Her recommendation: Try different positions when feeding and be sure to burp frequently, as often as after every ounce (if bottle feeding).

You can also try different nipples if you bottle feed. "There are many to choose from, and there isn't one that works best for all babies," Jonides says.

■ **CUT THE COW JUICE.** Some child-care specialists believe that colic is caused when cow's milk is transmitted from mother to infant through breast milk. Though some research refutes this, experts agree that a maternal diet free of cow's milk may be worth a try, especially in families with a history of allergies. "I recommend that mothers start by eliminating cow's milk from their diets and see what happens," Graff-Radell says. "If that does it, you don't have to go any further, but if not, you may need to cut back other dairy products."

■ **CHECK THE DIET CONNECTION.** "Sometimes certain foods the mom eats can set off a bout of colic for a breastfeeding baby," says pediatrician John D. Rau, M.D. Suspect foods may include chocolate, bananas, citrus fruits, strawberries, spicy foods, and caffeinated drinks. "Watch for a link between the mommy's diet and baby's colic," Dr. Rau says. Gassy foods such as broccoli and cabbage could also be culprits, Graff-Radell says.

■ **TRY A WRAP SESSION.** "I recommend holding and swaddling a colicky baby," Jonides says, "or using a backpack to hold the baby so you have your arms free to do other things." Wrapping a baby snugly in a blanket has a calming effect. It's very popular in some cultures, and it does sometimes stop colic attacks. It does not spoil an infant, says Jonides.

■ **USE A VACUUM INSTEAD OF A LUL-LABY.** Colicky babies seem to love the sound of a vacuum cleaner. Science has failed to explain this mystery. "The white noise of a vacuum cleaner or other appliances such as a dishwasher seems to calm a colicky baby," Dr. Rau says. Some parents record the sound of a vacuum cleaner and play it back when baby gets fussy. Others simply start vacuuming the carpet and hope the child outgrows colic while there's still some rug left.

Another option is to incorporate both vibration and white noise together. "Take baby for a car ride," Dr. Rau suggests. "It's worked for me and many families."

Graff-Radell offers a more aggressive approach: "Put baby in a front pack and

vacuum at the same time—it's a win-win. That colicky baby goes out like a light, and you have a clean house."

■ **DO THE DRYER DRIBBLE.** "Put the baby in an infant seat and rest it against the side of a running clothes dryer so the baby gets that buzzing sound and vibration through the seat," suggests pediatric nurse Helen F. Neville, R.N. "There's something about the vibration that really soothes a colicky baby." Sound too farfetched? Wait until the baby fusses for another 3 hours—you'll try anything.

■ **WARM THAT TUMMY.** "A hot-water bottle or heating pad *set on low* and placed on the baby's tummy sometimes helps," Jonides says. (Place a towel between the baby and the hot-water bottle so she doesn't get burned.)

■ **LOG IT IN.** "Keeping a log would be a very good idea," Neville says. "Often, when it seems like the baby was fussing for 2 hours straight, it was really only 45 minutes. A log will help you determine just how long the baby's crying, and—more important—what might be bringing it on."

■ **SWING INTO ACTION.** "Motion-type things are good for colic," says Jonides. "Swinging may quiet many babies at least long enough for you to get through dinner."

■ **TRY A LITTLE MASSAGE.** "Many infants will calm with a gentle massage of their tummy, legs, or back," Jonides says. "Make sure your hands are soft and warm, and just apply a gentle pressure."

■ **TOUR THE HOUSE.** "I like to walk around the house telling the baby all about the artwork, photos, pets, and other random items of home," Graff-Radell says. Baby calms down from the constant motion, interesting visuals, and an engaging voice. "Babies love when you talk to them," she says.

PANEL OF ADVISORS

SHARON GRAFF-RADELL IS VICE PRESIDENT OF THE INTERNATIONAL NANNY ASSOCIATION, FOUNDER OF WWW.FINDTHEBESTNANNY.COM, AND OWNER OF TLC FOR KIDS IN ST. LOUIS, ONE OF THE FIRST NANNY AND CHILD-CARE AGENCIES IN THE UNITED STATES.

LINDA JONIDES, B.S., R.N., C.P.N.P., IS A PEDIATRIC NURSE PRACTITIONER IN ANN ARBOR, MICHIGAN.

HELEN F. NEVILLE, R.N., IS A PEDIATRIC NURSE AT KAISER PERMANENTE HOSPITAL IN OAKLAND, CALIFORNIA, AND AUTHOR OF *TEMPERAMENT TOOLS* AND *IS THIS A PHASE?*

JOHN D. RAU, M.D., IS A DEVELOPMENTAL BEHAVIORAL PEDIATRICIAN AND AN ASSOCIATE PROFESSOR OF CLINICAL PEDIATRICS AT INDIANA UNIVERSITY SCHOOL OF MEDICINE. HE IS ALSO THE DIRECTOR OF THE RILEY CHILD DEVELOPMENT CENTER IN INDIANAPOLIS.

Conjunctivitis

10 Remedies for Pinkeye

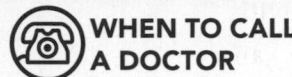 **WHEN TO CALL A DOCTOR**

Conjunctivitis is an easily treatable problem that will usually go away on its own in about a week. You should, however, avoid taking a wait-and-see attitude. See your doctor if:

■ The infection is worse, not better, after 5 days

■ You have a red eye that is associated with significant eye pain, change in vision, or a copious amount of yellow or greenish discharge.

■ The redness is caused by an injury to your eye. "Sometimes infections can get in the eye if you've scratched the cornea," says Robert Petersen, M.D.

Aside from it being an irritating condition, pink eye can be very contagious, so the sooner you take care of it the better you—and those around you—will be.

Conjunctivitis is inflammation of the conjunctiva, a membrane that lines the inside of the eyelid and covers the white of the eye. Red and irritated, infected eyes feel as if they're bedeviled by stray grains of sand. There's often a discharge, too. The culprits behind all that itching? Viruses, bacteria, or allergies. While conjunctivitis won't threaten an adult's sight, it's unsightly. And it's no fun. Here's what you can do.

■ **SOOTHE THE RED AWAY.** "A warm compress applied to the eyes for 5 to 10 minutes three or four times a day will make you feel better," says Robert Petersen, M.D.

■ **KEEP EYES CLEAN.** "A lot of times conjunctivitis gets better by itself," says Dr. Petersen. "To help the healing process along, keep your eyes and eyelids clean by using a cotton ball dipped in warm water to wipe the crusts away."

■ **BABY YOURSELF.** A warm compress works well for children, but sometimes adults need a little something more. "Adults who have a lot of discharge should make a solution of 1 part baby shampoo to 10 parts warm water," says Peter Hersh, M.D., FACS. "Dip a sterile cotton ball into the solution and use it to clean off your eyelashes. It works very well. The warm water loosens the crust and the baby shampoo cleans off the junction of your eyelid and eyelash." An over-the-counter solution called Eye-Scrub, used the same way, is just as effective.

■ **THROW IN THE TOWEL.** Toss your towel, washcloth, and anything else that came in contact with your eyes into the washer. "This infection is highly contagious. Don't share a towel or washcloth with anyone, because it will easily spread the disease," says Dr. Petersen.

■ **DE-CHLORINATE.** Does swimming in a pool leave you seeing pink? "The chlorine in swimming pools can cause conjunctivitis, but without the chlorine, bacteria would grow—and that could cause it, too," says Dr. Petersen. "If you're going to go swimming and you're susceptible to conjunctivitis, wear tight-fitting goggles while in the water."

Cures from the Kitchen

 Try these culinary-based tips to help remedy conjunctivitis.

BE A LITTLE FISHY. Cold-water fish contain omega-3 fatty acids—a good kind of fat, and one that can help with the puffiness of pinkeye. "These fatty acids help manage symptoms by reducing inflammation," says nutritionist Linda Antinoro, R.D. She suggests eating up to three 4-ounce servings of fatty fish, such as salmon or canned light tuna, every week.

CURB IT WITH HERBS. According to botanist James Duke, Ph.D., ancient herbalists based many of their treatments on the physical resemblance that plants bore to parts of the body—enter chamomile's eyelike flowers and the eyebright plant. Make a warm compress of chamomile tea to help heal a sore eye, or use eyebright instead for its astringent and antibacterial actions to reduce eye irritation and fight an infection. You can also make a mild, cool tea from either of these to use as an eyewash.

■ **PUT ALLERGIC CONJUNCTIVITIS ON ICE.** If you survive the summer swim but not the summer pollen, your conjunctivitis may be caused by allergies. "If your eye itches like a mosquito bite and you have red eyes with stringy mucus, most of the time that's the sign of allergic conjunctivitis," says J. Daniel Nelson, M.D. "Taking an over-the-counter antihistamine will help that, and use cold, not warm, compresses. A cold compress will really relieve the itch." Dr. Nelson also suggests trying over-the-counter allergy eyedrops, one drop twice a day.

■ **CATCH SOME ZZZS.** Putting your pink eyes to bed can help ease discomfort and speed healing. "Adequate sleep gives the eyes a break," says Rubin Naiman, Ph.D. "During sleep, complex changes occur that replenish the eye's moisture and protection." Aim to sleep at least 8 hours each night.

■ **MEDICATE AT NIGHT.** "Germ-caused conjunctivitis intensifies when your eyes are closed. That's why it tends to get worse at night when you're asleep," says Dr. Petersen. "To combat that, put any prescribed antibiotic ointment in your eyes before you go to bed. That way it will prevent crusting."

■ **TRY MASSAGE.** "Nasal massage can help to unblock the duct that drains the eye's tears into the nose," says Ken Haller, M.D. "A blockage can cause eye irritation or prevent a small infection from clearing itself up." Place your thumb and index finger just below the bridge of the nose—where the pads of eyeglasses would rest—and gently massage the area.

PANEL OF ADVISORS

LINDA ANTINORO, R.D., IS SENIOR NUTRITIONIST AT BRIGHAM AND WOMEN'S HOSPITAL IN BOSTON.

JAMES DUKE, PH.D., HELD SEVERAL POSTS IN HIS MORE THAN THREE DECADES WITH THE USDA, INCLUDING CHIEF OF THE MEDICINAL PLANT RESOURCES LABORATORY. HE IS AUTHOR OF *THE GREEN PHARMACY*.

KEN HALLER, M.D., IS ASSISTANT PROFESSOR OF PEDIATRICS AT SAINT LOUIS UNIVERSITY IN MISSOURI.

PETER HERSH, M.D., FACS, IS THE DIRECTOR OF THE CORNEA AND LASER EYE INSTITUTE AND A PROFESSOR OF CLINICAL OPHTHALMOLOGY AT THE UNIVERSITY OF MEDICINE AND DENTISTRY OF NEW JERSEY. HE IS ALSO A FORMER INSTRUCTOR OF OPHTHALMOLOGY AT HARVARD MEDICAL SCHOOL.

RUBIN NAIMAN, PH.D., IS THE DIRECTOR OF SLEEP PROGRAMS AT MIRAVAL RESORT IN TUCSON.

J. DANIEL NELSON, M.D., IS AN OPHTHALMOLOGIST WITH HEALTHPARTNERS MEDICAL GROUP AND A PROFESSOR OF OPHTHALMOLOGY AT THE UNIVERSITY OF MINNESOTA, BOTH IN MINNEAPOLIS.

ROBERT PETERSEN, M.D., IS AN ASSISTANT PROFESSOR OF OPHTHALMOLOGY AT HARVARD MEDICAL SCHOOL. HE IS ALSO A PEDIATRIC OPHTHALMOLOGIST AND DIRECTOR OF THE EYE CLINIC AT CHILDREN'S HOSPITAL IN BOSTON.

Constipation

20 Solutions to a Common Problem

Constipation is an uncomfortable, exceedingly common problem, affecting more than 4 million Americans and accounting for an estimated 2.5 million doctor visits each year. Women appear to experience more constipation than men, and older people more than younger people.

There are many causes of constipation, including a lack of fiber in the diet, insufficient liquid intake, stress, medications, lack of exercise, and bad bowel habits, says Paul Rousseau, M.D.

We take a look at all of these factors, as well as suggest ways to remedy the situation.

■ **DETERMINE IF YOU ARE *REALLY* CONSTIPATED.** Madison Avenue bombards us with laxative advertisements that give the impression that a daily bowel movement is essential to good health, and that just isn't so, says Marvin Schuster, M.D.

Many Americans, he says, are subject to *perceived constipation*—they think they're constipated when they are not. In reality, the need to defecate varies greatly from individual to individual. For some, a bowel movement three times a day may be considered normal, for others three times a week may suffice.

■ **FINE-TUNE YOUR FLUID AND FIBER INTAKE.** Our experts agree that the first thing you should do if you're constipated is check your diet. The foremost menu items for battling constipation are foods rich in dietary fiber such as fruits, vegetables,

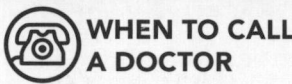

WHEN TO CALL A DOCTOR

Constipation itself usually isn't serious, says Marvin Schuster, M.D. However, you should call your doctor when symptoms are severe, last longer than 3 weeks, are disabling, or if you find blood in your stool, he says. Although it's rare, constipation can signal a serious underlying disorder.

In addition, contact your doctor if your constipation accompanies an enlarged or bulging abdomen, which may signal an intestinal obstruction, says Paul Rousseau, M.D.

beans and other legumes, and liquids, which are essential to keeping the stool soft and helping it pass through the colon.

How much liquid and fiber do you need? Let's start with the liquid. A minimum of six glasses of liquid, preferably eight, should be part of every adult's diet, says Patricia H. Harper, M.S., R.D., L.D.N. While any fluid will do the trick, the best is water, she says.

■ **EAT LOTS MORE FIBER.** Most Americans don't get enough fiber in their diets, says Harper. The American Dietetic Association recommends 20 to 35 grams of dietary fiber daily for all adults and at least 30 grams for those who experience constipation.

Whole grains, fruits, and vegetables are the best fiber sources, says Harper. It's not difficult to get 30 grams in your daily diet if you choose foods carefully. A half cup of green peas, for example, gives you 5 grams, one small apple supplies 3 grams, and a bowl of bran cereal has as much as 13 grams. Tops among the fiber heavyweights are cooked dried beans, prunes, figs, raisins, popcorn, oatmeal, pears, and nuts. One word of caution, though: Increase your fiber intake slowly to avoid gas attacks.

■ **WORK YOUR TRIGGER POINTS.** "Animal studies suggest that acupuncture may spur contractions in the colon, moving your bowels," says Steven Tan, M.D. "If your episode is minor, you could be helped by a single treatment; chronic sufferers may need about 10. Acupressure may help, too."

To try acupressure for constipation, it takes only two fingers and less than 2 minutes. Using your index and middle fingers, apply firm pressure on the outside of your leg, about 3 inches below the kneecap, for 5 seconds and then release for 10 seconds. Repeat five times. Visit www.aaaomonline.org, the Web site for the American Association of Acupuncture and Oriental Medicine, to search for an acupuncturist near you.

■ **TAKE TIME TO GO TO THE GYM.** Exercise is good for your heart, but it's also good for your bowels. In general, regular exercise tends to combat constipation by moving food through the bowel faster, says Edward R. Eichner, M.D.

■ **TAKE A WALK.** Any form of regular exercise tends to alleviate constipation, but the one mentioned most often by our experts is walking. This activity is particularly helpful to pregnant women, many of whom experience constipation as their inner workings are compressed to accommodate the growing fetus.

Everyone, including mothers-to-be, should walk a hearty 20 to 30 minutes a day, suggests Lewis R. Townsend, M.D. Pregnant women should take care not to get too winded as they walk.

■ **LEARN NEW HABITS.** Throughout our lives, many of us condition ourselves to go to the bathroom not when nature calls but when it's convenient. Ignoring the urge to defecate, however, can eventually lead to constipation. It's never too late to improve your bowel habits, says Dr. Schuster. "The most natural time to go to the toilet is after a meal," he adds. So pick a meal, any meal, and every day following that meal sit on the toilet for 10 minutes. In time, says Dr. Schuster, you will condition your colon to act as nature intended.

■ **LEARN TO RELAX.** "Patients with chronic or severe gastrointestinal woes tend to have more anxiety and stress," says Lin Chang, M.D. "Behavioral techniques like relaxation training can decrease symptoms, and calming breaths help regulate the nervous system and relax the digestive tract."

To ease discomfort, focus on how your stomach moves as you inhale for a count of 4 and exhale. Do this twice daily for 15 minutes.

Try yoga two or three times a week. The breathing is similar, and exercise helps you clear your bowels.

■ **HAVE A HEARTY LAUGH.** It may sound funny, but a good belly laugh can help with constipation in two ways. It has a massaging effect on the intestines, which helps foster digestion, and it's a great stress reliever, says Alison Crane, R.N.

■ **RECONSIDER USING LAXATIVE TABLETS.** Chemical laxatives often do what they're intended to do, but they're terribly addicting, warns Dr. Rousseau. Take too many of these chemical laxatives, and your bowel gets used to them, and your constipation can get worse. When should you take laxatives from a bottle? "Almost never," he says.

■ **KNOW THAT NOT ALL LAXATIVES ARE THE SAME.** In most drugstores, right next to the chemical laxatives, you'll find another category of laxatives, often marked "natural" or "vegetable" laxatives, whose main ingredient is generally crushed psyllium seed. This is a concentrated form of fiber, which, unlike the chemical laxatives, is nonaddictive and generally safe, even if taken over long periods, says Dr. Rousseau. He cautions, however, that these must be taken with lots of water (read the instructions on the package), or they can gum up inside you.

■ **TRY THIS SPECIAL RECIPE.** Psyllium-based laxatives can be expensive. So make your own by buying psyllium seeds in a health food store and crushing them yourself. Grind 2 parts psyllium with 1 part flaxseed and 1 part oat bran (also available in health food stores) for a high-fiber concoction. Mix the ingredients up with water, and have it as a little mash every night around 9 p.m. Psyllium absorbs liquid in the intestines, making a softer stool that's easier to pass.

■ **REVIEW YOUR MEDICATIONS AND SUPPLEMENTS.** There are a number of medications that can bring on or exacerbate constipation, says Dr. Rousseau. Among the common culprits are antacids containing aluminum or calcium, antihistamines, anti-Parkinsonism drugs, calcium supplements, diuretics, narcotics, phenothiazines, sedatives, and tricyclic antidepressants.

■ **BEWARE OF CERTAIN FOODS.** Some things may constipate one person but not another. Milk, for example, can be extremely

An Apple a Day...

If you're constipated, apples are a great food choice because they contain both insoluble fiber and soluble fiber.

■ **Insoluble fiber** is found in the skin of apples, which contains most of their fiber. Soluble fiber forms a coating inside your digestive tract to help things move through easily.

■ **Soluble fiber** in apples is good roughage and also helps prevent other digestive disorders, such a diverticulitis and possibly even colon cancer. Insoluble fiber soaks up water as it passes through your intestines, helping to bulk up and weigh down your stool, helping gravity do its job.

For a good clean-out, eat three or four small apples a day until your constipation clears. But be sure you eat them with the skins on.

constipating to some, while causing diarrhea in others. Foods that tend to produce gas, such as beans, cauliflower, and cabbage, can be problematic for people whose constipation is the result of a spastic colon, says Dr. Schuster. You should suspect a spastic colon and avoid gas-producing foods if your constipation is sharply painful.

■ **USE DIETARY OILS SPARINGLY.** By avoiding dietary oils, such as vegetable, olive, or soy oil, you may be less constipated, says Grady Deal, Ph.D., D.C. "It's not oil per se, but eating it in its free state causes constipation and many other digestive problems," says Dr. Deal. He bases his theory on the work of the turn-of-the-century health reformer John Henry Kellogg, M.D.

The problem with these oils, Dr. Deal explains, is that they form a film in the stomach, which makes it difficult to digest carbohydrates and proteins there and in the small intestine. Adequate digestion is delayed up to 20 hours, causing putrefaction, gas, and toxins, which back up the colon and large intestine, he says. But oils eaten in their natural form found in whole nuts, avocados, and corn are released slowly into the body, so no oil slicks occur to block digestion and create constipation problems. These oils, as opposed to the separated kind, are "a wholesome and nutritious element of food," he says.

■ **TUNE IN TO YOUR BODY.** "In biofeedback, sensors display the activity of your pelvic floor muscles on a screen as you learn to relax them, making it easier for you to pass your stool," says Jeannette Tries, Ph.D. A recent study found that in some cases, biofeedback may be more effective than laxatives.

Find a licensed biofeedback practitioner in your area by visiting www.bcia.org, the Web site of the Biofeedback Certification Institute of America. You may need 8 to 10 visits over the course of 3 to 4 months to get relief.

■ **BE CAUTIOUS ABOUT HERBS.** Herbal remedies for dealing with constipation abound. Among those touted are aloe juice, senna, medicinal rhubarb, cascara sagrada, dandelion root, and plantain seeds. Some, such as cascara sagrada, can be very effective, but you need to be careful. Herbal laxatives, just as chemical ones, should be carefully chosen and not overused.

■ **DON'T STRAIN.** Forcing a bowel movement is unwise. You risk giving yourself hemorrhoids and anal fissures, which are painful and can aggravate your constipation by narrowing the anal opening. Straining can also raise your blood pressure and lower your heartbeat, which can be dangerous, especially in the elderly.

■ **GET FAST RELIEF—ONCE IN A WHILE.** If you're really miserable, nothing works faster to move your bowels than an enema or a suppository. For occasional use, they are perfectly all right, says Dr. Rousseau. Use them too often, however, and you risk creating a lazy colon, exacerbating your constipation problem.

Use clear water only or saline-solution enemas, *never* soapsuds, which can be irritating, says Dr. Rousseau. And when shopping for a suppository, stick with glycerin, avoiding the harsher chemical selections on the market.

PANEL OF ADVISORS

Cough

21 Throat-Soothing Strategies

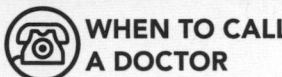
WHEN TO CALL A DOCTOR

If you cough up blood or if your cough lasts more than 2 weeks, see a doctor, says Robert Sandhaus, M.D., Ph.D.

Cancer and heartburn are both common causes of persistent coughs, he says. So are asthma, chronic obstructive pulmonary disease (COPD), and other respiratory diseases.

"You have to worry about pneumonia, especially if the cough is accompanied by sharp chest pains, chills, or a fever higher than 101°F," says Dr. Sandhaus.

Other warning signs include wheezing, shortness of breath, and leg swelling. When accompanied by a persistent cough, these symptoms could be a sign of heart failure, which requires immediate medical attention.

Have your doctor take a throat culture in order to rule out strep throat, which requires an antibiotic, says Stuart Ditchek, M.D.

It's no accident that the wracking coughs that accompany allergies, colds, and other respiratory problems never seem to go away. Coughing is the body's way of removing irritating substances from the airways. Too much coughing, though, can make it impossible to sleep or even relax. Some people have even broken ribs during severe coughing fits.

Mucus-filled "productive" coughs are usually caused by allergies, colds, or other respiratory tract infections. Buildup of mucus in the airways makes it hard to breathe, and the body responds by trying to remove it. "Dry" coughs, on the other hand, are caused by irritation due to smoking, for example, or from inhaling fumes, dust, or other airborne irritants.

Most coughs clear up on their own within a week to 10 days. In the meantime, here are a few ways to reduce the discomfort and help the cough pass more quickly.

■ **ENJOY SLIPPERY ELM LOZENGES.** Available in drugstores and health food stores, slippery elm is loaded with a substance that soothes the throat and helps reduce coughing. These lozenges even taste pretty good, says pediatrician Stuart Ditchek, M.D. Suck on a maximum of five or six lozenges per day.

■ **TRY THIS SLIPPERY SOLUTION.** The next time you have a wracking cough, try this helpful formula. Add 1 teaspoon of slippery elm powder or liquid to 2 cups of hot water. Stir in 1 tablespoon of sugar and a sprinkling of cinnamon, and drink it down, suggests Dr. Ditchek. If you use slippery elm liquid extract, use $\frac{1}{2}$ teaspoon for kids 2 to 4 years old and 1 teaspoon for those 5 years and older, he advises.

■ **SIP GINGER TEA.** Ginger acts as a potent natural anti-inflammatory herbal agent. Most people use ginger tea as a way to soothe their painful throats, although fresh ginger from the produce section of your local supermarket is also good.

■ **TRY ZINC LOZENGES.** The research isn't conclusive, but some studies suggest that sucking on zinc lozenges can reduce the discomfort of a scratchy throat. Most zinc lozenges contain 22 milligrams of zinc, but not all of it is absorbed, says Dr. Ditchek. Don't take more than the amount recommended by your doctor. Zinc can be toxic in large doses.

■ **DRINK LOTS OF WATER.** The body naturally loses fluids when you have a cold or flu. In addition, the accompanying congestion forces mouth breathing, which increases throat dryness and coughing, says Robert Sandhaus,

M.D., Ph.D. Try to drink at least eight 8-ounce glasses of water each day. This will moisturize tissues and help calm the cough.

Here's another reason to drink more water. Mucous membranes kept moist are better able to resist cold-causing viruses, says Dr. Sandhaus. "If mucus is too thick, this barrier doesn't work as well."

■ **TAKE VITAMIN C.** Nothing prevents the occasional cold, but studies have shown that taking vitamin C at the first sign of infection can cut the severity of symptoms, including cough, by about 50 percent, says Dr. Ditchek. Megadoses like those used in years past are no longer commonly advised, he adds. While the Daily Value for vitamin C is 60 milligrams, doses between 100 and 500 milligrams per day can be beneficial.

A dose for a small child at the start of a cold should be 100 milligrams a day, says Dr. Ditchek. For older kids, go with 200 milligrams. "Foods high in vitamin C—such as citrus fruits, strawberries, broccoli, bell peppers, and melon—are also a good option," he says.

■ **ADD SOME ECHINACEA.** Available in health food stores and most drugstores, echinacea helps the immune system battle cold viruses. It also may reduce the duration and severity of coughs and other cold symptoms, says Dr. Ditchek. While clinical studies vary on the effectiveness of echinacea, many people include this herb in their wintertime regimens.

For children, Dr. Ditchek advises 6 to 7 drops of standardized liquid extract in a small

Cures from the Kitchen

"One thing that can trigger coughs is throat irritation," says Robert Sandhaus, M.D., Ph.D. Sucking on hard candy increases saliva flow. The combination of saliva and ingredients in the candy soothes irritated tissues, he says.

amount of water or juice. This can be safely done three to five times a day. "For older children, 8 to 15 drops should do the trick," he says.

Take 12 drops of echinacea tincture four times a day. In capsule form, take one or two capsules three or four times a day for 10 days to 2 weeks. People with autoimmune diseases or ragweed allergies should not take echinacea, says Dr. Ditchek.

■ **DRINK SOMETHING HOT.** A cup of chamomile tea works well, especially if it's flavored with honey and lemon. "Hot liquids are soothing when you have a cough," says Dr. Sandhaus. Adding honey to tea may provide additional relief because the thick sweetener soothes irritated tissues and cough receptors in the throat, he says. Drinking plenty of broth, tea, or other warm fluids is particularly helpful for "dry" coughs.

■ **EAT RAW OR LIGHTLY COOKED GARLIC.** It's rich in chemical compounds that help inhibit cough-causing viruses in the respiratory tract, says Dr. Ditchek. Garlic is a wonderful natural antibiotic that can assist in fighting off colds and common upper-respiratory infections. "Extracts of aged garlic can be used as well," he says.

Try to eat two to four garlic cloves each daily, Dr. Ditchek says. Or use garlic supplements, following the directions on the label. But avoid garlic supplements at least 7 to 10 days prior to any surgery. Using these supplements can increase the risk of bleeding, especially when used for long periods of time, he says.

■ **SWIG CHICKEN SOUP.** And be sure to add lots of hot, pungent spices like pepper, garlic, and curry powder. The warm fluid and the pungent spices will help break up stagnant mucus in your beleaguered lungs, and these natural expectorants will help get rid of the mucus.

■ **HUMIDIFY THE AIRWAYS.** Once or twice a day, take a long, hot shower or bath. Or plug in a vaporizer or humidifier. Breathing steam reduces airway irritation and makes mucus easier to cough up.

Humidifying the air is a good way to prevent cough-causing colds and other infections, says Dr. Ditchek. Air that's too dry takes moisture from the nose, throat, and lungs, making it easier for viruses to take hold.

■ **FLUSH IT OUT.** Using a salt and water solution to flush out the nasal cavity can do wonders to relieve a productive cough. A popular option is the neti pot—a ceramic pot that looks like a cross between a small teapot and a magic lamp. The salt solution in the neti pot is drained into each nostril. Nasal irrigation using this technique has been around for centuries, originating in Ayurvedic medicine.

"Older kids and teens can use a neti pot to rinse out their nasal passages and relieve congestion," Dr. Ditchek says. Neti pots are available at most drugstores.

■ **STAY AWAY FROM CIGARETTE SMOKE.** Even if you don't smoke, breathing secondhand smoke almost guarantees that you'll have

Chronic Cough Cause

After a cold, you feel okay but the cough hangs around. Sound familiar? Each year, people schedule 30 million visits to the doctor because of a chronic cough (one that lingers for more than 3 weeks). Often doctors can't offer much help, but a Mayo Clinic study found that in one-third of cases, there may be an easy fix.

When researchers examined CT scans of the sinuses of 132 patients with chronic coughs, they discovered that 37 percent actually had chronic sinusitis, an infection or inflammation that can cause coughing and sneezing. Sinusitis can be treated with antibiotics, decongestants, or a nasal steroid spray.

an irritated throat. Smokers often have persistent coughs, because the body responds to the irritation by producing enormous amounts of mucus, says Dr. Sandhaus.

If you're a smoker, the best thing to do is quit. Insist that friends or family members keep their cigarette smoke away from you.

■ **CONSIDER A COUGH SUPPRESSANT.** Over-the-counter medicines that contain dextromethorphan (such as Triaminic DM or Robitussin DM) aren't a cure for coughs, but they will help blunt the "cough reflex" in the brain. Doctors recommend these products for temporary relief only—when a cough keeps you up at night, for example.

Cough suppressants should be used only if you have a dry cough, Dr. Sandhaus says. Productive coughs should be encouraged, not suppressed, because it's important to clear secretions from the airways.

■ **USE AN EXPECTORANT.** One way to make productive coughs even more productive is to take an over-the-counter expectorant that contains guaifenesin (such as Robitussin). Expectorants make mucus thinner and easier to expel, says Dr. Sandhaus.

■ **BLOW YOUR NOSE.** For productive coughs, blowing your nose frequently helps eliminate mucus before it has a chance to stimulate the cough reflex, says Dr. Ditchek. "Postnasal drip is by far the most common cause of hacking coughs in young children," he says. And these coughs worsen when you lie flat. "Teach kids from a very young age how to blow their noses to help relieve many episodes of cough," Dr. Ditchek says. Gravity helps, too, so try elevating the head of the bed.

■ **CONTROL HEARTBURN.** It's a common cause of persistent coughs, says Dr. Ditchek. The same stomach acids that cause heartburn (also called gastroesophageal reflux) can also trigger coughing fits when the acids irritate the esophagus or airways. If you cough mainly at night, after meals, or while lying down, there's a good chance that stomach acids are to blame.

Bad Cough? Try This African Flower

South African tribes have long used the pelargonium flower (*Pelargonium sidoides*) to treat coughs and congestion. Known as umckaloabo, which in Zulu roughly means "chest cold and pain," this member of the geranium family has deep burgundy flowers and heart-shaped leaves.

Studies have shown that pelargonium shortens the severity and duration of sore throats and acute bronchitis. In a study conducted by U.S., Russian, and German researchers, 85 percent of those who took this herb were almost or completely symptom-free after 1 week. Pelargonium contains polyphenol compounds known to stimulate the immune system, helping it target viruses and bacteria.

To try this natural remedy, look for *Umcka ColdCare* by Nature's Way, available at health food stores and at www.naturesway.com. Follow dosage instructions on the label.

One of the easiest strategies to keep stomach acids where they belong is to elevate the head of your bed a few inches by putting wood blocks under the legs. It's also helpful to eat four or five small meals a day instead of two or three large meals. Finally, stay on your feet—or at least sit upright in a chair—for at least 2 hours after eating. Avoid food triggers, such as dairy, that aggravate symptoms.

If you want to try an herbal heartburn remedy, suck on licorice lozenges. Always use the deglycyrrhizinated form (DGL), which doesn't generally cause blood pressure elevation. Always check your blood pressure if you use licorice lozenges for more than a few days, says Dr. Ditchek. The DGL lozenges come standard at 380 milligrams of licorice—suck on two a day before meals. Some taste better than others, so try out different brands. DGL is not approved as safe for children.

■ **CHECK YOUR BLOOD PRESSURE.** If you take an ACE inhibitor (such as Vasotec) for high blood pressure and you have a persistent cough, the cause could be your medication. ACE inhibitors can cause cough, so talk to your doctor about testing a different antihypertensive medication, says Dr. Sandhaus.

■ **GET ALLERGIES UNDER CONTROL.** If you're sensitive to pollen, mold, or other allergens, even a brief exposure can stimulate mucus production—followed by days or weeks of coughing as your body tries to remove it, says Dr. Ditchek.

"Air purifiers at home or work are very important," he says. "After a day of school or a few hours of outdoor play, children should bathe or shower immediately to remove any pollen. This will help tremendously."

Once you know what allergy is causing your cough, avoidance is the best approach. If you get hay fever, for example, stay indoors during the morning and evening hours, when pollen concentrations are highest. For quick relief from symptoms, take an over-the-counter antihistamine, such as diphenhydramine (Benadryl), loratadine (Claritin), or cetirizine hydrochloride (Zyrtec). "The prescription medication montelukast sodium (Singulair) is a safe, effective seasonal allergy treatment," says Dr. Ditchek.

Of all of these medications, diphenhydramine is the only one that can cause either drowsiness or hyperactivity, so use it with caution. Over-the-counter decongestants should not be used by children younger than 8.

"The rapid relief from antihistamines is helpful when you're having bad days," says Dr. Ditchek. "I actually love recommending stinging nettles. It is often as or more effective than medications, and it doesn't cause drowsiness or behavioral side effects. It simply takes longer to achieve therapeutic effect."

■ **CHECK FOR ASTHMA.** One of the most common causes of unexplained cough is undetected asthma, says Dr. Sandhaus. "Asthma often shows up as a cough that lasts for weeks after a minor respiratory infection has cleared up," he explains. Ongoing airway inflammation caused by asthma can be treated with inhaled steroids to quiet things down. The good news? "You'll know what caused the cough and what to do about it, and inhaled steroids have little or no side effects when taken as directed," Dr. Sandhaus says.

■ **GET SOME REST.** It's the oldest—and probably the most ignored—advice for combating cold symptoms like coughing. "People want to keep going, but you have to try to get some rest," Dr. Sandhaus says. Otherwise, that "minor" cold and cough might progress to something a lot more serious, like pneumonia.

PANEL OF ADVISORS

STUART DITCHEK, M.D., IS A PEDIATRICIAN AND CLINICAL ASSISTANT PROFESSOR OF PEDIATRICS AT NEW YORK UNIVERSITY SCHOOL OF MEDICINE IN NEW YORK CITY. HE IS COAUTHOR OF THE BOOK *HEALTHY CHILD, WHOLE CHILD* AND FOUNDER OF WWW.DRDITCHEK.COM, A PARENTING WEB SITE.

ROBERT SANDHAUS, M.D., PH.D., IS A PULMONARY SPECIALIST, DIRECTOR OF ALPHA-1 CLINIC, AND PROFESSOR OF MEDICINE AT NATIONAL JEWISH HEALTH IN DENVER. HE IS ALSO EXECUTIVE VICE PRESIDENT AND MEDICAL DIRECTOR OF ALPHA-1 FOUNDATION IN MIAMI AND WWW.ALPHANET.ORG.

Cuts and Scrapes

22 Ways to Soothe a Sore

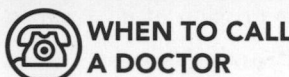 **WHEN TO CALL A DOCTOR**

First aid isn't always enough. See a doctor when:

■ Bleeding is bright red and spurting. You may have punctured an artery.

■ You can't wash all the debris out of the wound.

■ The cut or scrape is on your face or any area where you want to minimize scarring.

■ Your wound develops red streaks or weeps pus, or the redness extends more than a finger's width beyond the cut.

■ The wound is large, and you can see inside it. You may need stitches. Never try to stitch a wound yourself, even if you are stranded far from medical help.

Mix one pair of roller skates with a sidewalk that boasts more cracks than Death Valley and voilà—a recipe for scraped knees and small cuts that seem anything but small to a frightened and hurting child.

While boys and girls seem to have a monopoly on boo-boos, adults trip and fall into their share of cuts and scrapes, too.

A finger gets in the way of a knife slicing bagels. A backpack carelessly tossed in the front hall sets the stage for a nasty fall. And every winter, ice lurks like a sinister prankster waiting for victims who fall, causing tears in their pants and their skin at the same time.

Life is rife with mishaps. Luckily, your kitchen and medicine cabinet are filled with the tools to manage them. Here's a crash course—pardon the pun—on what to do.

■ **STOP THE BLEEDING.** The fastest way to stop bleeding is to apply direct pressure. Place a clean, absorbent cloth over the cut, then firmly press your hand against it. If you don't have a cloth, use your fingers. If blood soaks through your first bandage, layer on a second one and press steadily. Add new bandages over old ones, because removing a cloth may tear off coagulating blood cells.

If applying pressure doesn't stop the bleeding, elevate the limb to heart level to reduce the pressure of blood on the cut. Continue applying pressure. This should take care of it.

■ **BE LIKE A DOG.** If you're out in the middle of nowhere with no way to clean a wound, just lick it. Scientists in Amsterdam have

Cures from the Kitchen

CLOVE. "The dried flower buds of this tropical tree can be found on your spice rack," says botanist James Duke, Ph.D., in his book *The Green Pharmacy*. "You can sprinkle powdered cloves on a cut to keep it from becoming infected." Clove oil is rich in eugenol, a chemical that's both an antiseptic and a painkiller. Ask your dentist or aromatherapist about it, too.

GARLIC. A flavor enhancer, garlic—and its relatives, onion and chive—is also a natural antibiotic with lots of antiseptic compounds. Tape a clove of garlic directly on a cut or scrape to help with healing. If this irritates your skin, remove it immediately.

HONEY. This natural sweetener contains three powerful wound-healing ingredients: sugar for absorbing moisture so bacteria can't survive, hydrogen peroxide to disinfect, and the nectar-based compound propolis to kill bacteria. An added bonus? Honey dries to form a natural bandage.

found that human saliva contains a protein that greatly speeds healing by acting as an antibacterial, antifungal, antiviral, and anti-inflammatory agent.

■ **STRAP IT UP.** When the bleeding stops or at least slows, tie the wound firmly with a cloth or wrap it with an elastic bandage so there is pressure against it, *but do not cut off circulation,* says emergency medical technician John Gillies.

■ **GO FOR EXTRA PRESSURE.** If the cut continues to bleed, it is more serious than you thought, and you probably need to see a doctor immediately. Until you get medical help, find the pressure point nearest the cut between the wound and your heart. Pressure points are places you might think of when taking a pulse: inside your wrists, inside your upper arm about halfway between the elbow and armpit, and in the groin where your legs attach to your torso. Press the artery against the bone. Stop pressing about a minute after the bleeding stops. If bleeding starts again, reapply pressure.

■ **DON'T USE A TOURNIQUET.** With most everyday cuts and scrapes, first aid is plenty. Tourniquets can be dangerous. "Once you apply a tourniquet, the person may end up losing that limb because you cut off circulation," cautions Gillies.

■ **WASH THE WOUND TWICE A DAY.** This is important to prevent infection and to decrease the chance of permanent discoloration. Wash the area with soap and water or just water, says Hugh Macaulay, M.D. The idea is to dilute the bacteria in the wound and remove debris. If you don't remove stones, dirt, or sand from the cut, they can leave color under the skin.

■ **CLEAN IT WITH MYRRH.** Another way to clean a cut or scrape is by using myrrh, a reddish-brown dried tree sap available in health food stores. Myrrh is a natural antiseptic and known for its "blood-moving" properties that help with healing. Use 1 teaspoon of myrrh extract in 4 ounces of water

Why Are Little Paper Cuts Such a Big Pain?

Office workers know it. Paper pushers of any kind can testify to it, too. Even though they're small, paper cuts pack a real pain punch. What is it about these small cuts that prompts such big reactions from us? In a word, particles.

If a woman cuts herself shaving her legs, the razor makes a clean cut, leaving behind few, if any, particles that trigger pain. A paper cut, on the other hand, leaves paper fibers coated with chemicals from the papermaking process. These fibers and bacteria remain in the wound and stimulate pain receptors in the skin. What to do?

■ If you can see the particles, remove them with a clean pair of tweezers.

■ Crazy as it sounds, consider Krazy Glue. The glue binds the outer skin together, allowing inner layers to heal faster. Fill your cut with a tiny amount of Krazy Glue using a toothpick or the rod portion of a cotton swab. Apply the glue so that it's flat and smooth, with no bumps. Take care not to stick your fingers to each other or to objects. Don't use Krazy Glue for anything but paper cuts and small cracks in the skin. Stay alert for the sign of an allergic reaction: red, inflamed skin.

and pour it over the wound, letting it air-dry before bandaging.

■ SMEAR ON AN OVER-THE-COUNTER ANTIBIOTIC OINTMENT. Broad-spectrum antibacterial ointments work best, according to James J. Leyden, M.D. (See "Choosing an Over-the-Counter Ointment," page 161.)

People who use a triple-antibiotic ointment and the right kind of bandage heal 30 percent faster, says wound researcher Patricia Mertz.

Still, Mertz warns, be wary of over-the-counter drugs that contain neomycin or ointments that contain a lot of preservatives. They can cause allergic reactions. If you have an allergic reaction to the ointment, your scrape will get red and itchy, and may become infected.

■ TRY TEA TREE OIL. This oil contains a powerful antiseptic compound and has long been popular worldwide for helping wounds heal. Botanist James Duke, Ph.D., suggests diluting several drops of tea tree oil in a couple tablespoons of vegetable oil and applying it to the cut or scrape.

■ HAVE A SWEET TREAT(MENT). Got a cut or wound? You can speed up the healing process with a little table sugar, says orthopedic surgeon Richard A. Knutson, M.D. He's treated wounds with a mixture of a topical iodine solution and sugar, healing a variety of mishaps such as cuts, scrapes, and burns. (Don't use raw iodine; it will burn the skin.) Sugar, he says, leaves bacteria without the nutrients necessary to grow or multiply. Wounds usually heal quickly, without a scab and often with little scarring. Keloids (irregular, large scars) are kept to a minimum.

To make Dr. Knutson's ointment, you must mix 1 part canola or olive oil with 3 parts of white table sugar, then add 3 tablespoons of first-aid antibiotic ointment (Betadine Antibiotic Ointment, for example). You can find the ointment in your local drugstore. Pack a cleaned wound with the homemade ointment and cover carefully with gauze. Four times a day, rinse the area gently with water and hydrogen peroxide and pack on fresh ointment. Taper off as healing progresses.

Choosing an Over-the-Counter Ointment

Confused about choosing the best product for your boo-boo? In one study, James J. Leyden, M.D., compared the effectiveness of nine over-the-counter products on wound healing. He found that some products mend minor cuts, scrapes, and burns faster than others. Here's what his research uncovered.

■ Polysporin (active ingredients: polymyxin B, bacitracin ointment): 8.2 days

■ Neosporin (active ingredients: neomycin, polymyxin B, bacitracin ointment): 9.2 days

■ Johnson & Johnson First Aid Cream (wound protectant with no antibiotic agent): 9.8 days

■ Mercurochrome (active ingredient: merbromin): 13.1 days

■ No treatment: 13.3 days

■ Bactine spray (active ingredient: benzalkonium chloride): 14.2 days

■ Merthiolate (active ingredient: thimerosol): 14.2 days

■ Hydrogen peroxide (3 percent): 14.3 days

■ Campho-Phenique (active ingredients: camphor, phenol): 15.4 days

■ Tincture of iodine: 15.7 days

Bandage Busters

Got a boo-boo but dread taking off the bandage? To minimize the consequences of this procedure, follow these tips for painless removal.

■ Use a tiny pair of scissors to separate the bandage part from the adhesive sections. Pull it gently away from your scrape. Then remove the adhesive strips.

■ If your scab is stuck to the bandage, soak the area in a mixture of warm water and salt—normally about a teaspoon of salt to a gallon of water should do it. Have patience. The dressing will eventually let go.

■ If the bandage is stuck on your forearm, leg, or chest hair, pull in the direction of hair growth. Use a cotton swab saturated in baby oil or rubbing alcohol to moisten the adhesive fully before pulling away from the skin.

Be sure the wound is clean, and the bleeding has stopped before applying the mixture. Sugar makes a bleeding wound bleed more. Dr. Knutson recommends applying a dry dressing for 24 to 48 hours to help stop the bleeding.

■ **THINK ZINC.** This essential mineral strengthens the immune system, which helps with wound healing. To help speed up the healing of a cut or scrape, add more zinc-rich foods to your diet. Good sources of zinc include oysters, meat, eggs, seafood, black-eyed peas, tofu, and wheat germ.

■ **KEEP IT UNDERCOVER.** When exposed to air, cuts form scabs, which slow down new cell growth, says Mertz. She recommends a plastic bandage similar to food wrap. They come in all sizes. Or look for gauze

impregnated with petroleum jelly. Both types of bandages keep healing moisture on the wound but allow only a little air to pass through. Cells regenerate more rapidly when moist.

■ **TOP IT OFF WITH A TETANUS SHOT.** If you haven't had a tetanus shot in the past 5 years, you need a booster, says Dr. Macaulay. Local health departments usually give them for a minimal fee or for free, he adds. If you don't remember when you had your last booster, it's a good idea to have one within 24 hours of the injury.

PANEL OF ADVISORS

JAMES DUKE, PH.D., HELD SEVERAL POSTS IN HIS MORE THAN THREE DECADES WITH THE USDA, INCLUDING CHIEF OF THE MEDICINAL PLANT RESOURCES LABORATORY. HE IS AUTHOR OF *THE GREEN PHARMACY.*

JOHN GILLIES, E.M.T., IS A FORMER EMERGENCY MEDICAL TECHNICIAN AND PROGRAM DIRECTOR FOR HEALTH SERVICES AT THE COLORADO OUTWARD BOUND SCHOOL IN DENVER.

RICHARD A. KNUTSON, M.D., IS A FORMER ORTHOPEDIC SURGEON AT DELTA MEDICAL CENTER IN GREENVILLE, MISSISSIPPI.

JAMES J. LEYDEN, M.D., IS AN EMERITUS PROFESSOR OF DERMATOLOGY AT THE UNIVERSITY OF PENNSYLVANIA IN PHILADELPHIA.

HUGH MACAULAY, M.D., IS AN EMERGENCY ROOM PHYSICIAN AT ASPEN VALLEY HOSPITAL IN COLORADO.

PATRICIA MERTZ IS AN EMERITUS PROFESSOR IN THE DEPARTMENT OF DERMATOLOGY AND CUTANEOUS SURGERY AT MILLER SCHOOL OF MEDICINE AT THE UNIVERSITY OF MIAMI IN FLORIDA. SHE IS ALSO THE FOUNDER OF MIAMI DERMATOLOGY RESEARCH INSTITUTE.

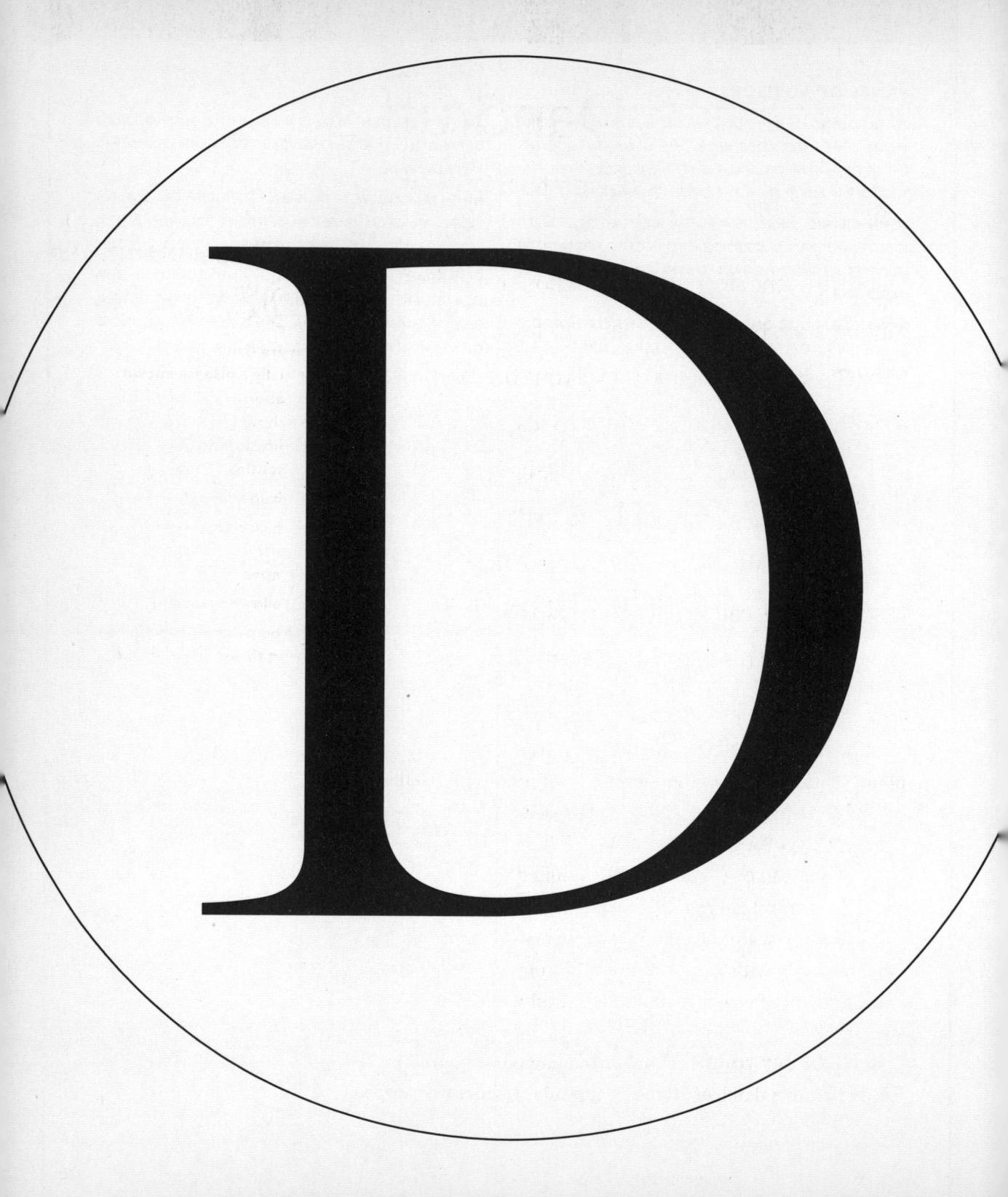

Dandruff

18 Tips to Stop Flaking

Dandruff—the single most common scalp complaint among stylists' clients—plays no favorites. Dermatologists say that just about everyone has the problem to some degree, often leading to a scratch-and-itch cycle, says Maria Hordinsky, M.D. Ignoring the condition lets the scaling build up. That, in turn, can cause itching, which can lead to scratching. Scratching too vigorously can wound the scalp and leave it open to infection. This vicious cycle can be avoided, however, with some simple home remedies.

■ **SHAMPOO OFTEN.** The experts are unanimous on this point: Wash your hair often—every day if necessary. "Generally, the more frequently you shampoo, the easier it is to control the dandruff," says Patricia Farris, M.D.

■ **START MILD.** Often a mild, nonmedicated shampoo is enough to control the problem. Dandruff is frequently caused by an overly oily scalp, says hair-care specialist Philip Kingsley. Washing daily with a mild brand of shampoo, diluted with an equal amount of water, can control the oil without aggravating your scalp.

■ **THEN GET TOUGH.** If regular shampoos aren't doing the job, switch to a dandruff-fighting formula. Dandruff shampoos

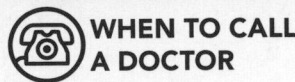

WHEN TO CALL A DOCTOR

Severe dandruff is actually a disease known as seborrheic dermatitis, which requires prescription medications. So, see a doctor if you have:

■ Scalp irritation

■ Thick scale despite regular use of dandruff shampoos

■ Yellowish crusting

■ Red patches, especially along the neckline

The Biology of Dandruff

Dandruff is characterized by accelerated cell turnover. In other words, the cells on the surface of your skin build up like crazy.

"Typically, it takes 21 days for new cells to migrate to the surface of your scalp, where they are shed," says Yohini Appa, Ph.D. "Ideally, it's an invisible process. But with dandruff, the cell reaches the surface in half the time." As a result, cells build up on your scalp in clumps before they're shed. And when they do shed, they look like tiny white flakes.

Another cause is yeast infection of the scalp, says Dr. Appa. And though hormonal and seasonal changes don't cause dandruff, they can exacerbate it, she says.

are classified by their active ingredients, which work in different ways, says Yohini Appa, Ph.D. The tar-based shampoos slow cell production, while salicylic acid–based shampoos slough off dead cells before they clump. And both shampoos have antifungal properties and help fight invading yeast microbes, which is one of dandruff's most persistent triggers. Zinc pyrithione and selenium sulfide reduce cell turnover, while sulfur is believed to cause slight skin irritation—just enough to lead to the shedding of flakes.

■ **BEAT THE TAR OUT OF IT.** "For very stubborn cases, I recommend tar-based formulas," says Dr. Farris. "Lather with the tar shampoo and then leave it on for 5 to 10 minutes so that the tar has a chance to work." Most people rinse dandruff shampoos off too quickly. Two brands to look for are Sebutone Tar Shampoo and MG 217 Medicated Tar Shampoo.

Today's newer tar formulas are much more fragrant than the smelly solutions of old.

■ **DON'T BE TOO HARSH.** If tar-based shampoos—or any other dandruff preparations—are too harsh for everyday use, alternate them with your regular shampoo, suggests Dr. Farris.

■ **DON'T MIX BLACK WITH BLOND.** If you have light-colored hair, think twice about tar-based shampoos. In rare instances, they can give white, blond, bleached, or tinted hair a temporary brownish discoloration, says Dr. Farris.

■ **LATHER TWICE.** Always lather twice with a dandruff shampoo, says R. Jeffrey Herten, M.D. Work up the first lather as soon as you step into the shower. Leave it on until you're just about finished with your shower, then rinse your hair very thoroughly. Follow that with a quick second lather and rinse. The second washing will leave just a bit of the medication on your scalp so that it can work until your next shampoo.

■ **CAP IT.** To improve the effectiveness of medicated shampoos, put a shower cap on over your wet hair after you've lathered up. Leave it on for an hour, then rinse as usual.

■ **SWITCH-HIT.** If you've found a brand of shampoo that works well for you, keep using it, says Howard Donsky, M.D. But don't stock up on one antidandruff shampoo. Your scalp may become immune to a shampoo's active ingredient, a condition called tachyphylaxis,

---

Cures from the Kitchen

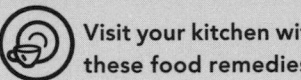 Visit your kitchen with towel in hand to try these food remedies for dandruff:

GREEN TEA. Douse dandruff with a cup of anti-oxidant-packed green tea, which will naturally exfoliate dry flakes without dehydrating skin. Steep two tea bags of green tea in 1 cup of hot water for 20 minutes to overnight. Once it's cooled, massage the strong tea into your scalp.

THYME. A common kitchen herb, thyme is reputed to have mild antiseptic properties that can help alleviate dandruff. Make an effective rinse by boiling 4 heaping tablespoons of dried thyme in 2 cups of water for 10 minutes. Strain the brew and allow it to cool. Pour half the mixture over clean, damp hair, making sure the liquid covers the scalp. Massage in gently. Do not rinse. Save the remainder for another day.

OLIVE OIL. Although excess scalp oil can cause problems, an occasional warm-oil treatment helps loosen and soften dandruff scales, says R. Jeffrey Herten, M.D. Heat a few ounces of olive oil on the stove until just warm. Wet your hair (otherwise the oil will soak into your hair instead of reaching your scalp), then apply the oil directly to your scalp with a brush or cotton ball. Section your hair as you go so that you treat just the scalp. Put on a shower cap and leave it on for 30 minutes. Then wash out the oil with a dandruff shampoo.

---

says Jerome Litt, M.D. Your only recourse is to switch to a new antidandruff shampoo with a different formulation.

■ **MASSAGE IT IN.** When shampooing, says Dr. Farris, gently massage your scalp with your fingertips to help loosen scales and flakes. But don't scratch your scalp, she warns. That can lead to sores that are worse than the dandruff.

■ **FLAKE OFF.** Joseph F. Fowler Jr., M.D., recommends one particular over-the-counter product called Psoriasin Scalp Multi-Symptom Psoriasis Relief Liquid for people with especially stubborn scaling and crusting. Apply it to your scalp at bedtime and cover your hair with a shower cap. Wash it out in the morning. Although you can use this preparation every night, Dr. Fowler recommends once-a-week treatments. "It's just too messy for daily use," he says.

■ **GET INTO CONDITION.** Although dandruff shampoos are effective on your scalp, they can be a little harsh on your hair, says Dr. Farris. So apply conditioner after every shampoo to counteract their effects.

■ **TAP INTO TEA TREE.** Tea tree oil is a natural antiseptic containing substances called terpenes that penetrate the top layers of the scalp, making their disinfectant powers absorb deeper than most. You should look for shampoos that contain tea tree oil, such as Nature's Gate Organics Tea Tree & Blue Cypress Shampoo.

■ **LET THE SUN SHINE.** "A little sun exposure is good for dandruff," says Dr. Fowler. That's because direct ultraviolet light has an anti-inflammatory effect on scaly skin conditions. And it may explain why dandruff tends to be less severe in summer.

But by all means, says Dr. Fowler, use sun sense. Don't sunbathe; just spend a little time outdoors. Limit sun exposure to 30 minutes or less each day. And wear your normal sunscreen on exposed skin. "You have to balance the sun's benefit to your scalp with its harmful effect on your skin in general," he advises.

■ **CALM DOWN.** Don't overlook the role emotions play in triggering or worsening skin conditions such as dandruff and other forms of dermatitis. These conditions are often made worse by stress, says Dr. Fowler. So if your emotions are overtaxed, look for ways to counteract the stress. Exercise. Meditate. Get away from it all. And don't worry so much about your dandruff.

Denture Troubles

20 Ideas for a More Secure Smile

The Etruscans of central Italy invented false teeth nearly 3,000 years ago. They made dentures out of ox teeth, held together with highly visible gold bands. For Etruscans, wearing dentures was nothing to be ashamed of—it was actually a status symbol.

False teeth have come a long way since Etruscan times. Today, with millions of Americans wearing at least partial dentures, choices in dental ware abound. There are partial and full dentures, those that can be removed, and those that are implanted into the bone like real teeth.

All dentures, like any artificial body part, take some getting used to, says George A. Murrell, D.D.S. He and other dental specialists have some helpful suggestions.

■ **LOOK IN THE MIRROR.** Smile. Frown. Be happy. Be sad. Be serious. Practice moving your teeth and lips in private so that you'll be more confident in front of other people, says Dr. Murrell.

■ **PRACTICE TALKING.** "Having dentures is like having a prosthetic limb," says Jerry F. Taintor, D.D.S. "You have to practice using it to use it well." Say your vowels. Recite your consonants. Read aloud to yourself, he says. Listen to your pronunciation and your diction and correct what doesn't sound right.

■ **START SOFT AND SLOW.** No, you're not doomed to baby foods for the rest of your life, but start soft, says Dr. Taintor. Gradually increase the texture and hardness of your food so that your

Cures from the Kitchen

What you put in your mouth (and your stomach) can help with common denture troubles. Try these tasty remedies:

MINT. If your dentures are causing you pain, try mint anything—gum, candies, tea. The herb has a numbing effect on whatever it touches, and can make sore gums feel better.

CHILE PEPPER. Considered the herbal equivalent of aspirin, chile pepper contains capsaicin, a compound that stimulates the release of pain-relieving endorphins. If you're bothered by mouth pain, eat fresh chile or season your food with red pepper flakes.

TEA. Real teeth or dentures, you still have plaque to fight, and doing so will keep your gums healthier and your breath fresher. Tea can help, since it contains numerous compounds that act as antibiotics. Drinking it is a great way to wash away bacteria. Black tea is best; rinsing your mouth with black tea several times a day fights plaque buildup better than swishing with just water.

Dentures and Drugs

Drugs that cause dry mouth can contribute to denture pain, says Gretchen Gibson, D.D.S. Without enough saliva, your dentures will rub against your gums and cause discomfort.

Medications that are used to control high blood pressure, like prazosin (Minipress), and antidepressants like amitriptyline (Elavil), are among the common drugs prescribed to seniors that can dry out the mouth and lead to denture discomfort, Dr. Gibson says. Denture pain may also be a side effect of:

- Diuretics such as chlorothiazide (Diuril) or furosemide (Lasix)

- Nitroglycerin (Nitrostat) and other drugs used to control angina

- Oxybutynin (Ditropan) and other drugs used to control urinary incontinence

- Oral steroids used for asthma, like beclomethasone (Beclovent)

gums and your ability to use the dentures build on good experience.

■ **USE AN ADHESIVE.** If you feel that your new teeth are a less-than-perfect fit, there's nothing wrong with using a denture adhesive during the adjustment period, says Dr. Taintor. It's when you have to use the adhesive all the time that you need to have the denture refitted. You can find over-the-counter denture adhesives—a type of soft paste that forms a vacuum between your gums and your dentures to temporarily "glue" them together—in any drugstore.

■ **TRY A LOZENGE.** One common complaint among denture wearers, says Dr. Murrell, is excess saliva during the first few weeks of wearing dentures. Solve this problem neatly by sucking on lozenges frequently for the first couple of days. This helps you swallow more frequently and gets rid of some of the excess saliva.

■ **GIVE YOUR GUMS A REST.** Don't leave your dentures in too long, especially when they're new. If you develop sore gums, take your dentures out and set them aside for a few days while your gums heal. Then try using the dentures again, suggests Flora Parsa Stay, D.D.S. Take your dentures out for at least 6 hours a day, either while you're sleeping or when you're at home doing household chores, says Dr. Stay.

■ **MAKE A CLEANING COMMITMENT.** If you wear implants, you'll need to set up a twice-daily cleaning ritual just like when you were caring for your original teeth, says Dr. Murrell. "We can do beautiful dentistry, but it won't last if it isn't taken care of."

■ **CLEAN 'EM RIGHT AT NIGHT.** Take your dentures out before bed, brush them thoroughly with a denture cleanser, then place them in a glass of water overnight. Avoid using regular toothpastes, because they are too abrasive for most dentures, according to Kenneth Shay, D.D.S. These pastes can damage your dentures to the point that they don't fit properly, which will cause sore gums.

■ **BABY YOUR MOUTH.** "Babies are born with plaque in their mouths," says Eric Shapira, D.D.S. "Even if you have no teeth, you need to wash your gums to remove the plaque." Use a soft brush and gently whisk your gums, but not too hard—you don't want to make the inside of your mouth sore. A good cleaning lowers the possibility of bad breath and helps your gums stay healthier, he says.

■ **MAKE A VIDEO.** A video is valuable for several reasons, says Dr. Murrell. It can give you a stranger's-eye view of how you look. Plus you can show the tape to a dentist, who can look at it to decipher problems in jaw muscles or lip movements.

■ **WATCH OUT FOR TOOTHPICKS.** Those tiny wooden spikes are especially dangerous for denture wearers, says Dr. Taintor. "You lose a lot of your tactile sense with dentures. You bite into a toothpick, but you don't know it because you can't feel it. You can get it accidentally lodged in your throat."

■ **MASSAGE YOUR GUMS.** Place your thumb and index finger over your gums (index on the outside) and massage them. This promotes circulation and gives your gums a healthy firmness.

■ **RINSE WITH SALTY WATER.** To help you to clean your gums, rinse your mouth daily with 1 teaspoon of salt in a glass of warm water, says Dr. Taintor.

■ **DOUSE THE ACHE.** Take out your dentures, then rinse your mouth three times a day with a ½ cup of rinse made with goldenseal, a potent herbal remedy, to help soothe denture pain, Dr. Stay says. To prepare the rinse, add ½ tablespoon of dried goldenseal and ½ teaspoon of baking soda to ½ cup of warm water. Cool and strain before using.

■ **SEEK HERBAL SOOTHING.** Dab a bit of aloe vera gel or eucalyptus oil on a cotton swab and apply it to the spots on your gums where the dentures are rubbing, suggests Dr. Stay. These products help soothe and heal sore gums. You can use them as needed, but for best results, avoid eating for at least 1 hour after application.

■ **RULE OUT ALLERGIES.** Some people are allergic to denture cleansers and adhesives, says Dr. Stay. A few are even allergic to materials in the dentures themselves. There may be a burning sensation in the mouth, and allergies can irritate the gums and cause mouth ulcers. If you suspect you have an allergy, ask your dentist about other cleansers and adhesives you can use. Try them out one by one and see whether the irritation subsides. If there's no change, leave your dentures out and see what happens. If the dentures are the cause of the pain, you may need new dentures that are made with different materials, Dr. Stay says.

■ **EXPECT CHANGE.** Over time, your dentures may not fit as well as they once did, says Dr. Shay. No matter what your age, your gums continue to change over time, and as they do, dentures that once fit like a glove may begin to feel like hippo teeth. These dentures will need to be adjusted or replaced.

PANEL OF ADVISORS

GRETCHEN GIBSON, D.D.S., IS DIRECTOR OF THE GERIATRIC DENTISTRY PROGRAM AT THE VETERANS ADMINISTRATION MEDICAL CENTER IN DALLAS.

GEORGE A. MURRELL, D.D.S., IS A RETIRED PROSTHODONTIST IN MANHATTAN BEACH, CALIFORNIA. HE ALSO HAS TAUGHT AT THE UNIVERSITY OF SOUTHERN CALIFORNIA SCHOOL OF DENTISTRY IN LOS ANGELES.

ERIC SHAPIRA, D.D.S., IS A DENTIST IN THE SAN FRANCISCO BAY AREA AND A SPOKESPERSON FOR THE ACADEMY OF GENERAL DENTISTRY.

KENNETH SHAY, D.D.S., IS CHIEF OF DENTAL SERVICES AT THE VETERANS AFFAIRS MEDICAL CENTER IN ANN ARBOR.

FLORA PARSA STAY, D.D.S., IS A DENTIST IN OXNARD, CALIFORNIA, AND AUTHOR OF *THE COMPLETE BOOK OF DENTAL REMEDIES*.

JERRY F. TAINTOR, D.D.S., IS FORMER CHAIR OF ENDODONTICS AT THE UNIVERSITY OF TENNESSEE COLLEGE OF DENTISTRY IN MEMPHIS AND UCLA SCHOOL OF DENTISTRY. HE IS AUTHOR OF *THE COMPLETE GUIDE TO BETTER DENTAL CARE*.

Depression

34 Mood Lifters

It would be nice if blue moods came only once in a blue moon. But life happens. The breakup of a relationship, the loss of a job, and other bumps and knocks on the road of life can make a mood shift from rosy to blue.

"We have a range of emotions, and feeling depressed at times, for short periods, is very normal," says Bernard Vittone, M.D.

But for the more than 20 million Americans who experience depression, the blues just don't go away.

If you and your doctor agree that your depression is mild, experts offer many ways to boost your mood. Even if you're being treated for chronic or severe depression, the following strategies just may help you.

■ **GET EDUCATED.** Learn more about depression and look for signs of wellness. Read books, listen to tapes, or watch videos. Education helps you realize that you're not alone and that the condition you have is really very common, says Edward M. Hallowell, M.D.

■ **EXPRESS YOURSELF.** The opposite of depression is expression. The blues often result from a pattern of suppressing and then repressing feelings, says Dr. Hallowell. Release your feelings through art, music, or anything creative.

■ **GET OUT.** Of the house, that is. Aim for a few hours out and about every day, says Dr. Vittone. Being in the same place too long, particularly if you're alone, is a breeding ground for depressive

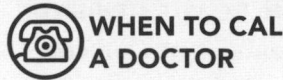 **WHEN TO CALL A DOCTOR**

See a doctor if you are depressed most of the time for 2 or more weeks, even though you haven't experienced a significant loss, such as the death of a loved one. Also seek help if you have experienced a loss and your depression continues for several months, or if you have intermittent bouts of depression for more than 2 years. Be sure to have a physical to rule out other possible illnesses such as hypothyroidism or anemia.

Symptoms of depression include feeling hopeless, helpless, sad, or blue; losing interest in previously enjoyable activities; or having an inability to be cheered by normally happy events. Other signs include insomnia, changes in appetite, low energy, poor concentration, irritability, a negative attitude, and frequent feelings of guilt. Know, too, that symptoms of depression and anxiety (page 27) often overlap.

thoughts and symptoms. Visit the library, go shopping, see a movie. Stimulation is important for people with depression, he says. Researchers speculate that stimulation keeps the brain's feel-good neurotransmitters, such as serotonin, flowing.

■ **BE WITH FRIENDS.** Socialize at least twice a week, Dr. Vittone says. Don't just schedule business meetings, client lunches, or conference calls. Get together with people to talk, laugh, and relax. You'll be firing up those feel-good neurotransmitters. Although researchers aren't sure *how* socialization affects nerve chemicals, says Dr. Vittone, they do know that they're helpful.

■ **GET YOUR CHUCKLES.** Watch a comedy show on TV, see a funny movie, or catch a comedian on stage. Happiness is contagious, says Dr. Vittone.

■ **LET IT BE.** It's okay to feel *anything*, says Dr. Hallowell. There are no "bad" feelings. Accepting how you feel helps you get past it. Similarly, remind yourself that feelings change and that you will survive.

■ **GET GOING.** Depression causes a huge amount of inertia. It makes it hard to get out of bed in the morning and may tempt you to become a couch potato. But don't, says Dr. Vittone. Instead, get moving. Exercise helps banish the blues.

Walk, jog, bicycle, swim, cross-country ski, or participate in other aerobic-type activities such as classes at your local fitness center. Aim for 20 to 30 minutes, four or five times a week. Or try yoga, tai chi, or stretching about three times a week to loosen your body, relieve stress, and get you smiling again. And even better, mix it up.

Some doctors believe that exercise, especially aerobic, produces endorphins, the body's natural antidepressants. "We don't really know why exercise works," says Dr. Vittone. "We only know that it does."

■ **TAKE TIME TO HEAL.** Be patient with yourself. Sometimes you'll take a step forward; other days you'll take two steps backward. Healing never occurs in a straight line. Remember that tomorrow is another day when you can try again.

■ **STICK TO A SCHEDULE.** Alternating rest with activity brings healing by restoring the body's natural rhythms. For example, go to sleep and get up at about the same time every day. When your inner world is chaotic, maintaining a schedule gives you some sense of order, says Dr. Hallowell.

■ **SLEEP.** Lack of sleep may cause depressive-like symptoms, such as lack of concentration and low energy, or exacerbate existing depression. Gauge how much sleep you need by how rested you feel.

■ **USE SOME COMMON SCENTS.** Well we've all heard the benefits of aromatherapy, but do you know which odors can actually lift your spirits? Research shows us that lemon, orange, peppermint, and lavender scents just may help remedy mild feelings of depression as much as an antidepressant.

Cures from the Kitchen

Stock up on sardines, herring, mackerel, wild salmon, kippers, and other fish from cold northern waters, says Andrew Weil, M.D. These fish are high in omega-3 fatty acids. Research shows that low levels of the fatty acids may underlie some psychiatric illnesses, such as depression. "In fact, there's some evidence suggesting that the rising levels of depression in the Western world in recent decades may be related to a low omega-3 intake," he says.

■ **BE AN OPTIMIST.** Be optimistic, even if you don't believe it at first, says Dr. Vittone. Your attitude is likely to become a self-fulfilling prophecy. If you expect a positive outcome, you're more likely to act in ways that make that happen, and other people are more inclined to respond favorably. The way we think directly affects our moods, he says.

■ **STAY CURRENT.** Tune in to the TV or radio news. Pick up a newspaper or magazine. Keeping up with current events helps you feel more involved in life around you, says Dr. Vittone. One caveat: Limit viewing or reading about traumatic events, such as September 11, to 30 minutes at a time. Viewing too much bad news, he says, isn't good.

■ **SEEK OUT A SIBLING.** A survey conducted by Kutztown University of Pennsylvania found that 60 percent of respondents who said they had close relationships with brothers or sisters were less lonely and depressed and had higher self-esteem compared with those who had poor sibling con-nections. Even those with few friends and who confessed to being lonely still tended to report healthy levels of well-being as long as they felt they could count on their siblings.

■ **DON'T DECIDE NOW.** Keep decision making to a minimum when you're feeling low. Decisions are less clear when you're depressed than when you're feeling your best.

■ **FORGIVE YOURSELF.** Even with mild depression, forgetfulness and clumsiness are common. Try to laugh at silly mistakes and keep in mind that your nervous system is not at its best.

■ **GET A MASSAGE.** When you're feeling blue, you may feel as if your mind and body are disconnected. A healing touch—once a week if possible—helps reconnect mind, body, and spirit, says Dr. Hallowell.

■ **WALK IT OFF.** Researchers found that a quick walk can temporarily boost your liveliness and improve your well-being. After only half an hour, your brain's levels of serotonin—a feel-good chemical—will increase, and you'll get an extra boost from knowing you've done something good for yourself.

■ **REAFFIRM BELIEFS.** Research shows that spirituality can improve mood, whether you pray, attend services, or read uplifting materials. Spirituality restores hope.

■ **DON'T LAY BLAME.** No matter what mistakes you think you've made, forgive yourself. Treat yourself with kindness, and never give in to regret. Everybody has failures. Guilt is self-punishment that you don't deserve.

Have a Cookie—Really

Scientists have an explanation for that burst of good cheer from eating your grandmother's cookies. Studies at MIT have shown that snacking on readily digested carbohydrates, such as those in a cookie or bagel, can raise the brain's level of the chemical serotonin, the very same target of modern antidepressant medications. "Cookies can brighten your spirits when eaten judiciously," says psychologist Thomas Crook, Ph.D.

Try this to raise your mood-lifting serotonin levels a couple of times a day:

Have a small carbohydrate snack about 3 or 4 hours after each meal and about 1 hour before your next meal. Make sure that your stomach is empty and that you eat no protein between meals. The carbohydrates should be easily digestible—such as one or two oatmeal cookies, a third of a bagel, or a slice of whole wheat bread. "This will cause tryptophan in your blood to enter the brain, where it's metabolized into serotonin, and elevated serotonin will improve your mood within 20 to 30 minutes," says Dr. Crook.

■ **TRY SHOCK THERAPY.** Consider taking a vacation, says Dr. Vittone. Even 3 days at the beach, for example, may be enough to jolt you out of a mild depression. Alternately, take mini vacations throughout the day. When your mood is low, find a minute or two to picture where you'd like to be. Immerse yourself in the sights, sounds, feelings, and scents of that special locale. "It will give you a little lift," he says.

■ **BE THANKFUL.** Remind yourself what's good in life. Each day, jot down five things for which you're grateful. "Try to find things, little or big, that you appreciate," says Dr. Vittone. When we feel blue, we tend to overlook the good things in life.

■ **MAKE SOMEONE'S DAY.** One way to feel good about yourself is to make someone else feel good. Give a compliment, create a bond, or smile at a stranger. "You'll walk away feeling better," says Dr. Vittone, "and the other person will feel good, too."

■ **FIND SOME FLOWERS.** A Harvard Medical School study showed that people who receive flowers feel a quick mood lift, and within a week feel a drop in sadness and anxiety. It's thought that the beauty of flowers is naturally inspiring and pleasing.

■ **LOOK FORWARD.** Try to have at least one substantial activity at the end of each week that you can anticipate with enthusiasm. Plan a day trip, a shopping excursion, or dinner at a favorite restaurant. When you feel blue, remind yourself of your plans.

■ **EAT HEALTHFULLY.** Choose a balanced diet rich in complex carbohydrates (such as

D

fruits, vegetables, and whole grains), lean protein, and some fat. These foods provide the nutrients our bodies need to produce the chemicals that help maintain normal mood states, says Dr. Vittone. Don't reach for too much or too little of anything. Moderation is the key.

■ **DRINK MORE WATER.** If you're suffering from low energy, make sure you're getting enough water. "Half of the people who come to me complaining of fatigue are actually dehydrated," says Woodson Merrell, M.D. Aim for six to eight glasses of water a day.

■ **B DILIGENT.** A lack of B vitamins is sometimes associated with depressive symptoms, such as fatigue, poor concentration, or moodiness. Take a multivitamin/mineral supplement that's high in the Bs, including folic acid, B_6, and B_{12}. Folic acid may even increase the effectiveness of antidepressant medications, says Andrew Weil, M.D. He recommends that your supplement contain about 400 micrograms of folic acid.

■ **TRY ST. JOHN'S WORT.** Many studies show that this herbal remedy improves mild depression, says Dr. Weil. The recommended dosage is 300 milligrams of standardized extract of 0.125 percent hypericum, three times a day with meals. "Be prepared to wait several months before you see the full benefit," he adds.

■ **SAMPLE SAM-E.** This dietary supplement, which is short for S-adenosylmethionine, helps regulate some hormones and the neurochemicals that are important to mood: serotonin, melatonin, dopamine, and adrenaline, Dr. Weil says. In Europe, where it is a prescription drug, SAM-e (pronounced "Sammy") is widely used to treat depression. Compared with antidepressant drugs, SAM-e works quickly, and patients often feel the effects within a week. But it's pricey and doesn't work for everyone, he notes. If you want to try SAM-e, take 1,600 milligrams of the butanedisulfonate form daily on an empty stomach. Because SAM-e may increase blood levels of homocysteine, a significant risk factor for cardiovascular disease, this supplement should be taken with folic acid and vitamins B_6 and B_{12} to keep homocysteine levels down.

■ **AVOID ALCOHOL.** Alcohol is a central-nervous-system depressant. After a drink, you may feel better at first. Later, depression may worsen, leading to a vicious cycle of drinking to chase away the blues, followed by more depressive feelings, followed by more drinking. Limit alcohol to one or two drinks at a time, Dr. Vittone says, "and definitely not every day."

■ **SPRUCE UP.** Spend time on grooming. Buy an outfit that enhances a positive outlook. "You'll feel better," Dr. Weil says. For women, add some color to your lips *and* your mood. Researchers have found that applying lipstick improves self-image and instantly makes you feel more vibrant. Colorful lips help you feel more attractive, and that feels good.

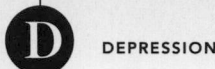

PANEL OF ADVISORS

THOMAS CROOK, PH.D., IS A CLINICAL PSYCHOLOGIST AND CEO OF COGNITIVE RESEARCH CORP. IN ST. PETERSBURG, FLORIDA. HE IS A FORMER RESEARCH PROGRAM DIRECTOR AT THE NATIONAL INSTITUTE OF MENTAL HEALTH.

EDWARD M. HALLOWELL, M.D., IS A PSYCHIATRIST AND FOUNDER OF THE HALLOWELL CENTERS FOR COGNITIVE AND EMOTIONAL HEALTH IN SUDBURY, MASSACHUSETTS, AND NEW YORK CITY. HE IS THE AUTHOR OF *WORRY: HOPE AND HELP FOR A COMMON CONDITION* AND *CONNECT: 12 VITAL TIES THAT OPEN YOUR HEART, LENGTHEN YOUR LIFE, AND DEEPEN YOUR SOUL.*

WOODSON MERRELL, M.D., IS A CLINICAL ASSISTANT PROFESSOR OF MEDICINE AT COLUMBIA UNIVERSITY COLLEGE OF PHYSICIANS AND SURGEONS AND EXECU- TIVE DIRECTOR OF THE CONTINUUM CENTER FOR HEALTH AND HEALING, BOTH IN NEW YORK CITY. HE IS AUTHOR OF *THE SOURCE: UNLEASH YOUR NATURAL ENERGY, POWER UP YOUR HEALTH AND FEEL 10 YEARS YOUNGER.*

BERNARD VITTONE, M.D., IS A PSYCHIATRIST AND FOUNDER AND DIRECTOR OF THE NATIONAL CENTER FOR THE TREATMENT OF PHOBIAS, ANXIETY, AND DEPRESSION IN WASHINGTON, D.C.

ANDREW WEIL, M.D., IS A CLINICAL PROFESSOR OF MED- ICINE AND DIRECTOR OF THE INTEGRATIVE MEDICINE PROGRAM AT THE UNIVERSITY OF ARIZONA IN TUCSON. HE IS THE AUTHOR OF SEVERAL BOOKS, INCLUDING *8 WEEKS TO OPTIMUM HEALTH* AND *NATURAL HEALTH, NATURAL MEDICINE.*

Dermatitis and Eczema

29 Clear-Skin Remedies

Eczema is sometimes called "the itch that rashes." That's because rather than a rash that itches, here the reverse is true: Scratching produces the rash. While eczema may look different from person to person, it usually shows up as dry, red, extremely itchy patches on the skin.

One of the most common forms of eczema is atopic dermatitis, which afflicts about 1 out of every 10 kids and becomes a chronic disease of adulthood that waxes and wanes in an unlucky few.

Although scientists still do not fully understand what causes eczema, it appears to be an abnormal inflammatory response of the immune system to an irritant, which can be anything from pet dander to rough fabrics to detergents. Some people can learn to avoid triggers, but for many the best strategy is to control the itching and dryness that typically accompany these physician-diagnosed skin conditions.

The experts tell us that, in general, the best way to treat the itching of eczema at home is to keep any patches of dry skin moist and well lubricated. For that reason, many of the remedies offered in Dry Skin and Winter Itch, on page 225, may help with this problem as well.

■ **BEWARE OF DRY AIR.** Eczema is aggravated by dehumidified air, especially during winter months when forced-air heat circulates in the home.

"Forced-air heat is a bit more drying than other types of heat,"

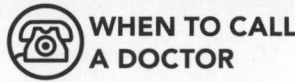
**WHEN TO CALL
A DOCTOR**

When eczema is severe or widespread, and lotions, home remedies, and over-the-counter medications don't relieve the itching, visit a dermatologist. Many prescription medicines can help. A physician will also be able to rule out other causes for your eczema. Lupus, an autoimmune disorder, is one such disease, leaving a patchy, red skin rash, roughly resembling a butterfly, on the cheeks or bridge of the nose. As one patch heals, a new one forms. These lesions itch and form scales. A person with lupus may experience severe arthritic joint pain, fever, and lung inflammation. If you recognize these symptoms, contact your physician immediately.

Also, if oozing eczema, also known as weeping eczema, does not respond quickly to cold compresses applied several times a day, consult your physician, says John F. Romano, M.D.

says dermatologist Howard Donsky, M.D. Because dry air tends to aggravate the itching of eczema or dermatitis, keeping indoor air moist should be a priority for sufferers and their families. "If you can counter dry air with a good humidifier, then forced-air heat is not as much of a problem," he notes.

However, don't expect a single-room humidifier to provide enough moist air for you entire home. Humidifiers are like air conditioners—you really need a big unit to do anything. If you have a room humidifier, sleep next to it for it to be effective. Try putting one next to your bed.

"A less expensive option is to set several shallow pans of water near the radiators in the bedroom," says dermatologist Nelson Lee Novick, M.D. "The heat will cause the water to evaporate and humidify the air."

■ **MAKE BATHWATER LUKEWARM.** A lukewarm bath helps to cleanse and moisturize your skin without overdrying. Baths or showers that are steamy or longer than 10 minutes will aggravate your condition. And always remember to use a moisturizer within 3 minutes of getting out of the tub.

■ **MOISTURIZE.** "You're better off using soapless soaps or cleansers labeled for sensitive skin," says Dr. Novick. "These nondetergent products are less likely to strip your skin of its all-important natural oils and moisturizing factors that lock water in."

It's also best to follow up with a moisturizer to keep your skin from drying out, Dr.

Novick adds. "You can't bathe too frequently if you grease up afterward," he says. "The moisturizer is what holds the water in, and dry skin is a function of water loss, not of oil loss."

Good options for after-bath lotions include Complex-15, Eucerin, Keri, Lubriderm Lotion, and Moisturel Lotion. If your skin still seems dry after using one of those products, move up to creams such as Lubriderm, Purpose, or Moisturel, or ointments such as Aquaphor, Eucerin, or Nivea.

For dry skin that's even more stubborn, Dr. Novick suggests trying some dermal lotions such as Amlactin or LacHydrin. These products contain 15 percent ammonium lactate, a powerful alpha hydroxy acid that holds on to water in the skin.

■ **TAKE AN OATMEAL BATH.** For an additional soothing treat, Dr. Donsky recommends adding colloidal oatmeal products such as Aveeno to the bath, and even using oatmeal as a soap substitute. For bathing, pour 2 cups of colloidal oatmeal (available at drugstores) into a tub of lukewarm water. The term *colloidal* simply means that the oatmeal has been ground to a fine powder that will remain suspended in water. For use as a soap substitute, wrap colloidal oatmeal in a handkerchief, place a rubber band around the top, dunk it in water, and use as you would a washcloth.

■ **SPRITZ YOURSELF.** To soothe skin instantly, spritz it with mineral water, says dermatologist Christopher Dannaker, M.D. Studies show that mineral-rich springwater relieves the

Cures from the Kitchen

 Relief from dermatitis and eczema may be as close as your pantry or refrigerator:

AVOCADO. The oil of the avocado is actually patented as a treatment for some forms of dermatitis, and some herbalists believe it helps relieve eczema, too. "Avocado oil is rich in vitamins A, D, and E, all of which help maintain healthy skin," says James Duke, Ph.D., in his book *The Green Pharmacy*. He suggests applying it directly to any itchy, red, or irritated areas.

CUCUMBER. "Cool as a cucumber? That's not just a figure of speech," says Dr. Duke. Cucumber has long been used for soothing dermatitis. Dr. Duke suggests blending peeled cucumbers (and maybe some avocados, too) in a blender or food processor and applying the puree directly to the affected area, leaving it on for 15 to 60 minutes.

MILK. Cold, wet compresses can help soothe and relieve the itching associated with eczema that gets so bad that it begins to ooze. "I tell people to try cold milk instead of water," says John F. Romano, M.D. "It seems to be a lot more soothing."

His recommendation: Pour milk into a glass with ice cubes and let it sit for a few minutes. Then pour the milk onto a gauze pad or thin piece of cotton and apply it to the irritated skin for 2 to 3 minutes. Resoak the cloth and reapply, continuing the process for about 10 minutes.

OLIVE OIL. "Soothe eczema flare-ups by applying olive oil directly to the irritated area," says Christopher Dannaker, M.D. "Rub in 1 teaspoon per square inch," he says. "It creates a seal so skin won't dry out." Olive oil is the basis of many moisturizers—but used alone, it lacks chemical irritants you may find in store-bought creams. For serious cases, cover oil-slathered skin with plastic wrap overnight.

TEA. If you have itchy eczema, try steeping, cooling, and splashing on a bit of Red Zinger tea, says Dr. Duke. The red color of this tea comes from hibiscus flowers, known to shamanistic healers in the Amazon as a powerful treatment for eczema.

pain, itching, and redness from rashes. "Mist it onto irritated skin and its trace minerals will work as anti-inflammatories," he says.

■ **AVOID ANTIPERSPIRANTS.** Metallic salts such as aluminum chloride, aluminum sulfate, and zirconium chlorohydrate are the active ingredients in many antiperspirants, and these can cause irritation in people with sensitive skin. "Usually it's the antiperspirant, as opposed to the deodorant, that's irritating," Dr. Donsky says. Look for products that do not contain aluminum zirconium, such as Tom's of Maine, Nature Gate's Organics, and Arm & Hammer Essentials Natural deodorant.

■ **TRY THIS OVER-THE-COUNTER CREAM.** Topical creams, ointments, and lotions containing cortisone are often used to alleviate the itching and inflammation of eczema. Hydrocortisone is the mildest member of the cortisone family of steroid hormones, and it's available in drugstores.

"Half-percent (0.5) hydrocortisone cream is available without a prescription," says Dr. Novick, "and that can help." If that doesn't give relief, he suggests trying 1 percent hydrocortisone cream (Cortaid, Cortizone 10), which is also available over the counter.

■ **TAKE VITAMIN E.** This popular supplement is widely touted for skin problems and is an ingredient in many skin creams and cosmetics. In particular, vitamin E has been shown to clear up dermatitis, according to James Duke, Ph.D. Try taking 400 IUs of vitamin E a day.

The Power of Prevention

Women who have atopic dermatitis may wish to protect their children from the same fate. An analysis by Israeli researchers of 18 scientific studies offers hope. The researchers found powerful evidence that, in families with a history of atopic dermatitis, exclusively breastfeeding for the first 3 months can go a long way to protect infants from developing the condition during childhood.

The preventive role of breastfeeding was less powerful in the general population and "negligible" in babies with no first-degree relatives who had experienced atopic dermatitis.

■ **COOL WITH CALAMINE.** "Calamine lotion is good for many types of rashes that ooze and may need to be dried out," says John F. Romano, M.D. "Also, calamine lotion with menthol or phenol added to it can be purchased over-the-counter, and that seems to help itching better than calamine lotion alone."

■ **TAKE COMFORT IN COTTON.** Cotton clothing worn next to the skin is much better than polyester, and especially better than wool, says Dr. Romano. The bottom line: Avoid synthetics or itchy fabrics as well as tight- or ill-fitting clothing.

■ **PUT YOUR DIET TO THE TEST.** "Food allergies can play a big role in atopic dermatitis during childhood," says Dr. Novick. "They are intimately related before age 6, and you can manipulate an infant's diet and do well in helping his skin."

Traditionally, eggs, orange juice, and milk have been implicated as eczema aggravators in children. But, says Dr. Novick, "I certainly wouldn't incriminate those foods wholesale."

That means parents should consult their physicians about trying elimination diets, just to be sure. Such diets seem to work best in children younger than 2 years old, he says. "After age 6, we've found that food plays a minimal role in most people."

For adults, Dr. Novick says that he leaves diet manipulation largely in the hands of his patients. If you find a food you eat has an adverse effect on your skin, avoid it and see what happens, he says. If your problem clears up, you may have a food allergy.

■ **TRY BOOSTING YOUR OMEGA-3 INTAKE.** Salmon, mackerel, and tuna contain omega-3s and other essential fatty acids that may help to prevent allergies and inflammation, both of which are associated with eczema.

■ **AVOID QUICK CHANGES IN AIR TEMPERATURE.** "If you have eczema," says Dr. Donsky, "rapid temperature changes can be a problem." Simply going from a warm room out into the cold winter air, or even from an air-conditioned room in to a hot shower, can trigger itching. Wearing layers of clothing—

cotton clothing—and avoiding hot baths or showers are the best ways to protect yourself, says Dr. Donsky.

■ **BEWARE OF BABY LOTIONS.** "Sometimes baby lotions aren't the best thing for childhood eczema," Dr. Romano says. "They have a high water content, and that can further dry and irritate the skin as evaporation takes place." Some of the fragrances and active ingredients in baby lotions (lanolin and mineral oil) are common causes of skin allergy.

"What you want instead are creams or ointments," explains Dr. Romano. "Something like Eucerin cream, Aquaphor, or Vaseline Dermatology Formula."

■ **READ LABELS FOR UREA.** "Emollients that contain urea are pretty good for relieving the itch of eczema or dermatitis," says Dr. Novick. "Urea is a sloughing agent, and it's a good product. We usually use it when the skin is a little thick from rubbing and scratching."

A couple of urea-containing products to try include Carmol 10 or 20 and Ultra Mide 25. Emollients that contain lactic acid (Lacti-Care 1 percent or 2 percent or Lac-Hydrin Five) are also recommended.

■ **GIVE YOUR SKIN LIPID SERVICE.** Tough cases of eczema deserve a trial with a new breed of over-the-counter moisturizers, according to Dr. Novick. Somewhat more expensive than their counterparts, these creams—which include Mymex, Epiceram, and Tricerim—replenish the skin with lost or depleted lipids. In addition, they appear to pos-

sess anti-inflammatory properties to help reduce irritation and itching, Dr. Novick adds.

■ **DRINK OREGON GRAPE TEA.** Oregon grape root, sold in health food stores, is known for its antihistamine, anti-inflammatory, and antifungal properties. Add 1 tablespoon of the dried root to 1 cup of boiling water. Continue boiling for 10 minutes. Strain and drink every morning, adding dried chamomile for extra flavor. Herbalists say that this remedy may take more than a year, or as little as 3 months, to have a significant benefit for the skin.

■ **USE ANTIHISTAMINES.** Antihistamines are used to block the release of histamine from mast cells, and this reduces such classic allergy symptoms as headache, runny nose, and itching. For that reason, "over-the-counter antihistamines such as Benadryl are good for eczema," says Dr. Romano.

Andy Spooner, M.D., recommends Children's Benadryl Allergy Fastmelts. Kids like the way they dissolve on the tongue (no swallowing required), and they're effective for adults, too. Check the label for dosage.

Antihistamines reduce itching by preventing histamine from reaching and swelling sensitive skin cells. Follow label directions and be aware that antihistamines can cause drowsiness, leading to possible problems with driving or handling machinery.

■ **WASH ONCE, RINSE TWICE.** When it comes to doing laundry for people with eczema or dermatitis, it's not the detergent so much as the rinse, says Dr. Romano.

Got a Nickel Rash?

Eczema, or atopic dermatitis, is one type of skin rash, and doctors aren't quite sure what causes it. Another type, called contact dermatitis, is clearly caused by, you guessed it, contact with an irritant. One example of contact dermatitis is poison ivy. Another, increasingly common type is nickel rash.

"Nickel dermatitis is probably the most common contact dermatitis going," says Howard Donsky, M.D. "But people often don't suspect that it's the problem—they believe they have a problem with gold."

Nickel dermatitis occurs 10 times more often in women than men and is often triggered by ear piercing. Strangely enough, having the ears pierced can cause rashes to occur in other areas of the body that touch nickel-containing metal. Suddenly, bracelets, necklaces, and other jewelry worn for years can bring on a contact rash.

If this sounds like what's happening to you, the following tips might help.

Buy posts of stainless steel. Newly pierced ears should be studded only with steel posts until the earlobes heal (about 3 weeks).

Stay cool. Since perspiration plays a big role in nickel dermatitis—it leaches out the nickel in nickel-plated jewelry—don't get overheated if you're wearing this type of jewelry. Or don't wear it if you're going out in the heat of the day.

Go for the gold. Buy only quality gold jewelry, says Dr. Donsky. "If it's less than 24-karat gold, there's some nickel in there," he says, "and the lower the karat, the higher the nickel."

Consider dietary changes. Some European dermatologists advise nickel-sensitive patients to watch what they eat. Having observed that nickel dermatitis can occur without any apparent contact with the metal, the doctors tell folks to avoid apricots, chocolate, coffee, beer, tea, nuts, and other foods high in nickel.

While intriguing, the theory hasn't garnered a great following on this side of the Atlantic. "The jury's still out on foods high in nickel causing a reaction," Dr. Donsky confirms. "But if you're highly sensitive to nickel, there might be some validity to it."

"You have to make sure the detergent is washed out thoroughly," he says. "Don't use too much detergent when washing, and always use a second rinse cycle to get all the soap out."

■ **GET TO KNOW YOUR EYE DOCTOR.** In a 20-year study of 492 people at the Mayo Clinic in Rochester, Minnesota, 13 percent of those with atopic dermatitis developed cataracts. "There is a higher incidence of cataracts in people with atopic dermatitis," Dr. Novick confirms. So see your ophthalmologist regularly.

PANEL OF ADVISORS

CHRISTOPHER DANNAKER, M.D., IS AN ASSISTANT PROFESSOR OF DERMATOLOGY AT THE UNIVERSITY OF CALIFORNIA IN SAN FRANCISCO AND A DERMATOLOGIST AT MONTEREY DERMATOLOGY AND LIPOSUCTION LASER MEDICAL CENTER IN MONTEREY AND BEVERLY HILLS.

HOWARD DONSKY, M.D., IS A CLINICAL INSTRUCTOR OF DERMATOLOGY AT THE UNIVERSITY OF ROCHESTER SCHOOL OF MEDICINE AND DENTISTRY. HE IS A DERMATOLOGIST AT THE DERMATOLOGY AND COSMETIC CENTER OF ROCHESTER IN NEW YORK AND AUTHOR OF *BEAUTY IS SKIN DEEP.*

JAMES DUKE, PH.D., HELD SEVERAL POSTS IN HIS MORE THAN THREE DECADES WITH THE USDA, INCLUDING CHIEF OF THE MEDICINAL PLANT RESOURCES LABORATORY. HE IS AUTHOR OF *THE GREEN PHARMACY.*

NELSON LEE NOVICK, M.D., IS A CLINICAL PROFESSOR OF DERMATOLOGY AT MOUNT SINAI SCHOOL OF MEDICINE IN NEW YORK CITY.

JOHN F. ROMANO, M.D., IS AN ASSISTANT PROFESSOR OF DERMATOLOGY AT THE WEIL MEDICAL COLLEGE OF CORNELL UNIVERSITY AND AN ATTENDING PHYSICIAN AT NEW YORK PRESBYTERIAN HOSPITAL AND ST. VINCENT'S HOSPITAL, ALL IN NEW YORK CITY. HE HAS A PRACTICE IN MANHATTAN.

ANDY SPOONER, M.D., IS DIRECTOR OF THE DIVISION OF GENERAL PEDIATRICS IN THE COLLEGE OF MEDICINE AT THE UNIVERSITY OF TENNESSEE HEALTH SCIENCE CENTER IN MEMPHIS AND A FELLOW OF THE AMERICAN ACADEMY OF PEDIATRICS.

Diabetes

55 Ways to Steady Blood Sugar

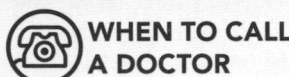

WHEN TO CALL A DOCTOR

Diabetes is a serious illness that requires a doctor's care, even when it is well controlled. In addition, three complications of diabetes require *prompt* medical attention:

■ Severe hyperglycemia (high blood sugar), characterized by frequent urination, fatigue, unexplainable weight loss, and increased thirst.

■ Hypoglycemia, which causes shakiness, dizziness, headache, confusion, sudden mood changes, and a tingling sensation around the mouth. Many people with diabetes experience hypoglycemia, but frequent or severe episodes require a doctor's care.

■ Ketoacidosis, the warning signs of which include increased thirst, nausea, frequent urination, fatigue, and vomiting. This is a serious, potentially life-threatening condition that occurs when ketones—acids that build up in the blood— become dangerously high.

Most people never give it a second thought—the food they eat is transformed into energy and that's that. Their bodies do all the work for them: digesting the food and converting carbohydrates into a type of sugar called glucose that enters the bloodstream. Next, the pancreas kicks out insulin, a hormone that travels through the body, attaching to receptors on the outside of cells. Once attached, insulin acts like a key that "unlocks" the cell so that glucose can enter it and be used for energy. If the body doesn't need the sugar for energy, it stores it as fat. Usually, this process hums along like a well-oiled machine. People take notice only when the process breaks down.

The monkey wrench that interrupts the flow is diabetes. Nearly 18 million people in the United States were diagnosed with this disease in 2007, a number that's more than tripled in the past 30 years—and may double again by 2050. And new evidence shows that at least 57 million Americans have prediabetes, a condition in which your blood sugar level is higher than normal, but not quite high enough to be classified as full-blown diabetes—not yet, that is.

Diabetes, also known as diabetes mellitus, comes in two forms. Type 1, previously called juvenile diabetes or insulin-dependent diabetes mellitus, is believed to be an autoimmune condition in which the pancreas fails to manufacture insulin. Though onset can occur at any age, patients are usually diagnosed in childhood or as young adults and require daily insulin injections throughout their lives.

People with the other form, type 2, usually develop the disease in adulthood, although more and more children and young adults also are developing type 2 diabetes now. In this case, the pancreas *produces* insulin, but the body does not use it properly, and the pancreas kicks into overdrive to make up for this "resistance." In time, the pancreas can't produce enough insulin to make up for the insensitivity, and diabetes follows. Inactivity, aging, obesity, or a diet high in saturated fat can contribute to insulin resistance. Type 2 diabetes, also known as adult-onset diabetes or noninsulin-dependent diabetes mellitus, accounts for 90 to 95 percent of all cases. With either form of diabetes, glucose builds up in the bloodstream. Left untreated, this can lead to serious complications, including kidney failure, limb amputation, heart disease, and blindness. But the good news is that type 2 diabetes often can be controlled through simple measures. Weight loss, proper nutrition, adequate exercise, and stress reduction all can improve blood glucose levels. Some experts believe that dietary supplements may help, too. Even people with diabetes who require medication will maintain better glucose control if they adhere to a healthy lifestyle. Here's our experts' advice.

NURTURE GOOD NUTRITION

No one nutrition prescription can apply to everyone with diabetes, says Marion Franz, M.S., R.D., L.D., C.D.E. "Each person with diabetes deserves to have an individualized meal plan." The American Diabetes Association (ADA) urges people to consider what ethnic and cultural foods they prefer, what other health concerns they may have (high cholesterol and high blood pressure, for example), and what changes they are realistically willing to make. Working within that framework, people should aim for the following goals.

■ **LOSE WEIGHT.** The most effective thing that an overweight person with type 2 diabetes can do is to drop some pounds, says Christopher D. Saudek, M.D.

Shedding excess pounds is sometimes all it takes to bring blood sugar under control. How much weight to lose varies for each individual, but even small drops can yield big results.

"You don't have to be skinny skinny, and you don't have to reach that ideal body weight," says Carla Miller, Ph.D., R.D. Losing as few as 10 to 20 pounds, or just 5 to 10 percent of your body weight, may be enough to attain glucose control. Of course, you'll have to maintain that weight loss, or your blood sugar will rise again.

And that's why how you trim down is especially important.

Avoid fad diets, says Dr. Saudek. Most are difficult to sustain, and some are not healthy. Your best bet is to combine exercise with a low-calorie diet. Work with a health care professional or a registered dietitian to determine how many calories are right for you.

■ **COUNT CARBS.** The ADA emphasizes that carbohydrates are an important part of a healthful diet. This food group includes cereals, baked goods, legumes, fruits, vegetables, low-fat milk, and starches such as whole grains.

Because carbohydrates have the biggest impact on blood sugar right after you've eaten, it's important to get enough at each meal. An average portion size consists of 15 grams of carbohydrates. That's equivalent to one slice of bread, $\frac{1}{3}$ cup of rice, a small piece of fruit, two small cookies, or $\frac{1}{2}$ cup of ice cream. Aim for three or four carbohydrate servings at each meal and one serving for snacks.

■ **READ LABELS.** The best way to figure out how many carbohydrates are in a meal is to look at food labels. Also, be sure to check the serving size. A serving of pasta, for example, is just $\frac{1}{2}$ cup, much less than most people typically eat at one time.

■ **MEASURE YOUR FOOD.** Don't guesstimate, says Dr. Miller. Use a measuring cup for foods such as rice and vegetables. Meats are often gauged in ounces, so you'll need a kitchen scale, available at most department stores, says Dr. Miller. When you're without a scale, such as

in restaurants, just remember that 3 ounces of meat is about the size of a deck of cards.

■ **WATCH YOUR SUGARS.** Sugars aren't as ominous as they would seem for people with diabetes. When eaten in equal amounts, starches and sugars have similar effects on blood sugar, Franz says. Still, foods containing sugars and sweets are often high in calories and low in nutritional value. If you do eat something high in sugar, it's important to substitute that for other carbohydrate foods in your menu.

■ **EAT FEWER FATS.** Keeping fats to about 30 percent of your total calories can reduce your chance of developing high cholesterol and heart disease, both risk factors of diabetes.

■ **EAT EVEN FEWER SATURATED FATS.** Saturated fats, from meats and cheeses, and polyunsaturated fats, in hydrogenated margarine, should account for only 10 percent of total daily calories. Switching to a diet higher in monounsaturated fats, found in olive oil and nuts, and lower in polyunsaturated fats may help reduce insulin resistance, according to Harry G. Preuss, M.D., M.A.C.N., C.N.S. Choose low-fat dairy products and lean meats, and avoid margarine and baked goods containing trans fats, coconut oil, or palm oil.

■ **PASS ON HIGH-PROTEIN DIETS.** Because foods high in animal protein, such as meats and cheeses, also tend to be high in fat and cholesterol, limit proteins to between 10 and 20 percent of your diet. It's true that you might lose weight following popular high-protein, low-carb diets, but keeping it off can be a problem. You're better off adopting a balanced diet that you can live with for a long time, says Franz.

Cures from the Kitchen

 Many foods and spices have been found to lower or help control blood sugar. Give these a try.

AVOCADO. This fruit is rich in a particular kind of monounsaturated fat called oleic acid, which has been found to improve fat levels in the body and help control diabetes.

BEANS. Many studies have shown that eating foods high in soluble fiber, particularly beans, reduces the rise in blood sugar after meals and delays the drop in blood sugar later on, which helps maintain blood sugar at close-to-desired levels.

CINNAMON. Some alternative practitioners think that cinnamon may be helpful in making insulin receptors work better. Stir 1 teaspoon daily into a food or beverage. Other spices found to help the body use insulin more efficiently include bay leaf, cloves, and turmeric.

COFFEE. Regular drinkers may be less likely to develop diabetes, reveals a study from the University of Minnesota. Diabetes experts suspect that compounds and minerals in coffee beans may improve the sensitivity of insulin receptors and help the body process blood sugar more efficiently.

ORANGE. Studies indicate the soluble fiber and pectin in oranges can help control changes in blood sugar as well as help lower cholesterol.

SWEET POTATO. Despite its name, and a flavor so divine it makes a good dessert, the sweet potato doesn't raise your blood sugar as high, or as fast, as a white potato.

TEA. Studies have shown that extracts of black tea may significantly reduce blood sugar levels. And enjoying a cup of chamomile tea may be more than a restful nighttime ritual—the herb may help reduce blood sugar fluctuations.

■ **SKIMP ON SODIUM.** Diabetes and high blood pressure sometimes go hand in hand, and people with diabetes can be more sensitive to the effects of excess sodium, says Franz. Limit sodium to less than 2,400 milligrams a day, which is the amount of sodium in 1 teaspoon of salt. The easiest way to do this is to eat less than 800 milligrams at each meal and no more than 400 milligrams in each food. Look for the amount of sodium on food labels.

■ **FEAST ON FIBER.** One small study of 13 people who ate 25 grams each of soluble and insoluble fiber—a total of 50 grams a day—found that they were able to achieve a 10 percent drop in blood sugar levels.

While that's encouraging news, Franz cautions that, from a practical standpoint, 50 grams a day may be a bit tough to stomach. "We really don't know if, in the long term, people *can* eat enough fiber to influence blood glucose levels," she says.

Nevertheless, high-fiber diets have other health advantages. They slow the absorption of fats and carbohydrates into the system, reducing their adverse effects on the glucose-insulin system. Also, high-fiber foods tend to be very filling, so you eat less. Shoot for 25 to 35 grams a day by eating lots of whole grains, beans, lentils, and vegetables.

■ **DRINK SPARINGLY.** You needn't become a teetotaler the moment you're diagnosed with diabetes. Moderate drinking has been shown to lower the risk of heart disease and may

DIABETES

Best and Worst Foods for Your Blood Sugar

What you eat (and don't) may play a major role in your risk of developing type 2 diabetes, according to a study from researchers at Tulane University and Harvard School of Public Health who tracked the eating habits of more than 71,000 women for 18 years. Here's how to help prevent the disease, based on their research.

Add: Leafy greens. For every additional serving of spinach, kale, or chard you eat, you may lessen your likelihood by as much as 9 percent.

Add: Whole fruit. For every three servings, you may slash your risk by up to 18 percent.

Avoid: Juice. Consuming one serving a day may raise your odds by nearly 18 percent. Some varieties are rich in antioxidants, but consider trading your daily glass of juice for whole fruit.

actually improve insulin sensitivity, according to some studies. To realize such benefits, however, don't drink too much. Women should cork the bottle after one drink a day (or fewer), and men after two or fewer. (One drink is 12 ounces of beer, 4 ounces of wine, or 1½ ounces of hard liquor.) If you choose beer, light is best since it contains fewer carbohydrates and calories.

■ **DO IT DRUG-FREE.** "Beating type 2 diabetes by getting tough about your diet (and exercising) works better than drugs," says researcher Christian Roberts, Ph.D. At the end of his small, controlled 3-week study at UCLA, Dr. Roberts found that 6 out of 13 overweight or obese men with type 2 diabetes were diabetes-free, with normal blood sugar levels. How? They ate meals low in fat (12 to 15 percent of calories), moderate in protein (15 to 25 percent), and high in carbs (65 to 70 per-

cent). Participants also walked 45 to 60 minutes a day, and cut out refined carbs—absolutely no pastries or brownies. These changes were critical to their success, says Dr. Roberts, who predicts that sticking to the diet long-term may undo heart damage already started by earlier diabetes.

■ **ENLIST YOUR SPOUSE.** Dr. Miller studied the eating patterns and food choices of 45 men and women with type 2 diabetes for 1 year. She found that those with the best blood sugar control were men whose wives prepared low-fat meals and walked with them. On the other hand, women without that level of support from another person didn't have good blood sugar control. Worst off were those women who prepared low-fat meals for themselves but made separate meals for their families. The moral: Persuade your family to get healthy along with you.

■ **PLAN AHEAD.** Diabetes requires a pretty intensive lifestyle overhaul, acknowledges Dr. Miller. You need to exercise, eat healthy, and monitor your blood sugar, which requires an enormous amount of organization and time. In her study, Dr. Miller discovered that the people most successful at controlling their blood sugar levels were those who did a lot of meal preplanning.

Decide at the beginning of the week which healthy foods you want to prepare. Then shop for these foods. If you make bag lunches and have healthy food on hand, you'll be less likely to rely on high-fat, fast-food meals or sugary snacks.

■ **VISIT A DIETITIAN.** A dietitian or nutritionist can design a customized nutrition plan just for you. This is especially important if you have other health issues, such as high cholesterol and high blood pressure, as well as diabetes, says Dr. Miller. Plan several sessions so that you can gradually incorporate changes.

GET YOUR HEART PUMPING

In addition to the obvious nutrition changes, experts recommend regular exercise for people with diabetes.

"Exercise acts just like medicine," explains diabetes educator Robert Hanisch, M.A., C.D.E., C.S.C.S. It lowers blood sugar as muscles turn glucose into energy.

According to the American College of Sports Medicine (ACSM), obese people with type 2 diabetes who exercise regularly achieve better glucose control. What's even better, studies find that increased physical activity, including walking, can reduce the risk of heart attack, stroke, and other complications in people with diabetes.

Even people dependent on insulin or oral medicines can reap the benefits of exercise. "At the very least, they will take less medicine. And the results are immediate," says Hanisch. You should check your blood glucose immediately before and after exercise. There will be individual variations, but on average there is a 1 to 2 point drop in blood sugar for every minute you exercise. This means 10 minutes of aerobic exercise will usually cut blood sugar 10 to 20 points. The glucose will remain lower until the next meal or snack.

Check with your doctor before beginning any exercise program. Here are some tips to get you going.

■ **START EASY.** Not accustomed to exercise? Don't sweat it. Begin with a low-impact, low-intensity workout, such as walking. "Walk at a comfortable pace," says Hanisch. If you push yourself too hard, you won't find it enjoyable, and you'll be less likely to continue. "Blood sugar can go down even when you are walking very slowly," he says.

■ **JOIN THE 1,000 CLUB.** The ACSM recommends that people with type 2 diabetes burn a minimum of 1,000 calories a week through daily activity and that everyone with diabetes should get *at least* 3 nonconsecutive days of exercise each week, for 10 to 15 minutes. Hanisch suggests a goal of gradually building up to a 30-minute workout on most days of the week. If you weigh about 150 pounds, you'll burn 166 calories in 30 minutes of brisk walking. Walk briskly for 30 minutes 5 days a week, and you'll come close to that goal. The rest of your daily activities will easily put you well over that minimum of 1,000 calories a week.

■ **STRIVE FOR FIVE.** "Consistency is the key," notes Hanisch. Whether you hike, bicycle, swim, or jog, a routine you can manage five times a week will produce optimum results, creating a long-term change in your body. After 2 to 3 months of consistent exercise, you likely will become more sensitive to insulin, and you'll need less medicine, Hanisch says.

■ **BE A MORNING PERSON.** An early workout will hold blood sugar down all day long. You will still see fluctuations in glucose levels after meals, but a 30-minute morning walk will keep levels 30 points lower than what they might otherwise be, says Hanisch.

■ **DRINK UP.** Dehydration can affect blood glucose levels, so staying well hydrated during exercise is especially important for people with diabetes. Drink 16 ounces of fluid—two glasses of water—2 hours before exercising, and sip throughout your workout.

■ **LIFT LIGHTLY.** Weight training can help build strength. But people with long-standing diabetes, and especially those with diabetes-related eye disease, need to limit themselves to multiple repetitions with very light resistance

in the range of 1- to 5-pound weights. Heavy weights can injure weakened eye muscles, says Hanisch. To know that the weight is light enough, you should be able to perform the correct strengthening techniques with minimal effort. If in doubt, use a lighter weight.

■ **TAKE CARE OF YOUR TOES.** People who have diabetes-related foot problems such as peripheral neuropathy (see "Take Care of Your Feet," page 193) should take special care before they go walking or jogging. "They may need to work with a podiatrist to get shoes that distribute the force differently when they land," says Hanisch.

STRESS LESS

When something gets you stressed out, sending your emotions on a roller coaster, your blood sugar goes along for the ride. That's because stress hormones, such as adrenaline, increase blood glucose. "Stress hormones mobilize glycogen that has been stored in the liver and metabolize it into glucose," says Angele McGrady, Ph.D.

The adrenaline and extra sugar released into the bloodstream give you a boost of energy. If you were undergoing physical stress—say, being chased by a pack of wild dogs—you'd respond by running away, and the extra blood sugar would be used up, Dr. McGrady points out. Today, however, most of our stressors are psychological. We sit and stew and don't use up all that blood sugar.

Since their bodies don't metabolize glucose

Take Care of Your Feet

Peripheral neuropathy is a complication of diabetes in which high blood sugar damages nerve cells over time, leading to a lack of sensation. Because the nerves in the feet are the longest in the body, the feet are usually most affected by this condition, making them prone to injury and damage. Sores on the feet that don't heal properly can become ulcerated and infected and, in serious cases, may lead to amputation. An estimated 6 out of every 1,000 people with diabetes have a limb amputated—and it often can be avoided. Here are some recommendations for protecting your feet.

See a podiatrist. Once you've been diagnosed with diabetes, have your feet checked frequently, recommends Marc A. Brenner, D.P.M. A podiatrist will determine if you have neuropathy and will help care for your feet if you do. Trimming toenails or self-treating calluses and corns, for example, can pose hazards for people with neuropathy and should be done by a podiatric physician.

Keep them covered. Wear a good pair of socks. The best are made of a combination of cotton and synthetic material. On very cold days, wear two pairs—a thin one next to your skin and a thick pair. "The more insulation you have between your foot and the ground, the better," says Dr. Brenner.

Make sure the shoe fits. Your shoe size should be determined by a certified pedorthist, a person specially trained to measure feet, says Dr. Brenner. Ask your podiatrist to recommend a shoe store that offers such services. Have your feet measured in the afternoon, when your feet are more likely to be swollen.

Step out in sneaks. You probably won't need custom shoes. A high-quality cross-trainer or running shoe will serve you well. Look for a type with a roomy toebox, a removable inlay to exchange for a custom orthotic, a padded tongue, and a cushioned heel and ball.

Wear an orthotic. A diabetic orthotic is a custom-made device that fits into your shoe. It's important to wear one since it keeps pressure off certain spots on the foot or spreads pressure across the entire foot. Your podiatrist can advise you and measure you for an appropriate orthotic.

Inspect daily. Check for swelling or sores, using a large mirror to see all angles of the foot. Better yet, ask a family member to look for discoloration and feel for warm spots—signs of possible infection.

Take them swimming. If you have neuropathy, exercise is still important. "Swimming is safest," says Dr. Brenner, because you don't have to put pressure on your feet. Carefully dry your feet afterward and sprinkle them with foot powder to avoid fungus or yeast.

effectively, it's especially important for people with diabetes to try to decrease their stress levels. In a small study that Dr. McGrady conducted, 18 people with diabetes reduced their blood sugar levels 9 to 12 percent by practicing simple relaxation exercises. Those who also had depression, however, did not benefit without additional treatment. Here are some stress busters worth trying.

■ **BREATHE DEEPLY.** "Deep breathing is a good way to start," says Dr. McGrady. Sit with your legs and arms uncrossed. Inhale deeply from your abdomen. Then breathe out as much air as you possibly can, relaxing your muscles as you do. Continue this relaxed breathing for about 15 minutes.

■ **PURCHASE A RELAXATION CD.** Can't settle down? A relaxation CD can help. "Most of us aren't used to sitting quietly with no thoughts in our heads," says Dr. McGrady. "It's very helpful to have sound in the background." Recordings of gentle noises from nature, such as ocean waves, enable you to pace your breathing and set a tone for you to relax. Or choose a guided imagery CD, in which a soothing voice mentally shepherds you through a pleasant scene, such as a walk in a forest. Look for them wherever CDs are sold.

■ **FOCUS ON SOMETHING PLEASANT.** Guided imagery works because it guides your senses of recall and concentration to help you relax. You can achieve the same effect by examining an art book or an illustration that you find pleasant. "Look at the picture for several minutes, then close your eyes and recall as much as you can," explains Dr. McGrady. "If you do it enough, you can eventually do it without even having the book in front of you." You could put a peaceful scene on your computer screensaver, too, she suggests.

■ **PRACTICE PROGRESSIVE RELAXATION.** Tensing and relaxing your muscles allows you to consciously control their tension. First, lie on your back in a comfortable position. Begin deliberately tensing and releasing one muscle—the fist is a good place to start. Move upward along your arms, to the neck and face, and then down the back and legs. Don't tense any muscle enough to make it hurt, Dr. McGrady cautions. CDs are available to talk you through this process.

■ **TRY BIOFEEDBACK.** Researchers at the Medical University of Ohio followed 30 diabetes patients, half of whom practiced daily tension-taming exercises such as muscle relaxation, and had their techniques monitored with weekly 45-minute biofeedback sessions. The others took diabetes education classes. After 10 weeks, those who relaxed saw about a 10 percent drop in fasting blood sugar and in their average blood glucose level—a sign that their glucose had stayed lower around the clock for the previous couple of months. Meanwhile, the education group's same levels rose slightly. But if that's not motivation enough, the stress management group also experienced a drop in depression and anxiety.

To find a biofeedback therapist in your area, visit the Biofeedback Certification Institute of America at www.bcia.org and click on Find a Practitioner.

SUPPLEMENT SAVVY

Some practitioners believe that dietary supplements can be helpful for people with diabetes. Consult your physician before trying them out. Here are a few that the experts recommend.

■ **CONSIDER CHROMIUM.** Some people with diabetes can benefit from chromium supplements, especially if they have a deficiency of this mineral. Dr. Preuss suggests 400 to 600 micrograms of chromium a day for 1 to 2 months under the direction of a physician.

■ **GET SOME AMERICAN GINSENG.** One small Canadian study found that patients with type 2 diabetes who took 3 grams of American ginseng 2 hours before eating 25 grams of sugar reduced their after-meal blood sugar levels by 20 percent. Talk with your doctor about the right dose for you.

■ **SEEK SIGHT-SAVING HERBS.** According to herbal experts, the herbs bilberry and ginkgo biloba may improve circulation, thereby lowering the risk of eye damage for people with diabetes. Both are available freeze-dried or as a tincture. Follow the manufacturer's directions.

■ **BABY YOUR ARTERIES WITH ASPIRIN.** Aspirin reduces heart attack risk by discouraging blood cells called platelets from sticking together in the arteries. Amazingly, it's even more effective for those with diabetes than for those without diabetes. That's good news, because the incidence of heart attack among women with diabetes has been rising in recent years. Ask your doctor how much aspirin is right for you, says Aaron I. Vinik, M.D., Ph.D.

■ **TRY A GOOD MULTI.** Look for a good multivitamin and mineral supplement that provides at least 25 percent of the Daily Values of magnesium, zinc, vitamin E, and vitamin C. Magnesium deficiency is thought to increase insulin resistance, high blood pressure, and cardiovascular disease in people with diabetes. Zinc deficiency also can negatively impact glucose levels. Vitamin E helps sensitize insulin receptors. Vitamin C assists the immune system and enables tissue repair, says Dr. Preuss.

TESTING, TESTING

Once diagnosed with diabetes, testing your blood sugar at home becomes an integral part of your life. Here are some techniques that experts advise.

■ **LOOK FOR PATTERNS.** Monitor your glucose levels by recording your levels five times a day for several weeks, suggests Dr. Miller. That helps you discern patterns, she says. Check first thing in the morning, 1 to 2 hours after meals, and right before bed.

■ **CHECK OUT CHANGES.** When making changes in your diet, test immediately before a meal, then 2 hours after. Before a meal, levels should range between 90 to 130 milligrams per deciliter (mg/dl). After a meal, levels should be no higher than 160 mg/dl.

■ **TEST WHEN YOU EXERCISE.** If you start a new exercise routine, test immediately before and immediately after your workout, says Hanisch. If your blood sugar is low before starting—100 to 120 mg/dl—eat a piece of fruit or drink half a cup (4 ounces) of juice. Both have about 15 grams of carbohydrates to elevate blood sugar about 25 points. Do the same if your levels drop after exercise.

■ **DO SPOT CHECKS.** Most people with diabetes habitually monitor first thing in the morning. That's not enough, says Dr. Miller. Do an occasional test after lunch or in the evening to achieve a better picture of what influences your blood glucose. Blood sugar values should be 110 to 150 mg/dl on average at bedtime.

■ **WRITE IT DOWN.** Keep a written record of your levels, and note what and when you ate as well as when you exercised and for how long. "Use a spiral-bound notebook, or make up a spread sheet on your computer," suggests Dr. Miller. Share the information with your doctor. The log can help you and your doctor better manage your care.

PANEL OF ADVISORS

MARC A. BRENNER, D.P.M., IS FOUNDER AND DIRECTOR OF THE INSTITUTE OF DIABETIC FOOT RESEARCH IN GLENDALE, NEW YORK. HE IS PAST PRESIDENT OF THE AMERICAN SOCIETY OF PODIATRIC DERMATOLOGY AND AUTHOR AND EDITOR OF VARIOUS BOOKS.

MARION FRANZ, M.S., R.D., L.D., C.D.E., IS FORMER DIRECTOR OF NUTRITION AND HEALTH PROFESSIONAL EDUCATION AT THE INTERNATIONAL DIABETES CENTER IN MINNEAPOLIS AND PAST COCHAIR OF THE AMERICAN DIABETES ASSOCIATION'S TASK FORCE TO REVISE NUTRITION PRINCIPLE RECOMMENDATIONS. SHE IS EDITOR OF THE *AMERICAN ASSOCIATION OF DIABETES EDUCATORS CORE CURRICULUM FOR DIABETES EDUCATION.*

ROBERT HANISCH, M.A., C.D.E., C.S.C.S., IS AN EXERCISE PHYSIOLOGIST AND GRADUATE PROGRAM INSTRUCTOR IN THE DIABETES DEPARTMENT OF THE HEALTH AND SCIENCES DIVISION AT MOUNT MARY COLLEGE IN MILWAUKEE.

ANGELE MCGRADY, PH.D., IS A PROFESSOR AND DIRECTOR OF MEDICAL EDUCATION IN THE DEPARTMENT OF PSYCHIATRY AT THE UNIVERSITY OF TOLEDO COLLEGE OF MEDICINE IN OHIO.

CARLA MILLER, PH.D., R.D., IS ASSOCIATE DIRECTOR OF THE DIABETES CENTER AT PENNSYLVANIA STATE UNIVERSITY MILTON S. HERSHEY MEDICAL CENTER AND AN ASSISTANT PROFESSOR OF NUTRITION AT PENNSYLVANIA STATE UNIVERSITY, BOTH IN HERSHEY.

HARRY G. PREUSS, M.D., M.A.C.N., C.N.S., IS A PROFESSOR AT GEORGETOWN MEDICAL CENTER IN WASHINGTON, D.C. AND A CERTIFIED NUTRITIONAL SPECIALIST. HE IS FORMER PRESIDENT AND A MASTER OF THE AMERICAN COLLEGE OF NUTRITION AND FORMER PRESIDENT OF THE CERTIFICATION BOARD FOR NUTRITION SPECIALISTS. DR. PREUSS IS COAUTHOR OF *THE NATURAL FAT-LOSS PHARMACY.*

CHRISTIAN ROBERTS, PH.D., IS AN ASSISTANT ADJUNCT PROFESSOR IN THE DEPARTMENT OF PHYSIOLOGICAL SCIENCE AT THE UNIVERSITY OF CALIFORNIA IN LOS ANGELES.

CHRISTOPHER D. SAUDEK, M.D., IS FORMER PRESIDENT OF THE AMERICAN DIABETES ASSOCIATION AND DIRECTOR OF JOHNS HOPKINS DIABETES CENTER IN BALTIMORE.

AARON I. VINIK, M.D., PH.D., IS A PROFESSOR OF MEDICINE AND SCIENTIFIC DIRECTOR OF THE DEPARTMENT OF INTERNAL MEDICINE AT THE STRELITZ DIABETES RESEARCH INSTITUTE AT EASTERN VIRGINIA MEDICAL SCHOOL IN NORFOLK.

Diaper Rash

9 Easy Solutions

Diaper rash can interrupt the peaceful routine of an otherwise carefree baby, and it won't do much for the parents' quality of life either. Babies have a knack for making their problems their family's problems, and if your baby has diaper rash, well, you'll know about it.

During the first 2 to 3 years of a baby's life, just about every parent shares in the diaper rash experience at least once. It's not surprising, given that the most common rash-triggering irritants come from what is typically found in baby's diaper: bowel movements and urine. Thankfully, nearly half of all diaper rashes go away by themselves within 1 day. But the other 50 percent can last 10 days or more (though it might seem longer).

Here's some other diaper rash trivia: In some babies, diaper rash may be a harbinger of future skin problems such as eczema or sensitive skin. Also, breastfed babies have less diaper rash than bottle-fed babies, and this resistance continues long after a baby is weaned.

Enough of the trivia. Here's some advice on how to help your little one feel better.

■ **CHANGE BABY OFTEN.** "If you keep baby in a clean, dry diaper she's less likely to develop diaper rash," says nanny industry expert Sharon Graff-Radell. Diaper rash most often occurs when a wet or soiled diaper is left on too long. "If baby's bottom becomes red and irritated, I suggest putting a barrier between her skin and

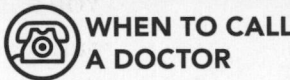
WHEN TO CALL A DOCTOR

There's a natural tendency to panic whenever something out of the ordinary happens to a baby. In the case of diaper rash, though, it very rarely is anything to worry about. It most commonly occurs after introducing solid foods, but it can affect any baby wearing diapers. Just treat the rash for a few days at home, and keep a watchful eye for the following:

■ The rash doesn't improve after 2 or 3 days.

■ The rash looks severe or is accompanied by blisters, boils, or pus.

■ Your baby develops a fever along with the rash.

■ The rash spreads beyond the area covered by the diaper

The "Bead Bottom" Mystery

A medical journal article tells of parents calling pediatricians to report a strange diaper rash that looks like "small, shiny beads" covering their babies' bottoms. Pediatricians investigating the mysterious outbreak of "bead bottom" noticed that the afflicted infants all wore superabsorbent disposable diapers. Was there a connection?

Yes. The "beads" are actually the gelling material that makes superabsorbent diapers "super." Apparently, small, loose quantities of the material may occasionally pass through a break in the top sheet of the diaper and transfer to the infant's skin. Doctors say the material is nontoxic and presents no reason for concern.

her diaper, such as Balmex or A&D Diaper Rash Ointment. In my experience, Balmex can work miracles in healing a baby's bottom." Cloth or disposable diapers work equally well, says Graff-Radell.

■ **KEEP IT NATURAL.** "Throw out the baby powder and bring in the cornstarch," says Graff-Radell. "Don't apply baby lotion and powder after every diaper change. If you prefer to use baby powder, try cornstarch instead." Baby powder contains perfume and additives, while cornstarch works naturally.

■ **GIVE IT SOME AIR—OR WATER.** The oldest advice is sometimes still the best. "Give a baby's bottom some air," says Graff-Radell. Simply take the baby's diaper off and lay her chest down, with her face turned to one side, on towels placed atop a waterproof sheet. Leave her resting on her chest as long as you're there to keep an eye on her. (An unwatched, undiapered baby is trouble waiting to happen.) Another option is a sitz bath: Place baby in a basin or tub of lukewarm water for several

minutes every time you change her diaper. "This keeps her bottom clean and may restore moisture to her skin," says Graff-Radell.

■ **LET SUPERDIAPERS COME TO THE RESCUE.** "Superabsorbent diapers with microbreathable liners have been shown to greatly reduce diaper rash by keeping a baby's bottom much drier," says pediatrician John D. Rau, M.D. "Many studies have proven that babies in superabsorbent diapers get fewer skin rashes." The absorbent gel material in these diapers reduces wetness and cuts down on skin infections that require moisture to grow. But don't take their super powers for granted. "Frequent diaper changes are still needed for a baby's bottom to stay as dry as possible," says Dr. Rau.

■ **CLEANSE GENTLY.** Don't use regular diaper wipes containing alcohol because they can burn irritated skin and worsen the condition. Instead, diapering experts recommend alcohol-free brands, or try cotton balls dipped in baby oil. Another option is to use warm water

The Dye May Be Why

That diaper rash that just won't go away may actually be caused by the dye used in disposable diapers or training pants.

University of Massachusetts Medical School researchers report that red, irritated skin that aligns with colored areas on diapers and training pants may be a sign of a dye allergy. Switch to diapers labeled dye-free, and the rash may disappear in a few days.

in a squirt bottle to rinse the baby's bottom.

■ **BLOW-DRY THAT BABY.** Keeping the diaper area clean promotes healing, but drying with a towel can irritate sensitive skin. Option? "Try a blow-dryer," says pediatric nurse practitioner Linda Jonides, B.S., R.N., C.P.N.P. Dry the diaper area with a hair dryer set on "low," which eliminates rubbing to wet skin. After the area is dry, apply a zinc oxide ointment such as A&D Diaper Rash Ointment or Desitin. Petroleum jelly such as Vaseline also provides a protective coating, even on sore, red skin. If you use cornstarch or baby powder, sprinkle carefully, as either one can trigger breathing problems in little ones.

■ **GIVE CLOTH DIAPERS A VINEGAR RINSE.** Diaper rash enzymes are most active in a high-pH environment, which often exists in cloth diapers after washing. To counter this, add 1 ounce of vinegar to 1 gallon of water during the final rinse to bring the pH of cloth diapers in line with the pH of baby's skin. "Actually, I believe there's a lot to be said for

diaper services," Graff-Radell notes. "They go to a lot of trouble to get the pH balance right, and they're not all that expensive."

■ **MAKE THE CRANBERRY CONNECTION.** When urine and feces mix in the diaper area, the result is a high pH that irritates the skin and promotes diaper rash. Unorthodox as it may sound, Jonides says that 2 to 3 ounces of cranberry juice given to older babies leaves an acid residue in the urine, helping lower pH and reduce irritation.

PANEL OF ADVISORS

SHARON GRAFF-RADELL IS VICE PRESIDENT OF THE INTERNATIONAL NANNY ASSOCIATION, FOUNDER OF WWW.FINDTHEBESTNANNY.COM, AND OWNER OF TLC FOR KIDS IN ST. LOUIS, ONE OF THE FIRST NANNY AND CHILD CARE AGENCIES IN THE UNITED STATES.

LINDA JONIDES, B.S., R.N., C.P.N.P., IS A PEDIATRIC NURSE PRACTITIONER IN ANN ARBOR, MICHIGAN.

JOHN D. RAU, M.D., IS A DEVELOPMENTAL BEHAVIORAL PEDIATRICIAN AND AN ASSOCIATE PROFESSOR OF CLINICAL PEDIATRICS AT INDIANA UNIVERSITY SCHOOL OF MEDICINE. HE IS ALSO THE DIRECTOR OF THE RILEY CHILD DEVELOPMENT CENTER IN INDIANAPOLIS.

Diarrhea

27 Strategies to Deal with It

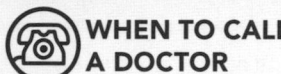
WHEN TO CALL A DOCTOR

Diarrhea should normally leave you only slightly worse for wear. In infants, small children, elderly people, or those already sick or dehydrated from another illness, however, acute diarrhea can be particularly severe and demands prompt medical attention.

Medical help is also needed if diarrhea doesn't subside in 1 to 2 days, if it's accompanied by fever and severe abdominal cramps, or if it occurs with rashes, jaundice (yellowing of the skin and whites of the eyes), or extreme weakness. If there's blood, pus, or mucus in your stools, call your doctor.

"The most immediate risk associated with acute diarrhea is dehydration," says Harris Clearfield, M.D. "If an individual is having a major bout of diarrhea and isn't taking in any food or drink during that time, you're looking at a medical emergency."

In the past when someone had diarrhea, doctors whipped out their prescription pads and dispensed antidiarrheal medication. Today, they think the best medicine is to simply let diarrhea run its course, if you'll pardon the pun.

"Acute diarrhea is one of your body's best defense mechanisms," says Lynn V. McFarland, Ph.D. "It's your body's way of getting something nasty out of your system."

That thought may or may not be of comfort to you right now, but it explains why doctors today tell you to "tough it out" instead of automatically trying to stem the tide of this annoying, but hopefully short-lived, illness.

"I don't recommend antidiarrheal medications when a patient has acute diarrhea unless he has an urgent need for control—like a very important business meeting that just can't be missed," says David A. Lieberman, M.D. "Otherwise, I think the purge is probably beneficial and helps speed recovery," he says.

Heeding that approach, most of the tips that follow are designed to help you weather the discomfort of diarrhea and make a quick recovery, rather than trying to halt the course of diarrhea and risk prolonging the illness. For those who may have "an urgent need for control" while stricken, we've listed some medications to help stem the tide while you take care of other business.

■ **MAKE THE MILK CONNECTION.** A leading cause of diarrhea in this country is lactose intolerance, says William Y. Chey, M.D.

"Lactose intolerance can have its onset when you're just a baby, or it can kick in suddenly during your adult years," says Dr. Chey. One day you could be drinking milk, and the next thing you know—bam!—you have gas, pain, and diarrhea.

The cure, of course, is to avoid lactose-containing foods, which means staying away from most dairy products, with the exception of yogurt, some aged cheeses such as Cheddar, and those cheeses specifically designed to be lactose-free, such as Lactaid.

■ **TAKE THE TOLERANCE TEST.** Given the dose-related nature of lactose intolerance, as well as its ability to kick in unexpectedly, how can you be sure that milk products are responsible for your tummy troubles?

First, completely abstain from milk and other dairy products for a week or two and see if that helps, says Dr. Lieberman. If it does, gradually add back dairy products with the knowledge that you may hit an intolerance point and the symptoms will return. Once you know what that point is, you can avoid lactose-induced diarrhea by eating fewer dairy products.

■ **THINK ABOUT YOUR MEDICATIONS.** Our experts say there's a good possibility that the diarrhea you have now was caused by the heartburn you had earlier today. It's not because of a direct connection between stomach and bowel, but because of the antacid you may have taken to soothe your burning belly.

"Antacids are the most common cause of drug-related diarrhea," says Harris Clearfield, M.D. "Maalox and Mylanta both have magnesium hydroxide in them that acts exactly like milk of magnesia, which makes these antacids a common cause of diarrhea."

To avoid future bouts of heartburn-related diarrhea, he suggests trying antacids that contain aluminum hydroxide, with no magnesium added, such as Gaviscon or AlternaGel. "These are less likely to cause diarrhea," Dr. Clearfield says, "but they're less effective, too."

Some antibiotics, quinidine, lactulose, and colchicine may also cause diarrhea. Consult your doctor if you suspect that these or any other medications may be causing problems for you.

Large doses of vitamin C can be a culprit behind diarrhea, too. Amounts over the Daily Value (60 milligrams) may cause diarrhea in some people, but most are fine with up to 2,000 milligrams per day as long as they divide their doses over the course of the day.

■ **EAT LIGHTLY.** "The less food that your system has to process, the fewer symptoms of cramping and diarrhea you will experience," says Sheila Crowe, M.D. But if you're hungry, eat bland, light foods such as toast, cooked rice, or bananas.

■ **CONSUME A CLEAR DIET.** "Start with a clear-liquid diet," says Dr. Chey. "By 'clear' I mean chicken broth, Jell-O, or other foods and

(continued on page 204)

Traveler's Diarrhea: The Globetrotter's Curse

Montezuma's revenge, Delhi belly, Tiki trots. Whatever you call it, traveler's diarrhea—the official name is turista—can dampen one's spirits on even the best of vacations.

"If you're going to be abroad for any length of time, you'll probably have some episodes of diarrhea," says Stephen Bezruchka, M.D., a frequent traveler. "Conceptually, it is totally preventable. In reality, it's rare if you don't get an occasional loose movement." In fact, you have a 50 percent chance of getting turista, even if you take the recommended precautions.

The most common cause is the *Escherichia coli* bacteria. This widespread little organism normally resides in your intestines and performs a role in digestion. But foreign versions of *E. coli*—and to a foreigner, the American version is foreign—can give you diarrhea by producing a toxin that prevents your intestines from absorbing the water you ingest in the form of fluid and food.

As the toxin prevents the absorption of water, you have all this extra water in there, and it's got to come out, Dr. Bezruchka says. "The toxin doesn't get absorbed. You don't usually feel sick, but you might feel you have to pass some gas. Only it isn't gas at all."

Shigella and salmonella bacteria can also produce turista, while a smaller number of cases are caused by rotavirus and the giardia parasite. Changes in diet, fatigue, jet lag, and altitude sickness have been blamed but without sufficient proof, and up to 50 percent of all turista cases are unexplained.

Luckily, there are ways to help your body fight turista. Here's what doctors suggest.

Drink water, water anywhere. When you have turista, your stools are mostly water. So why would the most important treatment be to drink plenty of the right fluids? Because dehydration, the loss of water and electrolytes, can kill.

"A lot of what you take in will be pumped right back out the other end," concedes Thomas Gossel, Ph.D., R.Ph. "But you'll reach a point where you stabilize and begin retaining it. If you didn't replace any fluids at all, you could become dehydrated in a day."

Put your bladder to the test. The yellower your urine, the more fluid you need. It should be clear or pale yellow.

Use a rehydration solution. An even better way to rehydrate is to drink an ORS, also known as an over-the-counter rehydration solution. These drinks contain sugar and salt and help replace important electrolytes that are lost through diarrhea. They also help your intestines absorb water better.

Over-the-counter rehydration solutions are readily available in the United States, so you can buy and take them with you. Brands include ReVital and Pedialyte.

Choose a backup beverage. If you didn't manage to pack an ORS, drink clear fruit juices or weak tea with sugar.

Get in the pink. Pepto-Bismol, the well-known over-the-counter stomach medication, can be the traveler's friend. It makes stools bulkier and firmer, and it kills bacteria.

Don't worry if your tongue and diarrhea turn black. It's a natural side effect of Pepto-Bismol.

Wine a little. No Pepto in sight? Knock back a glass of wine (red or white). One study found it worked as well or better than the pink stuff. The alcohol's antibacterial properties killed off bacteria that cause traveler's diarrhea within 20 to 30 minutes. But no need to overindulge—one glass is probably enough. Researchers estimate that 6 ounces of wine is all it takes to get the benefits.

Do a little coaxing. Natural fiber-based laxatives for relieving constipation, such as Metamucil and Citrucel, also help with diarrhea. Some can absorb up to 60 times their weight in water to form a gel in the intestine. "You're still going to expel excess water," Dr. Gossel says, "but it won't be so runny." Other brands are Equalactin, FiberCon, and Konsyl.

Of course, it's best not to have to worry about traveler's diarrhea in the first place. Here's how to protect yourself.

■ Avoid uncooked vegetables, especially salads, fruits you can't peel, undercooked meat, raw shellfish, ice cubes, and drinks made from impure water (the alcohol in drinks won't kill the turista bug).

■ Ask if the dishes and silverware you use have been cleaned in purified water.

■ Drink only water that's been carbonated and sealed in bottles or cans. Clean the part of the container that touches your mouth with purified water. Boiling water for 3 to 5 minutes purifies it, as does adding iodine liquid or tablets.

■ Drink acidic drinks like colas and orange juice when possible. They help keep down the *E. coli* count, the bacteria most responsible for digestive distress.

■ Drink acidophilus milk or eat yogurt before your trip. The bacterial colonies established in your digestive system before your trip and maintained during it will help you reduce the chance of a turista invasion.

fluids you can look 'clear' through." This helps your bowel to rest during the diarrhea, rather than forcing your system to handle more than it really should have to.

After you've tested the waters with broth and Jell-O, you can gradually introduce rice, bananas, applesauce, and yogurt into your diet as your symptoms improve.

■ **CUT BACK ON MEAT.** "Fatty foods are hard to digest and may often lead to diarrhea," says Barbara Frank, M.D. So avoid high-fat snacks, and eat lean meat and nonfat dairy products, not full-fat versions.

■ **KEEP LIQUID LEVELS HIGH.** "The type of food you eat doesn't really matter as much as drinking enough," says Dr. McFarland. "The most serious thing is to make sure your fluid intake is high." Though many folks don't feel like consuming large amounts of liquids during bouts of diarrhea, all our experts agree that increasing your fluid intake is vital to ward off dehydration.

Fluids that contain salt and small amounts of sugar are particularly beneficial, because they help the body replace glucose and minerals lost during diarrhea. A good "rehydration fluid" can easily be made by adding 1 teaspoon of sugar and a pinch of salt to 1 quart of water.

A more complex but tastier mix can be made by adding ½ teaspoon of honey or corn syrup and a pinch of table salt to 8 ounces of fruit juice. Stir well and drink often.

Or just buy Gatorade. It contains glucose and electrolytes in sufficient quantities to replace those your body is losing.

■ **AVOID THESE FOODS.** While eating may not be as important as drinking for riding out diarrhea, some foods should be avoided. Obvious ones to pass up include beans, cabbage, and brussels sprouts.

Other foods containing large amounts of poorly absorbed carbohydrates can aggravate diarrhea. A short list includes bread, pasta, and other wheat products; apples, pears, peaches, and prunes; corn, oats, potatoes, and processed bran.

And, just in case you were reaching for that carton of ice cream, all our experts say that you should avoid dairy products (with the exception of yogurt) during a bout of diarrhea. Even if milk products didn't trigger diarrhea, they tend to aggravate diarrhea after you have it.

■ **STAY AWAY FROM ARTIFICIAL SWEETENERS.** Sorbitol, an artificial sweetener found in sugarless gum and mints and in many diet sodas often leads to the runs, because it's not easily digested, says Ann Ouyang, M.D.

■ **AVOID SOFT DRINKS.** "I'd suggest avoiding carbonated beverages as well," cautions Dr. Clearfield. "The gas they contain may add additional explosiveness to a delicate situation."

■ **STAY OUT OF THE KITCHEN.** While we're still on the subject of food, you or any member of your family with diarrhea should not prepare food for other members of the household until the diarrhea subsides. Also, good hand-washing helps keep a parasitic infection from spreading. (If your job involves contact with large numbers of people or food handling, state law may require that you stay off the job until all symptoms subside.)

■ **IF YOU MUST, TAKE SOMETHING TO STEM THE TIDE.** Our experts insist that letting diarrhea "run its course" is the best medicine going. If, however, you absolutely must go someplace and be in control while you're there, the over-the-counter product Imodium, which is available in capsule or liquid form, is probably your best bet for slowing down the flow.

"Imodium is very effective," says Dr. Clearfield. "It works by causing the bowel to tighten up, and by doing so, prevents things from moving along."

But Imodium isn't your one and only choice. Hydrophilic (*hydro* means water, and *phili* means love) products, such as Kaopectate and Pepto-Bismol, may also help treat mild diarrhea.

■ **TRY SOME TEA.** Tea is rich in tannins, which help bind stools and hold back bowel movements. Evangeline Lausier, M.D., suggests drinking a cup of chamomile tea. The herb has an antispasmodic effect that stops contractions in the lower intestine.

■ **CONSIDER THIS HONEY OF AN IDEA.** "Stir some honey into your iced or green tea and get double the health benefits—in the honey and in the tea," says Janet Maccaro, Ph.D., C.N.C. "I try to steer people away from artificial sweeteners, and honey is a wonderful healthful alternative," she says. "Honey contains all the vitamins and minerals necessary for proper metabolism and the digestion of glucose and other sugars. It's a natural sweetener with antibiotic and antiseptic properties."

Dr. Maccaro recommends using from a teaspoon to a tablespoon in a cup of hot tea or glass of iced tea, depending on your preferred level of sweetness. Not a tea drinker? Drizzle a tablespoon of honey over some fresh fruit for a tasty treat, she says.

■ **CALM AND SOOTHE.** When diarrhea strikes his family, Gannady Raskin, M.D., N.D., cures it with herbal concoctions. "Tea made from pomegranate skin will help an upset stomach," he says. Set aside the leftovers of your next purchase; you can store dried pomegranate skin for up to 6 months. Steep a tablespoon's worth in a cup of boiling water for 3 to 4 minutes. Oak bark (available at health food stores) works, too: Boil for 3 minutes, let sit for half an hour, and then strain. Both recipes are rich in tannins, which help the body produce mucus to line the stomach and lessen irritation. Drink 2 tablespoons, four to six times a day.

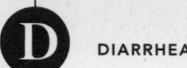

PANEL OF ADVISORS

STEPHEN BEZRUCHKA, M.D., IS A SENIOR LECTURER IN THE SCHOOL OF PUBLIC HEALTH AND COMMUNITY MEDICINE AT THE UNIVERSITY OF WASHINGTON IN SEATTLE.

WILLIAM Y. CHEY, M.D., IS DIRECTOR OF THE ROCHESTER INSTITUTE FOR DIGESTIVE DISEASES AND SCIENCES AND A PHYSICIAN IN ROCHESTER, NEW YORK. HE HOLDS POSITIONS OF PROFESSORSHIP AT NUMEROUS UNIVERSITIES IN CHINA AND KOREA, AND IS A FELLOW OF THE AMERICAN GASTROENTEROLOGICAL ASSOCIATION.

HARRIS CLEARFIELD, M.D., IS A PROFESSOR IN THE DEPARTMENT OF MEDICINE AT DREXEL UNIVERSITY COLLEGE OF MEDICINE AND SECTION CHIEF IN THE DEPARTMENT OF GASTROENTEROLOGY AT HAHNEMANN UNIVERSITY HOSPITAL, BOTH IN PHILADELPHIA.

SHEILA CROWE, M.D., IS A PROFESSOR OF MEDICINE IN THE DIVISION OF GASTROENTEROLOGY AND HEPATOLOGY IN THE DIGESTIVE HEALTH CENTER OF EXCELLENCE AT THE UNIVERSITY OF VIRGINIA IN CHARLOTTESVILLE.

BARBARA FRANK, M.D., IS A CLINICAL PROFESSOR OF MEDICINE IN THE DIVISION OF GASTROENTEROLOGY AND HEPATOLOGY AT DREXEL UNIVERSITY COLLEGE OF MEDICINE IN PHILADELPHIA.

THOMAS GOSSEL, PH.D., R.PH., IS FORMER DEAN OF THE COLLEGE OF PHARMACY AT OHIO NORTHERN UNIVERSITY IN ADA.

EVANGELINE LAUSIER, M.D., IS A CLINICAL ASSISTANT PROFESSOR OF MEDICINE AT DUKE INTEGRATIVE MEDICINE IN DURHAM, NORTH CAROLINA.

DAVID A. LIEBERMAN, M.D., IS HEAD OF THE DIVISION OF GASTROENTEROLOGY AT OREGON HEALTH AND SCIENCE UNIVERSITY IN PORTLAND.

JANET MACCARO, PH.D., C.N.C., IS A HOLISTIC NUTRITIONIST IN CENTRAL FLORIDA.

LYNN V. MCFARLAND, PH.D., IS A MEDICINAL CHEMISTRY ADJUNCT ASSOCIATE PROFESSOR AND EPIDEMIOLOGIST AT THE UNIVERSITY OF WASHINGTON IN SEATTLE AND COAUTHOR OF *THE POWER OF PROBIOTICS*.

ANN OUYANG, M.D., IS A PROFESSOR OF MEDICINE AT PENNSYLVANIA STATE COLLEGE OF MEDICINE AND FORMER CHIEF OF THE DIVISION OF GASTROENTEROLOGY AND HEPATOLOGY AT PENNSYLVANIA STATE UNIVERSITY MILTON S. HERSHEY MEDICAL CENTER IN HERSHEY, PENNSYLVANIA.

GANNADY RASKIN, M.D., N.D., IS DEAN OF THE SCHOOL OF NATUROPATHIC MEDICINE AT BASTYR UNIVERSITY IN SEATTLE.

Diverticulosis

17 Self-Care Techniques

Once upon a time—say, before 1900—diverticulosis was just another of the many "rare" medical conditions that doctors had heard about but seldom had seen. Even today, diverticulosis is rare in Third World countries.

But not in the United States, land of the Big Mac. Studies indicate that more than half of all Americans over the age of 60 have diverticulosis—characterized by tiny, grapelike pouches or sacs (diverticula) along the outer wall of the colon. Almost everyone over age 80 has the condition.

These pouches show up on x-rays, but many people never have this area x-rayed and don't even know that they have the condition, says Samuel Klein, M.D.

Of those who do have diverticulosis, Dr. Klein says, only about 10 percent will ever progress to diverticulitis—a painful inflammation that can become serious. So having diverticulosis does not mean that you're destined for severe pain or a hospital stay.

Fortunately, you can take an active role in treating and preventing diverticulosis, and avoiding the pain of diverticulitis. Here's what our experts suggest.

■ **BULK UP ON FIBER.** "Diverticulosis is a problem that is acquired," says surgeon Paul Williamson, M.D. "It's come about with the advance of processed foods—foods that are low in fiber."

The average American gets about 16 grams of fiber daily,

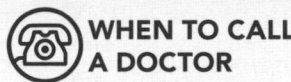

WHEN TO CALL A DOCTOR

If you live long enough, chances are you will get diverticulosis. Even so, odds are you won't get *diverticulitis*—a painful inflammation that is potentially serious. Still, you should be aware of the warning signs.

Fever, tenderness, or pain in the lower left abdominal region are good indicators that diverticulosis has advanced to diverticulitis, according to the National Digestive Diseases Information Clearinghouse.

This change shouldn't be taken lightly. Diverticulitis can lead to infection or bleeding. You should call your doctor *any* time you see blood after a bowel movement. And if you've been diagnosed with diverticulosis and develop left-sided belly pain that doesn't go away, you should do the same.

If you have an infection, it can be treated with antibiotics. For something more serious, like a tear, your doctor can determine the right plan of care.

which is not enough. According to health authorities like the American Dietetic Association, our optimal fiber needs are between 25 and 30 grams every day. This may sound like a lot—but it does a lot of good.

Fiber helps the colon expand when eliminating waste. Fiber also draws water into the stool, making bowel movements smoother. Whole wheat bread (check the label to be sure) and all-bran cereals are excellent sources of bran fiber, which appears to be the most effective type of fiber in preventing diverticulosis. Sprinkling raw bran on your foods is also an option.

Vegetables and fruits are other good sources of fiber, says Dr. Klein. Fruit and vegetable juices contain very little fiber, however, so reach for an apple instead of its juice.

■ **TRY TO RELAX.** Research published in the *British Journal of Surgery* showed that people with diverticulosis who scored high on an anxiety test were more likely to have pain. Lin Chang, M.D., suggests that a regular relaxation practice could help. "Patients with chronic or severe gastrointestinal woes tend to have more anxiety and stress," she says. "Behavioral techniques like relaxation training can decrease symptoms. Calming breaths help regulate the nervous system and relax the digestive tract."

When you are having abdominal discomfort, focus on how your lower belly expands as you inhale for a count of 4 and moves back in as you exhale. Do this twice daily for 15 minutes—or more often, if you find it helpful. You may also want to take a gentle yoga class or follow a yoga video two or three times a week. The breathing is similar, and the low-impact physical activity will help you digestive activity.

■ **EAT HIGHLY PROCESSED FOODS IN MODERATION.** This is good general-health advice, but it also applies to treating diverticulosis. If you eat a lot of low-fiber processed foods, says Dr. Klein, you won't have room to eat the high-fiber foods you need.

■ **DON'T SAY "SO LONG" TO SEEDS.** Until recently, many doctors told their patients to avoid tomatoes, strawberries, and other foods with small seeds. They believed that the seeds could lodge in the diverticula and trigger inflammation. Today, this is a controversial point among doctors. The National Institutes of Health says that there's no evidence to support the ban on seeds and that many of these foods are good sources of fiber. So go pick that tomato from your garden.

■ **INCREASE YOUR FIBER INTAKE SLOWLY.** Take 6 to 8 weeks to gradually increase your fiber intake to the recommended 30 to 35 grams each day, Dr. Klein suggests. "You need time for your digestive system to adapt."

You can expect bloating and gas in the first few weeks. But most people will get over this.

■ **IF YOU CAN'T GET ENOUGH FIBER IN YOUR DIET, TAKE A SUPPLEMENT.** The best are psyllium seed supplements (such as Metamucil).

■ **DON'T USE SUPPOSITORIES.** While they may offer a quick fix, suppositories aren't the best choice for stimulating bowel movements. "Your system can get addicted to them," Dr. Klein explains. "And then it becomes a vicious cycle—you need more suppositories."

■ **DRINK LOTS OF LIQUIDS.** "Drink six to eight glasses of water a day," advises Dr. Klein, adding that the liquid is an important partner to fiber in combating constipation, which is associated with diverticulosis. Straining during a bowel movement tends to expand the diverticula through the walls of the colon, making the problematic pockets bigger.

■ **GO WHEN YOU HAVE TO GO.** If you don't yield to nature's call, you defeat the purpose of adding more fiber to your diet and drinking more liquids. "Don't suppress the need to move your bowel," Dr. Williamson advises.

■ **EXERCISE.** It tones more than your legs and hips. Exercise also tones the muscles in

Cures from the Kitchen

This homemade remedy for constipation can be beneficial for anyone who wants to get more fiber: Mix ½ cup of unprocessed bran, ½ cup of applesauce, and ⅓ cup of prune juice. Refrigerate. Eat 2 to 3 tablespoons of the mixture after dinner, then drink a full glass of water. If you need to, you can increase your dose to 3 to 4 tablespoons.

Whole prunes, prune juice, and herbal teas are also very effective natural laxatives. Specially formulated teas can be found in most health food stores.

your colon. "It helps bowel movements; you don't have to strain as much," says Dr. Klein.

■ **SOOTHE YOUR PAIN WITH HEAT.** To relieve tenderness or cramping, hold a heating pad against the left side of your abdomen.

■ **APPLY A LITTLE PRESSURE.** Steven Tan, M.D., recommends this ancient healing art to encourage natural, normal digestive system activity, easing constipation that can make diverticulosis worse. "Animal studies suggest that acupuncture may spur contractions in the colon, moving your bowel," he says. "If your episode is minor, you could be helped by a single treatment; chronic sufferers may need about 10. Acupressure may help, too."

To try acupressure for constipation, it takes only two fingers and less than 2 minutes. Using your index and middle fingers, apply firm pressure on the outside of your lower leg, about 3 inches below the kneecap. Press in firmly for 5 seconds and then release for 10 seconds. Repeat five times. To find an acupuncturist for more treatment, visit www.aaaomonline.org, the Web site for the American Association of Acupuncture and Oriental Medicine, to search for an acupuncturist near you.

■ **AVOID CAFFEINE.** "Coffee, chocolate, tea, colas—they all tend to irritate," Dr. Williamson says.

■ **LOOK FOR A PATTERN.** Certain foods may disrupt your bowel habits or cause loose stools, Dr. Williamson says. Try to identify these foods and avoid them.

Strive for 35

You know that getting enough fiber in your diet (30 to 35 grams daily) is the most important thing you can do to treat and prevent diverticulosis. But what you may not know is how much fiber is in the recommended high-fiber foods or how to inject more fiber into your diet without sitting down to a bowl of raw bran.

Here are some of the top foods that can help you reach your fiber gram goal:

- 1 medium apple with skin = 3.3 grams
- 1 whole wheat English muffin = 4.4 grams
- ½ cup of green peas = 4.4 grams
- 1 medium sweet potato with skin = 4.8 grams

- ½ cup of black beans = 7.5 grams
- ½ cup of navy beans = 9.5 grams
- ½ cup of All-Bran cereal = 9.6 grams

■ **TAKE IT EASY WITH IBUPROFEN AND ACETAMINOPHEN.** Avoid high doses of ibuprofen, a common painkiller that is known as a nonsteroidal anti-inflammatory drug (NSAID). Regular and consistent use of acetaminophen is also associated with increased symptoms of diverticular disease. One study of more than 35,000 men found that those who took NSAIDs or acetaminophen at least two times a week were twice as likely to develop diverticular disease as men who didn't take the drugs regularly. NSAIDs inhibit prostaglandins, fatty acids that protect the cells in the intestinal tract.

PANEL OF ADVISORS

LIN CHANG, M.D., IS CODIRECTOR OF THE CENTER FOR NEUROVISCERAL SCIENCES AND WOMEN'S HEALTH AT UCLA IN LOS ANGELES.

SAMUEL KLEIN, M.D., IS A WILLIAM H. DANFORTH PROFESSOR OF MEDICINE AND NUTRITIONAL SCIENCE AND DIRECTOR OF THE CENTER FOR HUMAN NUTRITION AT WASHINGTON UNIVERSITY SCHOOL OF MEDICINE IN ST. LOUIS.

STEVEN TAN, M.D., IS CHAIRMAN OF THE CALIFORNIA STATE BOARD OF ACUPUNCTURE IN BEVERLY HILLS.

PAUL WILLIAMSON, M.D., IS A CLINICAL ASSOCIATE PROFESSOR OF SURGERY AT THE UNIVERSITY OF FLORIDA IN GAINESVILLE AND A COLON AND RECTAL SURGEON IN ORLANDO.

Dizziness

18 Tips to Stop the Spinning

Dizziness is certainly disorienting—but if you suffer from it, you certainly are not alone. At the top of the list with back pain and headaches, dizziness is one of the most common health complaints that bring people to the doctor's office. More than 2 million people seek help for dizziness each year. Older people usually experience dizziness or balance disorders more frequently, but these problems can affect people of all ages. It may be comforting to know that the Mayo Clinic says that dizziness is most often not a sign of a serious problem.

The sensation that the world is spinning is a type of dizziness called vertigo. Inner-ear problems such as injury, viral infections, inflammation, floating debris, and bleeding can all cause vertigo, says Terry D. Fife, M.D.

But not all dizziness is from inner-ear problems, Dr. Fife says. Dizziness may also result from poor circulation, side effects from medications, and a condition called orthostatic hypotension, in which blood pressure temporarily drops when you're in the upright position or after you suddenly get up.

Dizziness often disappears on its own, but it can have long-term

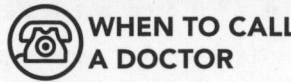

WHEN TO CALL A DOCTOR

Everyone gets dizzy from time to time—when getting out of bed, for example, or standing up after working in the garden—and it isn't always a problem.

"If it is mild, occurs rarely, and was clearly provoked by a particular activity, it is probably harmless," says Terry D. Fife, M.D. Dizziness that occurs often, however, or is accompanied by other symptoms is potentially serious.

Dizziness that's followed by fainting could be a warning sign of heart disease. Vertigo or dizziness accompanied by slurred speech, blurred or double vision, or numbness or tingling in the arms or legs may be a stroke.

If vertigo comes on completely out of the blue or is accompanied by any of these other symptoms, you need to see a doctor right away, Dr. Fife says.

consequences, especially when it leads to a loss of balance or falls. "People can become so frightened of falling that they stop being physically active," says Dr. Fife.

To get dizziness under control, here's what experts advise.

■ **STOP MOVING IMMEDIATELY.** If you feel an attack coming on, stay absolutely still for a few minutes. Don't move your head at all. Holding still allows your blood pressure to stabilize and helps the inner ear regain its normal equilibrium.

■ **THEN SIT DOWN.** Dizziness and vertigo usually occur when you change position or stand. Sitting down right away often causes the symptoms to subside—and it's a lot safer than trying to stay on your feet when the world is spinning.

■ **REACH OUT AND TOUCH SOMETHING.** When you feel an attack of dizziness or "spin-

---

Favorite Fixes

WHAT IT IS: To prevent vertigo, Alicia Fagan of Glen Mills, Pennsylvania, recommends keeping your eyes closed when changing position from upright to lying down.

WHY IT WORKS: Closing your eyes seems to keep confusing visual signals from bringing on dizziness or making it worse.

HOW TO USE IT: When lying down or flopping on the couch first sit on the edge and close your eyes before reclining. Similarly, when you rise, sit up with you eyes closed, then open them once you are upright.

---

ning" coming on, lightly rest your fingers on objects around you—a bookcase, for example, a table, or the back of a chair.

Spinning sensations occur when the brain receives conflicting messages, Dr. Fife says. Your eyes may be convinced that you're whirling, while your feet know very well that you're standing still. This conflict in sensations makes the vertigo worse. "If you make contact with enough objects, your sensory nerves start to adjust," he says.

■ **TRY THE TILTING TRICK.** The Epley maneuver, a simple series of head and neck movements that takes about a minute, has been shown to help vertigo. In one study, 94 percent of dizziness sufferers experienced relief after just one week of daily tilting sessions.

To learn the moves, watch a short instructional video clip at www.prevention.com/links (look for the November 2008 link list), or go to www.youtube.com and search for "Epley." You can also visit www.vestibular.org to find a knowledgeable doctor. The tilting exercises work by putting floating calcium crystals in motion and sending them back to the inner ear, where they can be reabsorbed.

■ **FLEX YOUR LEGS.** If you have orthostatic hypotension, the blood tends to pool in the legs and feet. This causes a reduction in brain bloodflow, which can result in dizziness. "Flexing your leg muscles before you stand up—by crossing and uncrossing your legs, for example—helps push blood back into circulation," says Joshua Hoffman, M.D.

Cures from the Kitchen

Dizziness often brings on nausea. Ginger, a traditional remedy for stomach upset, has been shown to ease this nausea, says Terry D. Fife, M.D. Fresh ginger, eaten by the slice or grated and used to make a tea, can be effective. Or try over-the-counter supplements, following the directions on the label.

■ **GET UP IN STAGES.** Don't leap out of bed in the morning. Instead, swing your legs over the side of the bed and slowly rise to a sitting position. Wait for a minute or two, then slowly stand up. This gives your blood pressure time to adjust, which may prevent dizziness, says Dr. Hoffman.

■ **KEEP MOVING.** It's normal for people who experience frequent dizziness to become increasingly afraid of falling. As a result, they become more and more sedentary. This reduces the ability of the brain to monitor and fine-tune the sense of balance—which will make falls even *more* likely.

It's important to stay physically active to maintain muscle strength as well as balance, says Dr. Hoffman. Take your usual walks. Go shopping. Jog or ride an exercise bike. As long as you move carefully at "high-risk" times— using handrails when walking down stairs, for example, or moving slowly after changing position—you're unlikely to lose your balance.

If you've already lost confidence in your balance, doctors advise that you should consult a balance specialist.

■ **KNOW YOUR TRIGGERS.** Dizziness and vertigo that occur at predictable times—first thing in the morning when getting out of bed, for example, or when you suddenly change position—may indicate an easy-to-treat inner-ear disorder.

A sudden drop in blood pressure can trigger dizziness, and this can be caused by a variety of things, including sudden temperature changes, such as when you go from a hot car into an air-conditioned building. "Hunger is another trigger for some people, and having just eaten is a trigger for others. Hunger-induced dizziness may be related to low blood sugar, while dizziness after a meal may be caused by digestive processes that 'steal' blood from the brain," says Dr. Fife.

If you've recently had a cold, don't be surprised if you start experiencing dizziness, he says. Cold viruses sometimes travel to the inner ear and cause a condition called vestibular neuritis, which causes inflammation and injury to the inner-ear balance mechanism, resulting in vertigo. "It usually clears up within a few months," says Dr. Fife.

■ **WEAR FLAT SHOES.** Apart from the fact that walking on heels is hazardous when the world seems to be spinning, flat shoes provide more contact with the ground. More contact makes it easier for your brain to process information about your posture. This prevents some inner-ear "confusion" and can help prevent falls, says Dr. Fife.

■ **THINK NONSKID.** Anyone who has a tendency to get dizzy should use only nonskid mats in the tub or shower, and on bathroom and kitchen floors. So skip the all-cotton throw rugs in these slip-prone areas—choose mats with a tacky rubber backing for safety.

■ **USE A NIGHT-LIGHT.** Darkness can be especially treacherous for those with inner-ear problems because the brain, which normally compensates for the lack of information from the ears by drawing on more information from the eyes, does not receive enough visual clues to help the body stay properly oriented. Simply using a night-light could help prevent dizziness or falls, says Dr. Fife.

"If you have significant inner-ear problems, never swim in the dark," Dr. Fife says. "When underwater, some people have found themselves unable to tell what's up and what's down. We have had a few patients nearly drown when they could not perceive which way to go to come up for air in the swimming pool, convinced that the bottom was the top."

■ **BE CAREFUL WALKING ON HEAVILY PADDED CARPETING.** Carpets with deep, soft padding may feel good on your feet, but the cushioning can make it harder for your body to stay properly oriented, says Dr. Fife. This is because the soft surface makes it harder for the nerves in the feet to detect changes in joint position used to maintain balance.

■ **TUCK AWAY WIRES.** Electrical cords and computer wires are like dangerous snakes lying in wait, particularly if you're struggling with dizziness. Prevent tripping by removing these hazards whenever possible. You can buy specialized wire covers at office supply stores that will keep all your wires neatly bundled together without tangles, and make them more visible in the process.

■ **BE CAUTIOUS WHEN YOU'RE IN BATHROOMS.** The bathroom is a high-risk area because the combination of slick surfaces and off-balance movements—bending over to brush your teeth, for example—makes falls more likely. In addition, bathing or showering causes blood vessels to dilate and triggers a drop in blood pressure. If you move too quickly, your brain may not get enough oxygen, making you feel light-headed and dizzy, says Dr. Hoffman. So install grab bars in the bath and shower and beside the toilet. Available in hardware stores, the bars provide something to stabilize you should dizziness strike as you're standing or stepping out of the bath.

■ **DRINK PLENTY OF WATER.** The sense of thirst declines over time, which means older adults tend to run a little on the dry side. Even mild dehydration can cause drops in blood pressure that result in occasional dizziness, says Dr. Fife.

Try to drink 8 to 10 glasses (8 ounces each) of water daily. "Water is good, but when someone is dehydrated, sports drinks are even better," says Dr. Fife. They contain sodium and other electrolytes that help the body retain fluids.

■ **CONSIDER MOTION-SICKNESS MEDICA-TION.** If you experience dizziness associated with motion (car sickness, airsickness, sea-sickness), your doctor may recommend an over-the-counter medication called Drama-mine or Bonine. These medications help reduce chemical signals from the inner ear to the brain's "vomiting center."

■ **REDUCE YOUR SALT INTAKE.** Vertigo is sometimes caused by a condition called Ménière's disease, which occurs when fluid accumulates in the inner ear. If you have been diagnosed with this condition, following a low-salt diet can help reduce fluid buildup that results in attacks of vertigo. Doctors usually advise no more than 2,000 milligrams of sodium daily.

When buying packaged foods, check the labels to see how much sodium they contain. Your best bet is to buy products that are labeled "low sodium" or "sodium-free." It's fine to add a bit of salt to foods at the table, but not during cooking, which some people find imparts less flavor.

■ **MAKE A LIST OF MEDICINES.** Then check it twice—first with your doctor, then with your pharmacist. Many prescription and over-the-counter drugs, including aspirin, antidepressants, and drugs for treating high blood pressure, cause dizziness. In some cases, switching drugs may be all that's needed to reduce or eliminate dizziness.

PANEL OF ADVISORS

TERRY D. FIFE, M.D., IS AN ASSOCIATE PROFESSOR OF CLINICAL NEUROLOGY AT THE UNIVERSITY OF ARIZONA IN TUCSON AND DIRECTOR OF THE ARIZONA BALANCE CENTER AT BARROW NEUROLOGICAL INSTITUTE IN PHOENIX.

JOSHUA HOFFMAN, M.D., IS AN INTERNIST AND MEDICAL DIRECTOR OF SUTTER MEDICAL GROUP HOSPITALIST PRO-GRAM IN SACRAMENTO, CALIFORNIA.

Dry Eyes

14 Moistening Ideas

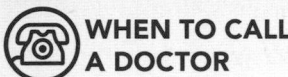

WHEN TO CALL A DOCTOR

If you notice that your eyes are drier than normal for more than a day or two, get some professional advice, says Ted Belheumer, O.D. The solution may be something as simple as changing your brand of contact lenses. Your doctor can help determine the cause of your dry eyes and if other steps are needed.

A treatment your doctor might recommend is the insertion of a tiny collagen plug into your tear drainage canal of each eye, says Anne Sumers, M.D. The plug helps conserve the tears that you naturally produce and also keeps artificial tears in your eyes longer.

Dry eye occurs when the eye doesn't produce enough tears to keep it moist and comfortable. This condition affects millions of Americans and is more common in women, especially after menopause, according to the National Eye Institute. As we age, the eyes usually produce fewer tears.

"Eye dryness is a common problem," says Anne Sumers, M.D., particularly if you are female. Half of all women older than age 40 experience dry eyes in some form, whether it's an intermittent or a persistent problem. Dry eyes are a part of aging, she says. "It's rotten, unfortunate, but true."

Blinking your eye creates a three-layered film of water, oil, and mucus. Around age 40, the tear glands begin to slow down, producing less of this soothing eye liquid. The problem is even worse for women after menopause because hormonal shifts dry up secretions, including tears, says Dr. Sumers.

Dry eye is a simple name for a complex and irritating condition that is characterized by redness, burning, itching, scratchiness, tearing, and sensitivity to light. Although usually just another hazard of aging, dry eyes may also be caused by exposure to environmental conditions, injuries to the eye, or general health problems. Sun, wind, cold, indoor heating and air-conditioning, glaring computer screens, and even high altitudes can cause further discomfort if you experience eye dryness.

In addition to postmenopausal women, those who are more prone to dry eye include contact lens wearers, people who have undergone LASIK surgery, and those with arthritis and diabetes. A wide variety of medications, including decongestants, antihistamines, diuretics, anesthetics, antidepressants, drugs for heart disease, ulcer remedies, chemotherapies, and drugs containing beta-blockers, can slow down your tear production and cause a case of dry eye.

The good news? With the right steps, it is possible to get those tears flowing again. Here's how.

■ **APPLY A WARM COMPRESS.** If your eyes become dry every now and then, try placing a clean, warm, damp compress on your eyelids for 5 to 10 minutes at a time, two or three times each day. The moist heat soothes dry eyes and can stimulate tears.

■ **OPT FOR OINTMENT.** To combat cases in which eye dryness gets unbearable while you sleep, apply a tear-replacement/moisture-sealing ointment at bedtime to help ease

Cures from the Kitchen

This "cure" comes straight from the kitchen sink. If your eyes seem dry, the rest of your body might be parched, as well. Do your best to drink more water, says optometrist Ted Belheumer, O.D. And cut back on beverages that have a diuretic effect, he says, such as coffee and alcohol.

your pain, says Dr. Sumers. These extra-thick, over-the-counter eye ointments contain white petroleum jelly and mineral oil, and they last longer than drops.

To apply the ointment, pull the lower eyelid down, look up and squeeze a dab of ointment in the trough between your lid and eye. Blink to spread the ointment around. These thick ointments can blur your vision for a while, so they're best applied when you're already in bed, Dr. Sumers cautions.

■ **EAT TO BEAT DRYNESS.** In one study, women who ate about 2,350 milligrams of omega-3s a week had a 68 percent lower occurrence of eye dryness than those who ate less than 500 milligrams. "These fatty acids help manage symptoms by reducing inflammation," says Linda Antinoro, R.D.

To try this nutritional remedy, take at least 500 milligrams daily of both DHA and EPA supplements. If you enjoy seafood, eat up to three 4-ounce servings of fatty fish like salmon or canned light tuna a week.

TAKE A CONTACT HOLIDAY. If you regularly wear contact lenses and are experiencing dry eyes, determine whether or not the lenses may in fact be the problem, says Ted Belheumer, O.D. "You need to determine if you have a physical problem, or a mechanical one related to having contact lenses in for many hours."

So pop out those contact lenses, and put on your glasses for the rest of the day. You will likely notice quite an improvement. If you find your eyes are more comfortable without your lenses in, you may want to take a "contact holiday" at least 1 day a week—or more often. Invest in a flattering pair of frames to feel stylish even when you give your eyes their much-needed rest.

■ **TRY ARTIFICIAL TEARS.** Available over-the-counter, artificial tears help soothe tender, gritty eyes, says Dr. Sumers. A mixture of saline and a film-forming substance such as polyvinyl alcohol or synthetic cellulose, artificial tears can be used throughout the day. They come in different thicknesses, so experiment to find the brand that's right for you, she says.

The thinner versions are less likely to blur your vision or leave a residue on your eyelashes, but they do require you to use more frequent applications.

Choose a preservative-free brand, because some preservatives can be toxic and damage the surface of the eye, Dr. Sumers says. Two good choices are GenTeal and Refresh Tears.

Whichever type you choose, here's how to insert the eyedrops. Gently pull down the lower lid and squeeze the drops into the corner of your eye near your nose. Keep the eye closed for a minute to make sure the drops stay in the eye.

Use them anywhere from 1 to 10 times per day, depending on how severe your dryness problem is, says Dr. Sumers.

■ **GET INTO THE SHADES.** Because wind and sun can further dry out your eyes, wear wraparound sunglasses, which extend past the sides of your eyes, suggests Dr. Sumers.

■ **STAY OUT OF THE DIRECT LINE OF FIRE.** A blast of heated air or air-conditioning might be just what the rest of your body needs to make the morning commute more bearable, but a direct flow of hot or cold air to your eyes can irritate them even more. If you have dry eyes, point your car's air vents downward, says Dr. Sumers. That way, you'll get the relief you need from the outdoor elements but without causing your already dry eyes any additional misery.

According to Dr. Sumers, the same principle applies in your home. Aim heating and cooling ducts away from areas where you spend a great deal of time. This is particularly important if you have a forced-air heating system, which causes your eyes to dry out more quickly.

When traveling by plane, make sure that the overhead air vents aren't spilling air directly at your eyes. "Airplanes are notoriously dry environments, so don't make matters worse on your eyes by having cool air blowing on your face," she says.

■ **GET FRESH.** Open a window and let in some fresh air, says Dr. Sumers. This will allow some much-needed moisture into the room as well, which could do your dry eyes a world of good, she says.

■ **MOISTEN THE AIR.** Try a home air humidifier unit to moisten dry air in your home, suggests Dr. Sumers.

■ **AVOID A COMMON MISTAKE.** Too many people take an antihistamine when they suffer dry and itchy eyes. This makes already dry eyes even drier, says Dr. Sumers.

■ **BLINK A LOT.** If part of your job description includes spending long hours in front of a computer screen, take occasional blink breaks, says Phillip J. Calenda, M.D. By constantly staring at the task at hand, you don't blink as much as you should, which causes eye moisture to evaporate more quickly. Taking a blink break will help restore the much-needed tear film over your eyes. Spending 5 minutes each hour looking off in the distance instead of reading or doing other close work will allow the eyes to blink more.

■ **REST YOURSELF—AND YOUR EYES.** Sleep expert Rubin Naiman, Ph.D., says, "During sleep, complex changes occur in the tear film—a thin layer of mucous, oil, and water that coats the eye, providing moisture and protection. Adequate sleep gives the eyes a break and replenishes the film."

Make it a goal to get at least 8 hours of literal shut-eye each night, without air blowing on your face from an open window, fan, air conditioner, or heater. If your bedroom air is dry (particularly in winter, when heating systems are on), use an air humidifier, says Dr.

Sumers. Some people slightly open their eyes while sleeping, and moist air in the bedroom can be very helpful.

■ **REARRANGE YOUR WORKSPACE.** The American Academy of Ophthalmology recommends the following changes in your workstation to minimize eye dryness and eyestrain while sitting in front of a computer.

- Screen distance: Sit about 20 inches from the computer monitor, which is a little farther than reading distance, with the top of the screen at or below eye level.

- Equipment: Choose a monitor that tilts or swivels and has both contrast and brightness controls.

- Furniture: Make sure you have an adjustable chair.

- Reference material: Place papers on a document holder so that you don't have to keep looking back and forth, frequently refocusing your eyes and turning your neck.

- Lighting: Modify your lighting to eliminate reflections or glare. A micro-mesh filter for your screen may help limit reflections and glare.

- Rest breaks: Take periodic breaks and be sure to blink often to keep your eyes from drying out.

PANEL OF ADVISORS

LINDA ANTINORO, R.D., IS A SENIOR NUTRITIONIST AT BRIGHAM AND WOMEN'S HOSPITAL IN BOSTON.

TED BELHEUMER, O.D., IS A DOCTOR OF OPTOMETRY AT TROY VISION CENTER IN TROY, NEW YORK. HE HAS BEEN IN PRIVATE PRACTICE FOR MORE THAN 30 YEARS.

PHILLIP J. CALENDA, M.D., IS AN OPHTHALMOLOGIST IN SCARSDALE, NEW YORK.

RUBIN NAIMAN, PH.D., IS DIRECTOR OF SLEEP PROGRAMS AT MIRAVAL RESORT IN TUCSON.

ANNE SUMERS, M.D., IS TEAM OPHTHALMOLOGIST FOR THE NEW YORK GIANTS AND THE NEW JERSEY NETS, AND HAS A PRACTICE IN RIDGEWOOD, NEW JERSEY. SHE SERVES AS SPOKESPERSON FOR THE AMERICAN ACADEMY OF OPHTHALMOLOGY.

Dry Mouth

16 Mouthwatering Solutions

Cotton balls, sawdust, and the Sahara are just three images that come to mind when you're suffering from dry mouth. The awful oral dryness can affect almost anyone, but certain people are more susceptible. No matter the cause, mouth dryness, officially known as xerostomia, can be debilitating. If left untreated, it can lead to painful mouth sores, rampant tooth decay and even tooth loss, and other oral health problems. Your mouth needs adequate saliva flow to coat and lubricate oral tissues, which in turn helps prevent tooth decay and gum disease.

According to Robert H. Hill II, D.D.S, dry mouth affects a wide variety of people, including older adults whose mouths naturally dry out over time, as well as people who have diabetes, depression, or an autoimmune disease known as Sjögren's syndrome. For cancer patients, dry mouth is often the result of chemotherapy or radiation therapy, and a consultation with both the oncologist and the dentist is advised.

Very often, mouth dryness is a side effect of prescription drugs, says Dr. Hill. Hundreds of medications cause mouth dryness, including commonly prescribed beta-blockers, diuretics,

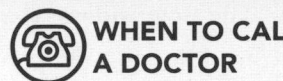 **WHEN TO CALL A DOCTOR**

Any time you notice that your mouth is dryer than usual for more than a few days (for instance, while getting over a cold), give your dentist a call, says Robert H. Hill II, D.D.S. "If there is any medical reason for the problem, your dentist can connect with your physician to go over your medications and health history," he says. There's no reason to wait until you *know* you have a problem.

anticholinergics, antihistamines, antidepressants, and some pain killers. As the population ages and prescription drugs become more common, dry mouth is more prevalent. "The good news is we are seeing patients who, at age 90, still have all their own teeth," says Dr. Hill. The downside is that the medications that are allowing us to live longer may be causing the discomfort of dry mouth.

Here are some suggestions to help relieve dryness, preserve soft tissue, and help prevent tooth decay.

■ **CHEW SUGARLESS GUM.** Chewing stimulates the salivary glands. Try sugarless gum that contains xylitol, a sweetening agent that reduces cavity-causing bacteria, says Dan Peterson, D.D.S. He also recommends Trident Advantage gum, which contains Recaldent, a remineralizing agent that adds calcium and phosphate to the teeth.

■ **DON'T FORGET TO DRINK.** Quenching your dry mouth with regular sips of water can make a big difference, says Dr. Hill. Swig on bottled water during the day to keep the fluid flowing.

Everyone should drink eight 8-ounce glasses of water each day, says Anne Bosy, M.Ed., M.Sc.. The more active you are, the more water you need. If you're exercising at the gym, take along a bottle of water. Have an all-day meeting with a key client? Put pitchers of water on the table.

■ **RINSE AWAY THE PAIN.** Chronic dryness will make your mouth more easily irritated and sore, because one of the primary chores of saliva is to neutralize the erosive acids from plaque. Rinse your mouth with a mixture of $1/4$ teaspoon of baking soda, $1/8$ teaspoon of salt, and 1 cup of warm water for some oral comfort. The soothing combination neutralizes acids and draws out infection from gum tissues.

■ **GIVE HARD CANDY A TRY.** Suck a piece of sugarless hard candy to stimulate saliva flow, says Dr. Peterson, who recommends citrus- or mint-flavored candies. They stimulate more saliva.

■ **MUNCH ON SOME VEGGIES.** Diets high in fiber and bulk also seem to stimulate salivary glands. Bosy suggests eating fibrous foods, such as raw carrots, celery, and apples at mealtimes and as snacks. These rough-textured foods also clean your tongue as you chew and swallow, which is good for overall oral hygiene.

■ **SAY NO TO SWEETS.** Limit your intake of sweet, sticky, sugary foods if you're experiencing dry mouth. Your lack of saliva will keep these foods stuck to your teeth, increasing your risk of cavities, says Dr. Peterson.

■ **DITCH THE COCKTAIL AND SKIP THE SMOKE.** Dr. Hill says that two common vices—alcohol and cigarettes—can make a bad thing worse. "You should certainly quit and see if it helps the dryness," he says.

■ **CHOOSE YOUR TOOTHPASTE WISELY.** When saliva production is low, your risk of cavities and gum disease is high. Dr. Peterson recommends brushing at least twice a day with an extra-strength fluoride toothpaste approved by the American Dental Association.

If you have mouth dryness, don't use toothpaste that contains the foaming agent sodium lauryl sulfate, because it can irritate gum tissue, says Dr. Peterson. He recommends trying Rembrandt's Natural or Biotene's Dry Mouth Toothpaste.

Here's a fluoride-treatment program Dr. Peterson recommends for extra tooth protection. After brushing and right before bed, apply toothpaste with your toothbrush or a cotton swab to your gums and teeth. Let it sit for 1 minute, then swish for 1 minute, moving the paste onto all your teeth and gums. Spit out the excess paste, but don't rinse your mouth. Go to bed with the fluoride residue on these surfaces. Do this again in the morning, and don't eat or drink anything for 30 minutes after this routine. This procedure should be done one or two times a day for 4 to 6 weeks.

Cures from the Kitchen

A dry mouth can make foods with little moisture go down like pencil shavings, so add sauces and gravies to perk up drier foods and make them more palatable, says Dan Peterson, D.D.S. Drinking fluids frequently throughout a meal will increase the moisture content of your mouth, make food easier to swallow, and improve taste.

■ **BE SELECTIVE ABOUT MOUTHWASH.** "If you have gum disease, your dentist may recommend that you use something antiseptic, like Listerine," says Dr. Hill. "But if you also have dryness, you'll want to avoid mouthwash containing alcohol." There are over-the-counter products that do not contain alcohol. For added tooth protection, look for an alcohol-free mouthwash that also contains fluoride, says Dr. Hill.

■ **CHANGE YOUR TOOTHBRUSH FRE-QUENTLY.** When your toothbrush has a buildup of toothpaste in between the bristles, it's time to make the investment in a new one, says Bosy. Over time, toothbrushes can harbor bacteria and infect your mouth with the bacteria that cause bad breath. Spending a few bucks for a new toothbrush every couple of months is a sound investment to keep bacteria and bad breath away.

■ **BRUSH AND FLOSS MORE FREQUENTLY.** Saliva plays many roles, from making it easier to speak to jumpstarting the digestion of the food we eat. Another key task of saliva is to keep the teeth clean and free of debris and plaque, says Dr. Hill. Saliva coats and lubricates the teeth, making it more difficult for plaque to attach and do its damage. If you are lacking in saliva, it's even more important to practice impeccable oral hygiene. "You may want to floss and brush up to three times a days," says Dr. Hill, "after every meal."

■ **SOAK YOUR DENTURES.** Dentures make people with dry mouth more susceptible to infection from yeast organisms, which adhere to the plastic. Soak your dentures overnight in 1 part chlorine beach to 10 parts water to prevent infection, says Dr. Peterson. Rinse thoroughly in the morning before putting them in.

■ **MOISTURIZE THE AIR.** Use a cool-air vaporizer in your bedroom to get some much-needed humidity in the air and to cut down on mouth dryness at night, says Dr. Peterson. If you're a mouth breather, make an effort to breathe through your nose at night to prevent saliva from evaporating while you sleep.

■ **MOISTEN UP WITH A MULTIVITAMIN.** A number of vitamin deficiencies, particularly riboflavin and vitamin A, can rob your mouth of moisture. Pernicious anemia from a vitamin B_{12} deficiency can also cause mouth dryness. If that's the case, try a daily multivitamin and mineral supplement to battle the dryness, says Dr. Peterson.

■ **IF ALL ELSE FAILS, FAKE IT.** For better overall comfort and lubrication of your mouth, Bosy suggests over-the-counter saliva substitutes in the form of rinses, gels, and sprays for people who have chronically dry mouth or little or no salivary action. These saliva substitutes include many of the same enzymes and minerals as real saliva and help keep mouth tissues lubricated. Use two or three times a day (one of those times being just before bedtime).

PANEL OF ADVISORS

ANNE BOSY, M.ED., M.SC., IS THE CHIEF SCIENTIST AND FOUNDER OF THE ORAFRESH SYSTEM IN TORONTO, CANADA. ALSO KNOWN AS THE "BREATH DOC," BOSY IS RECOGNIZED INTERNATIONALLY AS A WORLD-CLASS EXPERT IN THE FIELD OF BAD BREATH RESEARCH AND HAS TREATED THOUSANDS OF PATIENTS WITH DRY MOUTH ASSOCIATED WITH BAD BREATH.

ROBERT H. HILL II, D.D.S., IS A DENTIST IN AVERILL PARK, NEW YORK. HE HAS BEEN IN PRIVATE PRACTICE SINCE 1978.

DAN PETERSON, D.D.S., IS A DENTIST IN GERING, NEBRASKA. HE HAS BEEN IN PRACTICE FOR MORE THAN 25 YEARS AND HAS TREATED HUNDREDS OF PATIENTS WITH DRY MOUTH SYNDROME.

Dry Skin and Winter Itch

10 Cold-Weather Options

Too often, the winter months are synonymous with dry, itchy skin. But it doesn't have to be. Even if you live in a cold, dry climate—or stay warm in a home with drying, forced-air heat—you can retain healthy skin that is soft and slightly moist. Because the dryness results from a lack of water, not oil, all you need to do is replenish that moisture.

Here's how.

■ **DON'T TRY TO DRINK DRYNESS AWAY.** Many beauty books and glamour magazines recommend drinking "at least seven or eight glasses of water per day" to keep your skin hydrated and prevent dryness. And while adequate water is essential for good health, just don't believe the hype that you'll see the results in your skin.

"If you're totally dehydrated, your skin will become dry," says Kenneth Neldner, M.D. "But if you are normally hydrated, you can't possibly counteract or correct dry skin by drinking water."

■ **DRY YOURSELF DAMP—THEN STOP.** "It's much more effective to apply moisturizer to damp skin immediately after bathing than to put it on totally dry skin," says Dr. Neldner.

That's not to say you have to hop from the tub or shower soaking wet and immediately apply lotion. "But a couple of pats with a towel will make you as dry as you want to be before you apply the

Favorite Fixes

WHAT IT IS: Lotion can form a protective layer to soothe and defend winter-dry hands. If the heavy, sticky feeling of hand cream prevents you from buttering up as often as you should, try this spray-on solution.

WHY IT WORKS: Jennifer Hoffmann of Huntington, New York, says spraying lotion onto her hands soaks into her skin faster and doesn't require a lot of massaging. An extra bonus: Your supply of hand lotion will go much further, because spraying it on uses less per application.

HOW TO USE IT: She recommends putting lotion in a recycled hairspray bottle. It sprays out lighter and it's easier to apply. "I took an empty bottle and filled it with hand lotion. Now I just pump a few sprays on my hands after washing the dishes or before putting on my gloves to go outside."

lotion," he says. "You're trying to trap a little water in the skin, and that's the fundamental rule of overcoming dryness."

■ **DON'T GET GREASED BY AD HYPE.** "Nothing beats plain petroleum jelly or mineral oil as a moisturizer," says Howard Donsky, M.D. In fact, if you don't mind the greasiness, virtually any vegetable oil (sunflower oil, peanut oil) can be used to combat dry skin and winter itch. They're effective, safe, and pure skin lubricants—and inexpensive as well.

These products do have one drawback, however. All tend to be greasy and don't particularly smell or feel "clean." So if you prefer a scented over-the-counter moisturizer, go for it. Just know that they're all basically the same.

■ **USE OATMEAL TO HEAL.** Some researchers believe that people first discovered the skin-soothing effects of oatmeal nearly 4,000 years ago. Many folks are still discovering it today. "Oatmeal can work in the bath as a soothing agent," says Dr. Donsky. Just pour 2 cups of colloidal oatmeal (such as Aveeno, available at drugstores) into a tub of lukewarm water. The term *colloidal* simply means that the oatmeal has been ground to a fine powder that remains suspended in water.

"You can also use oatmeal as a soap substitute," he says. Tie some colloidal oatmeal in a cotton handkerchief, submerge it in lukewarm water, squeeze out the excess water, and use as just like you would use a normal washcloth.

■ **SELECT SUPERFATTED SOAPS.** People with dry skin should reach for "superfatted" soaps like Basis, Neutrogena, or Dove. Superfatted soaps have extra amounts of fatty substances—cold cream, cocoa butter, coconut oil, or lanolin—added during the manufacturing process.

■ **WASH ONLY WHAT'S DIRTY.** Any soap can be too cleansing for already dry skin, and may be unnecessary. When bathing, use soap or body wash only on areas that need it—your face, underarms, feet, groin, and buttocks. "Rinsing with water is enough to get other spots clean and prevent you from unnecessarily stripping skin of its natural oils," says Amy Wechsler, M.D.

■ **GET WET BEFORE YOU WASH.** Before you lather up, be sure your skin is sufficiently wet. Applying any kind of cleanser or soap, especially the foaming or gel types, to dry skin is more likely to cause you irritation, says Mary Lupo, M.D.

■ **PRACTICE SKY-HIGH MOISTURE TRICKS.** Airplane air can be super arid, with humidity levels as low as 5 percent, drying out even the dewiest skin, says Leslie Baumann, M.D. Take these simple steps to keep your skin supple and beautiful at 35,000 feet *and* on the ground. Skip the makeup mask when you travel so you can moisturize often, she says. Once you are onboard, spritz with a face mist every hour and apply your choice of face lotion to seal in the moisture.

■ **BEAT DRYNESS IN BED.** Did you know you can fight dry skin by keeping your house clean? Exposure to dust mites—microscopic insects that feed on dust and create irritating droppings—makes it harder for dry skin conditions to heal. To rule out this culprit, vacuum floors and wash bedding weekly in hot water at least 130°F.

■ **TRY TO HUMIDIFY.** If you use a humidifier in your bedroom, Dr. Neldner says, close the door to keep in moisture. It might also help to leave the bathroom door open when you take a shower. "Every little bit of humidity helps," he says.

PANEL OF ADVISORS

LESLIE BAUMANN, M.D., IS A PROFESSOR AND THE DIRECTOR OF COSMETIC DERMATOLOGY AT THE MILLER SCHOOL OF MEDICINE AT THE UNIVERSITY OF MIAMI AND AUTHOR OF *THE SKIN TYPE SOLUTION.*

HOWARD DONSKY, M.D., IS A CLINICAL INSTRUCTOR OF DERMATOLOGY AT THE UNIVERSITY OF ROCHESTER SCHOOL OF MEDICINE AND DENTISTRY. HE IS A DERMATOLOGIST AT THE DERMATOLOGY AND COSMETIC CENTER OF ROCHESTER IN NEW YORK AND AUTHOR OF *BEAUTY IS SKIN DEEP.*

MARY LUPO, M.D., IS A *PREVENTION* MAGAZINE ADVISOR AND A CLINICAL PROFESSOR OF DERMATOLOGY AT TULANE UNIVERSITY IN NEW ORLEANS.

KENNETH NELDNER, M.D., IS PROFESSOR EMERITUS IN THE DEPARTMENT OF DERMATOLOGY AT TEXAS TECH UNIVERSITY SCHOOL OF MEDICINE AND A DERMATOLOGIST AT DERMATOLOGY ASSOCIATES, BOTH IN LUBBOCK.

AMY WECHSLER, M.D., IS A CLINICAL ASSISTANT PROFESSOR OF DERMATOLOGY AT SUNY DOWNSTATE MEDICAL CENTER IN NEW YORK CITY.

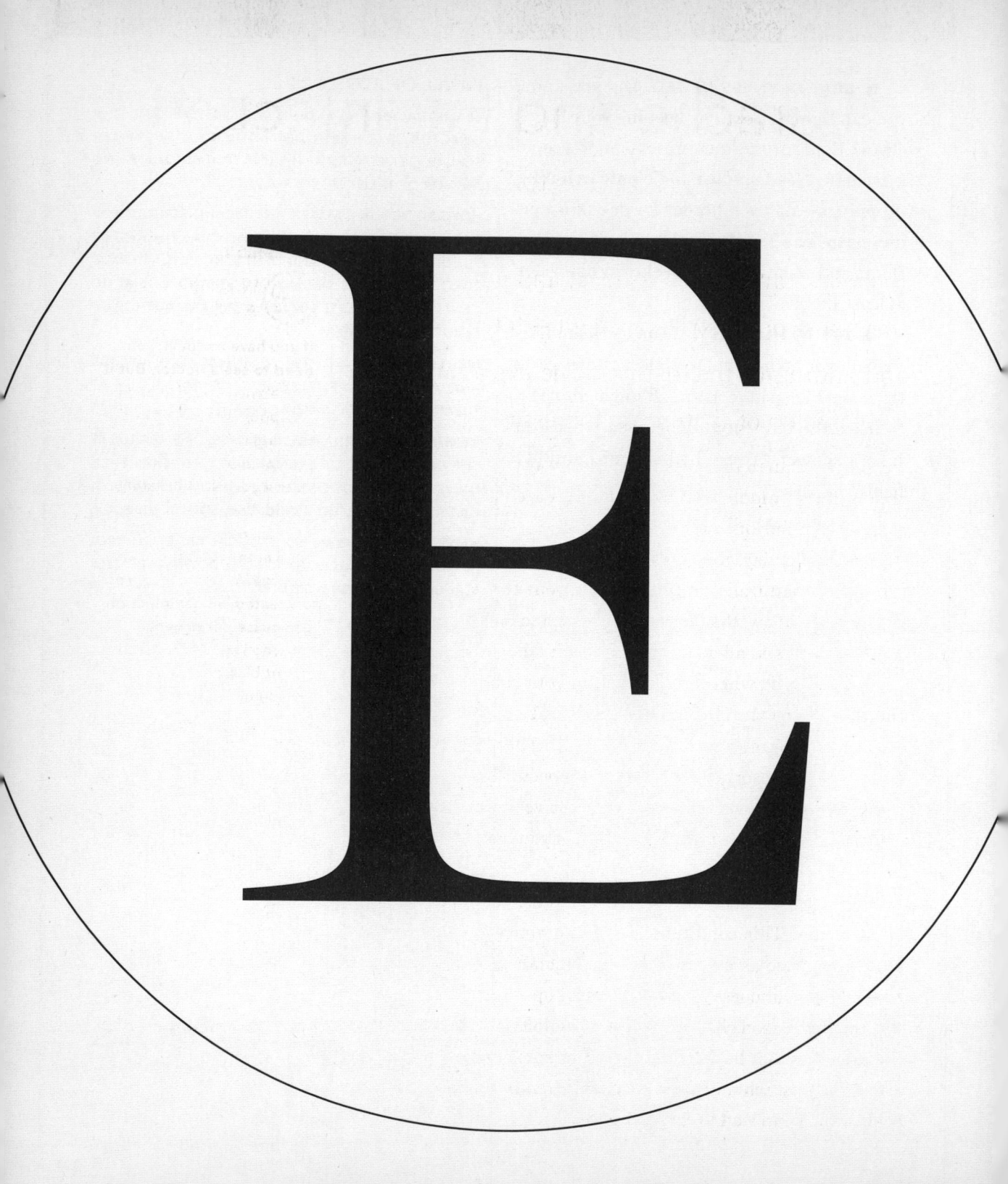

Earache and Ear Infection

25 Ways to Stop the Pain

Earaches can be very painful, and unfortunately, they most often strike at night—disrupting sleep and adding to the distress. The explanation is a combination of anatomy and pressure.

The eustachian tubes are the passageway from the back of the throat to the middle ear. Clogged tubes are the most common cause of earache for children and adults.

During the day, you hold up your head, and your eustachian tubes drain naturally into the back of your throat. Also, as you chew and swallow, the muscles of the eustachian tubes contract, opening them and allowing air into the middle ear.

But at night when you sleep and your head isn't upright, the tubes can't drain as easily. And you're not swallowing as often, so they aren't getting as much air. The air already in the middle ear is absorbed, and a vacuum occurs, sucking the eardrum inward. Several hours after you've fallen asleep, your eustachian tubes may clog, especially if you have a cold, a sinus infection, or an allergy.

Sometimes earache pain signifies a middle-ear infection, called otitis media. This condition is more common in children than adults, because as we grow, our eustachian tubes become narrower, longer, and less prone to plugging up.

Another reason children get ear infections is that the nerves to the area may not be fully developed in some babies, which can affect the eustachian tubes. Also, children in daycare get more colds, which can lead to ear infections.

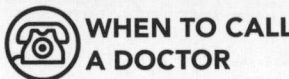

WHEN TO CALL A DOCTOR

If you have ear pain, you need to see a doctor. But if there's no pain, also make an appointment if you have hearing loss or if your ears stay plugged up for more than a couple of days after a cold. You could already have an ear infection or fluid in the middle ear, says George W. Facer, M.D. Left untreated, an ear infection can cause permanent hearing loss. Ten to 14 days of antibiotics is the usual course of treatment.

In adults, the stage is set for a middle-ear infection when sinuses get clogged as a result of allergies or a head cold, or when the eustachian tubes become blocked by air pressure during an airplane descent.

Even though the usual symptoms of a middle-ear infection are pain and hearing loss, adults and children can get ear infections without pain, says George W. Facer, M.D. Once infection hits, the best way to cure it is with antibiotics, although some infections clear up on their own, usually in a week to 10 days.

Other things cause earaches, too. Infections of the ear canal, known as external otitis or swimmer's ear, can trigger pain. Atmospheric pressure from airplane travel and deep-sea diving can cause ears to ache even if they aren't infected. Odd things, such as tiny clippings from a haircut, can fall into the ear canal and irritate your eardrum. Then there's

referred pain—a problem that exists somewhere else—that makes your ears tingle. These earaches can originate in your teeth, tonsils, throat, tongue, or jaw.

When your ears ache, you need to see a doctor. But until you get there, here are some quick pain stoppers.

■ **TRY ACETAMINOPHEN.** If you have an earache, the pain-reliever acetaminophen is a doctor's first choice. A dose at bedtime may be enough to let you sleep.

■ **SIT UP.** A few minutes upright decreases swelling and starts your eustachian tubes draining. Swallowing once you are sitting up also helps ease the pain. If it's possible, prop your head up slightly while you sleep to encourage better drainage.

■ **TAKE A DRINK.** Swallowing triggers the muscular action that helps your eustachian tubes open and drain. Open tubes mean less pain.

■ **WIGGLE YOUR EAR.** Here's a test to help determine whether you have otitis externa (an external problem like swimmer's ear) or otitis media (an internal middle-ear infection). Take hold of your outer ear, says Donald B. Kamerer Jr., M.D. If you can gently wiggle it without pain, the problem is probably in the middle ear. If moving your outer ear causes pain, then the infection is probably in the outer ear canal.

■ **TAKE AN HERBAL APPROACH.** Herbalists commonly recommend garlic and mullein oils for ear infections. Mullein is antimicrobial,

---

Favorite Fixes

 WHAT IT IS: For an aching ear, you can try a hot plate.

WHY IT WORKS: Lisa Orloff of South Orange, New Jersey, says, "I swear by this for earaches. The heat feels really good as it radiates inward."

HOW TO USE IT: "Microwave a small ceramic plate or saucer for a couple of seconds. It's ready when it's not too hot to the touch to take it out of the oven. Then place the plate gently cupped over the ear that hurts and hold it there."

An Ounce of Prevention

Ear infections are the most common cause of hearing loss in children, according to the American Academy of Otolaryngology-Head and Neck Surgery. Although you can't really prevent ear infections, there are some things you can do that may help lower the chances of your child getting them.

Choose child care carefully. Children exposed to large groups of other children are more likely to come into contact with the bugs that cause ear infections. Research has shown that children who attend daycare are more likely to come down with upper-respiratory infections that can lead to ear infection. If your child is prone to ear infections and must attend daycare, you may want to consider a smaller setting such as in-home family daycare.

Breastfeed. The American Academy of Pediatrics cites "strong evidence" from six major scientific studies that breastfeeding protects infants from otitis media.

In a study of 306 infants being seen in general pediatric practices, twice as many formula-fed infants as breastfed infants developed ear infections between the ages of 6 months and 1 year. In fact, formula feeding was the most significant factor associated with ear infections, even more important than being in daycare.

An earlier study of 237 infants in Helsinki, Finland, showed that 6 percent of breastfed babies and 19 percent of formula-fed babies had developed middle-ear infections by the end of their first year. By age 3, only 6 percent of those breastfed developed an infection compared with 26 percent of those fed formula.

Why the big difference? Researchers believe that breastfed infants have an enhanced immune response to respiratory infections.

If you bottle-feed your infant, experts advise holding your baby in your arms during feedings with the head above the stomach level. This semi-upright position will help keep the eustachian tubes from becoming blocked and reduce the risk of ear infections.

Quit smoking. Smoking can push an adult with ear problems toward an infection by littering the air with irritants, which, in turn, lead to eustachian tube congestion. Second-hand smoke, which is also pollutant-filled, can be just as troublesome on children prone to ear problems.

Douse the fire in your wood-burning stove. For the same clean-air reasons that you should quit smoking, put out the fire in your woodstove. Soot and smoke from the fire in your stove load the air with hard-to-breathe and hard-to-tolerate toxins.

Be patient. Some children outgrow ear infections by age 3, says George W. Facer, M.D.

and garlic works like an antibiotic. The oils will also migrate past the eardrum and help prevent further infections. You can buy garlic oil, mullein oil, or a combination of the two in most health food stores or drugstores. Apply 2 to 4 drops in the affected ear. Cover the ear with a little wad of cotton to keep the oil from running out. Apply more drops every 6 to 8 hours as needed. Use fresh cotton with each application.

Caution: If you suspect that the eardrum may be ruptured or perhaps punctured, never drop fluids into your ear.

■ **CHEW GUM.** Most people know this is one way to open their ears on an airplane flight, but have you considered it at midnight? The muscular action of chewing may open the eustachian tubes.

Cures from the Kitchen

This culinary tip to ease an ear infection may not be medically proven, but it's certainly safe. Marina Ormes, a nondenominational minister and doula, says, "This remedy was passed on to me by a fellow student in herb school. Take a medium- to large-size onion and cut it in half across the middle—the layers of the onion appear in concentric circles. Bake the onion half at 350°F until the onion is soft. Allow the onion to cool until it will not burn the skin and hold it over the affected ear with a towel."

You can rewarm the onion half and use it every couple of hours as needed, she says. The heat appears to help draw out the infection and the onion contains antimicrobial properties. Plus it feels good, Ormes says. "It works great on babies and kids."

■ **YAWN.** Yawning moves the muscle that opens the eustachian tube even better than chewing gum or sucking on mints.

■ **HOLD YOUR NOSE.** If you're flying at 32,000 feet when your ears begin to ache, pinch your nostrils shut, suggests the American Academy of Otolaryngology-Head and Neck Surgery. Take a mouthful of air and then, using your cheek and throat muscles, force the air into the back of your nose as if you were trying to blow your fingers off the end of your nose. A pop will tell you when you have equalized the pressure inside and outside your ear.

■ **DON'T SLEEP DURING AN AIRPLANE DESCENT.** If you must doze off while flying, close your eyes at the beginning, not at the end of the trip, the Academy recommends. Rapid changes in air pressure occur during ascent as well, but ear pain is typically more acute during descent because atmospheric pressure increases as you move closer to the ground. Since you don't swallow as often when you're asleep, your ears won't be able to keep up with the pressure changes during descent, and you might wake up in pain.

■ **HEAD OFF TROUBLE.** Before you get into trouble, use an over-the-counter decongestant. For instance, if you have to fly and you know your sinuses are going to back up and block your ears, take a decongestant or use nose drops an hour before you land. At home, if you have a stuffy head, use a decongestant at

Drying-Out Cures for Swimmer's Ear

All it takes to come down with a stubborn bout of swimmer's ear is a set of ears and unrelenting moisture. "It's like keeping your hands in dishwater. The skin gets macerated and leathery," says Brian W. Hands, M.D. "The ears are constantly bathed in water—swimming, showering, shampooing. Then people try to dry the ear with a cotton swab. That takes the top layer of skin off, along with protective bacteria. Then the bad bacteria win."

Swimmer's ear begins as an itchy ear. Left untreated, it can turn into a full-blown infection. The pain can be excruciating. Once infection sets in, you'll need a doctor's help and a round of antibiotics to squelch it. But there are plenty of things you can do to keep the pain from getting worse, and even more to stop it before it starts.

Try an over-the-counter remedy. Most drugstores carry ear drops that can help dry up swimmer's ear. If ear itchiness is still your only symptom, one of these preparations might be enough to head off infection. Use it each time your ear gets wet.

Soothe away pain with heat. Warmth—a towel fresh from the dryer, a covered hot-water bottle, a heating pad set on low—also helps ease the pain.

Leave your earwax alone. Earwax serves several purposes, including harboring friendly bacteria, says John House, M.D. Cooperate with your natural defenses by *not* swabbing the wax out. Wax coats the ear canal, protecting it from moisture.

Make substitute wax. Since the irritation of swimmer's ear wears away earwax, you can manufacture your own version using petroleum jelly. Moisten a cotton ball with the jelly, says Dr. Hands, and tuck it gently, like a plug, just in the edge of your ear. It will absorb any moisture, keeping your ear warm and dry.

Take a drop. Several fluids are great for killing germs and drying your ears at the same time. If you're susceptible to swimmer's ear or if you spend a lot of time in the water, use a drying agent every time you get your head wet. Any of the following homemade solutions works well.

A squirt of rubbing alcohol. Put your head down, with the affected ear up. Pull your ear upward and backward (to help straighten the canal) and squeeze a dropperful of alcohol into the ear canal. Wiggle your ear to get the alcohol to the bottom of the canal. Then tilt your head to the other side and let the alcohol drain out.

A kitchen solution. Ear drops of white vinegar or equal parts alcohol and white vinegar kill fungus and bacteria, says Dr. House. Use it the same way you would rubbing alcohol.

Mineral oil, baby oil, or lanolin. These can be preventive solutions before swimming. Apply as you would the alcohol.

Plug up the problem. Wear earplugs when you swim, shampoo, or shower to keep the water out, says Dr. House. Wax or silicone plugs that can be softened and shaped to fit your ears are available at most drugstores.

night before you climb into bed to help prevent the middle-of-the-night ache.

■ **AVOID AGGRAVATING THE SITUATION.** If you're prone to ear problems when you have a cold or allergies, consider delaying air travel or diving until your head clears.

PANEL OF ADVISORS

GEORGE W. FACER, M.D., IS AN OTOLARYNGOLOGIST AT THE MAYO CLINIC IN ROCHESTER, MINNESOTA.

BRIAN W. HANDS, M.D., IS AN OTOLARYNGOLOGIST WITH VOX CURA VOICE CARE SPECIALISTS IN TORONTO.

JOHN HOUSE, M.D., IS A CLINICAL PROFESSOR OF OTOLARYNGOLOGY AT THE UNIVERSITY OF SOUTHERN CALIFORNIA SCHOOL OF MEDICINE IN LOS ANGELES. HE SERVES AS A NATIONAL TEAM PHYSICIAN FOR UNITED STATES SWIMMING, THE NATIONAL GOVERNING ASSOCIATION FOR COMPETITIVE AMATEUR SWIMMING THAT SELECTS THE OLYMPIC TEAM.

DONALD B. KAMERER JR., M.D., IS AN OTOLARYNGOLOGIST AT CHARLOTTE EYE EAR NOSE AND THROAT ASSOCIATES IN CHARLOTTE, NORTH CAROLINA.

MARINA ORMES, IS A NONDENOMINATIONAL MINISTER AND DOULA FROM EUGENE, OREGON.

Earwax

4 Steps to Clean Ears

Earwax, also known as cerumen, protects your eardrum from dust and debris. Left alone, it does its job quite nicely, migrating harmlessly to the outer ear as it dries, only to be replaced by fresh wax that forms in the ear canal.

Occasionally, the wax forms a hard, little plug next to the eardrum that has to be removed by a doctor, says David Edelstein, M.D. Here's how to prevent that from happening.

■ **STICK NOTHING IN YOUR EAR.** That old cliché, "Never put anything smaller than your elbow into your ear," is one that ear doctors swear by. Never stick anything sharp—a bobby pin, a pencil tip, a paper clip—into your ear, because you could tear your eardrum. Don't use a cotton swab or finger either, says George W. Facer, M.D. Even though you think you're cleaning out your ear, you are actually ramming the wax deeper so that it acts like a cap over your eardrum.

■ **DROP IN A SOFTENING FLUID.** A few drops of a liquid that you probably already have at home can soften your earwax. Try hydrogen peroxide, mineral oil, or glycerin for inexpensive cleaning, says Dr. Facer.

Or buy an over-the-counter cleaner such as Debrox or Murine Ear Drops, says Dr. Edelstein.

Add a drop or two of one of the liquids to each ear. Allow the excess to flow out of your ear. The liquid left inside will bubble away at the wax and soften it. Try this for a couple of days.

Favorite Fixes

WHAT IT IS: You can prevent hardened earwax buildup with a light swipe of petroleum jelly.

WHY IT WORKS: The lubricant works by preventing earwax from drying out and accumulating in crusty layers.

HOW TO USE IT: John Heiser of Albany, New York, says he regularly swirls a light coating of Vaseline inside the opening of each ear canal with a fingertip.

Once the wax is soft, you're ready to rinse. Fill a bowl with body-temperature water, says Dr. Facer. Then fill a rubber bulb syringe with the water and, holding your head over the bowl, squirt the water *gently* into your ear canal. The stream of water should be under very little pressure. Turn your head to the side and let the water run out.

■ **BLOW-DRY YOUR EARS.** Don't rub your ears dry, say doctors. Instead, dry your ears with a hair dryer or drop a little alcohol in each ear to complete the drying. Do this once you have rinsed your ears to clean them, as described above, and also every time you shower.

■ **LET NATURE DO ITS WORK.** A once-a-month ear wash is plenty for anyone, says Dr. Edelstein. More than that, and you're washing away the protective layer of earwax that's supposed to be in there.

PANEL OF ADVISORS

DAVID EDELSTEIN, M.D., IS AN OTOLARYNGOLOGIST AT MANHATTAN OTOLARYNGOLOGY AND CLINICAL PROFESSOR OF OTORHINOLARYNGOLOGY AT THE WEILL MEDICAL COLLEGE OF CORNELL UNIVERSITY, BOTH IN NEW YORK CITY.

GEORGE W. FACER, M.D., IS AN OTOLARYNGOLOGIST AT THE MAYO CLINIC IN ROCHESTER, MINNESOTA.

Emphysema

22 Tips for Easy Breathing

Emphysema is a degenerative disease, developing gradually after many years of exposure to toxins or smoke, which destroy the alveoli, or small air sacks, in the lungs. Over time, the lungs lose their elasticity, making breathing difficult.

Although it develops slowly, the toll emphysema exacts on the lungs is anything but minor. The alveoli, which normally stretch as they transport oxygen from the air to the blood and then shrink as they force out carbon dioxide, lose their effectiveness. Patients with emphysema have difficulty exhaling because their damaged lungs trap air and can't exchange the old air for fresh air.

While there is no cure for emphysema, there are plenty of steps you can take to ease symptoms, prevent progression of the disease, and enjoy life. Here's how to save your energy for the things you really want to do.

■ **STAY AWAY FROM SMOKING.** People with emphysema need to be especially aware of airborne irritants that will only make matters worse. "Any irritants, whether cigarette smoke or environmental irritants, can exacerbate your symptoms," says Robert B. Teague, M.D. Simply put, if you smoke, quit. And if your spouse or anyone else in the household smokes, talk about your health concerns to motivate them to break the habit as well.

■ **KEEP IN THE CLEAR.** Keep out of smoky or fume-filled environments, such as bars, auto-repair shops, or freshly painted buildings. The irritation to your lungs just isn't worth it. For the same reason, you may want get rid of car air fresheners and those

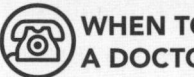

WHEN TO CALL A DOCTOR

See a doctor if you experience any of the following symptoms:

■ Confusion or disorientation during an acute respiratory infection

■ Sleepiness or slurred speech during an acute respiratory infection

■ Presence of blood or any other change in color, thickness, odor, or the amount of mucus that you cough up

■ Shortness of breath, coughing, or wheezing that worsens

■ Shortness of breath that wakes you more than once a night

■ Fatigue that lasts more than 1 day

■ Swollen ankles that remain even after a night of sleeping with your feet elevated

■ Elevation with pillows or the need to sleep in a chair instead of a bed to avoid shortness of breath

■ Morning headaches, restlessness, and dizzy spells

scented household plug-ins. Another good idea: Swap aerosols, like deodorants and hairsprays, for nonaersol products.

■ **TAKE SYMPTOM-CONTROLLING STEPS.** Managing emphysema is often mostly about controlling and minimizing your symptoms, says Dr. Teague. "Doing the sort of things that make you feel better is a good idea," says Dr. Teague.

Feel better when the fresh air is flowing? Keep a window open. Does the smell of city pollution or your neighbor's cooking make you uncomfortable? You might want to invest in a small but high-quality air filter. If the unit is not large enough to effectively treat your entire home (the manual should indicate the square footage), just keep it in your bedroom and enjoy clean air while you sleep.

■ **TAKE ACTION AGAINST ALLERGIES.** Allergies will be worse for people with emphysema. "If you happen to have allergies, that's a problem," says Dr. Teague. Let your doctor know so you can keep any allergic reactions on the radar and take quick action if needed. (For more on allergy control, see Allergies on page 14.)

■ **CONTROL WHAT YOU CAN.** You can't repair your airways. What you can do, says Robert Sandhaus, M.D., Ph.D., is increase how efficiently you breathe, use your muscles, and organize your work. You can rearrange your kitchen, for instance, so that you can do in 5 steps what used to take 10.

The American Lung Association suggests that you obtain a three-shelf utility cart to help with your housework. Small changes like these pay back with extra energy.

■ **EXERCISE.** All our experts agree that regular exercise is vitally important to people with emphysema. What kinds are best?

"Walking is probably the best overall exercise," says Dr. Teague. "You should also exercise to tone the muscles in your upper body. Try using 1- or 2-pound hand weights, and work the muscles in your neck, upper shoulders, and chest." This is important, he says, because people with chronic lung diseases use their neck and upper-respiratory chest muscles more than other people do.

People who have asthma and emphysema seem to really benefit from swimming, because the activity allows them to breathe very humidified air, says Dr. Teague.

■ **EAT LESS—BUT MORE OFTEN.** As emphysema progresses and there is more obstruction to airflow, the lungs enlarge with trapped air. These enlarged lungs push down into the abdomen, leaving less room for the stomach to expand.

Six small meals will leave you feeling better than three large ones—you won't be left so full. Your best bet, says Dr. Teague, is to reach for foods that pack a lot of calories into a small volume, like high-protein selections.

Be aware, too, that prolonged digestion draws blood and oxygen to the stomach and away from other parts of the body, which may need them more.

■ **TRY VITAMINS C AND E.** Dr. Sandhaus advises his emphysema patients to take a minimum of 250 milligrams of vitamin C twice a day, and 500 IU of vitamin E twice a day. (Of course, don't practice this or any vitamin therapy without your doctor's okay and supervision.)

Dr. Sandhaus says that the vitamin therapy can't hurt. He thinks that vitamins C and E may be helpful because they're antioxidants. "We know that the oxidants in cigarette smoke are what damage the lungs," he says.

■ **MAINTAIN YOUR IDEAL BODY WEIGHT.** Some people with emphysema gain a lot of weight and tend to retain fluid, says Dr. Teague. It takes more energy to carry extra body weight. The closer you are to your ideal weight, the better for your lungs.

Other emphysema patients tend to be very skinny, adds Dr. Teague. "Because they have to breathe harder, they expend more energy." If you're underweight, conscientiously add calories, says Dr. Teague. High-protein foods are a good source of calories.

■ **BECOME A CHAMPION BREATHER.** There are several things you can do to get the maximum oomph from each breath you take. They include:

■ **Make your breathing uniform.** When Dr. Teague and his colleagues studied 20 patients with advanced emphysema, they found that even under normal conditions their subjects had very chaotic breathing patterns.

"Their breathing was all over the map—big breaths, little breaths. We taught them normal breathing patterns, and it helped, at least in the short term," Dr. Teague says.

■ **Breathe from your diaphragm.** This is the most efficient way to breathe. Babies do it naturally. If you watch them, you'll see their bellies rise and fall with each breath.

Not sure whether you're breathing from your diaphragm or your chest? Francisco Perez, Ph.D., tells his patients to test by lying on the back, putting a phone book on their belly, and watching what happens with every breath. If you're breathing from your diaphragm, the book will rise with each inhalation.

■ **COORDINATE YOUR BREATHING TO YOUR LIFTING.** According to the American Lung Association, lifting will be easier if you lift while you exhale through pursed lips. Inhale while you rest. Similarly, if you have to climb steps, climb while you exhale through pursed lips and inhale while you rest.

■ **EXERCISE YOUR AIRWAYS.** To build up the abdominal muscles involved in exhaling, buy a device from the drugstore that offers resistance when you blow against it. "It looks like a little plastic mouthpiece with a ring on the end," says Dr. Sandhaus. "When you turn the ring, the opening at the mouthpiece changes size. You start with the largest opening, inhale and blow out. Once you master one setting, you move on to another one."

■ **LET LOOSE.** On your clothing, that is. Choose clothing that allows your chest and abdomen to expand freely. This means forget about tight belts, bras, or girdles, says the American Lung Association.

■ **ALLOW YOURSELF TO GRIEVE.** Your life with emphysema won't be the same as your life before emphysema. Allow yourself to move through each stage of the grieving process, says Dr. Perez. "There are some losses, but then you recognize that you have control over it."

■ **RELAX.** "If you cognitively view the disease as a threat, you'll arouse some physiological mechanisms that can make your emphysema worse," says Dr. Perez. "When you're in a constant state of alarm, you're demanding a lot of oxygen in the process. Alarm is created by the thought process, which you can control. In this way you can also control the physiological mechanisms."

■ **SHIFT YOUR FOCUS TO THE PRESENT.** When you find yourself feeling guilty that you brought on your disease, shift your orientation to the present and concentrate on what's happening now, says Dr. Perez. "You can't deal with events that happened in the past, you can only learn from them."

■ **SET SMALL GOALS.** One way to shift your focus from "emphysema is incapacitating" to "emphysema is something I can live with" is to set realistic small goals for yourself, says Dr. Perez.

Exercise is a great way to boost your confidence, he says. "Set some real objective goal based on the physical evidence. Use charts and graphs to measure your progress."

■ **FIND STRENGTH—AND SUPPORT—IN NUMBERS.** Those with emphysema should seek out an empathetic ear for their feelings, such as

a support group or counselor. Meeting others who face the same challenges you do can be remarkably inspiring and encouraging. Support groups can also be excellent sources of shared information on new treatments and coping strategies. To find a local meeting, contact your nearby American Lung Association chapter.

■ **HAVE A FAMILY MEMBER PLAY "COACH."** Have your significant other become your coach and help you through those times when you're short of breath, suggests Dr. Perez.

■ **DON'T ISOLATE YOURSELF SOCIALLY.** "You need to avoid generalizing about the shortness of breath," says Dr. Teague. "Some people with emphysema think, 'Well, I probably can't do this.' Because they're scared they might get out somewhere and get short of breath, they quit going places they'd normally enjoy." Don't let it isolate you.

■ **PACE YOURSELF.** "The other thing people with emphysema have to learn to do is to take their own time," says Dr. Teague. "They really can do what they want to do, but they have to do it at their own pace. That is not an easy thing to do."

PANEL OF ADVISORS

FRANCISCO PEREZ, PH.D., IS A CLINICAL ASSOCIATE PROFESSOR OF NEUROLOGY AND PHYSICAL MEDICINE AT BAYLOR COLLEGE OF MEDICINE IN HOUSTON.

ROBERT SANDHAUS, M.D., PH.D., IS A PULMONARY SPECIALIST, DIRECTOR OF ALPHA-1 CLINIC, AND PROFESSOR OF MEDICINE AT NATIONAL JEWISH HEALTH IN DENVER. HE IS ALSO EXECUTIVE VICE PRESIDENT AND MEDICAL DIRECTOR OF ALPHA-1 FOUNDATION IN MIAMI (WWW.ALPHANET.ORG).

ROBERT B. TEAGUE, M.D., PRACTICED PULMONARY MEDICINE FOR 20 YEARS IN THE HOUSTON AREA BEFORE RETIRING.

Erectile Dysfunction

12 Secrets for Success

Once upon a time, problems in the bedroom stayed in the bedroom. Today, sexual difficulties have come out in the open thanks to drug commercials, advances in treatments, and expert endorsements. Impotence, now commonly called erectile dysfunction or ED, is no longer a hushed-up diagnosis, and for good reason. It's treatable at any age, and many men who seek treatment are returning to normal sexual activity.

Doctors define ED as the consistent inability to obtain or maintain an erection sufficient for sexual intercourse.

It's more common than many people realize, affecting somewhere between 15 and 30 million American men. It's more prevalent with age. According to the National Kidney and Urologic Diseases Information Clearinghouse, about 5 percent of 40-year-old men experience ED, but for 65-year-old men that number jumps to 15 to 25 percent.

And even more of men have an occasional problem achieving an erection.

"If men are honest, every one of them will tell you they've experienced impotence at least one time in their lives," says Neil Baum, M.D. "Not every intimate encounter is a '10.' It can be devastating when ED occurs," he says. "A man's whole concept of his masculinity may be undermined."

Until the early 1970s, experts thought underlying problems in

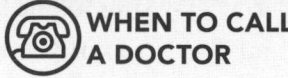 **WHEN TO CALL A DOCTOR**

Men of every age can be treated for impotence, or erectile dysfunction. When lifestyle changes fail to help, a urologist can assess your problem and offer an array of therapies that may resolve the problem. Here are the main avenues of treatment identified by the National Kidney and Urologic Diseases Information Clearinghouse.

■ Drug therapy, including testosterone replacement and drugs that allow more bloodflow into the penis, such as Viagra, Levitra, and Cialis

■ Vacuum devices that draw blood into the penis and hold it there to achieve an erection

■ Surgically implanted devices that can be mechanically expanded when an erection is desired

■ Counseling to deal with the emotional effects of erectile dysfunction

the psyche caused most erection problems. Today, the medical community recognizes that most ED is actually caused by medications conditions, lifestyle choices, or an injury.

Here's what our experts advise.

■ **GIVE YOURSELF TIME.** "As a man gets older, it may take a longer period of genital stimulation to get an erection," says Dr. Baum. "For men ages 18 to 20, an erection may take a few seconds. In your thirties and forties, maybe a minute or two. But if a 60-year-old doesn't get an erection after a minute or two, that doesn't mean he's impotent. It just takes longer."

The time period between ejaculation and your next erection tends to increase with age. In some men ages 60 to 70, it may take a whole day or longer to regain an erection. "It's a normal consequence of aging," says Dr. Baum.

■ **CONSIDER YOUR MEDICATION.** Prescription drugs might be at the root of the problem. Or it might be that over-the-counter antihistamine, diuretic, heart medication, medication for high blood pressure, or sedative you're using. Realize, of course, that not every individual reacts to medications the same way.

Drug-induced ED is most common in men older than 50, says Dr. Baum, with almost 100 drugs identified as potential causes of erectile dysfunction. If you suspect your medication, consult your doctor or pharmacist and ask about changing the dosage or switching to a different drug. Do not, however, attempt to do this on your own.

■ **GO EASY ON THE ALCOHOL.** Shakespeare was right when he said in Macbeth that alcohol provokes desire but takes away the performance. This happens because alcohol is a nervous-system depressant. It inhibits your reflexes, creating a state that's the opposite of arousal. Even two drinks during cocktail hour can be a cause for concern.

Over time, too much alcohol can cause hormonal imbalances. "Chronic alcohol abuse can cause nerve and liver damage," says Dr. Baum. Liver damage results in an excessive amount of female hormones in men. Without the right proportion of testosterone to other hormones, you won't achieve normal erections.

■ **KNOW WHAT'S GOOD FOR THE ARTERIES.** The penis is a vascular organ, says Irwin Goldstein, M.D. The same things that clog your arteries—dietary cholesterol and saturated fat—also affect bloodflow to the penis. In fact, he says, all men over age 38 have some narrowing of the arteries to the penis.

So watch what you eat. "High cholesterol is probably one of the leading causes of ED in this country," says Dr. Goldstein. "It appears to affect erectile tissue."

■ **DON'T SMOKE.** Studies show that nicotine can be a blood vessel constrictor, says Dr. Baum.

In a study at the University of Texas, researchers had a group of nonsmoking men chew gum with nicotine or a placebo gum. Those who chewed the nicotine gum had a 23 percent reduction in sexual arousal compared with the group who chewed the placebo gum.

■ **LOSE WEIGHT.** Studies show that men who are overweight are more likely to have difficulties maintaining an erection. If you are at least 20 percent heavier than your ideal weight, think about taking off a few pounds. Consider karate or a weight training program. Not only will a fitter body lessen the likelihood of ED, but it will also boost self-confidence. The better a man feels about his body, the better he'll feel for "the event," says Dr. Goldstein. But avoid going overboard if you're a cyclist. . . .

Cures from the Kitchen

Those heart-shaped boxes of chocolate have some competition. The red, juicy flesh of the watermelon may be the newest romantic food. Researchers at Texas A&M Fruit and Vegetable Improvement Center, in College Station, found that phytonutrients in watermelon have a Viagra-like effect. In particular, this juicy fruit contains citrulline, a compound that causes the body to relax the blood vessels. Unlike Viagra, watermelon doesn't target one particular organ. Citrulline encourages blood vessels throughout the body to relax, which benefits the heart, circulatory system, and immune system.

The watermelon rind contains more citrulline than the flesh. Because people don't eat the rind, researchers are working to develop a new breed with higher citrulline concentrations in the flesh. In the meantime, enjoy a generous slab to enhance all of your bodily systems.

■ **DON'T OVERDO BIKE RIDING.** Riding a bicycle on a narrow saddle puts excessive pressure on the area between your legs, where the nerves and blood vessels flow to your penis. If you ride, either get off your seat often, or ride on a wide seat with no nose. "If you get numb in your penis today, you may lose all ability to have an erection tomorrow," says Dr. Goldstein.

■ **HAVE MORE SEX.** A 5-year study of almost 1,000 Finnish men between the ages of 55 and 75 found that those who reported having intercourse less than once a week had twice the incidence of ED than those men who had intercourse once a week. The researchers conclude that regular intercourse appears to protect men against ED.

■ **RELAX.** A relaxed frame of mind is crucial to maintaining an erection. Here's why. Your nervous system operates in two modes: the sympathetic nervous system and the parasympathetic nervous system. When the sympathetic nerve network is dominant, your body is literally "on alert." Adrenal hormones prepare you to fight or take flight. Nervousness and anxiety undermine attaining an erection by pulling blood away from your digestive system and penis to your muscles.

Being anxious will turn on your sympathetic nervous system, says Dr. Baum. For some men, the fear of failure is so overwhelming that it floods the body with norepinephrine, an adrenal hormone. This is the opposite of it takes to have an erection.

The key is to relax and let your parasympathetic nervous system take over. Signals that travel along this network will direct the arteries and sinuses of the penis to expand and let more blood flow in.

■ **AVOID WHOLE-BODY STIMULANTS.** This means caffeine and certain questionable substances touted as potency enhancers. It's important to be relaxed during sex, says Dr. Goldstein, and stimulants tend to constrict the smooth muscle that must relax before an erection occurs.

■ **REFOCUS YOUR ATTENTION.** One way to relax is to focus with your partner on the more sensual aspects of intimacy. Experience foreplay and enjoy each other without worrying about having an erection.

"The skin is the largest sexual organ in the body," says Dr. Goldstein, "not the penis."

PANEL OF ADVISORS

NEIL BAUM, M.D., IS A CLINICAL ASSOCIATE PROFESSOR OF UROLOGY AT TULANE UNIVERSITY SCHOOL OF MEDICINE AND A STAFF UROLOGIST WITH TOURO INFIRMARY, BOTH IN NEW ORLEANS.

IRWIN GOLDSTEIN, M.D., IS DIRECTOR OF SEXUAL MEDICINE AT ALVARADO HOSPITAL AND CLINICAL PROFESSOR OF SURGERY AT THE UNIVERSITY OF CALIFORNIA AT SAN DIEGO.

Eyestrain

10 Tips to Avoid It

Asthenopia sounds like the name of a foreign country, but in fact, it's the technical term for a very familiar eye condition—otherwise known as eyestrain. People who spend as little as 2 hours a day staring at a computer screen can experience classic symptoms of eyestrain, including blurred vision, headaches, and dry eyes. Our eyes simply weren't designed to focus for hours on end at such close distances.

If you find your eyes straining to read your birthday cards or your vision blurring as you try to focus on your computer screen, here are some suggestions that may help.

■ **REST YOUR EYES.** Our experts say that it's the best way to relieve eyestrain. And that's easier than you may think. "You can do it while you're on the phone," says Samuel L. Guillory, M.D. "If you don't need to read or write, just close your eyes while you're talking. Depending on how much time you spend on the phone each day, you may be able to rest your eyes for almost an hour or two daily. People who practice this technique say that their eyes really feel better, and it helps rid them of eyestrain."

■ **PAY ATTENTION TO LIGHTING.** "It doesn't hurt your eyes to read in dim light, but you can strain them if the light doesn't provide enough contrast," says Dr. Guillory. "Use a soft light that gives contrast, but not glare, when you read. And don't use any lamp that reflects light directly back into your eyes."

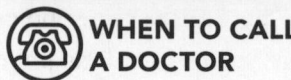

WHEN TO CALL A DOCTOR

Sometimes the cause of eyestrain is a lot more serious than just passing your 40th birthday. "Strain can also be caused by eye misalignment, where one eye starts to turn in or out," says David Guyton, M.D. "If that's the case, the problem needs to be treated by an ophthalmologist who can suggest specific exercises, prescribe special prism glasses, or, if necessary, perform eye muscle surgery to realign the eyes."

All the experts agree that if you have pain in your eye or sensitivity to light, you need to see an ophthalmologist right away.

EYESTRAIN

Insight with Yoga

For Meir Schneider, Ph.D., yoga wasn't only the key to gaining spiritual insight. It also was the key to simply gaining sight. "Yoga helped cure my blindness," claims Dr. Schneider, who was born blind. He credits daily yoga exercises for helping bring back his vision, which he says is now 20/60. And it's still improving. While it might be straining science a bit to say it cures blindness, some of his techniques may be helpful in handling eyestrain.

Try another sort of eye-hand coordination. If you want to help your eyes, Dr. Schneider says, you need to lend them a hand. "Take your hands and rub them together until they are warm. Then close your eyes and put your palms over your eye orbits. Don't press on your eyes; just cover them. Breathe deeply and slowly and visualize the color black. Do this for 20 minutes every day."

Put your eyes "on the blink." Your eyes have their own massage therapist—the eyelids. "Make it a point to consciously blink your eyes 300 times every day and not squint," says Dr. Schneider. "Each blink cleanses your eyes and gives them a tiny little massage." And it's free.

■ **TRY READING GLASSES.** You can get them from your doctor or at the drugstore. "If you have good distance vision in both eyes but have trouble seeing up close, go to your local drugstore and buy reading glasses," says David Guyton, M.D. They're commonly available, cost from $10 to $20, and are impact-resistant.

■ **RAISE YOUR BLINK RATE.** Under normal conditions, we blink our eyes about 15 times a minute. When staring at a computer screen, however, that rate drops to about half, exposing the eyes to more fluid evaporation, says Ted Belheumer, O.D. "Being aware of blinking may help," he says. If you know you'll be spending more time than usual in front of the screen, post a sticky note nearby reminding yourself to close your lids now and then.

■ **INTERRUPT YOUR WORK.** "If you use the computer for 6 to 8 hours," says Dr. Guillory, "take a break every 2 to 3 hours. Do some other work, get coffee, go to the bathroom—just take your eyes off the screen for 10 to 15 minutes." Also consider working from a printout instead of reading on the screen.

■ **DARKEN YOUR SCREEN.** Those aren't just letters and numbers on your screen. They're also tiny lightbulbs that send light directly into your eyes. You need to turn the wattage down, so to speak. "Don't make the screen too bright," advises Dr. Guillory. "Turn the brightness down to a dim level and then adjust the contrast to make up the difference."

■ **WORK IN THE SHADE.** When it comes to relieving eyestrain, it's best to keep your computer in the dark. "Shade your screen by creating a hood over it," Dr. Guillory suggests. "Go to an art supply store and buy a sheet of heavy black cardboard. Put it on top of your screen and fold both sides down over it. That will allow you to slide it back and forth. What you've done, essentially, is put your machine in a black box. So now you can turn the brightness down to a very low level."

■ **BREW A POT OF EYEBRIGHT TEA.** Cool it slightly and then soak a towel in the still-warm tea, says Meir Schneider, Ph.D. Lie down and place the warm towel over your closed eyes, leaving it there for 10 to 15 minutes. It will make your eyestrain go away. Be very careful not to pour tea into your eyes, though.

PANEL OF ADVISORS

TED BELHEUMER, O.D., IS A DOCTOR OF OPTOMETRY AT TROY VISION CENTER IN TROY, NEW YORK. HE HAS BEEN IN PRIVATE PRACTICE FOR MORE THAN 30 YEARS.

SAMUEL L. GUILLORY, M.D., IS AN OPHTHALMOLOGIST AND CLINICAL ASSOCIATE PROFESSOR OF OPHTHALMOLOGY AT MOUNT SINAI SCHOOL OF MEDICINE OF NEW YORK UNIVERSITY IN NEW YORK CITY.

DAVID GUYTON, M.D., IS THE KRIEGER PROFESSOR OF PEDIATRIC OPHTHALMOLOGY AND DIRECTOR OF THE KRIEGER CHILDREN'S EYE CENTER AT THE WILMER INSTITUTE AT JOHNS HOPKINS UNIVERSITY SCHOOL OF MEDICINE IN BALTIMORE.

MEIR SCHNEIDER, PH.D., IS FOUNDER OF THE SCHOOL FOR SELF-HEALING IN SAN FRANCISCO. HE IS THE AUTHOR OF *SELF-HEALING: MY LIFE AND VISION* AND *MOVEMENT FOR SELF-HEALING,* AND COAUTHOR OF *THE HANDBOOK OF SELF-HEALING.*

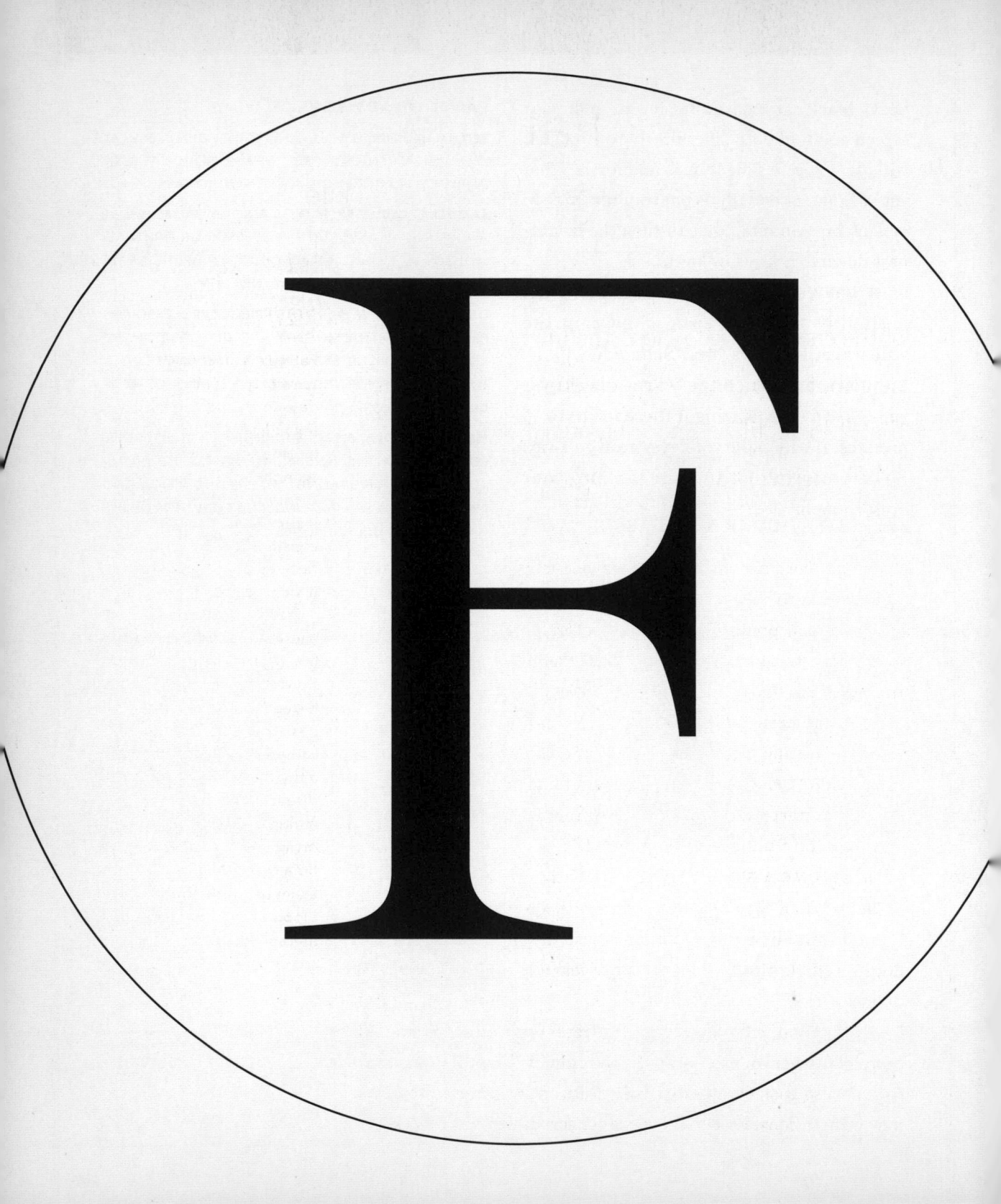

Fatigue

30 Hints for a High-Energy Life

Energy equals excitement, fun, and youth. Think of the energetic gal who is the life of the party, the neighbor who puts so much energy into her yard that it looks like something out of a magazine, or your "energizer bunny" grandson. Energy is what drives life and helps make life worth living.

But at one time or another, everyone feels fatigued. And who wouldn't like to have more energy than they now have?

The broad prescription from doctors is still the same: Get plenty of rest, eat a balanced diet, and exercise. But here authorities on fatigue go beyond these generalities and offer more specific, high-octane suggestions.

So, ladies and gentlemen, start your engines.

■ **WARM UP.** "Give yourself an extra 15 minutes in the morning before you start your day," says Vicky Young, M.D. "That way you don't start off feeling rushed and tired."

■ **BECOME A BREAKFAST EATER.** Fatigue can be a side effect of dieting or of regularly skipping meals, says Nita Parikh, M.D. If you habitually run out of your house in the morning without taking a single bite, "you may have to learn to eat breakfast every day," she says.

Even cereal (a complex carbohydrate) with milk (a source of protein) can get your day off to a good start. Wheat toast and muffins are also good complex-carbohydrate options. For protein, you may want to consider low-fat yogurt or scrambled egg whites.

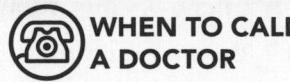
WHEN TO CALL A DOCTOR

Fatigue is most often temporary, lasting a few days to a couple of weeks. If you find that you've been unusually tired for longer than that, or if your fatigue is combined with weight loss or gain, diarrhea, constipation, hair loss, skin rash, or shortness of breath, it's time to call the doctor.

"Whenever fatigue causes new changes in your life, it's time to pay attention," says Nita Parikh, M.D. Extended, extreme tiredness could be a sign of something serious, such as a thyroid problem, cardiac disease, depression, multiple sclerosis, or even a malignancy. Your doctor will do a thorough physical exam and probably order blood tests to gather more information.

Guard against eating an ultra-high-carbohydrate breakfast laden with simple sugars. This can create a surge in insulin and a corresponding drop in blood sugar, leading to a jittery crash. So avoid the doughnut shop between home and the office.

■ **KNOW WHERE YOU'RE GOING.** If you don't know where you're going, you'll probably be too tired to get there. "Take time each morning to set specific goals for the day," says Dr. Parikh. "Determine what you want to do; don't let the routine control you."

■ **CONSIDER A LIFESTYLE CHANGE.** If fatigue has become a serious issue and you've ruled out any health conditions, you may need to assess your life and consider making some changes, says Dr. Parikh. "If you are doing the impossible and it is draining you, you need to come to grips with that and be open to changing."

It could be that second job you have—you might want to look at quitting or at least cutting back your hours. Or if you are the caregiver for both your children and your parents, you might need to get some help around the house. Try to think of these changes as positive—getting the help you need to do a better job—rather than throwing in the towel.

■ **GET IN THE ZONE.** TV is famous—make that infamous—for lulling human beings into lethargy. Try reading, knitting, or some other hobby that fully engages your attention. It's more energizing.

■ **WORK OUT TO REV UP.** "Exercise actually gives you energy," Dr. Young says. Study after study supports these words, including one by NASA. More than 200 federal employees were placed on a moderate, regular exercise program. The results: 90 percent said they had never felt better. Almost half said they felt less stress, and almost one-third reported that they slept better.

Dr. Young recommends giving yourself a dose of energetic exercise—brisk walking is enough—three to five times a week for 20 to 30 minutes each time, and no later than 2 hours before bedtime.

■ **BE CAREFUL NOT TO OVERDO.** For all the good that exercise can do, it can be addictive. And you can overdose if you're not honest about what your body is telling you.

"I have to work at telling myself that it will be good for me, that I will gain by taking time off," says endurance athlete Mary Trafton.

■ **DO THE WORST FIRST.** Many times, people feel fatigued because they think, "I have so much to do, and I don't know where to start." By setting priorities and charting your progress as you make your way through the list, you can remain focused and energetic.

■ **TAKE ONE A DAY.** If you're guilty of missing meals, dieting, and not eating properly, Dr. Young says, taking one multivitamin-mineral supplement a day is a good idea.

■ **TEACH YOUR BODY TO TELL TIME.** Circadian rhythms act as our bodies' internal clocks, raising and lowering blood pressure

Open Your Mind to Energy

When your mind goes, your body follows. That the mind can influence the body is now generally accepted. Here are some new attitudes that can affect your energy level.

Think positively. Championship athletes do it, successful CEOs do it, so you should do it. "It's important to think positively," says Mary Trafton, an avid hiker and marathoner. "If I step in a huge puddle while hiking, I don't think, 'Ah, I'm going to be cold and tired.' I think about the wool socks I have on for protection and warmth."

Be motivated. When you think about it, it's pretty hard to do much of anything if you're not motivated. But it's next to impossible to accomplish tasks that require mega energy if your spirit just isn't in it.

Take E. Drummond King, for example. He has participated in the grueling Ironman competitions in Hawaii—competitors swim, bicycle, and run long distances for hours on end. He says that when he's too far behind to win his age group, he finishes the race by walking instead of running. But when there's a chance to win or a bet is riding on his finish time, he somehow finds the energy to continue running.

Be confident. Chances are, if you feel you can do it, you'll have the energy to do it. And once you've proven to yourself that you have the energy, you'll become even more confident.

and body temperature at different times throughout the day. This chemical action causes the "swings" we experience—from feeling alert to feeling mentally and physically foggy.

So why are some people's natural peak times so inconvenient—like late at night? "I think sometimes people, perhaps without even knowing it, work themselves into a particular time cycle," says exercise physiologist William Fink.

Fink suggests changing your schedule as much as practically possible to complement your circadian rhythms. Start by getting up a little earlier or a little later—say, 15 minutes— until you feel comfortable. Keep it up until you reach your desired schedule.

■ **PUT OUT THE FIRE.** Doctors always advise giving up smoking, but add this to the list of reasons: Smoking reduces the amount of oxygen available in your body. The result is fatigue.

When you first quit, however, don't expect an immediate energy boost. Nicotine acts as a stimulant, and withdrawal may cause some temporary tiredness.

■ **JUST SAY NO.** Ease your load—and your fatigue level—by learning to delegate. If too many obligations or commitments are wearing you out, learn to say, "No, thank you."

■ **SHED.** As in pounds. "If you're obese—if you need to drop 20 percent of your weight or more—losing weight will be a great help," Fink says. Of course, make sure you follow a sensible diet in combination with exercise. Losing more than 2 pounds a week isn't healthy and will wear you down.

■ **GET FEWER ZZZS.** You can get too much of a good thing, even sleep. "If you oversleep, you tend to be groggy all day," Fink says. "Usually, 6 to 8 hours of sleep a night is enough for most people."

■ **BLOW OUT THE CANDLE.** Burning the candle at both ends—not going to bed until 2:00 a.m. and getting up at 5:00 a.m., for

Favorite Fixes

WHAT IT IS: When your legs and feet are exhausted from standing or walking all day, try this simple and revitalizing yoga pose.

WHY IT WORKS: Viparita karani, or "legs-up-the-wall," is a passive pose that combines the healing benefits of relaxation and inversion, says Gale Maleskey of Bridgewater, New Jersey.

HOW TO USE IT: "You just sit on the floor with one shoulder and hip near a wall," she says. "Lean back a bit and swing your legs up to lean on the wall, then let your upper body rest back on the floor. Stay in this position about 15 minutes, if possible." It's best to use a folded blanket or hard pillow to raise your hips 8 to 12 inches off the floor. This releases tension on your lower back. You might also want a 1- to 2-inch folded blanket under your head. If getting down on the floor is difficult, try it in bed.

example—will leave you feeling burned out. Don't shortchange yourself on sleep.

■ **GET 20 WINKS.** Naps aren't for everybody, but they might help recharge older people who aren't sleeping as soundly as they used to. Younger people with very hectic schedules and short nights also might consider taking naps. If you do decide to take naps, try taking them at the same time each day and for no more than an hour.

■ **BREATHE DEEPLY.** It's one of the best ways to relax and energize at the same time, according to doctors and athletes.

■ **HAVE JUST ONE.** Alcohol is a depressant and will slow you down more, not rev you up. If you seem to be drinking more in response to life stresses, cut back—or cut it out completely, says Dr. Parikh.

■ **EAT A LIGHT LUNCH.** Some doctors advise a light lunch to avoid a severe case of the postlunch I-want-to-crawl-under-my-desk-and-take-a-nap blues. If you're too tired too often, this advice is worth trying. Soup and salad and a piece of fruit make a light but nutritious meal.

■ **MAKE LUNCH YOUR BIG MEAL OF THE DAY.** If a light lunch doesn't satisfy you, Dr. Young suggests eating your largest meal of the day at lunch and following it up with a 20-minute walk. Eating most of your calories early in the day gives you the fuel you need to keep perking. But you have to be selective in the type of fuel you choose. Carbohydrate, for example, is a fast burner. Fat, on the other hand, burns slowly, so it'll slow you down.

■ **DIVERT YOUR ENERGY.** Strong emotion is mentally draining, but it can be physically draining, too, says Dr. Young. Redirect strong emotions, such as anger, and apply that energy to your job or a workout.

■ **SOOTHE YOUR STRESS.** A 25-year study by the Swedish medical university the Karolinska Institute showed that persistent anxiety can raise the risk for a medical condition called chronic fatigue syndrome. The research suggests that, over time, steady stress may wear down the body's resistance to fatigue. To alleviate an existing problem and prevent fatigue from getting out of hand, practice stress-reducing techniques such as deep breathing, yoga, meditation, and guided imagery. CDs and DVDs of these practices can be found at bookstores and online.

■ **TRY SOME MUSIC THERAPY.** When it's time to vacuum the house or tackle a pile of mind-numbing bills, crank up some energizing tunes. The best part of this fatigue fixer: You get to customize to your heart's content. Listen to Frank Sinatra one day, Led Zeppelin the next.

■ **GIVE YOURSELF A TARGET.** Some people simply need deadlines to keep moving forward. If that sounds like you, give yourself both short and long deadlines—so neither becomes too routine.

■ **MAKE A SPLASH.** When fatigue starts to drop one New York stockbroker, he doesn't buy or sell. He stops—long enough to hit himself in the face with splashes of cold water.

But if he were home, a cold shower might restore his energy even better. Cascading water emits negative ions in the air. Negative ions are thought to make some people feel happier and more energetic.

■ **DRINK UP.** Dehydration can cause fatigue. Drink at least eight 8-ounce glasses of water each day, even more when you're active. The day before a busy day out in the hot sun—say, a day at Disney World with your kids—doctors advise drinking plenty of water and continuing to do so the day of the activity.

E. Drummond King, an over-50 triathlete, learned the hard way that it's best to start drinking a lot of fluids the day before his body is going to need them.

"The major problem is dehydration and the fatigue that comes with it," he says. "Now I spend the day before a competition walking around with a water bottle in my hand."

■ **RETHINK YOUR MEDICATIONS.** Do you really need to take all those prescription and over-the-counter medicines? If not, you may be shocked at what eliminating or reducing dosages of certain medications may do for you.

Sleeping pills, for example, are notorious for their next-day hangover effects. But also among the villains, according to doctors, are high blood pressure medicines and cough and cold medicines.

If you suspect a medication is guilty of grand theft energy, discuss it with your doctor. Maybe you can get a new prescription or, better yet, quit the medicine altogether. But never stop taking a prescription medication without your doctor's approval.

■ **COUNTERACT SIDE EFFECTS WITH COQ10.** If you must take certain medications, check to see if they have energy-sapping side effects—then do something about them, says Chris D. Meletis, N.D. Statins and beta-blockers for lowering cholesterol can deplete the body of coenzyme Q10. With your doctor's okay, try supplementing with 30 to 60 milligrams of CoQ10 daily and see if your energy rises.

■ **IF IT FEELS GOOD, DO IT.** There's no denying the pleasures of massages, whirlpools, and steam baths. "It's hard to study scientifically whether or not they lessen fatigue," says Fink. "But there are those who swear by them. I'm convinced, too—if people feel better, they'll perform better."

■ **TRADE COFFEE FOR TEA.** Research shows that the combination of caffeine and the amino acid L-theanine, both found in regular black tea, can improve mental alertness and decrease fatigue. So the next time you need a caffeinated pick-me-up, try a cup of tea instead of that cappuccino.

Fever

10 Cooling Tactics

Think of fever not so much as a menace, but as your body's early warning system. It's the way your body fights infection—and a tool it uses to enhance its natural defense mechanisms.

The mechanics are rather simple. Your brain tells your body to move blood from the surface of your skin to the interior of the body. With blood so far from the skin, the body loses less heat and your temperature rises. Voilà! You have a fever.

Before you take steps to douse the fire, listen to what doctors say.

■ **MAKE SURE YOU HAVE A FEVER.** Although 98.6°F is considered the norm, that number is not etched in stone. "Normal" temperature varies from person to person and fluctuates widely throughout the day. Food, excess clothing, emotional excitement, and vigorous exercise can all elevate temperature.

If your temperature goes up to 100°F, consider it a mild fever. "You may watch it for a few days, and treat yourself with ibuprofen or acetaminophen if you are uncomfortable," says Nita Parikh, M.D. Restful waiting is the smart course for a mild fever.

Temperatures of 102°F or higher may be serious, particularly if you are also feeling sick—vomiting, headache, coughing. At this point, you have a good reason to call your doctor.

■ **DON'T FIGHT IT.** If you do have a fever, remember this: Fever itself is not an illness—it's a symptom of one. When your body senses a bacterial or viral invasion, it releases substances that tell your brain to raise your internal temperature, causing a fever. An elevated body temperature makes it harder for bacteria and viruses

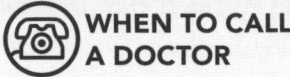

WHEN TO CALL A DOCTOR

See a doctor if you have fever and:

■ Stiff neck

■ Severe coughing or vomiting, or pain on taking a deep breath

■ Yellow or green discharge from the nose, and facial pain

■ Temperature higher than 101°F that lasts more than 3 days or fails to respond at least partly to treatment

■ Temperature higher than 103°F under any condition

Adults with chronic illnesses, such as heart or respiratory disease, may not be able to tolerate prolonged high fevers.

to reproduce and spread. So, in essence, your body's natural defenses can actually shorten an illness with its quick response and increase the power of antibiotics. These natural processes should be weighed against the discomfort involved in not medicating a slight fever and letting it run its course, says Stephen N. Rosenberg, M.D.

If you feel the need for extra relief, try the following steps.

■ **LIQUEFY YOUR ASSETS.** When you're hot, your body perspires to cool you down. But if you lose too much water—as you might with a high fever—your body turns off its sweat ducts to forestall further water loss. This makes it more difficult for you to cope with your fever. The moral of this story: Drink up. In addition to plain water, doctors favor the following:

■ **Watered-down Juice.** Straight juice, no matter how nutritious, is too concentrated to drink in any quantity when you have a fever, and may cause diarrhea. Always dilute 100 percent fruit or vegetable juice with 1 part juice to 1 part water to make it easier for your body to absorb.

■ **Try Tea.** Although any tea will provide needed fluid, several are particularly suited for fever, says Gale Maleskey, M. S., R.D. One combination she likes is thyme, linden flowers, and chamomile flowers. Thyme is antibacterial, linden promotes sweating, and chamomile

reduces inflammation, she says. Steep 1 teaspoon of the mixture in 1 cup of freshly boiled water for 5 minutes. Strain and drink warm several times a day. These herbs are available in most health food stores. Here are some more favorites.

■ **Linden Tea.** This tea by itself is also good, she says, and can induce sweating to break a fever. Use 1 tablespoon of the flowers in 1 cup of freshly boiled water for 5 minutes. Strain and drink hot often.

■ **Willow Bark.** This bark is rich in salicylates (aspirin-related compounds) and is considered "nature's fever medication," Maleskey says. Brew into a tea and drink in small doses.

■ **ICE.** If you're too nauseated to drink, you can suck on ice. For variety, freeze diluted fruit juice in an ice-cube tray.

■ **GET COMPRESSED RELIEF.** Wet compresses help reduce the body's temperature output. Ironically, hot, moist compresses can do the job. If you start to feel uncomfortably hot, remove those compresses and apply cool ones to the forehead, wrists, and calves. Keep the rest of the body covered.

But if the fever rises above 103°F, don't use hot compresses at all. Instead, apply cool ones to prevent the fever from getting any higher. Change them as they warm to body temperature and continue until the fever drops.

Thermometer Ins and Outs

Mothers are famous for the skill in gauging temperatures just by feeling their children's foreheads. If you didn't inherit the knack, you'll need to rely on thermometer readings. Here's how to get the safest, most accurate results.

■ First, consider the many types available. Some of the options are digital thermometers, ear thermometers, and glass galinstan thermometers, which are very similar to mercury thermometers except they contain gallium, indium, and tin.

■ All of these are very good alternatives to old-fashioned mercury thermometers, which can cause neurological problems if the glass breaks and the mercury vapor is inhaled. In fact, the concern about mercury thermometers is so great that several cities in the United States have banned the sale of mercury thermometers altogether. (One important environmental note: If you do have mercury thermometers at home, don't rush to toss them in the trash can. Instead, ask your local poison control center to provide tips on safe disposal.)

■ Wait at least 15 minutes after eating or drinking anything or after smoking before taking an oral reading. These activities alter mouth temperature and will cause inaccurate readings. Hot baths can also lead to inaccurate readings.

■ Before using a glass thermometer, hold it by the top end (not the bulb) and shake it with a quick snap of the wrist until the colored dye is below 96°F. If you're concerned about dropping and breaking the thermometer, do this over a bed, suggests Stephen N. Rosenberg, M.D.

■ Place the digital or glass thermometer under your tongue in one of the "pockets" located on either side of your mouth rather than right up front. These pockets are closer to blood vessels that reflect the body's core temperature.

■ Hold the thermometer in place with your lips, not your teeth. Breathe through your nose rather than your mouth so that the room temperature doesn't affect the reading. Leave the thermometer in place for at least 3 minutes (some experts favor 5 to 7 minutes).

■ After use, wash a glass thermometer in cool, soapy water. Never use hot water. And never store it near heat.

■ **SPONGE OFF.** Evaporation also has a cooling effect on body temperature. Mary Ann Pane, R.N., recommends cool tap water to help the skin dissipate excess heat. Although you can sponge the whole body, she says, pay particular attention to spots where heat is generally greatest, such as the armpits and groin area. Wring out a sponge and wipe one section at a time, keeping the rest of the body covered. Body heat will evaporate the moisture and cool the skin.

■ **DON'T SUFFER.** If you're very uncomfortable, take an over-the-counter pain reliever. For adults, aspirin, acetaminophen, or ibuprofen can be taken according to package directions. The advantage of acetaminophen and ibuprofen over aspirin is that fewer people experience side effects.

So which one should you take? All are effective, but some work better for particular ailments. For example, aspirin and ibuprofen are common nonsteroidal anti-inflammatory drugs (NSAIDs), so they're effective at reducing muscle pain and inflammation. Acetaminophen is recommended if you have gastrointestinal sensitivity or are allergic to aspirin. It doesn't work as well as NSAIDs for inflammation and muscle aches; however, it's a safer drug to use and has minimal side effects, as long as it's taken in the proper dosage.

■ **DRESS THE PART.** Use common sense as far as clothing and blankets go, says Pane. If you're very hot, take off extra covers and clothes so that body heat can dissipate into the air. But if you have a chill, bundle up until you're just comfortable.

■ **DROWN A FEVER.** Don't fret over whether you should feed a fever or starve one. Just drown it. "Most people don't want to eat when they have a fever, so the important thing is fluids," Maleskey says. Once your appetite starts to return, eat what appeals to you. Toast, scrambled eggs, chicken soup, and vanilla pudding all go down easy as part of your recuperation.

PANEL OF ADVISORS

GALE MALESKEY, M.S., R.D., IS A CLINICAL DIETITIAN, NUTRITION EDUCATOR, AND SPEAKER. SHE PRACTICES NUTRITION COUNSELING IN BRIDGEWATER, NEW JERSEY, WHERE SHE SEES CLIENTS FOR A WIDE VARIETY OF HEALTH PROBLEMS.

MARY ANN PANE, R.N., IS A NURSE CLINICIAN IN PHILADELPHIA. SHE WAS FORMERLY AFFILIATED WITH COMMUNITY HOME HEALTH SERVICES, AN AGENCY CATERING TO PEOPLE WHO REQUIRE SKILLED HEALTH CARE IN THEIR HOMES.

NITA PARIKH, M.D., IS AN INTERNAL MEDICINE SPECIALIST WITH COMMUNITY CARE PHYSICIANS IN LATHAM, NEW YORK.

STEPHEN N. ROSENBERG, M.D., IS AN EMERITUS CLINICAL PROFESSOR OF HEALTH POLICY AND MANAGEMENT AT COLUMBIA UNIVERSITY MAILMAN SCHOOL OF PUBLIC HEALTH IN NEW YORK CITY. HE IS ALSO THE AUTHOR OF *THE JOHNSON & JOHNSON FIRST-AID BOOK*.

Flatulence

8 Gas-Reducing Ideas

It's tough to be serious about flatulence, though we promise to try. It's tough because even the scientists who study the subject poke fun at their own research, writing of failed experiments that ended "without even a whiff of success."

Yes, of course, the pun was intended, and, yes, it was in bad taste, but such is the nature of this science—even at the highest levels. Consider Michael D. Levitt, M.D., one of the top researchers in the field. His peers know him as "the man who brought status to flatus and class to gas." In his own words, Dr. Levitt describes his work as "an attempt to pump some data into the field filled largely with hot air."

Hot air, perhaps, and a colorful history as well. Hippocrates investigated flatulence extensively, and ancient physicians who specialized in it became known as "pneumatists." In early American history, such great men as Benjamin Franklin taxed their minds seeking a cure for "escaped wind."

Yes, it's tough to be serious about flatulence, but here's our attempt. Read on.

■ **LAY OFF THE LACTOSE.** "If you are lactose intolerant, you could have flatulence problems from eating dairy foods," says Gale Maleskey, M.S., R.D. (For more tips, see Lactose Intolerance on page 391.) Lactose-intolerant people have a low intestinal level of the enzyme lactase, which is needed to digest lactose, the type of

Cures from the Kitchen

Sugar-coated fennel seeds are served after meals in India just as Americans would have an after-dinner mint. Look for them in gourmet shops and Asian food markets. Fennel is known as a carminative—an agent that can disperse gas from the intestinal tract, says nutritionist Gale Maleskey, M.S., R.D. The plain seeds (found in the spice aisle at the grocery store) can also be brewed as tea. Just cover 1 tablespoon with 1 cup of boiling water, strain, and sip.

sugar found in many dairy foods. It's easy enough to get around this by taking supplemental lactase, which can be found in products such as Lact-Aid.

But you don't necessarily need to be diagnosed as lactose intolerant to have unwanted repercussions. Some people can handle only certain amounts and different kinds of milk products with comfort. If you or your doctor suspects that your favorite dairy product is causing your problem, try eating it in smaller servings or along with a meal for a day or two until you notice where gas begins to be a problem.

■ **AVOID GAS-PROMOTING FOODS.** The primary cause of flatulence is the digestive system's inability to absorb certain carbohydrates, says Samuel Klein, M.D.

Though you probably know that beans are surefire flatus producers, many people don't realize that cabbage, broccoli, brussels sprouts, onions, cauliflower, whole wheat flour, radishes, bananas, apricots, pretzels, and many more foods can also be highly flatugenic.

■ **FIGHT OFF FIBER-INDUCED FLATUS.** "Although we often encourage fiber in the diet for digestive health, some high-fiber vegetables and fruits may increase gas," says Richard McCallum, M.D.

If you're adding fiber to your diet for health reasons, start with a small dose so that the bowel gets used to it. That lessens the increase of flatus, and doctors have found that most

people's flatus production returns to normal within a few weeks of adding fiber.

■ **USE CHARCOAL TO HELP YOU REACH YOUR GOAL.** Some studies have found that activated charcoal tablets are effective in eliminating excessive gas. "Charcoal absorbs gases and may be useful for flatulence," says Dr. Klein. "It's probably the best available treatment—after appropriate dietary changes have been made and other gastroenterological diseases have been treated or ruled out." Check with your doctor if you're taking any medication, because charcoal can soak up medicine as well as gas.

■ **GET QUICK RELIEF FROM POPULAR PRODUCTS.** While many physicians recommend activated charcoal for relief of intestinal gas, pharmacists say that simethicone-containing products are still the most popular with consumers. Among the over-the-counter favorites: Gas-X, Extra Strength Maalox, and Maximum Strength Mylanta.

Unlike activated charcoal's absorbent action, simethicone's defoaming action relieves flatulence by dispersing and preventing the formation of mucus-surrounded gas pockets in the stomach and intestines.

■ **BUY BEANO.** The plant enzyme–derived dietary supplement Beano is worth trying. Available over-the-counter in tablets or drops, take this plant enzyme is taken at the beginning of meals to help break down the gas-producing elements of foods such as beans, broccoli, and grains.

Bean Cuisine: Getting the Gas Out

If you love beans and legumes but hate living with the consequences, there is a solution. Clearly, beans and legumes cause flatulence, although the better they're cooked, the less the problem. Indeed, beans seem to lose a lot of their gas-producing properties in water. Studies show that soaking beans for 12 hours or germinating them on damp paper towels for 24 hours can significantly reduce the amount of gas-producing compounds. In fact, soaking followed by 30 minutes of pressure cooking at 15 pounds per square inch reduced the compounds by up to 90 percent in one study.

PANEL OF ADVISORS

SAMUEL KLEIN, M.D., IS A WILLIAM H. DANFORTH PROFESSOR OF MEDICINE AND NUTRITIONAL SCIENCE AND DIRECTOR OF THE CENTER FOR HUMAN NUTRITION AT WASHINGTON UNIVERSITY SCHOOL OF MEDICINE IN ST. LOUIS.

MICHAEL D. LEVITT, M.D., IS A GASTROENTEROLOGIST AND ASSOCIATE CHIEF OF STAFF AT THE MINNEAPOLIS VA MEDICAL CENTER.

GALE MALESKEY, M.S., R.D., IS A CLINICAL DIETITIAN, NUTRITION EDUCATOR, AND SPEAKER. SHE PRACTICES NUTRITION COUNSELING IN BRIDGEWATER, NEW JERSEY, WHERE SHE SEES CLIENTS FOR A WIDE VARIETY OF HEALTH PROBLEMS.

RICHARD MCCALLUM, M.D., IS A PROFESSOR OF MEDICINE AND DIRECTOR OF THE CENTER FOR GASTROINTESTINAL NERVE AND MUSCLE FUNCTION AND THE DIVISION OF GI MOTILITY AT THE UNIVERSITY OF KANSAS MEDICAL CENTER IN KANSAS CITY.

Flu

20 Remedies to Beat the Bug

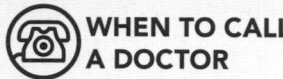
Getting the flu is sort of like taking a multiple-choice quiz. That's because there are three main types of influenza: A, B, and C. Within these types, though, the pesky viruses have unlimited ability to mutate into many forms.

Because the flu is a viral infection, antibiotics are powerless against it. But if you get to your doctor within the first 48 hours of symptoms, prescription antiviral drugs, such as zanamivir (Relenza) or oseltamivir (Tamiflu), may help you recover quicker. Both are considered 60 to 90 percent effective—but they are useless if you take them more than 2 days before or after exposure. So, the fact remains that the best defense is avoidance. (See "Outsmart the Flu Bug" on page 264.)

If avoidance didn't work, and you've succumbed to the bug, take these steps to help ease the symptoms.

■ **STAY HOME.** The flu is a very infectious disease that spreads like wildfire. So don't be a workaholic or a martyr. Stay home from work—and anywhere else—until at least 1 day after your temperature returns to normal. And keep your children home from school until they have fully recovered.

■ **BE PROPERLY DIAGNOSED.** When you feel sick and aren't sure why, the big question is: Is this infection caused by a virus (and therefore, flu) or a bacteria (and so, a cold)? Two FDA-approved tests can—in a matter of hours—tell your doctor if

Is It Really the Flu?

How can you tell a cold from the flu? This isn't a riddle. Or maybe it is. Although similarities exist between the two illnesses—and their treatment—they're caused by entirely different viruses. The worst part of a cold might last longer, but the flu generally causes more discomfort. Here is a comparison of common symptoms and the differences between them, depending on whether they are caused by a cold or the flu.

Fever. Prominent with flu, coming on suddenly; possible with a cold, though usually mild

Headache. Prominent with flu; rare with a cold

General aches. Prominent and often severe with flu; slight with a cold

Fatigue. Extreme with flu, lasting 2 to 3 weeks; mild with a cold

Runny nose. Occasional with the flu; common with a cold

Sore throat. Occasional with the flu; common with a cold

Cough. Common and possibly severe with the flu; mild to moderate with a cold

your misery is viral. This testing can potentially help you get the right treatment faster—and prevent inappropriate (and ineffective) antibiotic use against the flu.

A throat swab is all it takes for the xTAG RVP test to screen for a dozen different viruses; results are available in 6 hours. The Pro-Flu+ is quicker (3 hours) but can detect only four kinds of viruses. Ask your doctor if a test makes sense for you.

■ **GET SOME REST.** You shouldn't have much trouble following this advice, since you'll probably be too sick to do much else. Bed rest is essential, because it lets your body put its energy into combating the flu infection. Being active while you're still quite ill weakens your defenses and leaves you open to complications.

■ **DRINK UP.** Liquids are especially important to prevent dehydration if you have a fever, says Jay Swedberg, M.D. In addition, fluids can provide needed nutrients when you're too sick to eat. Thin soups are good, as are pure fruit and vegetable juices. Check the labels to be sure you are getting 100 percent juice. Dr. Swedberg recommends diluting fruit juice with water. "A little sugar provides necessary

Cures from the Kitchen

A sore or scratchy throat is apt to accompany the flu. Get some relief—and wash out any secretions collecting in your throat—by gargling with a saltwater solution, says Mary Ann Pane, R.N. Dissolve 1 teaspoon of salt in 1 cup of warm water. This concentration approximates the pH level of body tissues and is very soothing, she says. Use as often as needed, but do not swallow the liquid because it's very high in sodium.

F FLU

Outsmart the Flu Bug

Individual immunity and the particular strain of flu virus circulating in a given year play a large role in determining who will knuckle under to the flu. Still, there are steps you can take to reduce your susceptibility to this bug.

Get a flu shot. Every year, scientists develop a vaccine against the most recently circulating strain of the virus. And for good reason: The single best way to protect against the flu is to get vaccinated as early as September, according to the Centers for Disease Control and Prevention (CDC). Early flu shots are particularly important for residents of nursing homes; those with chronic conditions such as heart or kidney disease, asthma or other ongoing lung problems, or a weakened immune system; anyone over 65; and most medical personnel. All other groups, including household members of high-risk people, healthy people ages 50 to 64, and those who wish to decrease their risk of flu infection, should begin vaccination no later than November.

In cases when the shot doesn't prevent the flu, it considerably lessens the disease's severity. Don't wait until the flu's in town before acting, because the vaccine takes about 2 weeks to work. And don't get a flu shot at all if you're allergic to eggs—the vaccine is made from them.

Keep 'em clean. Hand washing really is key to keeping germs from entering your eyes,

glucose, but too much can cause diarrhea when you're ill," he says. "Also dilute ginger ale and other sugar-sweetened soft drinks. And allow them to go flat before drinking, because their bubbles can create gas in the stomach and make you more nauseated."

■ **REACH FOR PAIN RELIEF.** Aspirin, acetaminophen, or ibuprofen can reduce the fever, headache, and body aches that so often accompany the flu. Follow label instructions. Because symptoms are often most pronounced in the afternoon and evening, take the medication regularly over this period.. Children and teenagers should not take aspirin without their doctor's consent.

■ **THINK TWICE ABOUT WHAT YOU TAKE.** Over-the-counter cold medicines may give you some temporary relief of symptoms. Those with antihistamines, for example, can dry up a runny nose. But be careful—these drugs may suppress your symptoms to the point that you feel better. Prematurely resuming your normal activities can bring on a relapse or trigger serious complications.

■ **DO SOMETHING SWEET.** Sucking on hard candy and lozenges keeps your throat moist, so it feels better, says Mary Ann Pane, R.N. If you're concerned about the calories these products contain, look for sugar-free brands. They're just as effective.

264

nose, or mouth where they can set up an infection. Wash your hands well, using soap and water—and often. "I'm not talking about just before dinner," says William Schaffner, M.D. "We have a rule in my house: Anytime you walk in the door, you hang your coat and march straight to the sink to wash your hands." Alcohol-based waterless hand cleansers will work, too.

Avoid those already afflicted. It's only common sense: Being around sick people raises your risk of becoming sick as well. The CDC recommends staying away from people who show signs of the flu to protect yourself from infection.

Sequester yourself. When the flu hits your community, it's time to hunker down until the storm passes. "When you read in the paper that flu is around or see it on the news, that's the time to rent a movie and watch it at home, instead of going out to the theater," says Dr. Schaffner. To get a flu surveillance report for your area, enter your ZIP code at www.flustar.com.

More reason to quit. Smokers are more susceptible to influenza, and more of them die from flu than nonsmokers. Do yourself a huge favor and quit smoking, whether it's flu season or not.

Stay strong. Keeping yourself in good health every day goes a long way toward combating the flu, says the CDC. Be physically active, get plenty of sleep, and eat well year-round—but especially during flu season.

■ **HUMIDIFY THE AIR.** Raising the humidity in your bedroom also helps reduce the discomfort of a cough, sore throat, and dry nasal passages.

■ **PAMPER YOUR NOSE.** If you've been blowing your nose a lot, it's probably pretty sore. So lubricate your nostrils frequently to decrease irritation, says Pane. A product such as K-Y Jelly is preferable to petroleum jelly, which dries out quickly.

■ **TAKE SOME HEAT.** One characteristic of the flu is tired, achy muscles. Warm them and ease their pain with a warm bath or heating pad, says Pane.

■ **EAT LIGHTLY AND WISELY.** During the worst phase of the flu, you probably won't have an appetite at all. But when you're ready to make the transition from liquids to more substantial fare, put the emphasis on bland, starchy foods, says Dr. Swedberg. "Dry toast is fine. So

What the Doctor Does

TRY ZINC. Neil Schachter, M.D., pops zinc before getting on an airplane, because studies have shown it can be an effective flu preventer when used shortly after exposure to the virus. Taken in lozenge form, like a cough drop, this is a convenient measure to take when traveling. Look for zinc gluconate or zinc acetate without citric or tartaric acid—they seem to blunt zinc's protective powers. Take it no more than twice a day for 1 week.

Favorite Fixes

WHAT IT IS: It's all well and good that you wash your hands regularly during flu season, but how do you guarantee your kids' hands are clean? Provide a quick spritz of hand sanitizer.

WHAT IT DOES: Spray-on hand sanitizer means you can get clean hands anywhere, anytime. It also saves time and money and even makes it fun for the kids.

HOW TO USE IT: Jennifer Hoffmann, mom of two in Huntington, New York, says, "Take a clean, empty spray bottle, like one from hairspray. [You can buy spray bottles in drugstores.] Fill your bottle with an alcohol-based gel hand sanitizer and store it in your purse. Before every restaurant meal and after every shopping stop, ask your kids to hold out their hands and give them a spritz or two."

are bananas, applesauce, boiled rice, rice pudding, cooked cereal, and baked potatoes, which can be topped with yogurt." For a refreshing dessert, peel and freeze very ripe bananas, then puree them in a food processor.

PANEL OF ADVISORS

MARY ANN PANE, R.N., IS A NURSE CLINICIAN IN PHILADELPHIA. SHE WAS FORMERLY AFFILIATED WITH COMMUNITY HOME HEALTH SERVICES, AN AGENCY CATERING TO PEOPLE WHO REQUIRE SKILLED HEALTH CARE IN THEIR HOMES.

NEIL SCHACHTER, M.D., IS A PROFESSOR OF PULMONARY MEDICINE AT THE MOUNT SINAI SCHOOL OF MEDICINE IN NEW YORK CITY AND AUTHOR OF *THE GOOD DOCTOR'S GUIDE TO COLDS & FLU.*

WILLIAM SCHAFFNER, M.D., IS CHAIR OF THE PREVENTIVE MEDICINE DEPARTMENT AT VANDERBILT UNIVERSITY SCHOOL OF MEDICINE IN NASHVILLE, TENNESSEE.

JAY SWEDBERG, M.D., IS A PHYSICIAN AND AN OWNER AND PARTNER AT WESTERN MEDICAL ASSOCIATES IN CASPER, WYOMING.

Food Poisoning

26 Solutions for Food Flu

If you stop to think about the food you eat—where it started out, how it got to you, and all that happened along the way—it's pretty amazing that we don't get food poisoning more often. The fact is, our bodies are normally capable of handling most of what we ingest. There are some unbreakable rules, however, when it comes to food safety. Taking shortcuts with those rules can be regrettable.

For example, eating raw or undercooked meat or poultry, enjoying improperly washed fruits and vegetables, indulging in sun-warmed potato salad, and feasting on a host of other foods can open the door to a potentially life-threatening case of food poisoning. Despite well-publicized guidelines about food safety and inspections at restaurants and food-processing centers, government researchers estimate that Americans have 76 million food-borne illnesses each year, sending 325,000 people to the hospital and killing 5,000 in the United States.

Even non-life-threatening cases of food poisoning can make you feel miserable, resulting in dizziness, queasiness, diarrhea, vomiting, abdominal cramps, headache, and fever.

Toxic bacteria get into food in a variety of ways, generally as a result of inadequate cooking or processing.

In any case, once inside you, these bad bugs attack your intestines. For a day or so, you feel wretched as your body battles

(continued on page 270)

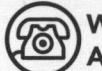

WHEN TO CALL A DOCTOR

With a normal case of food poisoning, the symptoms—cramps, nausea, vomiting, diarrhea, and dizziness—disappear in a day or two.

Call a doctor immediately if your symptoms are also accompanied by:

■ Difficulty swallowing, speaking, or breathing; changes in vision; muscle weakness or paralysis, particularly if this occurs after eating mushrooms, canned food, or shellfish

■ Fever higher than 100°F

■ Severe vomiting—you can't hold down even any liquids

■ Severe diarrhea for more than a day or two

■ Persistent, localized abdominal pain

■ Dehydration

■ Bloody diarrhea

Don't Let It Happen Again!

You can't always blame the diner across town for your stomach troubles. The truth is, says Daniel C. Rodrigue, M.D., many cases of food poisoning probably come from carelessness in your own home. Despite a 25 percent drop in the number of *Escherichia coli* infections and a 41 percent drop in shigella infections on account of improved government food-safety programs, food-borne illnesses demand consistent vigilance.

Follow these commonsense rules to significantly decrease your chances of poisoning yourself.

■ Wash your hands with warm water and soap for at least 20 seconds before and after preparing food to avoid passing on bacteria such as staphylococcus. This is especially important before and after handling raw meat and eggs. If you have an infection or a cut on your hands, wear plastic or rubber gloves. Be sure to wash your gloved hands just as often as you would wash your bare hands.

■ Heat or chill raw food. Bacteria can't multiply above 150°F or below 40°F.

■ Don't leave food at room temperature for more than 2 hours, and avoid eating anything that you suspect may have been unrefrigerated for that long. Bacteria thrive in warm protein food made with meat or eggs, and in cream-filled pastries, dips, potato salad, and so forth.

■ Raw food can harbor bacteria. Don't eat raw protein food like fish, fowl, meat, or eggs. Avoid sushi, oysters on the half shell, Caesar salad prepared with raw eggs, and unpasteurized eggnog. Don't use eggs if they have hairline cracks—harmful salmonella bacteria may have already set up shop. Don't sample raw cookie dough that you've made with eggs. (Commercially prepared cookie dough is not a food hazard.)

■ Don't buy cooked seafood, such as shrimp, if it's displayed in the same case as raw fish.

■ Buy fresh seafood only from reputable dealers who keep the products properly refrigerated or on ice and at a constant temperature.

■ If you are a recreational fisher and you eat your catch, follow state and local government announcements about fishing areas and frequency of consumption.

■ Cook meat until a meat thermometer inserted into the thickest part registers 160°F and the pink disappears, chicken with a bone until the thermometer registers 170°F and there are no red joints, chicken without a bone until the thermometer registers 160°F, turkey breast until thermometer registers 170°F, other turkey (ground or whole) until thermometer registers 165°F, and fish until it flakes easily. Complete cooking is the only way to ensure that all potentially harmful bacteria have been killed.

■ Don't taste-test foods before they're cooked, especially pork, fish, and eggs.

■ Don't let raw meat juice drip onto other food. It can taint otherwise harmless food.

■ Use a separate chopping board and utensils when handling raw meat, and sanitize them with hot, soapy water and a bleach solution after use to prevent cross-contamination.

■ Scrub fruits and vegetables thoroughly. Peel nonorganic produce, such as cucumbers, and remove the outer leaves of leafy vegetables.

■ Scrub can openers and countertops and always clean out crevices to prevent bacteria from hiding and growing there. For all areas that come in contact with food, use hot water and soap, followed by a bleach solution.

■ Replace sponges often and use paper towels to wipe off counters.

■ Thaw meat in the refrigerator. Or thaw it in the microwave and cook it immediately after it's thawed. Bacteria can multiply on food surfaces while the center is still frozen. When using the microwave to defrost, follow the instructions and leave at least 2 inches of space around the item to allow air to circulate.

■ Immediately refrigerate leftovers, even if they are still hot. Cool down large pots of food faster by refrigerating in smaller portions.

■ Never pick and eat wild mushrooms. Some carry toxins that attack the nervous system and can be deadly. Picking wild mushrooms should be left to the experts.

■ Never taste home-canned food before boiling for 20 minutes. If not properly canned, food contains bacteria that can produce a dangerous toxin.

■ Use common sense and don't taste any food that doesn't smell or look right. Avoid cracked jars or swollen, dented cans or lids; clear liquids that have turned milky; and cans or jars that spurt or have an "off" odor when opened. They could contain dangerous bacteria. Make sure you discard them carefully so that pets don't come in contact with them.

back. Here's what the experts say to do to help your body fight a case of food "flu."

■ **FILL UP ON FLUIDS.** The bacteria irritate your intestinal tract and trigger a great deal of fluid loss from diarrhea, vomiting, or both. Drink lots of fluids to prevent dehydration. Water is best, followed by other clear liquids such as apple juice, broth, or bouillon.

Soft drinks are okay, too, if you drink them flat, says Gale Maleskey, M.S., R.D. Otherwise, the carbonation can further irritate your stomach. Defizzed cola and ginger ale will also settle your stomach—just choose the flavor you prefer. Get the bubbles out of soft drinks quickly by pouring the soda back and forth between two glasses, she suggests.

■ **SIP A LITTLE, SLOWLY.** Trying to gulp down too much at once may trigger more vomiting, says Maleskey.

■ **REPLENISH ELECTROLYTES.** Vomiting and diarrhea can flush out important electrolytes—potassium, sodium, and glucose.

Cures from the Kitchen

Love lemon? You may want to pass on the puckery citrus slices the next time you're dining or drinking out. According to a recent study, nearly 70 percent of restaurant lemon wedges harbor nasty germs from saliva, skin, and—yuck—feces. The bacteria may have originated from dirty hands, indiscreet coughs and sneezes, or contaminated cutting boards and knives. Instead of ordering your beverage with a fruity twist, skip it or keep individual packets of lemon juice in your purse.

Experts suggest that you replace them by sipping commercially prepared electrolyte products such as Gatorade. Or try this rehydration recipe: Mix a cup of fruit juice (for potassium) with $\frac{1}{2}$ teaspoon of honey or corn syrup (for glucose) and a pinch of table salt (for sodium).

■ **DON'T INTERFERE WITH PROGRESS.** Your body is trying to flush the toxic organism out, explains Daniel C. Rodrigue, M.D. In some cases, taking antidiarrheal products (such as Imodium, Kaopectate, and Lomotil) may interfere with your body's ability to fight the infection. So stay away from them and let nature take its course. If you feel it's necessary to take something, consult your doctor first.

■ **REINTRODUCE BLAND FOODS.** Usually within a few hours to a day after the diarrhea and vomiting have subsided, you'll be ready for some "real" food. But go easy. Your stomach is weak and irritated. Experts suggest starting with easily digestible foods. Try cereal, pudding, saltines, or broth. Avoid high-fiber, spicy, acidic, greasy, sugary, or dairy foods that could further irritate the stomach. Do this for a day or two. After that, your stomach will be ready to get back to its routine.

■ **MIND YOUR PEAS AND CORNS.** They say an ounce of prevention is worth a pound of cure, and this may never be truer than when you are dealing with the aftermath of eating spoiled food. To keep yourself and your family safe from food poisoning, remember that produce is much more likely to cause trouble than poultry or beef, according to the Center for Science in the Public Interest. Be sure to rinse *all* fruits and vegetables (peelable or not): Bacteria on the surface can be transported inside by a knife when slicing or chopping. And never wash produce until just before you plan to eat it. Damp veggies will harbor mold and other microbes that can make you sick.

PANEL OF ADVISORS

GALE MALESKEY, M.S., R.D., IS A CLINICAL DIETITIAN, NUTRITION EDUCATOR, AND SPEAKER. SHE PRACTICES NUTRITION COUNSELING IN BRIDGEWATER, NEW JERSEY, WHERE SHE SEES CLIENTS FOR A WIDE VARIETY OF HEALTH PROBLEMS.

DANIEL C. RODRIGUE, M.D., IS AN INFECTIOUS DISEASE SPECIALIST AT LEXINGTON INFECTIOUS DISEASE CONSULTANTS IN LEXINGTON, KENTUCKY.

Foot Aches

16 Feet Treats

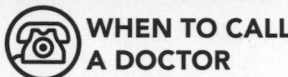

WHEN TO CALL A DOCTOR

According to Mark D. Sussman, D.P.M., you should definitely see a doctor if:

■ You have pain in your feet that continually increases during the day.

■ Your feet get to the point where you can't keep your shoes on.

■ You have trouble walking first thing in the morning.

Also be aware that painful burning in the feet can be a sign of poor circulation, athlete's foot, a pinched nerve, diabetes, anemia, thyroid disease, alcoholism, or other critical problem, and always warrants a call to the doctor.

The American Podiatric Medical Association reports that an overwhelming majority of Americans—75 percent—experience problems with their feet at some point during their lifetimes.

It's no wonder, considering the complexity of the foot. Each foot contains 26 bones, 33 joints, 107 ligaments, 19 muscles, and many tendons that hold the foot together and help it move in various directions. The average person takes 8,000 to 10,000 steps a day, at times putting so much pressure on the feet that it exceeds his or her body weight.

Amazingly, it's not really the workout that batters feet, it's most often a combination of ill-fitting shoes and neglect. Fortunately, much can be done to ease foot pain. Here's what our experts recommend.

■ **ELEVATE YOUR FEET.** The best thing you can do for your feet when you get home is to sit down, put your feet up, and exercise your toes to get the circulation going again. Elevate your feet at a 45-degree angle to your body (straight out from your hips) and relax for 20 minutes.

■ **SOAK THEM IN SALTS.** A tried-and-true foot revitalizer is to soak your feet in a basin of warm water containing 1 to 2 tablespoons of Epsom salts, says Mark D. Sussman, D.P.M. Rinse with clear, cool water, then pat your feet dry and massage with a moisturizing gel or cream.

■ **RUN HOT AND COLD.** Dr. Sussman recommends this treatment, popular at European spas. Sit on the edge of the bathtub and hold your feet under running water for several minutes. Alternate 1 minute of comfortably hot water with 1 minute of cold, repeating several times and ending with the cold. The contrasting bath will invigorate your whole system. If you have a shower-massage attachment, use that to give your feet an even more stimulating workout.

If you have diabetes or impaired circulation, however, don't expose your feet to extremes of temperature.

■ **MASSAGE AWAY YOUR ACHES.** "A really nice thing is to have somebody massage your feet with baby oil," says Dr. Sussman. Or you can do some soothing self-massage. With both hands, work over the whole foot, squeezing the toes gently, then press in a circular motion over the bottom of your foot. One really effective movement is to slide one thumb firmly up and down the arch of the foot.

■ **REACH FOR OVER-THE-COUNTER RELIEF.** Custom-made orthotics can help foot pain, but they can be quite pricey—and there is no guarantee they will work. For the acute heel pain that comes from plantar fasciitis (an inflammation of the plantar fascia, which runs along the sole of your foot), try a store-bought heel cup, says Marlene Reid, D.P.M. They cost only a few dollars. Select a firm one, she suggests.

■ **EXERCISE.** We don't mean aerobics or any other heavy-duty activity. But many doctors recommend that you exercise your feet and leg muscles periodically throughout the day to ward off aches and keep the circulation going. Try these ideas from experts at the Kinney Shoe Corporation.

■ If your feet feel tense and cramped any time during the day, give them a good shake, as you would your hands if they felt cramped. Do one foot at a time, and then relax and flex your toes up and down.

■ If you must stand for long periods of time, walk in place whenever you can. Keep changing your stance, and try to rest one foot on a stool or step occasionally. If possible, stand on carpeting or a spongy rubber mat.

■ To relieve stiffness, remove your shoes, sit in a chair, and stretch your feet out in front of you. Circle both feet from the ankles 10 times in one direction, then 10 times in the other, pointing your toes down as far as possible, then flexing them up as high as you can. Repeat 10 times. Now grasp your toes and gently pull them back and forth.

■ **ROLL AWAY THE PAIN.** For an easy and free mini massage that encourages your arch to stretch and relax, remove your shoes and roll each foot over a golf ball, tennis ball, or soup can for a minute or two. To cool achy foot pain, try rolling your feet, one at a time, over a bottle of frozen water.

■ **SAVE YOUR SOLES.** Wear shoes with thick, shock-absorbing soles to shield your feet

Cures from the Kitchen

Pour yourself a cup of tea to relax, and while drinking soak your feet in warm tea to sooth pain. Try a strong peppermint or chamomile tea. Steep four tea bags in 2 cups of boiling water. Add the brew to 1 gallon of comfortably hot water. Soak your feet for 5 minutes. Slosh your feet in the water and let the tea's warm scent relax you. Drain the water and pour some cold water over your feet. Follow that with hot water from the tap and then more cold.

from rough surfaces and hard pavements. Don't let your soles become too thin or worn, because they won't do the job they're supposed to do. Women's thin-soled, pointy-toed high heels are classic villains. If you must dress up for work, ease foot strain by wearing walking or athletic shoes to and from the job and switching to heels at the office.

■ **CHANGE HEEL HEIGHTS.** Wearing high heels tightens the calf muscles, which leads to foot fatigue, says John F. Waller Jr., M.D. Changing heel heights from high to low during the day is an excellent idea.

■ **WEAR INSOLES.** High heels have the added disadvantage of causing your feet to pitch forward as you walk, putting painful pressure on the balls of your feet, says Dr. Waller. To prevent this discomfort, wear a half-insole in each shoe to help keep your foot in place. And be sure to take the insoles with you to the shoe store to ensure that they'll fit comfortably in your new shoes.

■ **SHOE SHOP IN THE AFTERNOON.** Your feet expand during the day, so you should buy shoes in the afternoon or with enough space to accommodate the slight swelling. Measure your feet while standing, and always try on both shoes. If one foot is a bit larger than the other, buy the pair that feels best on the bigger foot, advises the American Podiatric Medical Association.

■ **STRETCH YOUR SHOES.** When you add insoles to your shoes, says Dr. Sussman, make sure they don't cramp your toes. If things are tight, you may be able to stretch the shoes to accommodate the insoles. Fill a sock with sand, stuff it into the shoe's toebox, and wrap the shoe with a wet towel. Let it dry out over the next 24 hours. Repeat once or twice, if needed.

PANEL OF ADVISORS

MARLENE REID, D.P.M., IS A BOARD-CERTIFIED PODIATRIST IN NAPERVILLE, ILLINOIS AND SPOKESPERSON FOR THE AMERICAN PODIATRIC MEDICAL ASSOCIATION. SHE IS ALSO VICE PRESIDENT OF THE AMERICAN ASSOCIATION FOR WOMEN PODIATRISTS.

MARK D. SUSSMAN, D.P.M., IS A WELLNESS CONSULTANT AND RETIRED PODIATRIST WHO FORMERLY PRACTICED IN WHEATON, MARYLAND.

JOHN F. WALLER JR., M.D., IS AN ORTHOPEDIC SURGEON SPECIALIZING IN THE FOOT AND ANKLE. HE IS ATTENDING SURGEON IN ORTHOPEDIC SURGERY AT LENOX HILL HOSPITAL IN NEW YORK CITY.

Foot Odor

15 Deodorizing Secrets

Your feet have more sweat glands per inch than any other part of the body—an average of 250,000 of them. They secrete sweat all the time, keeping your skin moist and supple. When you put your feet in a pair of shoes, the confinement allows fungi and bacteria to thrive. The teaming bacteria produce a substance called isovaleric acid, which emits the characteristic locker room stench associated with foot odor.

"The fungi and bacteria, which are a normal part of our skin's flora, proliferate in the dark, moist, warm environment of the shoes," says Paul Langer, D.P.M. "Foot odor tends to be worse in warm weather and in active people." About 25 percent of us have issues with foot odor, according to an American Podiatric Medicine Association survey of 1,700 adults.

The key to eliminating foot odor is good foot hygiene.

■ **WASH DAILY.** Keep your feet scrupulously clean. Use warm, soapy water and wash your feet every day, says Dr. Langer. Scrub gently with a soft brush, even between your toes, and be sure to dry your feet thoroughly.

■ **POWDER.** After washing, apply foot powder or cornstarch to help sweating feet stay drier, says Dr. Langer.

■ **SPRINKLE YOUR SHOES.** Another good method for keeping feet cool and dry is to treat your shoes—sprinkle the insides with talcum powder or cornstarch, says Suzanne M. Levine, D.P.M., P.C.

Cures from the Kitchen

A lot of intriguing remedies for foot odor have made the rounds over the years. To determine which ones actually work and which don't, we turned to Thom Lobe, M.D., founder and medical director of the Beneveda Medical Group in Beverly Hills.

JELL-O. "Many deodorants work by creating a gel that fills and obstructs the sweat glands, so they cannot excrete," he says. "Jell-O forms a gel, so you get a similar effect." Make Jell-O as you normally would, and soak your feet in it as it sets.

VODKA. "We sterilize wounds with alcohol. Vodka—which is odorless—will work just fine to get rid of the odor-producing microbes," Dr. Lobe says. "You could also use tequila, which doesn't have an odor, either."

ZINC. "Foot odor is one of many symptoms of zinc deficiency," Dr. Lobe explains. You can replenish your zinc levels with foods such as oysters, nuts, peas, eggs, whole grains, oats, and pumpkin seeds.

■ **USE AN ANTIPERSPIRANT.** The key to controlling odor is to use either an antiperspirant or a deodorant on your feet. You can buy foot deodorants or simply use your underarm brand. Keep in mind that deodorants eliminate odor, but they don't stop perspiration. Antiperspirants take care of both problems. Dr. Levine recommends products that contain aluminum chloride hexahydrate.

Don't use an antiperspirant if you have athlete's foot, says Stephen Weinberg, D.P.M., because it will sting. "I recommend roll-on products rather than sprays, because most of a spray's antiperspirant action is lost in the air," he says. "Use the product two or three times a day in the beginning, then gradually cut back to once a day."

■ **CHANGE YOUR SOCKS—OFTEN.** Always wear clean, dry socks. Change them when they get sweaty—as frequently as necessary—even a few times a day, says Glenn Copeland, D.P.M.

■ **AVOID COTTON SOCKS.** Cotton holds moisture next to the skin and can make foot odor worse, says Dr. Langer. Wool is a better choice because wool fibers wick moisture away from the skin. Synthetic fibers also have wicking properties.

■ **TRY SOME METAL THREADS.** There are now socks and insoles available that are made with copper or silver threads woven into the fabric. "Copper and silver have been shown to have antimicrobial properties," says. Dr. Langer.

■ **SHOW SHOE SENSE.** "Closed shoes aggravate sweaty feet and set up a perfect environment for bacteria to grow, leading to more odor and more sweat," says Dr. Levine. Choose sandals, open-toe shoes, and those with mesh uppers when appropriate, but stay away from rubber and plastic shoes, which don't allow feet to breathe easily.

■ **GIVE THEM A DAY OFF.** Never wear the same shoes two days in a row, says Dr. Levine. Air them out. It takes at least 24 hours for shoes to dry thoroughly.

■ **TAKE FREQUENT SOAKS.** Various soaking agents can help keep the feet dry, which may also control odor.

■ **Tea.** Tannin, which can be found in tea bags, is a drying agent. Boil three or four tea bags in 1 quart of water for about 10 minutes, then add enough cold water to make a comfortable soak, suggests Diana Bihova, M.D.

Soak your feet for 20 to 30 minutes, then dry them and apply foot powder. Do this twice a day until you get the problem under control. After that, repeat it twice a week to keep odor from recurring.

■ **Sodium bicarbonate.** This makes the foot surface more acidic, which cuts down on the amount of odor produced, says Dr. Levine. Dissolve 1 tablespoon of baking soda in 1 quart of water. Soak for 15 minutes twice a week

■ **Vinegar.** Another acid footbath that Dr. Levine recommends is ½ cup of vinegar

Do Your Feet Work Harder Than You Do?

Sometimes feet perspire a lot because they simply *work* harder than they should, says Neal Kramer, D.P.M. A structural defect (such as flat feet) or a job that keeps you hopping all day could be the underlying culprit. Either would increase the activity of your foot muscles. And the harder your feet work, the more they perspire in an attempt to cool themselves.

"If you correct the underlying problem with an arch support or some other orthotic shoe insert," says Dr. Kramer, "you can actually cut down on the amount of sweat produced. If the muscles don't have to work as hard, they just don't give off as much heat."

---

in 1 quart of water. Soak for 15 minutes twice a week.

■ **HEED SAGE ADVICE.** Europeans sometimes sprinkle the fragrant herb sage into their shoes to control odor, says Dr. Levine. Perhaps a dash of dry, crumbled sage leaves will do the trick.

■ **SUN YOUR SHOES.** Exposing the insides of the shoes to sunlight can kill some of the fungus and bacteria that cause foul odors, says Dr. Langer.

■ **STAY COOL.** The sweat glands in your feet, like those in your armpits and palms, respond to emotions, says Richard L. Dobson, M.D. Stress can trigger excessive sweating. That, in turn, can increase bacterial activity in your shoes, leading to extra odor. So try not to get frazzled.

■ **WATCH WHAT YOU EAT.** As bizarre as it may sound, says Dr. Levine, when you eat spicy or pungent foods (such as onions, peppers, garlic, or scallions), the essence of these odors can be excreted through the sweat glands in your feet. So, yes, your feet can end up smelling like your lunch.

PANEL OF ADVISORS

DIANA BIHOVA, M.D., IS A DERMATOLOGIST AFFILIATED WITH THE DERMATOLOGY DEPARTMENT AT THE COLUMBIA UNIVERSITY COLLEGE OF PHYSICIANS AND SURGEONS IN NEW YORK CITY.

GLENN COPELAND, D.P.M., IS A PODIATRIST AT THE WOMEN'S COLLEGE HOSPITAL IN TORONTO. HE IS ALSO CONSULTING PODIATRIST FOR THE CANADIAN BACK INSTITUTE AND PODIATRIST FOR THE TORONTO BLUE JAYS BASEBALL TEAM.

RICHARD L. DOBSON, M.D., IS A PROFESSOR EMERITUS OF THE DEPARTMENT OF DERMATOLOGY AT THE MEDICAL UNIVERSITY OF SOUTH CAROLINA COLLEGE OF MEDICINE IN CHARLESTON.

NEAL KRAMER, D.P.M., IS A PODIATRIST IN BETHLEHEM, PENNSYLVANIA.

PAUL LANGER, D.P.M., IS A CLINICAL ASSISTANT PROFESSOR AT THE UNIVERSITY OF MINNESOTA MEDICAL SCHOOL IN MINNEAPOLIS AND AUTHOR OF *GREAT FEET FOR LIFE*.

SUZANNE M. LEVINE, D.P.M., P.C., IS A PODIATRIC SURGEON AND CLINICAL PODIATRIST AT NEW YORK–PRESBYTERIAN HOSPITAL IN NEW YORK CITY. SHE IS AUTHOR OF *YOUR FEET DON'T HAVE TO HURT*.

THOM LOBE, M.D., IS FOUNDER AND MEDICAL DIRECTOR OF THE BENEVEDA MEDICAL GROUP IN BEVERLY HILLS.

STEPHEN WEINBERG, D.P.M., IS DIRECTOR OF THE RUNNING CLINIC AT THE WEIL FOOT AND ANKLE INSTITUTE IN DES PLAINES, ILLINOIS, AND DIRECTOR OF PODIATRIC SERVICES FOR THE CHICAGO MARATHON.

Frostbite

19 Safeguards against the Cold

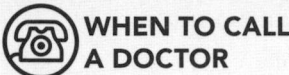

WHEN TO CALL A DOCTOR

Frostbite demands professional medical attention. Tissue is dying. And that opens the door to some dark possibilities—infection and loss of fingers or toes, and in extreme cases, loss of an arm or a leg.

With deep frostbite, the skin is cold, hard, white, and numb. When rewarmed, the skin may turn blue or purple. It also may swell, and blisters might form. The idea, of course, is to treat frostbite quickly and effectively so none of this happens.

When Tod Schimelpfenig was 18, he and a friend wanted a winter adventure. So they went hiking and mountain climbing in the northern Vermont wilderness.

"We were out trying to be mountaineers and ended up going to the school of hard knocks," Schimelpfenig says now, nearly 40 years later.

Schimelpfenig, in fact, took an advanced course in frostbite. The toes of his right foot turned white and hard. "They looked like a frozen steak," he recalls with a laugh.

Of course, he wasn't laughing then. Fortunately, he and his companion found a place to camp for the night, and he was able to stay off the frozen foot for a while. To prevent even more serious injury, he had to make sure that the foot didn't thaw and refreeze. So while keeping the rest of his body in a warm sleeping bag, he kept the frostbitten foot outside the bag and frozen. And he had to stay awake all night to do it.

"I walked out 8 miles the next morning, and I was fine," he says. "I still have all my toes."

Schimelpfenig, who is now curriculum director for the Wilderness Medicine Institute of the National Outdoor Leadership School in Lander, Wyoming, and a volunteer emergency medical technician, admits he put himself in a dangerous situation. Yet less severe forms of frostbite can occur quickly in much less extreme conditions. A review of frostbite cases in the *Journal of the American Board of Family Practitioners* found that in 90 percent of the cases, frostbite occurred on the hands and feet. Fingers, toes, the ears, and the tip of the nose are most susceptible to frostbite. Exposed to cold temperatures, your body goes into survival mode to preserve its core temperature by constricting the bloodflow in your extremities. With up to 90 percent less bloodflow to your fingers and toes, the skin and underlying tissues begin to freeze.

"Frostbite is the body's way of trying to preserve heat by shutting down circulation to an extremity," says Ruth Uphold, M.D. "Unfortunately, as you develop frostbite," she warns, "you might not even know that you have it because of the numbness."

Frostbite requires immediate treatment in a medical facility. Here are tips on how to prevent it and what to do until you can get help.

■ **LAYER ON PROTECTION.** Wear several layers of loose-fitting, lightweight, warm clothing, says Schimelpfenig. Trapped air between the layers will insulate you. Remove layers to avoid sweating and subsequent chill. Outer garments should be tightly woven, water repellent (not waterproof—it doesn't breathe and traps moisture), and hooded. Wear a hat, because half of your body heat can be lost through your head. Cover your mouth to protect your lungs from extreme cold. Mittens, snug at the wrist, are better than gloves.

■ **INSULATE YOUR FEET.** Wear insulated, waterproof boots that fit properly—snug, but not too tight. Wool socks are best because wool is the only fiber that keeps you warm even when

it is wet. Beware of doubling up on socks. It may actually make your feet colder by making your shoes too tight and cut off circulation.

■ **REMOVE METAL JEWELRY.** Because metal readily conducts cold, Schimelpfenig recommends removing all metal jewelry before heading out on winter adventures. Rings, in particular, are a problem because they can also constrict circulation.

■ **KNOW THE SIGNS.** Symptoms of frostbite progress from an initial feeling of coldness to stinging, burning, and throbbing sensations followed by numbness. Any tissue that remains numb for more than a few minutes may become frostbitten, says David Cheng, M.D. Frostbitten tissue looks white and feels firm to the touch. If you notice signs of frostbite, seek medical attention.

■ **DON'T DELAY.** Schimelpfenig learned the hard, cold way. "You can get into a trap saying, 'Well, my feet or my hands are kind of cold, but I'm going to get inside in a little while anyway.' Now I make sure I can honestly say my feet and hands are still *warm*."

■ **FACTOR IN THE WIND.** The windchill factor describes what the air temperature feels like to your skin and body when it's cold and windy outside. As wind increases, heat is carried away from the body at a faster rate, driving down both skin temperature (which can cause frostbite) and eventually the internal body temperature (which can kill). This is why you can get frostbite even when the temperature is above freezing, especially when participating in

Another Cold-Weather Danger—Hypothermia

The human body was designed to operate at an internal temperature of 98.6°F. Just a 6.5°F drop could be enough to kill. Below 92°F, cardiac arrest can occur

Hypothermia, simply defined as low body temperature, begins in its mildest stage at about 96°F. Symptoms include shivering, slow pulse, lethargy, and a general decrease in alertness. If body temperature drops low enough, muscles turn rigid, and the person may lose consciousness.

Falling into an icy pond would bring on hypothermia in less than an hour, but most cases result from prolonged exposure to cold temperatures. Elderly people are at increased risk for hypothermia because their bodies regulate temperature less effectively.

If hypothermia occurs, follow these tips and get the victim to a doctor as soon as possible.

- Move the person to a warmer place.

- Wrap the person with blankets.

- Give the person warm liquids, but not anything that contains alcohol. Alcohol just creates an artificial feeling of warmth.

activities like skiing or snowmobiling, which have a built-in windchill factor.

■ **KNOW YOUR RISK.** People from warm climates have a higher risk of developing frostbite, as well as people who have circulation problems (such as diabetes) and those who've had frostbite previously. Drinking alcohol and smoking also increase your risk, says Dr. Uphold.

■ **KEEP MOVING.** Don't stay in the same position for long periods of time; it slows circulation.

■ **USE YOURSELF.** If you can't get inside, take advantage of your own body heat. To warm fingers and hands, for example, place them in your armpits. "Rolling yourself into a ball also makes you more energy efficient," Schimelpfenig says.

■ **DON'T RUB WITH SNOW.** Or anything else for that matter. "It just causes friction with the skin and further tissue damage," Dr. Uphold says. "Plus, you lose more heat when you get wet."

■ **STAY DRY.** Heat loss is greatly accelerated by contact with water, says Bruce Paton, M.D. Wet clothing loses 90 percent of its insulating value, according to the National Safety Council (NSC). Replace wet and constrictive clothing with dry, loose clothing.

■ **USE THE "BUDDY SYSTEM."** You watch a friend's face—specifically the ears, nose, and cheeks—for any noticeable change in color, and he does the same for you. Keep in mind, superficial frostbite is characterized by white, waxy, or grayish-yellow patches on the affected areas, according to the NSC.

■ **STAY IN YOUR VEHICLE.** If you get stranded in your vehicle on a subfreezing night, it's best to stay put and not venture out into the unknown, says Schimelpfenig. You risk developing hypothermia or an abnormal drop in body temperature. "Many of the people we've found who were stranded and tried to walk for help were dead," he says.

■ **REWARM IN WARM WATER.** If you have superficial frostbite and can't get medical help for more than 1 hour, soak the frostbitten area in warm (102°F to 106°F) water for 20 to 40 minutes until the skin appears flush. Gently move the affected area while rewarming, says Dr. Cheng. The most common error, he says, is removing the injured area from the warm water too soon because the final few minutes typically are pretty painful. Never rewarm an area if there is a chance it may freeze again.

■ **DRINK WARM FLUIDS.** Be sure to consume only nonalcoholic, noncaffeinated beverages, such as broth.

■ **NO DRY HEAT.** Don't expose skin to a dry, radiant heat, such as that from a heat lamp or campfire, if it looks frostbitten, Dr. Paton says. Frostbitten skin is easily burned.

■ **DON'T ALLOW A FROSTBITTEN BODY PART TO REFREEZE.** "Never," says Dr. Uphold. "The water crystals are bigger when the part refreezes, which causes even more tissue damage."

■ **USE YOUR HEAD TO SAVE YOUR FOOT.** It's not advisable to walk on frozen feet, but it's better than allowing a frozen foot to thaw and refreeze. If you think walking may be your only route to survival, leave your shoe or boot on the frostbitten foot, says Dr. Paton. "The foot could blister and swell if you take it off, and you wouldn't be able to get the boot back on."

PANEL OF ADVISORS

DAVID CHENG, M.D., IS AN ASSISTANT PROFESSOR OF EMERGENCY MEDICINE AT THE UNIVERSITY OF ARKANSAS MEDICAL SCIENCES IN LITTLE ROCK.

BRUCE PATON, M.D., IS A FORMER CLINICAL PROFESSOR OF SURGERY AT THE UNIVERSITY OF COLORADO IN DENVER AND FORMER PRESIDENT OF THE WILDERNESS MEDICAL SOCIETY IN COLORADO SPRINGS.

TOD SCHIMELPFENIG IS CURRICULUM DIRECTOR OF THE WILDERNESS MEDICAL INSTITUTE FOR THE NATIONAL OUTDOOR LEADERSHIP SCHOOL IN LANDER, WYOMING.

RUTH UPHOLD, M.D., IS MEDICAL DIRECTOR OF THE EMERGENCY DEPARTMENT AT FLETCHER ALLAN HEALTH CARE IN BURLINGTON, VERMONT.

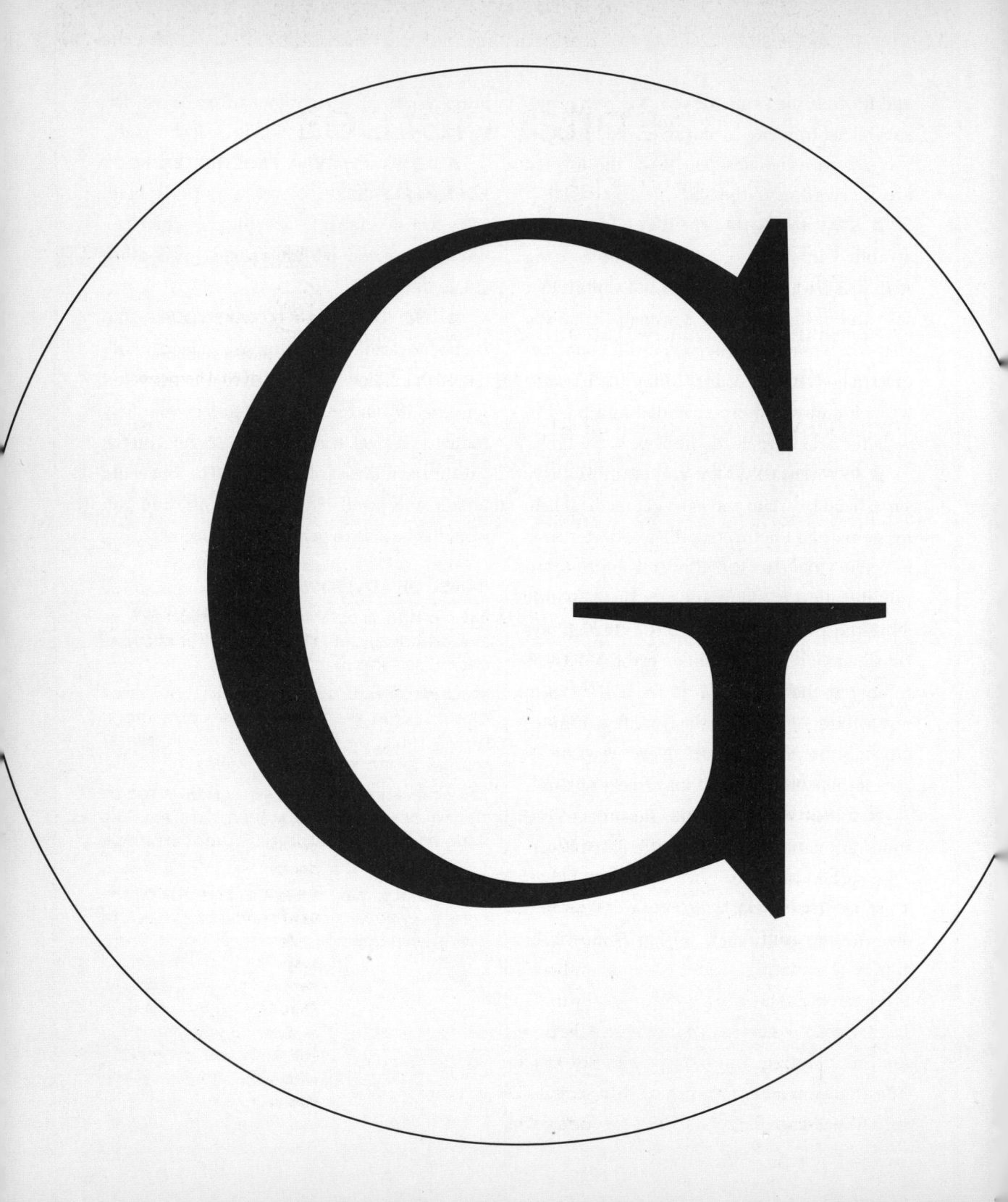

Genital Herpes

19 Managing Strategies

Genital herpes, caused by the herpes simplex virus, is an incurable sexually transmitted disease that sounds dire but that, in fact, can be treated and managed with medication. Most cases result from herpes simplex type 2 (HSV-2), but some are caused by HSV-1, which also causes most cold sores.

About one in five adults in the United States has genital herpes—however, close to 90 percent are unaware of it. Often it's because their symptoms are too mild to notice or mistaken for another condition, according to the American Social Health Association (ASHA). Women may think they have vaginitis, urinary tract infections, or hemorrhoids, when in fact it's herpes. A recent study of 5,400 adults from relatively affluent suburban areas around Atlanta, Baltimore, Boston, Chicago, Dallas, and Denver found HSV-2 infections in 36 percent of the women ages 40 to 49 and in 30 percent of women ages 50 to 59.

A typical attack begins with inflammation, followed by a small cluster of blisters on the genitals that break and weep after a few days, leaving painful ulcers. You may experience fever, headache, and difficulty urinating. Once the initial outbreak of herpes (which is often the worst) comes and goes (usually in 2 to 3 weeks), the virus lies dormant—a sleeping giant—most of the time. Subsequent attacks are usually infrequent and generally not as severe as the first one. The average number for a person with genital HSV-2 is four or five a year. The average for genital HSV-1 is one a year.

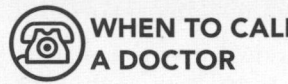 **WHEN TO CALL A DOCTOR**

If you have a stubborn case of genital herpes or are experiencing many recurrences, you may want to consider seeing your doctor for a prescription of valacyclovir (Valtrex), a drug that reduces frequency of attacks, limits their severity, and speeds healing time. This drug, approved by the FDA in 2001, stays in the body longer than acyclovir (Zovirax), so you have to take only one pill a day to fight off recurrences.

If you are having your first attack or your recurrences are frequent, or if you believe them to be frequent, talk to your doctor. If you are pregnant, be sure to tell your doctor that you have herpes, since the virus can infect newborns.

A strong link was once suspected between genital herpes and cervical cancer. That link is not as strong as once thought, but it's still important for women with herpes to get a yearly Pap test.

There is no cure for the disease, but medications and lifestyle measures can help manage symptoms and reduce outbreaks. Here's what the experts recommend:

■ **TAKE TIME TO UNDERSTAND YOUR DIAGNOSIS.** For most people, the social and emotional impact of herpes is greater than the physical distress, at least in the beginning. Society tends to have a judgmental attitude about sexually transmitted diseases. Many people feel embarrassed or isolated after they are diagnosed. With time, accurate information, and support, most people put herpes in perspective, says Mitch Herndon, program manager of the Herpes Resource Center and National Herpes Hotline at ASHA.

■ **CONSIDER AN ORAL ANTIVIRAL MEDICATION.** Talk to your doctor about antiviral medications such as Famvir (famciclovir), Zovirax (acyclovir), and Valtrex (valacyclovir). They can be taken either at the first sign of an outbreak to reduce the severity and duration or every day to suppress outbreaks, says Mary Jane Minkin, M.D.

MANAGING OUTBREAKS

■ **USE PLAIN SOAP AND WATER.** You may be inclined to bombard your newly discovered sores with everything in your medicine cabinet. As with any sores, you do need to be concerned about developing a secondary (bacterial) infection, but soap and water is all you need or want to keep the area sufficiently germ-free.

■ **STEER CLEAR OF OINTMENTS.** Genital sores need lots of air to heal. Petroleum jelly and antibiotic ointments can block this air and slow the healing process. *Never* use a cortisone cream, which can inhibit your immune system and actually encourage the virus to grow.

■ **WARM WATER EASES THE DISCOMFORT.** During your primary attack or bad secondary attacks, a warm bath or shower three or four times a day may provide soothing relief to the genital area.

■ **USE TWO TOWELS.** During an outbreak use a separate towel on your genitals than the one you use on the rest of your body. Wash the towel after each use.

■ **BLOW DRY.** When you get out of the shower or bath, blow dry the genital area with a hair dryer set on low or cool, taking care not to burn yourself. The air from the dryer also proves soothing and may possibly speed up the healing process by helping to dry out the sores.

■ **WEAR LOOSE-FITTING COTTON UNDERWEAR.** Because air is essential to healing, wear only underpants that allow your skin to breathe—that is, cotton, not synthetic, says Judith M. Hurst, R.N. If you wear nylon panty hose, make sure the crotch is made of cotton. If you want to wear a bathing suit without compromising fashion, consider cutting the cotton crotch out of a pair of undies and sewing it into the swimsuit, says Hurst.

■ **DON'T TOUCH.** Although the disease is called *genital* herpes, it is possible, though not very common, to pass the virus to other parts of the body by touching a genital ulcer and then rubbing, say, your mouth or eyes. For this reason, it's important to wash your hands if there's contact with a sore, says Herndon. If you think you might scratch at night, cover the inflamed area with protective, breathable material such as gauze, he says.

■ **LEARN YOUR TRIGGERS.** The factors that contribute to a recurrence are highly individual, but with time, many people learn to recognize, and sometimes avoid, factors that seem to reactivate HSV for them. Illness, poor diet, emotional or physical stress, friction in the genital area, prolonged exposure to ultraviolet light (a common trigger for oral herpes) like a beach trip or skiing weekend for example, surgical trauma, and steroidal medication (such as asthma treatment) may trigger a herpes outbreak. The frequency of outbreaks can often be managed through effective stress management, and adequate rest, nutrition, and exercise.

■ **TRY AN HERBAL APPROACH.** Try echinacea to stimulate your immune system and burdock root as a gentle cleansing tonic. Here's a recipe by herbalist Aviva Romm. Toss 1 ounce each of dried echinacea and burdock root into a quart of boiling water. Let the herbs steep for 4 to 8 hours, then strain the liquid. To treat an outbreak, drink 4 cups a day until the blisters disappear. To prevent recurrent outbreaks, drink ½ cup two to four times a day. You can use this infusion for up to 3 months. After that, take a 3-day break after each 27-day stretch.

■ **CONSIDER THESE SUPPLEMENTS WITH CAUTION.** The amino acid lysine healed sores and prevented their recurrence in laboratory studies at UCLA in Los Angeles. Other potential supplements that may fight off herpes attacks include zinc, in topical form or capsules, or the food additive butylated hydroxytoluene (BHT), taken as a supplement. But despite mixed studies on their effectiveness, these two are unproven remedies, say most doctors. If you decide to try either, know that high dosages may be dangerous and should be taken only under a doctor's supervision.

PREVENTING TRANSMISSION

■ **CALL FOR HELP.** If you have any questions about HSV, help is available, says Herndon. ASHA runs two hotlines that offer free advice to people with herpes. Call the National Herpes Hotline at 919-361-8488, Monday through Friday, 9:00 a.m. to 7:00 p.m. (EST); or the toll-free National STD Hotline at 800-227-8922, 24 hours a day, 7 days a week. ASHA also offers an e-mail response service, www.ashastd.org, where you can send in your questions about herpes. Or just go to the ASHA Web site, www.ashastd.org.

■ **TALK FIRST, LOVE LATER.** Explain to your partner what herpes is and the steps you're willing to take to avoid passing on the virus. Telling your partner shows respect and concern, allows the person to make an informed choice, and may build intimacy and trust, says Herndon.

■ **PRACTICE SAFE SEX.** "You don't have to give up sex," says Dr. Minkin. "But you do need to make some changes in how and when you have it. The herpes virus can be transmitted by both sexual intercourse and oral-genital sex.

■ **AVOID SKIN-TO-SKIN CONTACT DURING OUTBREAKS.** When there are signs or symptoms of HSV around the genital or anal region, refrain from sexual activity until all signs have healed. This includes oral, vaginal, and anal sex, says Dr. Minkin.

■ **USE PROTECTION BETWEEN OUTBREAKS.** Although you are most contagious when you have sores, you can spread the virus even when there are no symptoms through "viral shedding"—small amounts of the virus come to the surface of the skin. Shedding can happen at any time. One study found that 70 percent of cases were contracted when the sexual partner was symptom-free. Latex condoms used between outbreaks for genital-to-genital contact can reduce the risk of transmission. Although condoms don't cover all the potential sites of viral shedding, they are useful against the virus by protecting or covering the mucous membranes most likely to be infected.

■ **TALK TO YOUR DOCTOR ABOUT SUPPRESSIVE THERAPY.** Valacyclovir (Valtrex) has been shown to lower the risk of herpes transmission to a virus-free partner by 50 percent. A daily regimen of 500 milligrams of valacyclovir has been effective for partners with a history of recurrent attacks. It's likely that a combination of suppressive valacyclovir and condoms provides greater protection than either method alone.

PANEL OF ADVISORS

MITCH HERNDON IS THE PROGRAM MANAGER AT THE HERPES RESOURCE CENTER AND THE NATIONAL HERPES HOTLINE AT THE AMERICAN SOCIAL HEALTH ASSOCIATION (ASHA) IN RESEARCH TRIANGLE PARK, NORTH CAROLINA.

JUDITH M. HURST, R.N., IS MEDICAL ADVISOR TO TOLEDO HELP, A SUPPORT GROUP FOR PEOPLE WITH HERPES IN THE TOLEDO, OHIO, AREA. SHE IS ALSO A RETIRED OBSTETRIC NURSE.

MARY JANE MINKIN, M.D., IS A CLINICAL PROFESSOR OF OBSTETRICS AND GYNECOLOGY AT YALE UNIVERSITY SCHOOL OF MEDICINE AND AN OBSTETRICIAN-GYNECOLOGIST IN NEW HAVEN, CONNECTICUT. SHE IS COAUTHOR OF *WHAT EVERY WOMAN NEEDS TO KNOW ABOUT MENOPAUSE* AND *A WOMAN'S GUIDE TO MENOPAUSE AND PERIMENOPAUSE.*

AVIVA ROMM IS A CERTIFIED PROFESSIONAL MIDWIFE, HERBALIST, AND PROFESSIONAL MEMBER OF THE AMERICAN HERBALISTS GUILD. SHE PRACTICES IN BLOOMFIELD HILLS, MICHIGAN, AND IS COAUTHOR OF *NATURALLY HEALTHY BABIES & CHILDREN: A COMMONSENSE GUIDE TO HERBAL REMEDIES.*

Gingivitis

23 Ways to Stop Gum Disease

A survey reported in the *Journal of the American Dental Association* found that a majority of adults have gingivitis, the first sign of periodontal disease and the major reason adults lose their teeth.

Gingivitis is simply inflammation of the gums. The gums' usual pale pink color turns bluish red. The tender gums swell between the teeth and bleed easily, especially during toothbrushing. Caused by plaque and tartar above and below the gumline, gingivitis, if left unchecked, can lead to periodontitis, in which pus collects in deep pockets of the gum, teeth become sensitive to pressure, loosen, and fall out. Research also suggests gum disease can boost the risk for other serious health conditions, including heart disease, stroke, diabetes, respiratory infections and premature birth.

But don't despair. Dentists have much to offer that will keep the false teeth away.

■ **BRUSH RIGHT.** You can help prevent gum disease by brushing twice a day and cleaning once a day between the teeth with floss or an interdental cleaner, says the American Dental Association. Block out 3 to 5 minutes two or three times a day for good oral hygiene, says Robert Schallhorn, D.D.S.

■ **BRUSH AT THE GUMLINE.** The plaque-catching area around the gumline is where gingivitis starts, and it is the most neglected area when we brush, says Vincent Cali, D.D.S. Place your brush at a 45-degree angle to your teeth so that half of your brush cleans your gums while the other half cleans your teeth. Then shimmy your brush by moving it in a forward and backward motion.

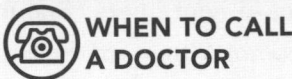
WHEN TO CALL A DOCTOR

You can risk more serious periodontal disease and the possible loss of your teeth if you ignore sore, bleeding gums. See your dentist if you notice:

■ Gums that bleed during brushing and flossing

■ Red, swollen, or tender gums

■ Gums that have pulled away from your teeth

■ Persistent bad breath

■ Loose or separating teeth

■ A change in your bite

■ Your partial dentures fit differently

■ Pus pockets between your teeth and gums

Also, if your gums still bleed when you brush your teeth and continue to be sore and swollen despite all your efforts at good oral hygiene, see your dentist again.

■ **HAVE TWO TOOTHBRUSHES.** Alternate between them, says Dr. Cali. Allow one to dry while using the other.

■ **KEEP THEM GERM-FREE.** Store your toothbrush in an upright position if possible. Don't routinely cover or store toothbrushes in closed containers. The moist environment promotes the growth of most germs. When storing more than one brush, keep them separated to stop germ transmission from one brush to another.

■ **CHOOSE YOUR TOOTHBRUSH.** Although studies show that using an electric toothbrush improves oral health, the American Dental Association reports that manual toothbrushes are just as effective. As long as you're brushing properly, it doesn't matter which toothbrush you use. Electric toothbrushes are advantageous for people who have limited manual dexterity or hand braces, because the rotating head can clean hard-to-reach areas.

■ **BANK SOME BONE.** Gingivitis is the beginning of what Dr. Cali calls periodontal osteoporosis. Just as the bones in the rest of your skeleton can shrink and become brittle, so, too, can your jawbone. You can strengthen the bones all over your body by exercising regularly and not smoking.

And don't forget your calcium! Getting at least 800 milligrams of calcium a day can reduce your chances of developing severe gum disease, according to a study from the State University of New York at Buffalo. Calcium strengthens the alveolar bone in the jaw, which helps hold your teeth in place. Dairy products are the best sources of dietary calcium, but you'll also get good amounts of the mineral from salmon, almonds, and leafy dark green vegetables such as kale and broccoli.

■ **USE A GUM STIMULATOR.** A rubber or specially designed triangular gum stimulator is better than a toothpick for massaging the gums, says Dr. Cali. It also cleans the surfaces between the teeth. Rest the rubber point between two teeth. Point the tip in the direction of the biting surface until the stimulator is at a 45-degree angle to the gumline. Apply a circular motion for 10 seconds, then move on to the next tooth.

■ **STOCK UP ON VITAMIN C.** Vitamin C won't cure gingivitis, but it can help check bleeding gums, according to a study at the USDA Western Nutrition Research Center in San Francisco. The National Institute of Health recommends a daily dose of 100 to 200 milligrams.

■ **CONSIDER VITAMIN D.** A study published in the *American Journal of Clinical Nutrition* examined data from 6,700 people who took the third National Health and Nutrition Examination Survey. Those with the highest levels of vitamin D were 20 percent less likely to show signs of gingivitis. Although the results don't necessarily mean vitamin D is responsible for healthier gums, it has been shown to have possible anti-inflammatory benefits, which might explain its association with reduced inflammation and bleeding between the gums.

■ **DRINK TEA.** Black and green teas contain polypenols, antioxidant compounds that prevent plaque from adhering to your teeth, which helps reduce your chances of developing gum disease, says Christine D. Wu, Ph.D.

■ **BRANDISH A PROXA BRUSH.** A proxa brush is a specially designed brush (available at most drugstores) that's shaped like a tiny bottle brush. It slides between your teeth or under your crown or bridge to get to those hard-to-reach places, says Roger P. Levin, D.D.S.

■ **USE LISTERINE.** In a study reported in the *Journal of Clinical Periodontology*, Listerine mouthwash inhibited the development of plaque and reduced gingivitis.

■ **SCRUTINIZE THE LABEL.** When buying generic mouthwash, look for the chemicals cetylpridinium chloride or domiphen bromide on the label. Research shows these are the active ingredients in mouthwash that reduce dental plaque.

■ **EXAMINE YOUR LIFESTYLE.** Too much stress? Too little relaxation? Do you work around toxic chemicals? Any of those factors can adversely affect your gums. Examine every aspect of your lifestyle to see what you can change to make living more healthy, suggests Dr. Cali.

■ **CUT YOUR VICES.** Excessive smoking and drinking can drain your body of vitamins and minerals vital to a healthy mouth, says Dr. Cali.

■ **SCRAPE YOUR TONGUE.** Remove the bacteria and toxins hiding there. It doesn't matter what you use to scrape with, as long as it isn't sharp, says Dr. Cali. He recommends a small spoon, a Popsicle stick, a tongue depressor, or your toothbrush. Or you may wish to buy a specifically designed tongue scraper. You will need to scrape from back to front 10 to 15 times.

■ **TAKE AN INTERMISSION.** Don't try to perform all these oral ablutions in one day. Stimulate your gums one day, and scrape your tongue the next, says Dr. Cali. If you do something different after you brush and floss, you won't bore yourself to death.

■ **SNUFF IT WITH H_2O_2.** Buy a 3 percent solution of hydrogen peroxide, mix it half-and-half with water, and swish it around your mouth for 30 seconds. Don't swallow. Use this wash three times a week to inhibit bacteria, says Dr. Cali.

■ **WASH WITH AN ORAL IRRIGATION UNIT.** Use an oral irrigation device to flush water around your teeth and gums, says Dr. Cali. To use it correctly, direct the stream of water between your teeth, not down into your gums.

■ **PACK A PORTABLE IRRIGATOR.** When you travel, carry an ear syringe (a rubber bulb with a long nose). Fill it with water, then flush your teeth, says Dr. Cali.

■ **EAT A RAW VEGETABLE A DAY.** It will keep gingivitis away, says Dr. Cali. Hard and fibrous foods clean and stimulate teeth and gums.

■ **TRY THE BAKING SODA AND WATER SOLUTION.** Take plain baking soda, mix it with a little bit of water, and apply it with your fingers along the gumline in a small section of your mouth. Then brush. You'll clean, polish, neutralize acidic bacterial wastes, and deodorize, all in one swoop, says Dr. Cali.

■ **SAY "ALOE" TO YOUR DRUGGIST.** Some people brush their gums with aloe gel, says Eric Shapira, D.D.S. "It's a healing agent, and it will reduce some of the plaque in your mouth."

PANEL OF ADVISORS

VINCENT CALI, D.D.S., IS A NEW YORK CITY DENTIST AND AUTHOR OF *THE NEW, LOWER-COST WAY TO END GUM TROUBLE WITHOUT SURGERY.* HE ALSO HAS A POSTGRADUATE DEGREE IN CLINICAL NUTRITION FROM THE FORDHAM PAGE INSTITUTE AT THE UNIVERSITY OF PENNSYLVANIA IN PHILADELPHIA.

ROGER P. LEVIN, D.D.S., IS THE CEO OF THE LEVIN GROUP, A DENTAL PRACTICE IN BALTIMORE.

ROBERT SCHALLHORN, D.D.S., IS A DENTIST IN AURORA, COLORADO, AND PAST PRESIDENT OF THE AMERICAN ACADEMY OF PERIODONTOLOGY.

ERIC SHAPIRA, D.D.S., IS A CLINICAL ASSISTANT PROFESSOR AND LECTURER AT THE UNIVERSITY OF THE PACIFIC SCHOOL OF DENTISTRY IN SAN FRANCISCO AND A DENTIST IN HALF MOON BAY, CALIFORNIA.

CHRISTINE D. WU, PH.D., IS A PROFESSOR AND DIRECTOR OF CARIOLOGY RESEARCH AT THE DEPARTMENT OF PEDIATRIC DENTISTRY AT THE UNIVERSITY OF ILLINOIS CHICAGO SCHOOL OF DENTISTRY. SHE CURRENTLY SERVES AS A CONSULTANT TO THE AMERICAN DENTAL ASSOCIATION'S COUNCIL FOR SCIENTIFIC AFFAIRS.

Gout

18 Coping Ideas

Gout is an excruciatingly painful form of arthritis—so painful that most patients can't even bear the weight of a bedsheet on the tender joint. Its throbbing pain strikes abruptly, often at night, turning the skin red-hot and leaving the affected joint swollen and tender for 5 to 10 days.

Gout is the most prevalent form of inflammatory arthritis. It occurs seven to nine times more often in men than women—each year striking an estimated 3.4 million American men older than age 40.

Gout is caused by excessive levels of uric acid, a waste product from body tissues. We all have uric acid in our blood, which is normally excreted in the urine. If you experience gout, you either produce too much uric acid or your kidneys don't excrete enough—the cause of about 90 percent all cases. And, the excess uric acid turns into tiny, needlelike crystals that collect in joints, causing intense inflammation, swelling, and pain.

In most cases gout strikes one joint, and 50 percent of the time the big toe is the prime target. Other frequent sites include the forefoot, instep, heel, ankle, and knee. While almost any joint can become a sore point, gout is uncommon in the upper body. Although only one small joint may be affected, the inflammation can be intense enough to cause fever, muscle aches, and other flu-like symptoms. To minimize pain and promote healing, heed these do's and don'ts from the experts.

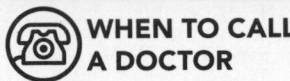 **WHEN TO CALL A DOCTOR**

If you experience sudden and intense pain in a joint, call your doctor. Even if the pain goes away in a day or two, it is important to see your doctor, because gout left untreated can lead to more pain and joint damage.

Your doctor may prescribe a number of prescription medications to help reduce inflammation and relieve pain during a gout attack, including corticosteroids such as prednisone.

Once an attack has passed, your doctor may prescribe a medication to lower your uric acid in an attempt to prevent future attacks. You also may receive colchicine, a medicine used for thousands of years to handle gout, sold under the names Allopurinol and Probenecid.

■ **GET SOME R AND R.** During an acute attack, be sure to rest and elevate the inflamed joint. You'll probably have little trouble following this advice to the letter because the pain will be so intense.

■ **REACH FOR IBUPROFEN AT THE FIRST SIGN OF PAIN.** It is the tremendous inflammation around the affected joint that causes the pain. So when you need a painkiller, make sure it's one that can reduce inflammation—namely ibuprofen, says Jeffrey R. Lisse, M.D. Follow label instructions. If those dosages don't give relief, he says, consult your doctor before increasing them.

■ **AVOID ASPIRIN OR ACETAMINOPHEN.** All pain relievers are not created equal. Aspirin can actually make gout worse by inhibiting excretion of uric acid, says Dr. Lisse, and acetaminophen doesn't have enough inflammation-fighting capability to do much good.

■ **SKIP SUGARY SODA.** In a 12-year Canadian study of men with no history of gout, University of British Columbia researchers found that men who drank two or more sugary sodas or other fructose-loaded soft drinks each day increased their risked of gout by 85 percent compared with men who drank one serving or less per month. Even moderate intake—five or six soft drinks a week—increased the risk significantly. If you must have your soda fix, drink the diet version, which doesn't increase the risk of gout.

■ **APPLY ICE.** If the affected joint is not too tender to touch, try applying a crushed-ice pack, says John Abruzzo, M.D. The ice has a soothing, numbing effect. Place the pack on the painful joint for about 10 minutes. Cushion it with a towel or sponge. Reapply as needed.

■ **DRINK LOTS OF WATER.** Large amounts of fluid can help flush excess uric acid from your system before it can do any harm. Uric acid levels are typically elevated for 20 to 30 years before they cause any trouble. For best results, drink five or six glasses of water a day.

As a bonus, lots of water may also help discourage the kidney stones that can affect people with gout.

■ **CONSIDER HERBAL TEAS.** Another good way to take in sufficient liquid is with herb teas. They're free of both caffeine and calories, so large amounts won't make you jittery or pile on unwanted pounds. Eleonore Blaurock-Busch, Ph.D., especially recommends sarsaparilla, yarrow, rose hip, and peppermint teas. Place 2 tablespoons of the dried herb in a pint of boiling water. Steep for 10 to 20 minutes, then strain before drinking.

■ **AVOID HIGH-PURINE FOODS.** "Foods that are high in a substance called purine contribute to higher levels of uric acid," says Robert Wortmann, M.D. Therefore, avoiding such foods is prudent.

Those foods most likely to *induce* gout contain anywhere from 150 to 1,000 milligrams of purine in each 3½-ounce serving. They include high-protein animal and fish products such as anchovies, brains, consommé, gravy, heart, herring, kidney, liver, meat extracts, meat-containing mincemeat, mussels, sardines, and sweetbreads.

■ **LIMIT OTHER PURINE-CONTAINING FOODS.** Foods that may *contribute* to gout have a moderate amount of purines (from 50 to 150 milligrams in 3½ ounces). Limiting them to one serving daily is necessary for

Cures from the Kitchen

Cherries have long been a folk remedy for gout. Now there is scientific evidence that eating cherries lowers uric acid levels. In a small study, 10 women ate about 1½ cups of cherries after an overnight fast. Researchers found that plasma levels of urate, found in uric acid, fell significantly over a 5-hour period after the cherries were eaten.

Although there is no hard scientific evidence that cherries help relieve gout, many people find them beneficial. If you are lucky enough to have fresh cherries, eating about a half dozen daily may relieve the symptoms of gout. When you feel an attack coming on, eat 20 to 30 cherries immediately. It doesn't seem to matter whether they are sweet or sour varieties or whether the cherries are canned, frozen, or fresh. Reported amounts vary from a handful (about 10 cherries) a day up to ½ pound. You can also try natural, concentrated black cherry juice and drink several tablespoons of the concentrate daily until the pain is relieved. People have also reported success with 1 tablespoon of cherry concentrate a day, says Agatha Thrash, M.D.

those with severe cases. These foods include asparagus, dry beans, cauliflower, lentils, mushrooms, oatmeal, dry peas, shellfish, spinach, whole grain cereals, whole grain breads, and yeast.

In the same category are fish, meat, and poultry. Limit them to one 3-ounce serving 5 days a week.

■ **SIP COFFEE.** The risk of gout was 40 percent lower for men who drank four to five cups of java a day, and 59 percent lower for men who drank six or more a day than for men who didn't drink coffee, according to a Harvard University study of 45,869 men older than age 40 with no history of gout. "Coffee consumption is associated with lower serum uric acid levels, but tea consumption is not," says lead researcher Hyon K. Choi, M.D., Dr.P.H. He speculates that components in coffee, other than caffeine, may be responsible for the beverage's gout-prevention benefits. Among those possibilities is phenol chlorogenic acid, a strong antioxidant.

■ **SKIP BEER.** Drinking two 12-ounce beers a day increases the risk of gout more than twofold, while consuming two drinks with hard liquor raises the risk 1.6 times, according to a follow-up study of 47,000 men from the Harvard School of Public Health. Drinking wine showed no influence. "Individuals with gout should try to limit or even cut out their beer consumption, but wine is allowed," says Dr. Choi.

■ **CONTROL YOUR BLOOD PRESSURE.** If you have high blood pressure and gout, you have double trouble. Certain drugs prescribed to lower blood pressure, such as diuretics, actually raise uric acid levels, says Branton Lachman, Pharm.D., J.D. So taking steps to lower your blood pressure naturally is wise. Try decreasing your sodium intake, losing excess weight, and exercising. But never discontinue any prescribed medication without consulting your doctor.

■ **LOSE 10 POUNDS AND KEEP IT OFF.** In a 12-year study of 47,150 men with no history of gout, Massachusetts General Hospital researchers found that men who lost 10 pounds and kept it off reduced their risk of gout by 39 percent.

■ **BEWARE OF FAD DIETS.** The same study showed that being overweight increases your risk of developing gout. Heavier people tend to have high uric acid levels. But stay away from fad diets, which are notorious for triggering gout attacks, says Dr. Lisse. Such diets—including fasting—cause cells to break down and release uric acid. So work with your doctor to devise a gradual weight-loss program.

■ **GET ENOUGH CALCIUM.** If you're a man older than 40 with a family history of gout, aim for 1,000 milligrams of calcium a day. That much daily calcium reduced the risk of gout 40 percent in a group of 48,000 men studied for 12 years, according to the American College of Rheumatology.

■ **CONSULT YOUR DOCTOR ABOUT SUPPLEMENTS.** Be careful when taking vitamins, says Dr. Blaurock-Busch, because too much of certain nutrients can make gout worse. Excess niacin and vitamin A, in particular, may bring on an attack, she says. So always consult a physician before increasing your vitamin intake.

■ **DON'T HURT YOURSELF.** For some unknown reason, gout often strikes a joint that's been previously traumatized. "So try not to stub your toe or otherwise injure yourself," says Dr. Abruzzo. "And don't wear tight shoes, which can also predispose your joints to minor injury."

PANEL OF ADVISORS

FORNIA LAW SCHOOL, AND THE CALIFORNIA PUBLIC SCHOOL SYSTEM.

JEFFREY R. LISSE, M.D., IS A PROFESSOR OF MEDICINE, HEAD OF CLINICAL OSTEOPOROSIS RESEARCH, AND ASSOCIATE CHIEF OF THE ARTHRITIS CENTER AT THE UNIVERSITY OF ARIZONA IN TUCSON.

AGATHA THRASH, M.D., IS A PATHOLOGIST WHO LEC-TURES WORLDWIDE. SHE IS ALSO COFOUNDER OF UCHEE PINES INSTITUTE, A NONPROFIT HEALTH-TRAINING CENTER IN SEALE, ALABAMA, AND AUTHOR OF MANY BOOKS.

ROBERT WORTMANN, M.D., IS A PROFESSOR OF MEDICINE AT DARTMOUTH-HITCHCOCK MEDICAL CENTER IN LEBANON, NEW HAMPSHIRE.

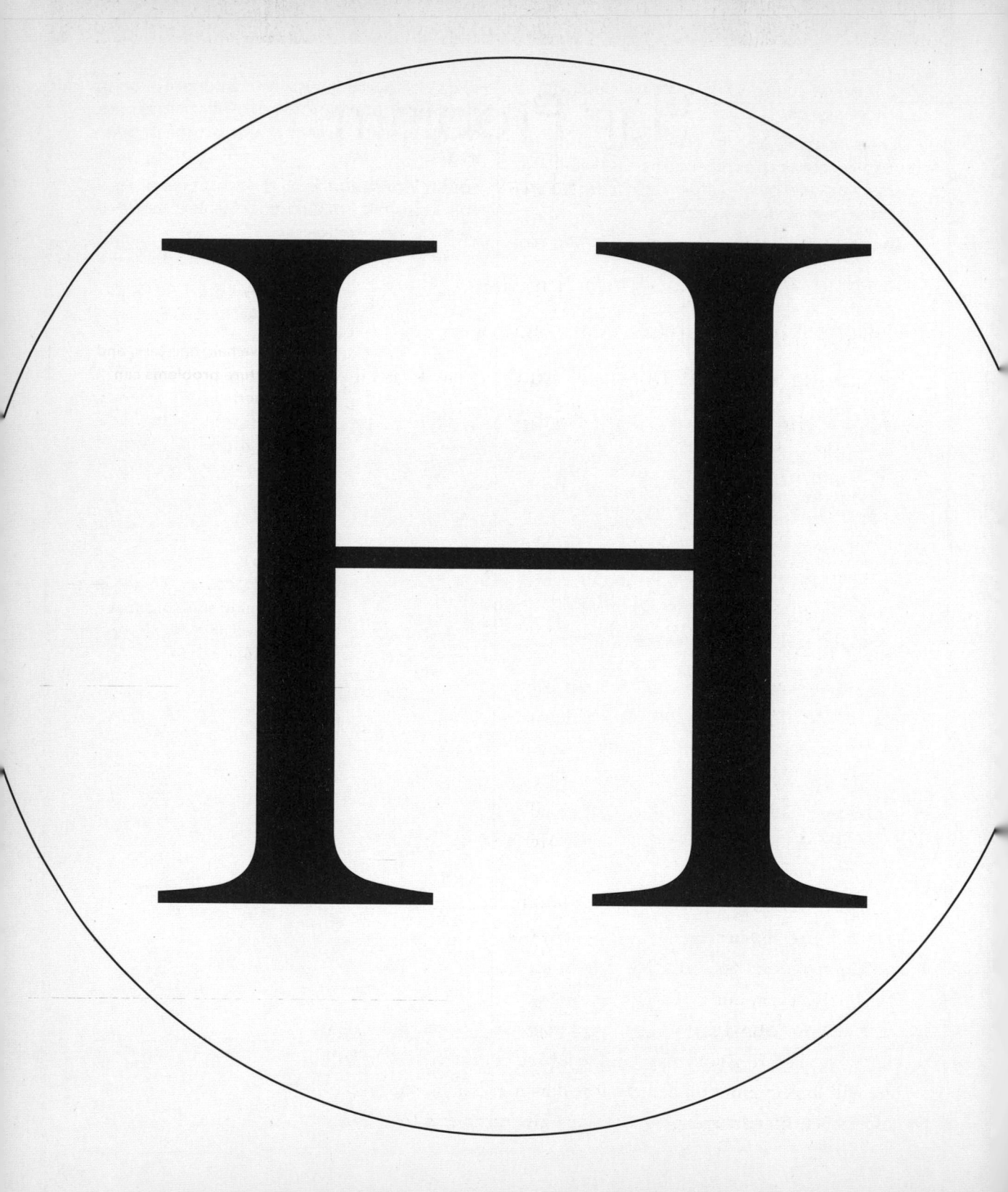

Hair Problems

22 "Bad Hair Day" Fixes

"I could announce one morning that the world was going to blow up in 3 hours and people would be calling in about my hair," said Katie Couric once of the constant attention her hair received from *Today* viewers.

Yes, we care about hair.

Although a really bad hair day can *feel* like the end of the world, most hair problems are solvable.

Here's what our experts have to say.

GRAY HAIR

Wash that gray out of your hair? More women are saying, "No way!" According to L'Oréal, nearly half of women older than 40 are no longer hitting the bottle. Besides being profoundly liberating (no more pesky roots!), going gray makes a statement of supreme confidence: This is who I am, and I'm proud of my natural beauty. Gray hair can also look fabulous: Think Meryl Streep's chic silver cut in *The Devil Wears Prada*.

If you want to give gray a try, here's how to avoid the awkward gray hair growing-in stage that keeps many women from returning to their roots. But fear not; this step-by-step guide will help you look terrific every minute of the way to gray.

■ **GO GRADUALLY.** Wait until your roots are at least 60 percent silver before giving up your dye job, so your new gray hair hue will look symmetrical and natural as it grows in, suggests colorist Jennifer Jahanbigloo. But don't give up color altogether

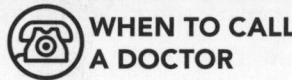
WHEN TO CALL A DOCTOR

Excessive hair, hair loss, and hair texture problems can signal hormonal imbalances, illness, nutritional deficiencies, or stress. See a doctor if you notice a sudden change in your hair, just to rule out a serious underlying cause.

Even if your problem is cosmetic, doctors can offer a number of solutions that aren't available as an over-the-counter product.

just yet. "The contrast in texture and tone as your hair grows can look unkempt," she says. During this phase, which can last up to a year, get a do-it-yourself highlighting kit or ask your colorist to weave in a few fine highlights or lowlights (darker streaks) to add dimension and blend in roots.

■ **CONSIDER A CUT.** Cropping your hair above your collarbone during the in-between period will lessen the contrast between silver and pigmented strands. Layers can help camouflage multiple hues. "A choppy cut looks youthful and helps hide your roots," says colorist Jonathan Gale.

■ **GO CONTEMPORARY.** When your gray has grown out, don't regress to a matronly 'do. "For gray to look glamorous and chic, your cut should be contemporary," says salon creative director Mark DeVincenzo. To enhance silver strands, which absorb light, making your mane look dull, style hair straight (use a flatiron or a dryer and a round brush) to promote shine. Once your hair is completely white, talk to your stylist about adopting an above-the-shoulder, layered style that provides movement and softly frames your face.

■ **PICK SILVER-SPECIFIC PRODUCTS.** When hair turns gray, the protective cuticle thins out, which can make strands coarse and prone to breakage. Keep tresses soft and healthy by using a moisturizing shampoo and using a formula geared for gray hair once a week to counteract yellowing. And apply a clear gloss or glaze each month to coat the cuticle and boost shine.

HAIR LOSS

A normal person has about 150,000 strands of hair on their head and loses 100 each day, but you have to lose much more—over 50 percent of your scalp hair—before hair loss becomes apparent, according to the American Academy of Dermatology.

More than half of men have heredity-driven male pattern hair loss by the age of 50. Women aren't immune either. About 40 percent of women notice that their hair is thinning by the time they reach menopause. Hair loss in women typically begins between ages 25 and 40, says Dominic A. Brandy, M.D. "Hair is very much a part of a woman's body image. Losing it can cause a great deal of stress and, in some cases, can make women lose a certain amount of self-respect," he says.

The most common cause of hair loss in women is a shift in the growth cycle, says Rebecca Caserio, M.D. In other words, at any given time, some of your hair is growing and some of it is done growing. Most hairs have a life expectancy of 3 to 6 years. These hairs go into a resting stage for 3 months and fall out. But then new hairs are produced from the exact same roots.

Hormone shifts, rapid weight loss, severe dandruff, iron deficiency, and a low protein intake can also speed up the normal rate of hair loss, says Dr. Caserio. Because some medical conditions and medications can cause hair loss, it's best to check in with your doctor if you notice your tresses thinning.

"Hair loss, particularly when it occurs at the crown, can also be caused by genetics," adds Dr. Caserio. Hereditary baldness is not just a male problem; women, too, can inherit a predisposition to baldness from either parent.

You can use proper nutrition to help prevent hair loss.

■ **GET ADEQUATE PROTEIN.** Eat at least two 3- to 4-ounce servings of fish, chicken, or other lean sources of protein every day, says S. Elizabeth Whitmore, M.D., Sc.M. Protein is needed by every cell in your body, including the cells that make the hair. Without adequate protein, the cells in your body don't work efficiently and can't make new hair to replace old hair that's been shed.

■ **MAINTAIN IRON LEVELS.** Iron-deficiency anemia can also cause hair loss, so make sure that you eat a well balanced diet that includes a daily serving or two of iron-rich foods, says Dr. Whitmore. Good sources of iron include lean red meat, steamed clams, cream of wheat, dried fruit, soybeans, tofu, and broccoli.

■ **TAKE VITAMIN B$_6$.** "I have no idea why it works, but 100 milligrams a day of vitamin B$_6$ seems to decrease hair shedding in some people," say Dr. Caserio. Just don't take any more than that without consulting a doctor, she cautions. Larger amounts can be toxic, especially over a prolonged time.

You can also try the following tips:

■ **MAKE A STYLING CHANGE.** Maximize the hair you have. If you have white hair, add some color so that it shows up better. If it's straight, a mild perm will help fill in the spaces. Consult your hairstylist for the newest, most gentle products, suggests Lenore S. Kakita, M.D.

■ **AVOID PULLING ON YOUR HAIR.** Don't use tight braids or rollers on thinning hair. These styling methods can break off thin hairs and make your situation worse.

■ **USE AN OVER-THE-COUNTER SOLUTION.** Minoxidil (Rogaine) is a hair-restoring treatment available in different strengths for men and women. Applied twice a day, it has

---

Cures from the Kitchen

 Try these expert-approved kitchen cures for dry hair.

GO HEAVY ON THE MAYO. "Mayonnaise makes an excellent conditioner," says Steven Docherty, former senior art director at the Vidal Sassoon Salon. He recommends leaving the oily, white goo in your hair for anywhere from 5 minutes to an hour before washing it out.

TRY A SUDSY SOLUTION. "Beer is a wonderful setting lotion. It gives a crisp, healthy, shiny look, even to dry hair," says Docherty. The trick is to spray the brew onto your hair using a pump bottle after you've shampooed and towel dried, but before you blow-dry or style. Don't worry about smelling like a lush—the odor of the beer quickly disappears, he says.

GO FOR NATURAL NUTRIENTS. Hairdresser Joanne Harris makes a nutrient-rich conditioner in her kitchen. "I take old bananas, rotten and black, and mash them together with mushy, rotten avocado," she says. Leave the tropical puree in your hair for 15 minutes, and then wash it out in the kitchen sink.

been shown to stop hair loss and regrow new hair in some people.

Be patient. Rogaine, like other solutions to thinning hair, takes a while to work. Expect it to take at least 6 months.

DRY DAMAGED HAIR

Dry hair is generally caused by overprocessing—bleaching, coloring, straightening, and perming. It's further aggravated by use of heat-intensive devices like blow-dryers and curling irons. Swimming, overshampooing, and too much exposure to wind and sun are also common causes of strawlike locks.

Normally, the cells in each strand of hair line up in straight rows like the shingles on a roof, explains Yohini Appa, Ph.D. But if tiny sections of your hair's outer layer have been chipped or stripped away by harsh chemicals or intense heat, exposing the inner layers of the hair shaft, the hair loses moisture. Also dry, damaged hair doesn't reflect light the way that healthy, smooth hair does, so hair looks dull and lifeless.

Here's a quick rescue course of action for dried-out hair.

■ **CONDITION BEFORE YOU WASH.** Coat dry hair with a prewash conditioner or a deep conditioner that contains jojoba, lavender, shea butter, or rosemary oils. Keep it on for up to an hour to trap moisture in the hair, says salon owner Carmine Minardi. Wear a shower cap over the conditioner-coated hair, and wrap a warm towel around the cap to help the conditioner penetrate the hair's outer layer. Do this once or twice a week.

■ **SHAMPOO WITH CARE.** Shampooing doesn't wash away only dirt, it also washes out the hair's protective oils, says Thomas Goodman Jr., M.D. If your hair is dry from too much lather, give it a needed break by washing less often. Use only a mild shampoo, one labeled "for dry or damaged hair."

■ **USE A CONDITIONER.** When hair becomes dry, the outer layers, called cuticles, peel off from the central shaft. Conditioners glue the cuticles back to the shaft, add lubricant to the hair, and prevent static electricity (which creates frizz). Pick a conditioner that contains ceramides, naturally occurring lipids that penetrate the cuticle and give strands shine and elasticity, suggests Minardi, and use it after every shampoo.

■ **PICK THE RIGHT BRUSH.** When styling your hair, if at all possible use a boar-bristle brush; it's less prone to static buildup than metal, plastic, or nylon bristle brushes, and it smooths the cuticle with the least trauma to the hair, says Minardi.

■ **AVOID STYLING PRODUCTS WITH ALCOHOL.** Many gels and mousses contain alcohol, which can make dry hair even drier, says Minardi. Better options include styling creams packed with emollients like panthenal, silicone, or essential oils to add shine and texture without drying out hair.

■ **SNIP OFF THOSE FRAYED ENDS.** Dry hair tends to suffer most at the ends. The answer? Snip 'em off. A trim once every 6 weeks or so should keep those frayed ends under control.

■ **CHILL OUT.** Hot curling irons and electric curlers can both contribute to dried-out hair, says hairdresser Joanne Harris. She suggests that you rediscover those unheated, plastic cylinder rollers from years gone by. For straightening, wrap slightly moist hair under and around rollers (like a pageboy hairdo) for about 10 minutes. For curling or adding wave, try sponge rollers overnight, or sleep with moist braids.

■ **PROTECT YOUR HAIR FROM THE ELEMENTS.** "Whipping wind can fray your hair just like a piece of fabric," says Steven Docherty, former senior art director at the Vidal Sassoon Salon. Sun, too, takes a mighty toll. Solution: Wear a hat, both on breezy, balmy summer days and gusty, frosty winter days.

■ **USE A SWIM CAP.** "Chlorine is one of the most destructive things to hair," says Docherty. So make a rubber cap part of your regular swim attire. For extra protection, he says, first rub a little olive oil into your hair.

PANEL OF ADVISORS

YOHINI APPA, PH.D., IS EXECUTIVE DIRECTOR FOR SCIENTIFIC AFFAIRS FOR NEUTROGENA CORPORATION IN LOS ANGELES.

DOMINIC A. BRANDY, M.D., IS MEDICAL DIRECTOR OF DOMINIC A. BRANDY AND ASSOCIATES, A PERMANENT HAIR RESTORATION PRACTICE IN PITTSBURGH, PENNSYLVANIA.

REBECCA CASERIO, M.D., IS CLINICAL ASSOCIATE PROFESSOR OF DERMATOLOGY AT THE UNIVERSITY OF PITTSBURGH.

MARK DEVINCENZO IS CREATIVE DIRECTOR AT THE FRÉDÉRIC FEKKAI SALON IN NEW YORK CITY.

STEVEN DOCHERTY IS THE FORMER SENIOR ART DIRECTOR OF NEW YORK CITY'S VIDAL SASSOON SALON. HE HAS CARED FOR THE HAIR OF SOME OF NEW YORK'S TOP MAGAZINE AND TV MODELS.

JONATHAN GALE IS A COLORIST AT THE JOHN FRIEDA SALON IN LOS ANGELES.

THOMAS GOODMAN JR., M.D., IS A DERMATOLOGIST AND FORMER ASSISTANT PROFESSOR OF DERMATOLOGY AT THE UNIVERSITY OF TENNESSEE HEALTH SCIENCE CENTER IN MEMPHIS. HE IS AUTHOR OF *SMART FACE*.

JOANNE HARRIS HAS CREATED CHARACTER HAIRSTYLES FOR SOME OF HOLLYWOOD'S TOP ACTORS AND ACTRESSES, INCLUDING RICHARD GERE (IN *SOMMERSBY*) AND GWYNETH PALTROW (IN *SEVEN*). SHE OPERATES THE JOANNE HARRIS SALON IN LOS ANGELES.

JENNIFER JAHANBIGLOO IS A COLORIST AND OWNER OF JUAN JUAN SALONS IN BEVERLY HILLS, CALIFORNIA.

LENORE S. KAKITA, M.D., IS A FORMER ASSISTANT CLINICAL PROFESSOR OF DERMATOLOGY AT UCLA SCHOOL OF MEDICINE IN LOS ANGELES AND A DERMATOLOGIST IN PASADENA, CALIFORNIA.

CARMINE MINARDI IS THE OWNER OF MINARDI SALON IN NEW YORK CITY.

S. ELIZABETH WHITMORE, M.D., SC.M., IS AN ASSOCIATE PROFESSOR OF DERMATOLOGY AT JOHNS HOPKINS UNIVERSITY SCHOOL OF MEDICINE IN BALTIMORE.

Hangover

19 Ways to Deal with the Day After

The key ingredient for a hangover is drinking until you're intoxicated. The quantity you drink is actually a less important part of the equation. In fact, studies suggest that light and moderate drinkers are more susceptible to hangovers than heavy drinkers.

"Hangover symptoms usually begin about 8 to 16 hours after drinking and can last many hours," says John Brick, Ph.D. Depending on your biology, you may get one or many of the physical symptoms that come with a hangover—fatigue, headache, thirst, dizziness, stomach upset, nausea, vomiting, insomnia, high or low blood pressure, sensitivity to light, and shaky hands. Some people also experience psychological symptoms in the form of anxiety, depression, remorse, or difficulty concentrating. Here's how to restore the balance.

■ **GET SOME PAIN RELIEF.** A headache is almost always a part of the package that goes with a hangover, and good old-fashioned aspirin may be your best bet at relief, says Dr. Brick. Avoid non-aspirin pain relievers that contain acetaminophen. Combining acetaminophen with the alcohol that's still in your system can wreak havoc on your liver. And if you regularly have more than three drinks a day, talk with your doctor to see which pain reliever is best for you. Aspirin may cause stomach bleeding in some people.

■ **REPLENISH THOSE LOST FLUIDS.** Alcohol increases urination by inhibiting a hormone that regulates the kidneys. "Alcohol causes dehydration of your body cells," says Dr. Brick. "Drinking plenty of water before you go to bed and again when you get up the morning after may help relieve discomfort caused by dehydration." The Institute of Medicine advises that men should consume roughly 3.0 liters (about 13 cups) of total beverages a day and women should consume 2.2 liters (about 9 cups) of total beverages a day.

■ **EAT.** Alcohol metabolism depletes blood sugar, leaving you weak and shaky. Plus, many people forget to eat when they drink, further lowering blood sugar. A balanced meal will gently boost levels back to normal, says Kenneth Blum, Ph.D. Try these healing foods.

- *Eggs* provide protein to help stabilize blood sugar, while the cystine in protein may help break down toxins.

- *Toast* furnishes fast fuel from carbohydrates to ease fatigue and soothe the tummy.

- *Bananas* replenish potassium for muscle function.

■ **SIP A SPORTS DRINK.** Sometimes water just isn't enough. Sports drinks such as Gatorade replenish the electrolyte—sodium, potassium, and chloride—levels in your body and help relieve that weak, shaky feeling. Want quicker relief? Drink it at room temperature; cold liquids are more difficult for your body to absorb.

■ **TAKE B-COMPLEX VITAMINS.** Drinking drains the body of these valuable vitamins. Research shows that your system turns to B vitamins when it is under stress—and overtaxing the body with too much booze, beer, or wine definitely qualifies as stress, says Dr. Blum. Replenishing your body with a B-complex vitamin can help shorten the duration of your hangover.

■ **EAT AMINO ACIDS.** Amino acids are the building blocks of protein. Like vitamins and minerals, they can be depleted by alcohol. Replenishing amino acids plays a role in repairing the ravages of a hangover, says Dr. Blum. Eating some carbohydrates will help get amino acids back into the bloodstream. Amino acids are also available in capsule or liquid form at most health food stores.

■ **DRINK FRUIT JUICE.** "Fruit juice contains a form of sugar called fructose, which helps the body burn alcohol faster," explains Seymour Diamond, M.D. A large glass of orange juice or tomato juice will help accelerate removal of the alcohol still in your system the morning after.

■ **TRY CRACKERS AND HONEY.** Honey is a very concentrated source of fructose, and eating a little the next morning will help your

How to Avoid a Hangover

A 2008 study in the journal *Addiction* found that 25 to 30 percent of people don't seem to get hangovers regardless of what they drink—but the fact remains that most of us do suffer when we overindulge.

"There's good evidence emerging that the chief cause of hangover is acute withdrawal from alcohol," says Mack Mitchell, M.D. "The cells in your brain physically change in response to the alcohol's presence, and when the alcohol's gone—when your body's burned it up—you go through withdrawal until those cells get used to doing without the alcohol."

Couple that with the effects alcohol has on the blood vessels in your head (they can swell significantly, depending on the amount you drink), and you end up living through a day after that you'd rather forget. So how do you avoid it all?

Drink slowly. The slower you drink, the less alcohol reaches the brain—even though you may actually drink more over the long haul. The reason, according to Dr. Mitchell, is simple math: Your body burns alcohol at a fixed pace—about 1 ounce an hour. Give it more time to burn that alcohol, and less reaches your blood and brain.

Drink on a full stomach. "This is probably the single best thing you can do besides drinking less to reduce the severity of a hangover," Dr. Mitchell says. "Food slows the absorption of alcohol, and the slower you absorb it, the less alcohol actually reaches the brain." The kind of food you eat doesn't matter much.

Avoid the bubbly. That doesn't mean just champagne. Anything with bubbles in it—and a rum-and-Coke is just as bad as champagne—is a special hazard, say Dr. Blum and Dr. Mitchell. The bubbles move the booze into your bloodstream much more quickly. Your liver tries to keep up but can't, and the overflow of alcohol pours into your bloodstream.

body flush out whatever alcohol remains, says Dr. Diamond. The crackers are just the delivery system for the honey.

■ **BARK BACK.** Willow bark is a natural alternative if you'd prefer an organic pain reliever, according to Dr. Blum. "It contains a natural form of salicylate, the active ingre-dient in aspirin," he says and suggests taking it in capsule form.

■ **DRINK SOME BROTH.** Eating a clear broth made from bouillon cubes or a home-made soup broth will help replace the salt and potassium that your body loses when you drink, Dr. Diamond says.

Drink the right drinks. What you drink can play a major role in what your head feels like the next morning, according to Kenneth Blum, Ph.D. The chief villains are congeners.

"Congeners are other kinds of alcohols (ethanol is what gets you drunk) found in essentially all alcoholic beverages," Dr. Blum says. "How they work isn't known, but they're closely related to the amount of pain you experience after drinking."

The least perilous concoction is vodka. The most perilous are cognacs, brandies, whiskeys, and champagnes of all kinds. Red wine is also bad, but for a different reason. It contains tyramine, a histamine-like substance that produces a killer headache. Anyone who's spent an evening entertained by a bottle of red wine knows what we're talking about.

Prickly pear cactus preemptive. Researchers at Tulane University found drinkers who took two capsules of an extract of prickly pear cactus 5 hours before imbibing had 50 percent fewer hangover symptoms than those who popped a placebo. One theory is that compounds in prickly pear cactus boost the body's production of heat-shock proteins, which limit inflammation caused by overimbibing.

Be size sensitive. With few exceptions, there's no way a 110-pounder can go one-on-one with a 250-pound drinker and wake up the winner. So scale down your drinks. To come out even, the 110-pounder can handle about half the alcohol of the 250-pounder.

Have an Alka-Seltzer cocktail at bedtime. "There's no hard scientific data on this, but my own clinical experience and that of a lot of others says that water and Alka-Seltzer before going to bed can make your hangover much less of a problem," says John Brick, Ph.D. Others claim that two aspirin tablets (which is really Alka-Seltzer without the fizz) can also help.

■ **CUT YOUR COFFEE IN HALF.** Since alcohol generally causes the blood vessels in the brain to swell, and caffeine constricts blood vessels, having a cup of java may help. "On the other hand, too much caffeine may sensitize an already-frazzled nervous system," says Dr. Brick.

Also, coffee is a diuretic, so it may make you more dehydrated. Limit your coffee (or tea) to half of your normal intake.

■ **LET TIME HEAL.** The best and only foolproof cure for a hangover is 24 hours. Treat your symptoms as best you can. Get a good night's sleep, and the next day, hopefully, your hangover is history.

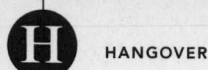

PANEL OF ADVISORS

KENNETH BLUM, PH.D., IS A RETIRED PROFESSOR OF PHARMACOLOGY AT THE UNIVERSITY OF TEXAS HEALTH SCIENCES CENTER AT SAN ANTONIO AND FORMER DIRECTOR OF THE NATIONAL INSTITUTE ON ALCOHOLISM AND ALCOHOL ABUSE. HE IS ALSO THE PRESIDENT OF SYNAPTAMINE, INC. IN SAN DIEGO.

JOHN BRICK, PH.D., IS A FELLOW IN THE AMERICAN PSYCHOLOGICAL ASSOCIATION AND FORMER CHIEF OF RESEARCH IN THE DIVISION OF EDUCATION AND TRAINING AT THE CENTER OF ALCOHOL STUDIES AT RUTGERS, THE STATE UNIVERSITY OF NEW JERSEY, IN PISCATAWAY. HE IS NOW THE EXECUTIVE DIRECTOR OF INTOXIKON INTERNATIONAL IN YARDLEY, PENNSYLVANIA.

SEYMOUR DIAMOND, M.D., IS DIRECTOR AND FOUNDER OF THE DIAMOND HEADACHE CLINIC AND THE INPATIENT HEADACHE UNIT AT ST. JOSEPH HOSPITAL IN CHICAGO. HE IS EXECUTIVE CHAIR AND FOUNDER OF THE NATIONAL HEADACHE FOUNDATION AND HAS WRITTEN SEVERAL BOOKS ON HEADACHES.

MACK MITCHELL, M.D., IS PRESIDENT OF THE ALCOHOLIC BEVERAGE MEDICAL RESEARCH FOUNDATION IN BALTIMORE, DIRECTOR OF GASTROENTEROLOGY AT JOHNS HOPKINS BAYVIEW MEDICAL CENTER, AND AN ASSOCIATE PROFESSOR OF MEDICINE AT JOHNS HOPKINS UNIVERSITY SCHOOL OF MEDICINE.

Headaches

32 Hints to Head Off the Pain

"It's a very rare—and lucky—person indeed who has never experienced a headache," says Seymour Solomon, M.D.

About 90 percent of all headaches are classified as tension headaches, according to the National Headache Foundation. The pain is typically generalized all over the head. You may feel a dull ache or a sense of tightness and perhaps experience a sense of not being clearheaded, says Fred Sheftell, M.D. Most people will describe it as feeling like a band is wrapped around their head. Stress, lack of sleep, hunger, bad posture, and eyestrain are the most common causes of tension headaches.

"Some people are born with biology that makes them headache prone," explains Joel Saper, M.D. For these people, headaches are a chronic problem.

An estimated 28 million Americans—nearly 10 percent of the population, and most of them women—suffer from migraines. Not "just a headache," migraine is a complex disease that causes severe and often disabling head pain, usually located on one side of the head, often accompanied by nausea, light and noise sensitivity, and other symptoms.

"Migraines can be crippling," says Patricia Solbach, Ph.D. So much so that they cause a loss of more than 157 million workdays each year.

For the migraine-prone, lots of things can set off an attack. Among the most common triggers are changing hormone levels, poor eating or sleeping habits, dehydration, stress, chemicals in

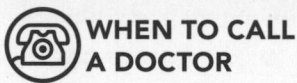

WHEN TO CALL A DOCTOR

Occasionally headaches are warning symptoms for serious disease. Here are the red flags to signal you to call your doctor.

■ You're older than 40 and have never had recurring headaches.

■ Your headaches have changed locations.

■ Your headaches are getting stronger.

■ Your headaches are coming more frequently.

■ Your headaches do not fit a recognizable pattern; that is, there seems to be nothing in particular that triggers them.

■ Your headaches have begun to disrupt your life; you've missed work on several occasions.

■ Your headaches are accompanied by neurological symptoms, such as numbness, dizziness, blurred vision, or memory loss.

■ Your headaches coincide with other medical problems or pain.

food, perfume, weather changes, seasonal changes, altitude, or low blood sugar.

HOME HEADACHE PREVENTION

People who get headaches know that an ounce of prevention is worth a pound of cure. Here's what our experts advise.

■ **KEEP A HEADACHE DIARY.** The first step in preventing headaches is to identify what triggers them. You are the one in the best position to recognize what habits and factors bring on your headaches. A headache diary does that by providing a daily log of factors that might relate to your headaches. Doctors at the New England Center for Headache suggest you record time of onset, intensity and duration, what you ate, medications you took, and any factors that might have triggered the headache. The American Headache Society offers free printable daily, weekly, and monthly headache diaries on its Web site, www.americanheadachesociety.org.

■ **EXERCISE PREVENTION.** "Exercise is useful as a preventive measure," says Dr. Solomon. It's a good way to chase away a tension-type headache. Daily exercise may also decrease your migraine attacks—but don't exercise during a migraine. An exercise schedule that involves some aerobic activity such as walking, running, cycling, or swimming 5 days a week for 20 to 30 minutes can make a big difference in reducing headaches and in promoting a general sense of improved well-being.

■ **DON'T OVERSLEEP.** Sleeping in may *feel* relaxing, but it's not a good idea. So no matter how tempting, avoid sleeping late on the weekend, says Ninan T. Mathew, M.D. "You're more likely to wake up with a headache." Same goes for napping.

■ **STAND TALL, SIT STRAIGHT.** Poor posture creates muscle tension that puts pressure on the nerves that cause headaches, says Seymour Diamond, M.D. For people who work at computers, a posture problem called forward head posture can develop. Every inch that your head moves forward feels like 10 extra pounds to the muscles in your upper back and neck, keeping them in constant contraction. Try this technique to correct forward head posture: Align your eyes over your shoulders. When you do this you will automatically straighten up.

■ **SLEEP LIKE A BABY—ON YOUR BACK.** Sleeping in an awkward position, or even on your stomach, can cause the muscles in your neck to contract and, consequently, trigger a headache. "Sleeping on your back helps," says Dr. Diamond.

■ **WATCH YOUR CAFFEINE INTAKE.** If you drink too much caffeine on a daily basis—three or more cups of coffee or large amounts of soda—your caffeine intake can cause or worsen your headaches. Moreover, suddenly stopping your caffeine will surely bring on a headache. But if you're not a regular caffeine consumer, one cup can go a long way toward providing headache relief. "Caffeine constricts the dilated blood vessels around your temples," says Alan Rapoport, M.D. "It also increases the efficacy of pain medicines. That's why it's in most headache medications."

■ **DON'T MISS A MEAL.** Fasting or skipping a meal can cause a dip in blood sugar and bring on a headache. To keep your blood sugar constant and minimize the effects of a missed meal, doctors at the New England Center for Headache recommend eating frequent mini meals throughout the day.

■ **PROTECT YOUR EYES.** Bright light—be it from the sun, fluorescent lighting, TV, or a computer screen—can lead to squinting, eyestrain, and, finally, headache. Sunglasses are a good idea if you're going to be outside. If you're working inside, take some rest breaks from the computer screen and also wear some type of tinted glasses, Dr. Diamond suggests.

■ **KNOW YOUR FOOD TRIGGERS.** "You can prevent migraine headaches at least 40 percent of the time just by making dietary changes," says Frederick Freitag, D.O. But to do this you have to avoid food triggers as well as eat healthfully. Fill up on whole, natural, unprocessed foods, especially vegetables and whole grains. Some foods known to trigger migraines are wine, cheese, citrus fruits, onions, tomatoes, and nuts.

■ **CURTAIL THE COCKTAILS.** "Alcohol is at the top of the list of food factors that affect the most people with migraines," says Dr. Rapoport. "It's a vasodilator, meaning that it expands blood vessels, which can trigger migraine." Although any type of alcohol can

do it, red wine more than white, beer, champagne, and eggnog are most frequently mentioned. And dark-colored alcohols such as scotch, rye, whiskey, brandy, bourbon, sherry, and cognac seem to trigger headaches more often than light-colored ones such as gin, vodka, and white wine.

■ **AVOID AMINES.** A hot fudge sundae studded with walnuts may sound like a midsummer night's dream. For people who get migraines, it could turn out to be a nightmare. "Chocolate may be the second biggest offender," says Dr. Rapoport. It contains an amine called phenylethylamine, which can cause your blood vessels to constrict and then dilate, triggering a headache. Experts believe the worst of the amines is tyramine, an amino acid found in aged cheeses, pickled herring, and liver. Other foods containing the dreaded amines include homemade yeast breads, lima beans, and snow peas.

■ **SAY NO TO MSG.** Monosodium glutamate (MSG) may bring out all those subtle and spicy flavors in wonton soup, but if you're one of the many people who are sensitive to this flavor enhancer, it might also bring on a whopping headache. Like other headache triggers, MSG launches its attack by dilating blood vessels and exciting certain nerves in the brain. If you get headaches and other symptoms from this aggravating additive, ask that MSG or seasoning salt (which contains MSG) be left out the next time you're when ordering Chinese. Many products are loaded with it, so read the labels carefully for additives with names like hydrolyzed protein, glutamate, and caseinate, all MSG in disguise.

■ **PASS ON THE HOT DOG.** Pounding headaches caused by nitrites are commonly called hot dog headaches. So stay clear of meat products that contain nitrates, such as hot dogs, bacon, ham, and salami, and stick to fresh, unprocessed meat. Nitrites dilate blood vessels, which can mean big-time head pain, says Dr. Mathew.

Try these basic stress reducers from several of the experts.

■ **BREATHE DEEPLY.** Deep breathing is a great tension reliever. "You're doing it right," Dr. Sheftell says, "if your stomach is moving more than your chest."

■ **DO THE BODY SCAN.** Dr. Sheftell suggests checking yourself for signs that you are tensing up and inviting a headache: clenched teeth, clenched fists, hunched shoulders.

■ **GO WITH THE FLOW.** Maybe older people are better at this. "We see more headaches in younger individuals," says Dr. Diamond. "And they're under more stress—trying to make a living, supporting a family. But it's important to not overdo."

Decreasing your expectations, both of yourself and others, wouldn't hurt, adds Dr. Sheftell.

■ **RELAX WITH IMAGERY.** "Imagine the muscle fibers in your neck and head to be all scrunched up," says Dr. Sheftell. "Then begin to *smooth* them out in your mind."

■ **HAVE A SENSE OF HUMOR.** "If people take life too seriously—and you can see who those people are—they're likely to be walking around with their faces all screwed up," says Dr. Sheftell. And probably wondering why they have another headache.

■ **SAY NO TO COLOGNE.** "Strong perfume can set off migraines," says Dr. Solbach.

■ **SEEK QUIET.** Excessive noise is a common trigger for tension headaches.

■ **FORGET ABOUT GUM.** The repetitive motion of simply chewing gum can tighten muscles and bring on a tension headache, says Dr. Sheftell.

■ **GO EASY ON THE SALT.** High salt intake can trigger migraines in some people.

■ **FISH OIL MAY FIGHT MIGRAINES.** A small study at the University of Cincinnati found that taking fish-oil capsules reduced frequency and severity of migraines compared with taking a placebo. While preliminary, these findings add to the mounting evidence of benefits from the omega-3 fatty acids in fish. Eating approximately 2 ounces of fatty fish daily would supply the amount of omega-3s used in the study.

■ **VITAMIN B$_2$ MAY HELP PREVENT MIGRAINES.** A European study found that high doses of vitamin B$_2$ (riboflavin), over time, reduced the frequency of migraines. But Dr. Diamond cautions, "We need longer and larger studies before we can recommend the use of vitamin B$_2$ in this dosage."

Cluster, Cluster Go Away

But please don't come back another day. Unfortunately, cluster headaches do tend to come back, even after long periods of remission. These headaches, which afflict about 1 million people—90 percent of them men—hit the unfortunate person with heavy-duty pain, typically around or behind one eye.

Cluster attacks may occur every day for weeks, or even months at a time. The cause is yet unknown, but "it's probably either hormonal or genetic," says Seymour Solomon, M.D. The male hormone testosterone is currently being studied for possible connections to cluster headaches.

Meanwhile, doctors have been able to isolate a common denominator. "For reasons we don't completely understand, men who have cluster headaches are typically heavy smokers," says Dr. Solomon.

So quit smoking, or at least cut back drastically. Then, maybe when the cluster headaches go away, they'll stay away.

HOME HEADACHE RELIEF

If, despite your best efforts, your brain is throbbing, here are some expert-recommended ways to get rid of the pain in your head.

■ **CATCH IT EARLY.** Don't ignore the early signs of a headache. At the first hint of pain, take the appropriate dose of aspirin, ibuprofen, naproxen sodium, or acetaminophen. Most pain relievers become less effective as the headache progresses, says Dr. Diamond.

■ **AVOID OVERUSE.** It's easy to overuse headache medication, and many headache sufferers do just that. Unfortunately, it can lead to rebound headache, a condition that requires medical attention. If you take over-the-counter or prescription pain medication 3 days a week, you are at risk for developing analgesic rebound headache, advises Dr. Sheftell.

■ **HYDRATE.** At the first twinge of pain, drink a cup or two of water. This tactic alleviated the headaches of 65 percent of sufferers within 30 minutes, reports a study in the journal *Headache*.

■ **SLEEP.** A lot of people sleep a headache off, says Dr. Mathew.

■ **GO HOT OR COLD.** "During a headache, some people like the feeling of cold against their foreheads or necks, and for them it seems to help," says Dr. Solbach. "But others prefer hot showers or heat on their necks."

■ **USE YOUR HANDS.** Both self-massage and acupressure can help, according to Dr. Sheftell. Two key pressure points for reducing pain with acupressure is the web between your forefinger and thumb (squeeze there until you feel pain) and under the bony bumps next to the ears on the back of the head (use each thumb to apply pressure there).

■ **PRETEND IT'S A ROSE.** "Put a pencil between your teeth, but don't bite," says Dr. Sheftell. "You *have* to relax to do that." The relaxation—and distraction—could help ease the headache.

■ **WEAR A HEADBAND.** "This old business of Grandmother tying a tight cloth around her head has some merit to it," Dr. Solomon says. "It decreases bloodflow to the scalp and lessens the throbbing and pounding of a migraine."

PANEL OF ADVISORS

SEYMOUR DIAMOND, M.D., IS DIRECTOR AND FOUNDER OF THE DIAMOND HEADACHE CLINIC AND THE INPATIENT HEADACHE UNIT AT ST. JOSEPH HOSPITAL IN CHICAGO. HE ALSO IS EXECUTIVE CHAIR OF THE NATIONAL HEADACHE FOUNDATION AND HAS WRITTEN SEVERAL BOOKS ON HEADACHES.

FREDERICK FREITAG, D.O., IS ASSOCIATE DIRECTOR OF THE DIAMOND HEADACHE CLINIC IN CHICAGO.

NINAN T. MATHEW, M.D., IS DIRECTOR OF THE HOUSTON HEADACHE CLINIC IN TEXAS. HE ALSO IS PRESIDENT OF THE INTERNATIONAL HEADACHE SOCIETY.

ALAN RAPOPORT, M.D., IS COFOUNDER AND CODIRECTOR OF THE NEW ENGLAND CENTER FOR HEADACHE IN STAMFORD, CONNECTICUT.

JOEL SAPER, M.D., IS DIRECTOR OF THE MICHIGAN HEAD PAIN AND NEUROLOGICAL INSTITUTE IN ANN ARBOR. HE ALSO IS THE AUTHOR OF *HANDBOOK OF HEADACHE MANAGEMENT.*

FRED SHEFTELL, M.D., IS DIRECTOR OF THE NEW ENGLAND CENTER FOR HEADACHE IN STAMFORD, CONNECTICUT.

PATRICIA SOLBACH, PH.D., IS A NEUROSCIENCE SCIENTIFIC LIAISON FOR ORTHO-MCNEIL PHARMACEUTICAL, A DIVISION OF JOHNSON & JOHNSON IN LAWRENCE, KANSAS, AND FORMER DIRECTOR OF THE HEADACHE AND INTERNAL MEDICINE RESEARCH CENTER AT THE MENNINGER CLINIC IN TOPEKA.

SEYMOUR SOLOMON, M.D., IS A PROFESSOR OF NEUROLOGY AT ALBERT EINSTEIN COLLEGE OF MEDICINE AT YESHIVA UNIVERSITY AND DIRECTOR OF THE HEADACHE UNIT AT MONTEFIORE MEDICAL CENTER, BOTH IN BRONX, NEW YORK.

Heartburn

26 Ways to Put Out the Fire

Eating too much food too fast is the most common cause of occasional heartburn, says Samuel Klein, M.D. But it's not the only one. Certain foods, prescription medications, and stress can also trigger it.

Heartburn occurs when the acidic digestive juices normally found in the stomach flow backward—or reflux—up into the esophagus, making your chest feel as though it's on fire. Normally, the lower esophageal sphincter (LES) keeps a lid on things. Like a pot on the stove that boils over, an overstuffed belly puts too much pressure on the LES. The result: heartburn, or *acid reflux*. The stomach has a protective lining that shields it from the acid, but the esophagus has no such lining. That's why upwardly mobile stomach acid burns, sometimes so badly that you may think you're having a heart attack.

To extinguish the fire, heed these tips from experts.

■ **EAT SMALLER MEALS.** Stomach acids can be forced up into the esophagus when there's too much food in your belly. Fill your belly more, and you'll force up more acid, says Dr. Klein.

■ **LIMIT FOODS THAT FAN THE FLAMES.** Certain foods are more likely to cause heartburn than others. Fatty foods, including meat and dairy, tend to sit in the stomach for a long time and foster surplus acid production, says Larry I. Good, M.D. It's also wise to stay away from citrus fruits and juices, onions, tomatoes, beer, wine, and other alcoholic beverages.

■ **SAY NO TO COCOA.** The number one food to avoid when you're experiencing heartburn is chocolate. The sweet confection

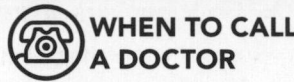 **WHEN TO CALL A DOCTOR**

If you're experiencing heartburn regularly for no apparent reason, it's time to call your doctor, says Samuel Klein, M.D.

How regularly? As a basic rule, two or three times a week for more than 4 weeks, says Francis S. Kleckner, M.D. Although heartburn is most usually caused by simple acid reflux, he cautions that it can also be a sign of an ulcer.

See a physician right away if any of the following symptoms accompany your heartburn, says Dr. Klein. It could mean you're having a heart attack or other serious disorder.

■ Difficulty or pain when swallowing

■ Vomiting with blood

■ Bloody or black stools

■ Shortness of breath

■ Dizziness or light-headedness

■ Pain radiating into your neck and shoulder

deals those with heartburn a double whammy. It is nearly all fat, *and* it contains caffeine. (For chocolate addicts, however, here's good news. White chocolate, while just as fatty, has little caffeine.)

■ **THINK MILD, FOR SPICE ISN'T ALWAYS NICE.** Chile peppers and their spicy cousins may seem like the most likely heartburn culprits, but they're not. Many people with heartburn can eat spicy foods without added pain, says Dr. Klein. Then again, some can't.

■ **IN THIS CASE, MILK DOESN'T DO A BODY GOOD.** Fats, proteins, and calcium in milk can stimulate the stomach to secrete acid. "Some people recommend milk for heartburn—but there's a problem with it," says Dr. Klein. "It feels good going down, but it stimulates acid secretion in the stomach."

■ **RETIRE THE SALT SHAKER.** A Swedish study of 3,153 acid reflux patients found that those who used extra table salt daily were 70

Cures from the Kitchen

An oft-touted remedy for heartburn is 1 teaspoon of apple cider vinegar in a half glass of water sipped during a meal. "I've used it many times—it definitely works," says home-remedy expert Betty Shaver. It may sound bizarre to ingest an acid when you have an acid problem, admits Shaver, but there are good acids and bad acids. For the best results, look for unfiltered apple cider vinegar that contains the sediment or the "mother."

percent more likely to develop the chronic form of heartburn, gastroesophageal reflux disease (GERD).

■ **STICK TO THE EIGHT O'CLOCK RULE.** No munchies or meals after 8:00 p.m. says Donald Castell, M.D. The stomach needs a full 3 hours to empty out before bedtime. Stomach acids can do more damage to the esophagus when you're lying down, increasing cancer risk.

■ **TAKE AN ANTACID.** "An over-the-counter antacid such as Maalox or Mylanta will generally bring fast relief from occasional heartburn," says Dr. Klein. These products help neutralize the acid in your stomach, while acid blockers like Pepcid AC, Zantac 75, and Tagamet can decrease the production of acid in the stomach for several hours. You can take these before a meal as well as after. (For more on antacids, see "Antacids Do Help," page 315.)

■ **CHEW GUM.** Chewing gum can provide temporary relief of heartburn, says Timothy McCashland, M.D. "It stimulates the flow of saliva, which neutralizes acid and helps push digestive juices back down where they belong. A small British study found that gum chewing doubles saliva production, and while it's not as efficient as taking an antacid, it is an all-natural remedy that's readily available in a pinch, says Dr. McCashland.

■ **LEAVE THE MINTS AT THE CASH REGISTER.** While it's often used as a tummy soother, peppermint makes heartburn worse because it lowers the pressure in the lower

Antacids Do Help

Over-the-counter digestive aids are generally effective and safe. One would hope so; Americans pay billions of dollars a year for these medications. The antacids that got the highest marks from our experts are many of the most common brands—all are made from a mixture of magnesium hydroxide and aluminum hydroxide. (One constipates and the other tends to produce diarrhea; combined, they counter each other's side effects.)

Although the mix may be relatively free of side effects, it still is not a good idea to stay on these antacids for more than a month or possibly two, says Francis S. Kleckner, M.D. They are so effective that they could mask a serious problem that requires a physician's care, he says. Our experts agree that liquid antacids, although not as convenient as tablets, are generally more effective.

esophageal sphincter allowing acid to rise into the esophagus.

■ **GO EASY ON THE CAFFEINE.** Caffeinated drinks such as coffee, tea, and cola may irritate an already inflamed esophagus. Caffeine also relaxes the sphincter.

■ **PASS ON FIZZY DRINKS.** A University of Arizona study of people with sleep troubles found that one in four experienced heartburn at night. A key reason: drinking soda. The acidity and carbon dioxide in soft drinks can overwhelm the muscle barrier between the stomach and the esophagus, allowing stomach acid to flow upward, says Ronnie Fass, M.D.

■ **CLEAR THE AIR.** "It doesn't matter whether it's yours or someone else's tobacco smoke—avoid it," says Francis S. Kleckner, M.D. It will relax your sphincter and increase acid production.

■ **CHECK YOUR WAISTLINE.** The stomach may be compared to a tube of toothpaste, says Dr. Kleckner. If you squeeze the tube in the middle, he says, something's going to come out of the top. A roll of fat around the gut squeezes the stomach much as a hand would squeeze a tube of toothpaste. But what you get is stomach acid.

■ **LOOSEN YOUR BELT.** Think again of the toothpaste analogy, says Dr. Kleckner. "Many people can get relief from heartburn simply by wearing suspenders instead of a belt."

■ **IF YOU'RE LIFTING, BEND AT THE KNEES.** If you bend at the stomach, you'll be compressing it, forcing acid upward. "Bend at the knees," says Dr. Kleckner. "It's not only a way to control acid, it's also better for your back."

■ **CHECK YOUR MEDS.** A number of prescription drugs may aggravate heartburn, including those used to treat asthma and

Herbal Heartburn Helpers

Walk into your health food store, and chances are you'll find a number of herbs reputed to fight heartburn. Herb researcher Daniel B. Mowrey, Ph.D., studied the evidence thoroughly and concluded that *some* herbal remedies do relieve and prevent heartburn.

Ginger. This, says Dr. Mowrey, is the most helpful. "I've seen it work often enough that I'm convinced," he says. "We're not sure how it works, but it seems to absorb the acid and has the secondary effect of calming the nerves." Take it in capsule form just after you eat. Start with two capsules and increase the dosage as needed. You know you've taken enough, says Dr. Mowrey, when you start to taste ginger in your throat.

Bitters. A class of herbs called bitters, used for many years in parts of Europe, is also helpful, Dr. Mowrey says. Examples of common bitters are gentian root and goldenseal. "I can vouch that they work," he says. Bitters can be taken in capsule form or as a liquid extract, just before you eat.

Aromatics. The aromatic herbs, such as catnip and fennel, are also reputed to be good for heartburn, but the research on these is sporadic, says Dr. Mowrey.

---

breathing difficulties, heart problems, blood pressure, arthritis and inflammation, osteoporosis, certain hormones, chemotherapy, and those that act on the nervous system, according to the National Heartburn Alliance. If you have heartburn and are on a prescription drug, review it with your physician, says Dr. Kleckner.

■ **TIME YOUR MEDS RIGHT.** Over-the-counter antacids and prescription drugs that decrease the flow of acid work better if you take them at bedtime, says Dr. Castell.

■ **DON'T LIE FLAT.** If you lie down, you'll have gravity working against you. "Water doesn't travel uphill, and acid doesn't either," says Dr. Kleckner. To create this effect, elevate the head of your bed 4 to 6 inches. Put blocks under the legs of the bed or slip a wedge under the mattress at the head of the bed. (Extra pillows, however, don't always do the trick.) Keeping the bed on a slant will discourage heartburn.

■ **SLEEP ON YOUR LEFT SIDE.** The esophagus enters the stomach on your right side. Sleeping on your left prevents remaining food in your stomach from pressing on the opening to the esophagus, which could cause reflux, says Dr. Castell.

■ **TAKE LIFE A LITTLER EASIER.** "Stress," says Dr. Klein, "may cause an increase in acid production in the stomach. Some good relaxation techniques may help reduce your level of tension, allowing you to rebalance your unbalanced body chemistry."

PANEL OF ADVISORS

DONALD CASTELL, M.D., IS A PROFESSOR OF MEDICINE IN THE DIVISION OF GASTROENTEROLOGY AND HEPATOLOGY, AND DIRECTOR OF THE ESOPHAGEAL DISORDERS PROGRAM AT THE MEDICAL UNIVERSITY OF SOUTH CAROLINA IN CHARLESTON.

RONNIE FASS, M.D., IS A PROFESSOR OF MEDICINE AT THE UNIVERSITY OF ARIZONA HEALTH SCIENCES CENTER IN TUCSON.

LARRY I. GOOD, M.D., IS A FORMER MEMBER OF THE LONG ISLAND GASTROINTESTINAL DISEASE GROUP IN MERRICK, NEW YORK. HE ALSO WAS AN ASSISTANT PROFESSOR OF MEDICINE AT THE STATE UNIVERSITY OF NEW YORK AT STONY BROOK.

FRANCIS S. KLECKNER, M.D., IS A GASTROENTEROLOGIST IN ALLENTOWN, PENNSYLVANIA.

SAMUEL KLEIN, M.D., IS A WILLIAM H. DANFORTH PROFESSOR OF MEDICINE AND NUTRITIONAL SCIENCE AND DIRECTOR OF THE CENTER FOR HUMAN NUTRITION AT WASHINGTON UNIVERSITY SCHOOL OF MEDICINE IN ST. LOUIS.

TIMOTHY MCCASHLAND, M.D., IS AN ASSOCIATE PROFESSOR OF INTERNAL MEDICINE AT THE UNIVERSITY OF NEBRASKA MEDICAL CENTER IN OMAHA.

DANIEL B. MOWREY, PH.D., IS A PSYCHOLOGIST WHO SPECIALIZES IN PSYCHOPHARMACOLOGY AND AUTHOR OF *HERBAL TONIC THERAPIES, SCIENTIFIC VALIDATION OF HERBAL MEDICINE,* AND *GUARANTEED POTENCY HERBS: NEXT GENERATION HERBAL MEDICINE.*

BETTY SHAVER IS AN HERBALIST AND A LECTURER ON HERBAL AND OTHER HOME REMEDIES WHO IS BASED IN GRAHAMSVILLE, NEW YORK.

Heat Exhaustion

24 Tactics to Stave Off Trouble

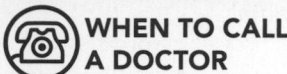 **WHEN TO CALL A DOCTOR**

If it's not treated, heat exhaustion can progress to heatstroke, which can be deadly. Yet it is sometimes difficult to distinguish between the two.

Of course, no one goes directly from feeling fine to the brink of death—no matter how hot it is, says Larry Kenney, Ph.D.

For this reason, a person who doesn't respond within 30 minutes to self-help measures for heat exhaustion should be taken to the doctor. It's important to get emergency care quickly, says Dr. Kenney, noting that possible complications such as shock and kidney shutdown could develop.

"If you have heat exhaustion, the worst you'll get is confused. If you have trouble walking or become unconscious, then you're getting into heatstroke," says Dr. Kenney.

Signs of heat exhaustion often begin suddenly, sometimes after excessive exercise, heavy perspiration, and inadequate fluid intake. Your body loses its ability to cool off, and your temperature starts to rise, sometimes as high as 104°F. The symptoms resemble the onset of shock. "You may feel weak, dizzy, or worried," says James L. Glazer, M.D. "You may have a headache or a fast heartbeat and feel nauseated."

Outdoor laborers, athletes, elderly people, and young children are the most frequently affected by heat-related illnesses. But no one is immune when the weather is hot and humid. Certain medications such as diuretics, blood pressure medicine, allergy medications, cough and cold medicines, laxatives, and benzodiazepines can decrease the body's ability to regulate its temperature—increasing the risk of heat exhaustion.

If you suspect that you or someone else has heat exhaustion, this is what to do.

■ **GET OUT OF THE HEAT—QUICKLY.** Move to a cool, shady place or an air-conditioned building. This is as critical as it is obvious, says Dr. Glazer. If body temperature continues to rise, heat exhaustion can rapidly progress to heatstroke, a more serious, potentially fatal condition. Even returning to the sun many hours later can cause a relapse in some cases.

■ **DRINK COOL WATER.** You need to get hydrated, so start drinking lots of water or other fluids, says Dr. Glazer. To stay hydrated in hot weather and prevent heat stress, the Occupational Safety and Health Administration recommends that you drink 1 cup of water every 15 minutes outdoors.

■ **REST.** Lie down with your legs and feet slightly elevated.

■ **LOOSEN YOUR CLOTHING.** This helps your body cool down faster.

■ **SPEED UP COOLING.** Have someone spray or sponge you with cool water, and then fan you with a folded newspaper. The evaporation of the water is very cooling, says Dr. Glazer.

■ **DO NOT DRINK ALCOHOL.** It may taste refreshing when you are so overheated, but it causes dehydration and can make heat exhaustion worse, says Dr. Glazer.

■ **MONITOR YOUR SYMPTOMS.** If you don't feel better in 30 minutes, seek medical help, says Dr. Glazer.

■ **WAIT ONE WEEK.** Having heat exhaustions makes you more vulnerable to hot conditions for about 1 week afterward, says Dr. Glazer. Be especially careful not to exercise too hard and avoid hot weather.

To avoid heat exhaustion, follow this advice from the experts.

■ **DON'T EXERCISE WHEN IT'S HOT AND HUMID.** Adjust your schedule to work out earlier or later in the day.

■ **DRINK DILUTED ELECTROLYTE BEVERAGES.** Gatorade, perhaps the best-known example, is widely used by professional sports teams. Football teams, for instance, often have twice-daily practices in July and August, and players who sweat heavily can lose a lot of potassium and sodium, says former New York Jets head trainer Bob Reese, Ph.D. "We have Gatorade and water available on the field at all times," he says.

■ **AVOID SALT TABLETS.** Once routinely handed out to athletes and anyone else who wanted them, they are now considered bad medicine by most doctors. "They do the opposite of what they're supposed to do," says Larry Kenney, Ph.D. "The increased salt in the stomach keeps fluids there longer, which leaves less fluid available for necessary sweat production."

■ **AVOID ALCOHOL.** Booze fast-forwards dehydration, says Danny Wheat, trainer for the Texas Christian University baseball club. The team often plays in 100°F-plus conditions in Fort Worth, Texas. "We stress to players that the night before a day game, they should limit their alcohol consumption," he says.

■ **AVOID CAFFEINE.** Like alcohol, it speeds dehydration and can make you sweat more than normal, says Dr. Kenney.

■ **DON'T SMOKE.** Smoking constricts blood vessels, and can impair your ability to acclimate to heat.

■ **ACCLIMATE SLOWLY.** If you travel to a place that is hotter than where you live, allow yourself 1 week to acclimate to the conditions before you exercise, says Dr. Glazer.

■ **TAKE IT EASY.** Whatever you're doing outside, you should do it more slowly than usual when it's extremely hot.

■ **POUR A COLD ONE—ON YOURSELF.** Dousing your head and neck with cold water will help if it's hot and dry outside, says Dr. Kenney, because the water evaporates and cools you off. "In humid conditions," he says, "there's much less benefit."

■ **BE YOUR OWN FAN.** Use a newspaper, a baseball cap—whatever you have—to give yourself a cool breeze.

■ **HIT THE SCALES.** Heat exhaustion doesn't necessarily develop in 1 day. You could be dehydrating gradually over several days. "During training camp, we check players' weight every day to make sure the water they sweat in practice is getting put back," Dr. Reese says.

■ **GIVE THE METEOROLOGIST A LITTLE CREDIT.** Granted, 2-inch snowfall predictions sometimes materialize as 10-inch snowfalls. But when it comes to summertime heat and humidity, the forecast is usually accurate. When they say it's going to be hot enough to fry an egg on Main Street, don't make that the day to begin painting your house.

■ **WEAR A HAT.** Choose a hat that shades your neck and is well ventilated. A wide-brimmed hat with lots of tiny holes, for example, is a good choice. "The blood vessels in your head and neck are close to the skin surface, so you tend to gain or lose heat there very quickly," says Dr. Kenney. "The top of the head is especially sensitive in people who are bald or balding."

■ **DON'T BARE YOUR CHEST.** "You pick up more radiant heat exposure with your shirt off," says Lanny J. Nalder, Ph.D. "Once you start perspiring, a shirt can act like a cooling device when the wind blows on the wet material," he says.

■ **WEAR LOOSE-FITTING, LIGHTWEIGHT CLOTHING.** Choose cotton/polyester blends. They breathe better than shirts that are 100 percent cotton or 100 percent tightly woven nylon.

■ **WEAR LIGHT COLORS.** They reflect the sun and therefore absorb less heat, says Dr. Nalder, while dark colors soak it up.

PANEL OF ADVISORS

JAMES L. GLAZER, M.D., IS ASSISTANT DIRECTOR IN THE DEPARTMENT OF FAMILY MEDICINE AND THE DIVISION OF SPORTS MEDICINE AT MAINE MEDICAL CENTER IN PORTLAND.

LARRY KENNEY, PH.D., IS A PROFESSOR OF PHYSIOLOGY AND KINESIOLOGY IN THE NOLL PHYSIOLOGICAL RESEARCH CENTER AT PENNSYLVANIA STATE UNIVERSITY IN UNIVERSITY PARK.

LANNY J. NALDER, PH.D., IS A PROFESSOR EMERITUS OF HEALTH, PHYSICAL EDUCATION, AND RECREATION AT UTAH STATE UNIVERSITY IN LOGAN.

BOB REESE, PH.D., IS THE FORMER HEAD TRAINER FOR THE NEW YORK JETS AND PAST PRESIDENT OF THE PROFESSIONAL FOOTBALL ATHLETIC TRAINERS SOCIETY. HE IS AN ASSOCIATE PROFESSOR AT THE JEFFERSON COLLEGE OF HEALTH SCIENCES IN ROANOKE, VIRGINIA.

DANNY WHEAT IS AN ATHLETIC TRAINER FOR THE HORNED FROGS BASEBALL TEAM AT TEXAS CHRISTIAN UNIVERSITY IN FORT WORTH.

Hemorrhoids

20 Tips to Find Relief

Hemorrhoids are among the most common of all health ailments. More than half of us will develop hemorrhoids, usually after age 30, according to the American Society of Colon and Rectal Surgeons. Even Napoleon had hemorrhoids. It is said the distracting pain of the emperor's hemorrhoids contributed to his defeat at Waterloo.

The swollen veins of hemorrhoids are in or around the anus. The condition becomes more prevalent as people age but are also associated with pregnancy and childbirth, chronic constipation, and chronic diarrhea. Heredity is a factor, but hemorrhoids can also be caused by—and remedied by—such things as diet and toilet habits.

Whatever the cause, the tissues supporting the vessels stretch. The vessels then dilate, their walls become thin, and they bleed. If the stretching and pressure continue, the weakened vessels bulge.

If you notice any of these symptoms, you could have hemorrhoids: pain, itching in the anal area, bleeding during a bowel movement, a protrusion in the anal area. Most hemorrhoids improve dramatically with simple measures. Here's what our experts suggest to relieve the pain and discomfort of this common problem.

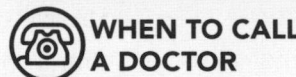 **WHEN TO CALL A DOCTOR**

If you've never had hemorrhoids, but all of a sudden you experience discomfort, it may well be related to something else. If discomfort is accompanied by itching and you've recently returned from a trip abroad, for example, you might have parasites. You will need medical treatment to get rid of them.

Bleeding from the rectum always warrants a trip to the doctor, says Edmund Leff, M.D. "Hemorrhoids can never become cancer, but hemorrhoids can bleed and cancer can bleed."

At other times, an enlarged vein in your anus can clot, creating a big, blue, swollen, hard area that's very painful. In most cases, your doctor can easily extract the clot.

■ **ADD FIBER TO YOUR DIET.** The American Gastroenterological Association suggests that drinking water and eating enough fiber are the two biggest ways to ease hemorrhoid flare-ups. "Fiber has a consistent beneficial effect," says Janelle Gurguis-Blake, M.D. Increased fiber in your diet can cause stools to soften and makes them easier to pass, reducing the pressure on your hemorrhoids. Boost fiber either by eating high-fiber foods or by taking a fiber supplement (such as Metamucil, Citrucel, or FiberCon), or both. Just make sure that you also drink plenty of fluids. High-fiber foods include broccoli, beans, wheat and oat bran, whole grains, and fruit.

■ **ADD IT SLOWLY.** Fiber can cause bloating or gas, so increase your daily amount slowly. Aim for 25 to 30 grams each day. As you increase your fiber, be sure to drink more water.

■ **EASE THE PASSAGE OF STOOLS.** Once you've increased the fiber and fluids in your diet, your stools should become softer and pass with less effort. You may help your bowels move even more smoothly by lubricating your anus with a dab of petroleum jelly, says Edmund Leff, M.D. Using a cotton swab or just your finger, apply the jelly about ½ inch into the rectum.

■ **EXERCISE.** Experts agree that you can keep your bowels moving with moderate aerobic exercise, such as 20 to 30 minutes of brisk walking each day.

■ **GO WHEN YOU GOTTA GO.** When the urge hits, head to the bathroom immediately; don't wait for a more convenient time. The stool can back up, which can result in increased pressure and straining.

■ **LIMIT YOUR TOILET TIME.** A British survey found that 40 percent of us read on the toilet. Not a good idea if you have hemorrhoids. Prolonged sitting on the toilet causes the blood to pool and enlarge the vessels.

■ **CLEAN YOURSELF TENDERLY.** It's extremely important to clean yourself properly and gently, says Dr. Leff. Toilet paper can be scratchy, and even contain chemical irritants. Buy only unscented white toilet paper, and dampen it under the faucet before each wipe, or use premoistened alcohol-free wipes.

■ **SIT IN A SITZ.** Most experts recommend a 20-minute sitz bath after each bowel movement (plus two or three additional times a day) to cleanse the anal area and relieve pain and irritation, says J. Byron Gathright Jr., M.D. Sit in a bathtub filled with 3 to 4 inches of warm water, or buy a plastic tub that holds the water and fits over your toilet seat.

■ **DRY GENTLY.** After a sitz bath, pat the anal area dry; don't rub or wipe hard. You can also dry the area with a hair dryer set on the cool setting.

■ **NO SCRATCHING.** Hemorrhoids can itch, and scratching can relieve it. But *don't* give in to the urge to scratch. You can damage the walls of these delicate veins and make matters much worse for yourself, says Dr. Leff.

■ **DON'T LIFT HEAVY OBJECTS.** Heavy lifting and strenuous exercise can act much like straining on the toilet, says Dr. Leff. If you're prone to hemorrhoids, get a friend to help or hire someone to move that piano or dresser.

■ **APPLY A HEMORRHOID MEDICATION.** There are many hemorrhoid creams and suppositories on the market, and while they generally will *not* make your problem disappear, most are designed as local painkillers and can relieve some of the discomfort, says Dr. Gathright. Limit their use to 1 week; they can cause the skin to get too thin.

■ **CHOOSE A CREAM.** Choose a hemorrhoid cream over a suppository, says Dr. Leff. Suppositories are absolutely useless for external hemorrhoids. Even for internal hemorrhoids, they tend to float too far up the rectum to do much good, he says.

■ **WORK WONDERS WITH WITCH HAZEL.** A dab of witch hazel applied to the rectum with a cotton ball is one of the very best remedies available for external hemorrhoids, especially if there's bleeding, says Marvin Schuster, M.D. Witch hazel causes the blood vessels to shrink and contract.

While anything cold, even water, can help kill the pain of hemorrhoids, icy cold witch hazel provides even more relief. Chill a bottle of witch hazel in an ice bucket or the refrigerator. Then take a cotton ball, soak it in the witch hazel, and apply it against your hemorrhoids until it's no longer cold, then repeat, suggests Dr. Schuster.

■ **FLAVONOIDS PREVENT FLARE-UPS.** These antioxidants, found primarily in dark berries, can help stop the thinning of veins, which can reduce the development of hemorrhoids. In a study of 120 people with frequent hemorrhoid flare-ups, those who received a twice-daily supplement of 500 milligrams of flavonoids had fewer and less severe hemorrhoid attacks. Another study, published in the British *Journal of Surgery,* looked at the effect of flavonoids on 100 patients facing surgery to fix their bleeding hemorrhoids. After 3 days of treatment with the flavonoids, bleeding stopped in 80 percent of the patients. Continued treatment prevented a relapse in nearly two-thirds of the patients.

■ **TRY STONEROOT.** "I have one patient who has found that collinsonia is the only thing that will control his hemorrhoids," says Grady Deal, D.C., Ph.D. Collinsonia, also known as stoneroot, is an old-fashioned herbal remedy, popular in the last century, although it can still be found in some health food stores today.

Herbalists describe *Collinsonia canadensis* as an herb that strengthens the structure and function of the veins. It is particularly good for the treatment of hemorrhoids, acting as an astringent that may help shrink the painful veins, says Dr. Deal.

Take two 375-milligram capsules twice a day with a full glass of water between meals for acute problems. Some people need to take a maintenance dose of two tablets daily indefinitely to control symptoms, says Dr. Deal. (But check with your doctor first.) "I keep them on hand for my hemorrhoid patients," he says.

■ **ENJOY SPICY FOOD.** A recent study shows that eating red hot chile pepper does not worsen hemorrhoidal symptoms. "There is no reason to prevent patients from occasionally enjoying a spicy dish if they so wish," says Donato F. Altomare, M.D.

■ **LIE ON YOUR LEFT SIDE IF YOU'RE PREGNANT.** Pregnant women are particularly prone to hemorrhoids, in part because the uterus sits directly on the blood vessels that drain the hemorrhoidal veins, says Lewis R. Townsend, M.D. A special hemorrhoid remedy if you are pregnant is to lie on your *left* side for about 20 minutes every 4 to 6 hours, he says. This helps decrease pressure on the main vein, draining the lower half of the body.

■ **GIVE IT A LITTLE SHOVE.** Sometimes the word *hemorrhoid* refers not to a swollen vein but to a downward displacement of the anal canal lining. If you have such a protruding hemorrhoid, try gently pushing it back into the anal canal, says Dr. Townsend. Hemorrhoids left hanging are prime candidates to develop into painful clots.

■ **BUY A SPECIAL PILLOW.** Sitting on hard surfaces can exacerbate hemorrhoids; a doughnut-shaped cushion (available in drugstores and medical supply stores) can take pressure off painful hemorrhoids, says Dr. Townsend.

Hiccups

18 Home-Tested Cures

It starts like you're taking a big breath. Your diaphragm suddenly contracts and pulls down. Your chest muscles go to work. A fraction of a second later—35 milliseconds to be exact—the narrow opening between your vocal chords snaps shut, and next comes that characteristic "hiccup" sound. Pretty funny? Not if you're the one hiccupping. Besides being somewhat annoying, hiccups are harmless and normally stop after several seconds or minutes.

"Hiccups appear to serve no purpose in humans or other mammals," says Garry Wilkes, M.B.B.S. Nobody is really sure what triggers the hiccup reflex. A common explanation is that it is caused by irritation or stimulation of the vagus nerve (which controls breathing) or phrenic nerve (which connects the brain and diaphragm). This may explain why hiccups frequently start from overeating, swallowing too much air, spicy food, carbonated beverages, sudden excitement, and stress. Interestingly, hiccups:

- Occur most often in the evening.

- Are more frequent in the first half of the menstrual cycle, especially several days before menstruation.

- Affect only half of the diaphragm—80 percent of the time, it's the left side, oddly enough.

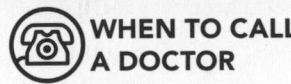

WHEN TO CALL A DOCTOR

See your doctor if your hiccups last more than 48 hours, or if they interfere with your ability to breathe or eat. There are several forms of medication that your doctor might use to treat hiccups, such as anticonvulsants and benzodiazepines. There also are treatments that involve massaging different locations on the body. Hiccups can sometimes be triggered by medications you are taking or an underlying health condition.

Though medical science has yet to nail down a sure cure for the hiccups, there are hundreds of home remedies out there. How most of these remedies work, however, is based on a few basic mechanisms of action: increasing carbon dioxide levels, disrupting the nerve impulses, or relaxing the diaphragm. Here are some cures from the experts.

■ **INHALE. INHALE. AND INHALE AGAIN.** Luc G. Morris, M.D., and his colleagues have had 100 percent success with a technique they developed that uses increased carbon dioxide levels, diaphragm relaxation, and positive

airway pressure to cure the hiccups. They call the method "supra-supramaximal inspiration." Here's how to do it. Take a full deep breath, and hold it for 10 seconds. Then, without breathing any air out, inhale a small breath and hold it for 5 seconds. Follow this with a third inhaled breath (again, without breathing any air out) and hold it for 5 seconds. The technique has worked with patients who've come to the emergency room with persistent hiccups, says Dr. Morris.

■ **BEND DOWN. DRINK UP.** "I cure my hiccups by filling a glass of water, bending forward, and drinking the water upside down," says Richard McCallum, M.D. "That always works, and I firmly recommend it for my normally healthy patients." This method may excite the nerves in the back of the throat and help the nervous system get out of its rut.

■ **SWALLOW SUGAR.** "One cure I find effective is a teaspoon of sugar, swallowed dry," says André Dubois, M.D., Ph.D. "That quite often stops the hiccups in minutes." The sugar is probably acting in the mouth to modify the nerve impulses that would otherwise tell the muscles in the diaphragm to contract spasmodically, he says.

■ **ADD IT UP.** Since the sugar cure isn't always practical, Dr. Dubois uses a mental-distraction remedy that can be done anywhere. Add two two-digit numbers in your head, for example 43 plus 77. "By the time you figure out the answer, your hiccups should be gone," he says.

Favorite Fixes

 WHAT IT IS: Put a piece of brown paper behind your ear to cure the hiccups.

WHAT IT DOES: This cure falls into the mental distraction category. Your brain is so busy thinking, "Huh?" that your hiccups go away.

HOW TO USE IT: On a trip to Vermont in 1968, Dana Kennedy had a case of hiccups so intense that she got a headache. Her husband stopped at a drugstore to get some aspirin. Looking at the brown paper bag containing the aspirin, Dana remembered a hiccup remedy her grandmother taught her—twist a piece of brown paper and put it behind your ear. Dana tore off a piece of the bag, put it behind her ear, and her hiccups were history. The next time she got the hiccups her husband asked, "Why don't you put a piece of paper behind your ear?" As soon as he asked the question, Dana's hiccups went away, and have gone away dozens of times since then just by being asked this strange question. Dana says the remedy has worked for numerous friends over the years. Maybe it will work for you.

■ **HOLD AND SWALLOW.** Hold your breath for as long as possible and, at the same time, swallow when you feel the hiccup sensation coming, says herbal expert Betty Shaver. Do that two or three times, then take a deep breath and repeat again.

■ **GO TO SLEEP.** Hiccups that are caused by stress will often resolve on their own if you get some sleep, says Wilkes.

■ **SEXUAL AROUSAL—IT'S WORTH A TRY.** A strong jolt to the nervous system in the form of an orgasm may work, suggests Roni Peleg, M.D., who reported a case study in the *Canadian Family Physician*. A 40-year-old man developed a bad case of hiccups after receiving a cortisone shot for his back pain. He tried various folk remedies. His doctors tried the standard medications. Nothing worked. On day 1, the man had sexual intercourse with his wife. His hiccups stopped immediately after he ejaculated. Dr. Peleg theorizes that the hiccups were caused by nerve stimulation similar to the startle response. "It's unclear whether orgasm in women would lead to a similar resolution. Under circumstances in which sexual intercourse with a partner is not possible,

The Laundry List

The truth must be told. Doctors approach the occasional bout of hiccups exactly the same way the rest of us do—by running through a list of favorite treatments until they find one that works. Thoughtfully, the *Journal of Clinical Gastroenterology* published a list of suggested hiccup cures to help doctors whose personal lists were a little weak. Here are the journal's recommendations.

■ Yank forcefully on the tongue.

■ Lift the uvula (that little boxing bag at the back of your mouth) with a spoon.

■ With a cotton swab, tickle the roof of your mouth where the hard and soft palate meet.

■ Chew and swallow dry bread.

■ Suck a lemon wedge soaked with Angostura bitters.

■ Compress the chest by pulling the knees up or leaning forward.

■ Gargle with water.

■ Hold your breath.

The journal didn't list these treatments, but you may want to give them a try.

■ Suck on crushed ice.

■ Place an ice bag on the diaphragm just below the rib cage.

Favorite Fixes

 WHAT IT IS: Pick up a Dixie cup full of water—with your fingers in your ears.

WHAT IT DOES: It's a physical challenge, and goes after hiccups in four different ways by making you do five things at once: It raises carbon dioxide levels, stimulates the vagus nerve, immobilizes the diaphragm, and provides mental distraction.

HOW TO USE IT: Dawn Horvath explains her cure like this: "Fill a Dixie cup with water and place it on the counter, then press your index fingers into your ears. Bend over at the waist and pick up the cup with the pinky finger and thumb of each hand and, while holding your breath, drink the water down in one or two gulps."

masturbation might be tried as a means of stopping intractable hiccups," says Dr. Peleg.

■ **IS IT ACID REFLUX?** A common cause of hiccups is gastroesophageal disease (GERD), a condition that allows stomach acid refluxes into the esophagus. See your doctor if you suspect GERD is the cause of your hiccups.

High Blood Pressure

26 Pressure-Lowering Strategies

High blood pressure is often called a "silent" disease—it causes no symptoms for years or even decades. In fact, 28 percent of the approximately 73 million Americans with high blood pressure don't know they have it.

But even in the absence of symptoms, high blood pressure, also called hypertension, can damage blood vessels and greatly increase the risk for stroke, kidney disease, and heart disease. That's because your arteries can take only so much force. When blood rushes through them at high pressure, it causes the arteries to thicken and harden over time. This, in turn, puts extra strain on the heart and increases the risk of blood-blocking clots, says Howard Weitz, M.D.

Smoking, obesity, and a sedentary lifestyle all contribute to high blood pressure, but in the majority of cases doctors don't know for sure what causes it. Studies have clearly shown, however, that most people with high blood pressure can control or eliminate it with some basic lifestyle changes, says Nilo Cater, M.D.

■ **CHECK YOUR PRESSURE—AT HOME.** The American Heart Association (AHA) encourages people with high blood pressure and those at risk for developing it to take their blood pressure at home, says Daniel W. Jones, M.D. Here's what you should do and why you shouldn't do it:

- Know your real numbers. Blood pressure fluctuates all the time, but you'll more likely get a true reading of your

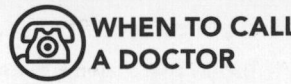

WHEN TO CALL A DOCTOR

Once you're diagnosed with high blood pressure, you should see your doctor regularly for blood pressure screenings. Ideally, they should be below 120/80 millimeters of mercury (mm Hg). If either of these numbers remains elevated despite lifestyle changes, your doctor may recommend medication.

The main classes of blood pressure-lowering drugs include diuretics, which reduce fluid in the body; beta-blockers, which slow heart rate; and ACE inhibitors, which cause blood vessels to dilate. The drugs are quite safe, but they can cause a variety of side effects, including dizziness or dehydration, says David M. Capuzzi, M.D., Ph.D. They can also cause blood pressure to drop too low in some cases.

Report side effects to your doctor right away, Dr. Capuzzi advises.

"normal" pressure at home. Up to 20 percent of people diagnosed with high blood pressure have white-coat hypertension, a temporary spike in blood pressure brought on by the stress of going to the doctor.

- Be in control. Those who take their blood pressure at home are more likely to have the condition under control than people who don't, says Dr. Jones. Of every 100 people with high blood pressure, 70 should be taking measures to lower their blood pressure. Check your blood pressure in the morning and in the evening for 1 week, then once or twice a month after that.

- Track your progress. You can't feel whether your blood pressure is getting better, so monitoring it at home gives you feedback that helps you stay on track with diet, exercise, and medication, says Dr. Jones.

- Pick the right machine. Make sure your BP monitor has a an upper-arm cuff that automatically inflates and records the pressure. And buy the right-size cuff—the inflatable portion should cover 80 percent of your upper arm. The AHA discourages wrist and finger home blood pressure monitors. "I usually ask patients to bring any home monitoring device into the office to check its accuracy," says Dr. Weitz.

- Perfect your technique. You can get a reading that's too high or too low if you use the wrong technique. To get the most accurate blood pressure reading, sit in a chair with your feet flat on the floor, support your arm at heart level, wrap the cuff around your bare upper arm, and follow the directions on your machine.

■ **LOSE WEIGHT IF YOU NEED TO.** It's the single most important thing you can do to manage high blood pressure, says Dr. Cater. If you're overweight, you're two to six times more likely to develop high blood pressure. The heavier you are, the worse your blood pressure is likely to be.

That's because the more you weigh, the more blood circulates through your arteries, causing an increase in pressure. As a result, both the heart and the circulatory system are under increased strain to move the blood throughout a larger body.

You don't necessarily have to lose a lot of weight to improve your blood pressure readings. In fact, research suggests that losing as little as 5 to 10 percent of your weight may be enough to lower your blood pressure to a healthier range.

Despite the plethora of weight-loss plans around, the basic approach is pretty simple: Consume fewer calories than you burn by practicing portion control, reduce your consumption of high-fat (and high-calorie) foods, and exercise regularly.

■ **GET SOME EXERCISE EVERY DAY.** Regular exercise can lower blood pressure by 5 to 10 percent, says David M. Capuzzi, M.D., Ph.D. This is often enough to keep high blood pressure from developing.

Research suggests that you'll get the most benefits by exercising 5 hours a week. Jogging, bicycling, and weight lifting are excellent exercises, as well as vigorous daily activities, such as brisk walking or yard work.

■ **GIVE UP CIGARETTES.** If you're a smoker, this is probably the last advice that you want to hear, but it makes a real difference. Every time you smoke, your blood pressure shoots upward, staying high for an hour or more. Put another way, even if you smoke only 10 cigarettes a day, your blood pressure may be constantly in the danger zone.

Cures from the Kitchen

The omega-3 fatty acids in fish may lower blood pressure slightly and reduce the risk of blood clots in the arteries. But what if you don't like fish? Try flaxseed. It has a pleasant, nutty taste, and it's loaded with omega-3s along with cholesterol-lowering fiber.

You can mix a tablespoon or two of flaxseed meal in a glass of water and slug it down once a day. A more flavorful option is to sprinkle the ground seeds on breakfast cereals or mix them into meat loaf, stews, and other dishes.

When you shop for flaxseed, get the ground variety—or buy whole seeds and grind them at home. Don't bother eating the whole seeds, because they'll pass through your digestive tract without being absorbed.

Smoking is probably the hardest habit to break. Some people succeed by going cold turkey, but you're more likely to be successful if you get some help by attending stop-smoking workshops, for example, or using nicotine patches or other medications to break tobacco's grip. (For more tips on how to beat smoking, see Addiction on page 6.)

■ **LEARN ABOUT DASH.** It stands for Dietary Approaches to Stop Hypertension. Apart from the use of medication, it's one of the most effective ways to keep blood pressure in a healthful range. The diet includes:

- 8 to 10 daily servings of fruits and vegetables
- 7 to 8 daily servings of whole grains
- 2 to 3 daily servings of low-fat dairy
- 2 or fewer servings of meat

People who follow the diet are often able to lower systolic pressure (the first number in your blood pressure measurement) by more than 11 points and diastolic pressure (the second number) by more than 5 points. Those are about the same improvements that some people get from taking medications. For many people who follow it, the diet is enough to keep blood pressure in the normal range without medicine.

"The DASH diet is a little difficult for people to follow, but it's ideal for the patient who is motivated to stick with it," says Dr. Weitz.

■ **SHAKE THE SALT.** There has been a lot of controversy about sodium's role in contributing to high blood pressure. Doctors have known for years that people who are "sodium-sensitive" have blood pressure spikes when they get too much salt in their diets. But what about the rest of us?

As it turns out, nearly everyone may benefit by eating less salt. Sodium attracts water, so too much dramatically increases your blood volume (much of which is water to begin with). This, in turn, raises blood pressure. The AHA suggests that everyone should limit salt consumption to no more than 2,400 milligrams daily by using low-sodium or sodium-free processed foods, for example, and avoiding pickles, sauerkraut, and other salty foods.

■ **ADD SALT AT THE TABLE, NOT IN THE KITCHEN.** Foods absorb a lot of salt when they cook, which reduces the intensity of the flavor. This means you have to keep sprinkling on the salt to get the taste you want. So add salt at the table to get the most flavor with the smallest sprinkle.

■ **READ FOOD LABELS.** Sodium hides in some unexpected places. Even healthful, whole grain breakfast cereals may contain 100 milligrams (or more) of sodium per serving. Snack foods, such as potato chips, are in a class by themselves: An 8-ounce bag of chips may contain 1,300 milligrams of sodium, more than 50 percent of the maximum daily limit recommended by the AHA. Checking labels while keeping a running tally of your daily sodium intake is the best way to maintain healthful limits.

■ **TAP THE POWER OF POTASSIUM.** Think of potassium and sodium as being at opposite ends of a seesaw. As your levels of potassium increase, sodium levels decline, leading to a reduction in blood pressure. Most Americans get barely half of the recommended amount of potassium—4,700 milligrams a day. Fruits, vegetables, beans, and some seeds are good sources. A medium-size baked potato with the skin has nearly 1,000 milligrams; and a medium banana, 425 milligrams. People who take diuretics—medications to control high blood pressure—may need a little more potassium, says Dr. Weitz.

■ **GET YOUR DAILY DAIRY.** In the National Heart, Lung, and Blood Institute's Family Heart study, the systolic blood pressure (the first number) of people who ate the most low-fat dairy—more than three servings per day—was almost 3 points lower than those who ate less than half a serving each day. New research suggests that eating dairy may also prevent high blood pressure. In a study of middle-age women, Harvard researchers found that those who ate the most low-fat dairy, 2 to 9.6 servings a day, were 11 percent less likely to have high blood pressure.

■ **PUT FISH ON THE MENU.** The omega-3 fatty acid, found in fish can help decrease blood pressure, reduce the risk of blood clots in the arteries, and lower the death rates in those who've already had heart attacks, says Dr. Cater. All fish contains omega-3s, but fatty fish, such as salmon, mackerel, tuna, and canned sardines, are the best source of omega-3s.

■ **GO FOR SOME GARLIC.** Evidence from numerous studies suggests that garlic can reduce blood pressure. A University of Alabama study showed compounds in garlic interact with red blood cells, causing a relaxation of the blood vessels. This response is a first step in lowering blood pressure and gaining the heart-protective benefits of garlic, says David Kraus, Ph.D. Aim to eat one to two cloves of raw garlic per day, or take a 300 milligram garlic supplement two or three times a day, or 7.2 grams of aged garlic extract.

■ **SUPPLEMENT WITH COQ10.** Coenzyme Q10 improves energy supplies to heart muscle cells, helping them pump more efficiently with less effort. That, in turn, helps lower blood pressure. Experts recommend taking about 100 milligrams a day.

■ **TRY HAWTHORN.** This herb boasts a long tradition as a remedy for heart ailments. European and Chinese doctors use it to lower blood pressure. Take 400 to 600 milligrams daily.

■ **DRINK MODERATELY.** Small amounts of alcohol don't affect blood pressure and may even be good for the heart. Too much alcohol, on the other hand, causes blood pressure to rise. For men, two drinks daily is the upper limit; women should have no more than one drink each day.

"We don't advise people who don't drink to start," Dr. Weitz adds. The benefits of alcohol for cardio protection are modest at best, but the potential risks from alcohol are significant.

■ **MANAGE STRESS.** Emotional stress doesn't cause long-term increases in blood pressure, but it can cause the numbers to rise temporarily. Stress can also trigger heart attacks in those with underlying cardiovascular problems, says Dr. Weitz.

Allow yourself time to slow down and relax—with meditation, exercise, deep breathing, or other stress-reduction techniques. "Stress is hard for people to eliminate in real life," Dr. Weitz says. "It often requires professional counseling or techniques such as biofeedback to get adequate results."

■ **BE AN OPTIMIST.** Keeping an optimistic outlook is proven to prevent a host of heart problems. According to Harvard researchers, highly pessimistic adults are up to three times as likely to develop hypertension as happier ones, and people with the most positive emotions have the lowest blood pressure.

■ **TAKE SNORING SERIOUSLY.** Frequent snoring may be a symptom of sleep apnea, a condition in which breathing intermittently stops during sleep. "It can definitely raise blood pressure, and it can also bring about heart irregularities called arrhythmias," says Dr. Weitz.

Apart from snoring, symptoms of sleep apnea include morning headaches or feeling tired when you get up. "If we suspect sleep apnea, we'll usually refer people to a sleep laboratory for evaluation," he adds.

■ **MIX IT UP WITH SOME MELODIES.** Thirty minutes of the right tunes every day can help lower your blood pressure, according to research from the University of Florence in Italy. Researchers found that those on a medication for hypertension further lowered their blood pressure after listening to music for 30 minutes daily while breathing slowly. Systolic readings (the first number) decreased an average of 3.2 points in a week; a month later, readings were down 4.4 points.

■ **KEEP AN EYE ON CHOLESTEROL.** High cholesterol doesn't cause high blood pressure, but it can make the arteries narrower, less flexible, and less likely to dilate during exercise or at other times when the heart needs more blood, says Dr. Weitz. Elevated cholesterol also results in fatty deposits, or plaque, on artery walls. Continued high blood pressure can cause the deposits to rupture, increasing the risk of dangerous clots. "Eighty percent or more of heart attacks are caused by the rupture of plaque," he says.

As part of your overall treatment plan for high blood pressure, you'll probably be advised to keep your total cholesterol under 200, but lower is better. Dietary changes, such as eating more fiber and reducing your consumption of saturated fat, can cause cholesterol to drop significantly. Getting regular exercise, losing weight, and, if necessary, taking medications are also important parts of long-term cholesterol control.

PANEL OF ADVISORS

DAVID M. CAPUZZI, M.D., PH.D., IS A PROFESSOR OF MEDICINE AND BIOCHEMISTRY AT JEFFERSON MEDICAL COLLEGE IN PHILADELPHIA AND DIRECTOR OF THE CARDIOVASCULAR DISEASE PREVENTION PROGRAM AT THE MYRNA BRIND CENTER OF INTEGRATIVE MEDICINE AT THOMAS JEFFERSON UNIVERSITY IN PHILADELPHIA.

NILO CATER, M.D., IS AN ASSISTANT PROFESSOR OF INTERNAL MEDICINE AND A NUTRITION SCHOLAR AT THE CENTER FOR HUMAN NUTRITION AT THE UNIVERSITY OF TEXAS SOUTHWESTERN MEDICAL CENTER AT DALLAS.

DANIEL W. JONES, M.D., IS VICE CHANCELLOR FOR HEALTH AFFAIRS, DEAN OF THE SCHOOL OF MEDICINE, AND PROFESSOR OF MEDICINE AT THE UNIVERSITY OF MISSISSIPPI MEDICAL CENTER IN JACKSON. HE IS PAST PRESIDENT OF THE AMERICAN HEART ASSOCIATION AND HELPED AUTHOR THE CURRENT GUIDELINES ON HYPERTENSION.

DAVID KRAUS, PH.D., IS AN ASSOCIATE PROFESSOR IN THE DEPARTMENTS OF ENVIRONMENTAL HEALTH SCIENCES AND BIOLOGY AT THE UNIVERSITY OF ALABAMA, BIRMINGHAM.

HOWARD WEITZ, M.D., IS CODIRECTOR OF THE JEFFERSON HEART INSTITUTE OF THOMAS JEFFERSON UNIVERSITY HOSPITAL AND DEPUTY CHAIR OF THE DEPARTMENT OF MEDICINE AT JEFFERSON MEDICAL COLLEGE, BOTH IN PHILADELPHIA.

High Cholesterol

31 Steps to Total Control

Your heart beats an average of 100,000 times a day. With every beat, it sends 2 to 3 ounces of blood whooshing through your vascular system—some 60,000 miles of arteries, veins, and capillaries.

The heart's an impressive organ, but its efforts won't do much good unless the vascular highway is free from obstructions. But for millions of Americans, buildups of cholesterol and other fatty substances in the arteries make them less flexible, restrict the flow of blood, and promote the development of blood clots. Over time, this can lead to heart attacks, strokes, and other vascular diseases.

Cholesterol itself isn't harmful. In fact, the body produces this waxy substance daily to manufacture cell membranes, bile acids, vitamin D, and a variety of sex hormones. Serious problems can occur when cholesterol levels in the blood rise to unhealthy levels.

We often talk about cholesterol as though it's a single substance, but there are two main types:

- Low-density lipoprotein (LDL) cholesterol is the most harmful form. High levels of LDL promote the development of a dense, fatty layer called plaque on artery walls. As the plaque layer gets thicker over the years, it's harder for blood to squeeze through. Plaque also promotes the development of blood clots that can impede or stop the flow of blood. It's best to keep your LDL cholesterol level well under 100.

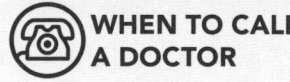

WHEN TO CALL A DOCTOR

Ideally, your levels of HDL "good" cholesterol should be above 40 (and better, above 60), and your levels of LDL "bad" cholesterol well below 100. The natural LDL levels of primates is 70, says David M. Capuzzi, M.D., so human levels should naturally be about the same. Your total cholesterol, which is the sum of HDL, LDL, and other blood fats, should be below 200.

If your numbers aren't as good as possible, your doctor may advise you to take cholesterol-lowering drugs. They are very effective but are usually recommended only when lifestyle changes aren't effective.

Your doctor will look at more than just cholesterol numbers when considering drugs. Other risk factors for heart disease, such as smoking or a family history of heart problems, will also determine whether or not you need medication.

335

- High-density lipoprotein (HDL) cholesterol is *beneficial*. Its job is to remove excess LDL from the blood and carry it to the liver for disposal. Strive to keep this level *above* 40.

In general, aim to keep your total cholesterol level, which is the sum of HDL, LDL, and other blood fats, below 200.

Medications are often required to bring cholesterol into a healthful range, but many people with borderline numbers can control it by making simple long-term changes in their diets and lifestyles.

■ **CUT WAY BACK ON SATURATED FAT.** Found in meats, butter, and a variety of packaged foods, saturated fat is converted by the liver into cholesterol. If your cholesterol is already hitting the danger zone, limit saturated fat to less than 7 percent of total calories, says Marisa Moore, R.D. That equals about 15 to 20 grams of saturated fat per day for most people.

"Choose lean meat and poultry without the skin, and limit servings to about the size of a deck of cards," she says.

Even if you make few other changes in your diet, cutting back on saturated fat could lower your total cholesterol as much as 20 points in 6 to 8 weeks, she says.

■ **EAT MORE FIBER.** Found in plant foods, dietary fiber—especially the soluble fiber in oats, beans, barley, and asparagus—is essential for lowering cholesterol. But, most Americans get only 12 to 14 grams of dietary fiber daily, not the recommended 25 to 35 grams.

Fiber lowers cholesterol in several ways, Moore says. It absorbs water and swells in the stomach, increasing your feeling of fullness. In addition, soluble fiber dissolves and forms a gel in the intestine. The gel traps cholesterol molecules before they get into the blood.

"Everyone should have at least one source of soluble fiber daily," Moore says. More is better: Researchers have found that people who get 7 grams of soluble fiber daily have lower blood cholesterol levels, which may help reduce the risk of heart disease.

■ **COOK WITH OLIVE OIL.** It's the oil of choice in the Mediterranean, and the payoff is clear. People in Greece, Spain, and other Mediterranean countries are about half as likely as Americans to die of heart disease, even when their cholesterol levels are fairly high.

Olive oil—along with canola, sunflower, and other oils high in monounsaturated fats—lowers levels of harmful LDL without lowering HDL at the same time. "Olive oil, especially extra-virgin, is also rich in phytochemicals, which help prevent cholesterol from sticking to artery walls," Moore says.

Olive oil isn't medicine, of course. It's still 100 percent fat, which means it can add a lot of excess calories to your diet. The idea is to use it in place of butter or other fats in the diet, not in addition to them.

■ **TRY A NEW MARGARINE.** Traditional margarine is made with hydrogenated fats, which can raise cholesterol as much as saturated fat does. "Margarine can be as unhealthy as butter," says David Capuzzi, M.D., Ph.D. But there is a healthful alternative. Some margarines, such as Benecol and Take Control, contain plant sterols, compounds that help prevent cholesterol from getting into the blood.

Something as simple as replacing your margarine with one that contains plant sterols can result in a 15 percent reduction in LDL.

■ **MAKE OVER YOUR PROTEIN.** Most of the saturated fat in the American diet comes from meat, which is why anyone with high cholesterol should reassess how large a role meat plays in their meals. "Try to limit your intake of animal protein to 5 to 7 ounces a day," suggests Dr. Capuzzi. In general, eat organ meats only on special occasions, he says.

■ **PUT FISH ON THE MENU.** Fish contains omega-3 fatty acids, healthful fats that lower

---

Cures from the Kitchen

When you're trying to lower cholesterol, beans are among the best foods you can eat. They're very high in soluble fiber, which "traps" cholesterol in the intestine and helps keep it out of the bloodstream.

All beans are high in fiber, but some varieties really stand out. Black beans, for example, have 7½ grams of fiber in a ½-cup serving. Lima and kidney beans have about 6½ grams, and black-eyed peas contain about 5½ grams.

The drawback to beans, of course, is that they take forever to cook. Make life easy and use canned beans. They're just as good at lowering cholesterol as the dried kind.

LDL and triglycerides—harmful blood fats that have been linked to heart disease—while raising HDL at the same time. Fatty fish such as salmon, mackerel, and tuna contain the most omega-3s, Moore says.

■ **DON'T SHY AWAY FROM EGGS.** Once upon a time, eggs were portrayed as vessel-clogging culprits and banned from many heart-healthy diets. Research has restored the good name of eggs. In a study by Dr. Capuzzi, two groups followed a low-calorie, low-fat diet. One group ate two eggs daily, while the other group ate none. After 12 weeks, both groups had similar LDL and HDL profiles. "The eggs didn't adversely affect lipid levels," says Dr. Capuzzi. "People shouldn't be afraid of eggs. They are a good source of protein when eaten in moderation."

■ **EAT FLAXSEED.** A nutty-tasting seed, flaxseed is loaded with cholesterol-lowering omega-3s. It's also rich in soluble fiber and phytoestrogens, which help with cholesterol control, Moore says.

"Don't use flax oil," she adds. "You'll be missing out on the fiber as well as some of the phytoestrogens." Also, the oil contains many more calories than the seeds, so using too much can lead to weight gain, and weight gain can raise your cholesterol levels.

Health food stores and most supermarkets sell whole or ground flaxseed. If you buy the whole form, grind it at home; the whole seeds aren't broken down during digestion, Moore says.

■ **FOLLOW THE "RULE OF FIVE."** Some breakfast cereals, especially the supersugary kind, are fiber lightweights, but others provide a real fiber kick. Check the labels. Buy only cereals that provide at least 5 grams of fiber per serving, Moore says.

■ **ENJOY WHOLE GRAINS.** Limit refined grains in your diet. Most of the fiber in these products has been stripped away during processing. Whole grains, on the other hand, are loaded with it. A slice of whole wheat bread, for example, has 2 to 3 grams of fiber, three times more than a slice of white bread.

■ **SWITCH TO BROWN RICE.** It takes longer to cook than the white varieties, but it's higher in fiber and contains more rice oil, which is thought to have cholesterol-lowering effects, Moore says. You can also buy instant brown rice, which cooks faster.

■ **SNACK ON NUTS.** Even though nuts almost drip with fat, they are a healthful snack high in monounsaturated and polyunsaturated fats. Replacing saturated fat in the diet with these "good" fats can cause a significant drop in LDL, says Dr. Capuzzi. In fact, studies find that people who eat nuts are less likely to develop heart disease.

■ **ADD MILK TO YOUR DIET.** While full-fat milk, cheese, and other dairy foods are higher in saturated fat, fat-free and low-fat dairy do not. Plus, studies suggest that the calcium in low-fat dairy foods can help high blood pressure, Moore says.

■ **ADD MUSHROOMS TO RECIPES.** Studies show that shiitake mushrooms can lower cholesterol and triglyceride levels. Health food stores and many grocery stores carry both dried and fresh shiitake mushrooms. Try sautéing them for tasty and healthful additions to soups, stews, sauces, omelets, and stir-fried meals.

■ **CRUNCH INTO AN APPLE.** Apples are rich in the soluble fiber pectin. Experts have found that pectin mops up excess cholesterol in your intestine, like a sponge soaks up spills, before it can enter your blood and gunk up your arteries. Then the pectin is excreted, taking fat and cholesterol along with it.

■ **DRINK GREEN TEA.** It's rich in polyphenols, antioxidants that may prevent hardening of the arteries, says Moore. Black tea contains some of the protective compounds, but green tea, which undergoes less processing, is a better source.

■ **ADD SOY TO YOUR DIET.** It's a staple in Asian cuisine, which may be one reason heart disease is much less common in Asian countries than in the United States. Soy foods such as tofu, tempeh, and soymilk contain chemical compounds called isoflavones, which appear to reduce the amount of cholesterol that the liver produces. People who eat about an ounce of soy protein daily can have drops in total cholesterol of about 10 percent.

"Soy is a good alternative to animal protein," says Dr. Capuzzi.

To incorporate more soy in your diet:

- Eat whole soybeans. They contain more of the beneficial compounds than processed soy foods. Soak the dried beans overnight, drain the water, and then cook them in a covered container for 2 to 3 hours. If this sounds like too much work, eat edamame (green soybeans), a favorite snack in Japan that is now available in specialty grocery stores in the United States.

- Add tofu to recipes. It has little flavor of its own, but it absorbs the flavors of other ingredients. Tofu is commonly added to stews, casseroles, and stir-fries in place of cheese or meat.

- Try tempeh. Along with miso, it's a fermented soybean product with a slightly smoky taste—and it's exceptionally high in isoflavones.

- Make a soy smoothie. A delicious way to get more soy in your diet is to blend 1 to 3 ounces of tofu, a variety of fresh fruits, and 1 cup of soymilk.

■ **TOAST YOUR HEALTH WITH WINE.** Dozens of studies suggest that drinking moderate amounts of red wine can reduce the risk of heart attack—by up to 68 percent, in some cases. Wine raises levels of HDL and helps prevent blood clots from forming in the arteries. It also contains antioxidant compounds that reduce cholesterol buildup in the arteries.

More isn't better, however. The risks of consuming too much alcohol vastly outweigh the cholesterol-controlling benefits. Men are advised to have no more than two drinks daily; for women, one drink is the upper limit.

■ **COOK WITH GARLIC.** It's loaded with sulfur compounds that may lower blood pressure and cholesterol and reduce the tendency of platelets—cell-like structures in blood—to form clots. There's even some evidence that garlic may reverse existing cholesterol buildup. "Garlic will not have a dramatic impact on cholesterol buildup in the arteries, but it has some potential health benefits," says Dr. Capuzzi.

Opt for fresh garlic instead of garlic tablets. The more garlic is tampered with, the more natural compounds you lose, all of which may play a role in protecting the heart, says Dr. Capuzzi.

■ **ADD MORE ONIONS.** They contain a powerful antioxidant called quercetin, which helps prevent LDL from accumulating in the arteries. In addition, the sulfur compounds in onions raise levels of beneficial HDL. Eating half of a raw onion a day may raise HDL as much as 30 percent.

All onions are helpful, but red and yellow onions contain the highest levels of other antioxidants called flavonoids.

■ **SHOP BY COLOR.** The next time you're in the produce section at the supermarket, make colorful choices: Fruits and vegetables with red, orange, and yellow hues are all rich in carotenoids, plant pigments that make cholesterol less likely to stick to artery walls, Moore says.

Carotenoid-rich foods include tomatoes, red peppers, sweet potatoes, and watermelon, among others. Studies find those who get at least 5 to 9 servings of fruits and vegetables a day—and get the most carotenoids—are less likely to develop heart disease than those who get smaller amounts.

■ **BE MINDFUL OF GRAPEFRUIT.** Incorporating fruit into your diet does a heart good. Some fruits, however, can interfere with the metabolism of certain medications. If you're on a calcium channel blocker or cholesterol-lowering medication, talk to your doctor before eating grapefruit, pomelos, Seville oranges, and any products made from these fruits, such as juice, marmalades, and compotes. If medication prevents you from enjoying these fruits, try others that are high in vitamin C, such as oranges and strawberries, says Dr. Capuzzi.

■ **CAN THE CANS AND JARS.** Choose fresh foods over canned or jarred. Preservatives used to maintain "freshness" compromise nutritional value. "Preservatives turn liquid fat into solid, and that's where trans fats come in," says Dr. Capuzzi. Preservatives also increase the carbohydrate content of food, and destroy B vitamins and ascorbic acids, which are important for cardiovascular health, he says.

■ **ASK YOUR DOCTOR ABOUT NIACIN.** Also known as vitamin B_3, niacin can raise levels of beneficial HDL by as much as 25 percent, while lowering LDL about 10 percent,

says Dr. Capuzzi. A compound of niacin called nicotinic acid appears to lower triglycerides, reduce LDL cholesterol, and increase HDL cholesterol.

Unfortunately, food and standard supplements don't contain the amount of nicotinic acid needed to reduce your risk of heart attack and stroke. "The dose you would need would qualify as a drug, not a vitamin," says Dr. Capuzzi. "It should be taken under the supervision of a physician." If dietary and lifestyle changes aren't improving your cholesterol profile, than talk to your doctor about prescription nicotinic acid.

■ **ADD A DASH OF TURMERIC.** Animal studies have shown that the Asian spice turmeric appears to lower cholesterol. Now studies are suggesting that turmeric has the same effect on humans. Scientists believe that curcumin, a powerful antioxidant component found in turmeric, prevents platelets from clumping together. More research needs to be done before doctors will prescribe turmeric to patients with high cholesterol. In the meantime, use this spice in the traditional way: Add $\frac{1}{4}$ to $\frac{1}{2}$ teaspoon to rice, couscous, and bean dishes.

■ **INQUIRE ABOUT CHINESE RED YEAST RICE.** If you have coronary heart disease, than a purified form of a Chinese staple called Chinese red yeast rice may reduce your cardiovascular risks. Researchers studied Chinese patients who had had heart attacks. Some patients received the red yeast rice extract and some received a placebo. Over the next 5 years, the group taking the extract had a nearly 50 percent drop in heart attacks. "The findings are very exciting because this is a natural product and there seems to be no side effects," says Dr. Capuzzi.

Although the news is encouraging, this doesn't mean you should treat yourself with over-the-counter Chinese red yeast rice supplements. The extract used in the study was made in the lab under controlled conditions, unlike the supplements in stores, says Dr. Capuzzi. Also, one of the compounds in red yeast rice is lovastatin, the same statin found in prescription medications, so the supplements work like, and should be considered, a drug. Talk to your doctor to see if the Chinese red yeast rice supplements available in stores are right for you.

■ **DIG SOME DANDELION.** The liver, which is home to cholesterol, secretes bile into the gallbladder and the small intestine. Bile emulsifies fats so they can be completely broken down by other enzymes in the small intestine. Dandelion helps facilitate this process by increasing bile flow and helping the body metabolize fat, including cholesterol. Take a cup or two of dandelion root tea before meals advises herbalist Betzy Bancroft.

■ **MAINTAIN A HEALTHY WEIGHT.** If you're overweight, your metabolism undergoes changes that can cause cholesterol levels to rise. If you change the composition of your diet in order to lose weight—by eating less fat and more fiber, for example—LDL will drop even more.

■ **GET REGULAR EXERCISE.** Walking, swimming, jogging, and even lifting weights can raise beneficial HDL as much as 10 to 15 percent for most people, says Dr. Capuzzi. And because people who exercise also may lose weight, it can cause a corresponding drop in LDL.

Any exercise is beneficial, but you'll get the most benefit if you do it regularly—say, for 20 to 30 minutes each day, 5 to 7 days a week.

■ **QUIT SMOKING.** Smoking lowers levels of HDL and increases LDL. It also damages LDL molecules in the blood, making them more likely to stick to artery walls. "There are 3,000 toxins in cigarettes," says Dr. Capuzzi. "Stay away from them at all costs."

PANEL OF ADVISORS

BETZY BANCROFT IS A PROFESSIONAL MEMBER OF THE AMERICAN HERBALISTS GUILD AND CODIRECTOR AND FACULTY MEMBER OF THE VERMONT CENTER FOR INTEGRATIVE HERBALISM IN MONTPELLIER.

DAVID M. CAPUZZI, M.D., PH.D., IS A PROFESSOR OF MEDICINE AND BIOCHEMISTRY AT JEFFERSON MEDICAL COLLEGE IN PHILADELPHIA AND DIRECTOR OF THE CARDIOVASCULAR DISEASE PREVENTION PROGRAM AT THE MYRNA BRIND CENTER OF INTEGRATIVE MEDICINE AT THOMAS JEFFERSON UNIVERSITY IN PHILADELPHIA.

MARISA MOORE, R.D., IS A REGISTERED AND LICENSED DIETITIAN IN ATLANTA, GEORGIA, AND A NATIONAL SPOKESPERSON FOR THE AMERICAN DIETETIC ASSOCIATION.

Hives

10 Ways to Stop the Itch

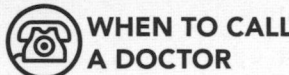
Hives are a common skin condition with itchy bumps known as wheals. They're usually surrounded by red, irritated skin. They shouldn't blister or become painful, and when you press one, it should look white, says Gary B. Carpenter, M.D.

Hives may be the first sign of an allergy to a drug, food, stinging or biting insect, or something inhaled, such as pollen, mold, dust mites, cockroaches, or animal dander. Some hives develop after physical contact with an allergen. A friendly dog lick can raise an angry hive on someone allergic to dog saliva.

Heat, emotions, exercise, and anything else that increases bloodflow to the skin can make hives more severe. The wheals invariably move up around the body and can occur anywhere. They spontaneously disappear and appear somewhere else. Once the allergen or infection is eliminated from the body, the hives will disappear within days or weeks. Here's what you can do in the meantime to relieve the itch and swelling.

■ **SEND ANTIHISTAMINES TO THE RESCUE.** Over-the-counter antihistamines cetirizine (Zyrtec) and loratadine (Alavert, Claritin) can effectively ease the itch, says Dr. Carpenter. Diphenhydramine (Benadryl) also works well, especially when it's taken before bedtime. It can cause drowsiness, so refrain from use if you must drive.

■ **COOL DOWN.** Cold compresses can make hives disappear by dousing the flames of heat, exercise, and emotions that make hives worse, says Dr. Carpenter. The cold shrinks the blood vessels, which decreases blood supply to the skin. Apply a cold compress for as long as is comfortable, usually 10 to 30 minutes.

■ **USE CALAMINE LOTION.** This astringent is famous for taking the itch out of poison ivy, but it may help temporarily soothe the itch of your hives as well. Just like cold compresses, astringents lessen blood supply to the skin, says Dr. Carpenter. Other astringents that may help hives are witch hazel and zinc oxide.

■ **TRY THE ALKALINE ANSWER.** Anything that's alkaline will usually help relieve the itch. So just dab some milk of magnesia on your hives, says Dr. Carpenter.

■ **HELP WITH HYDROCORTISONE.** If you have just a few small hives, a hydrocortisone cream like Cortaid applied directly may relieve the itching for a while, says Jerome Z. Litt, M.D.

■ **TAKE A BATH.** Soaking in a lukewarm tub of water with colloidal oatmeal can help temporarily, says Dr. Carpenter. Tepid water between 70°F and 95°F is cooler than normal body temperature and, when combined with evaporation from the skin, will reduce blood-flow and itching. The colloidal oatmeal is a good general anti-itch therapy, says Dr. Carpenter.

PANEL OF ADVISORS

GARY B. CARPENTER, M.D., IS A BOARD-CERTIFIED ALLERGIST-IMMUNOLOGIST AND CLINICAL ASSOCIATE PROFESSOR OF INTERNAL MEDICINE AND COMMUNITY AND FAMILY MEDICINE AT THE SOUTHERN ILLINOIS UNIVERSITY SCHOOL OF MEDICINE. HE IS CURRENTLY PRACTICING AT THE QUINCY MEDICAL GROUP IN QUINCY, ILLINOIS.

JEROME Z. LITT, M.D., IS A DERMATOLOGIST AND ASSISTANT CLINICAL PROFESSOR OF DERMATOLOGY AT CASE WESTERN RESERVE UNIVERSITY SCHOOL OF MEDICINE IN CLEVELAND AND AUTHOR OF *YOUR SKIN: FROM ACNE TO ZITS*.

Hostility

11 Soothers for Seethers

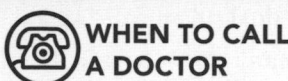

WHEN TO CALL A DOCTOR

If you can't control your hostility and it's affecting your relationships, then it's a good idea to see a therapist who can help you rein in those emotions. A psychologist or other licensed professional will teach you ways to express your anger without damaging relationships with others or hurting yourself.

Some psychologists have reported that highly hostile patients can significantly improve the quality of their lives with anger management therapy in 8 to 10 weeks.

Fits of rage and hostility are so common these days that terms such as *going postal* and *smackdown* have, sadly, become part of our everyday language. If left unchecked, however, hostility is serious business. It can blot out the lucrative deal landed at work, sabotage your efforts as a parent, and destroy everyday good deeds.

Anger is an instinctual response that allows us to defend ourselves against threats. It's a completely normal and healthy emotion, unless it's beyond our control. Then anger can become destructive to you and the people around you.

It doesn't take a degree in subatomic physics to know that explosive anger eventually takes its toll on a person. Numerous research studies have shown that angry people face heart disease in record numbers compared with their calmer counterparts. Hostility can also affect lungs in otherwise healthy young adults. In the first nationwide study to examine a link between hostility and lung function, researchers discovered that the more hostile a person is, the more compromised his lung function is. Uncontrolled anger has also been linked to other conditions, including white-blood-cell-count abnormalities, asthma, diabetes, and anorexia nervosa, as well as to everyday complaints such as backaches.

If the toll on your body isn't big enough for you, consider how it affects the quality of your everyday life. Anger, when it's not expressed appropriately or if repressed, can be the dynamite that explodes an important relationship or gets you fired from a job.

No one is suggesting that you never get angry. How you handle that charged energy, though, is what separates hotheads from those who keep their cool.

ANGER AVOIDANCE

The real secret to controlling your rage is to never let yourself get to the exploding point. Here's what our experts suggest to keep your anger from building.

■ **EXERCISE AT LUNCH.** Anger and tension tend to build up as the day progresses. By swimming laps or walking at lunch, you'll relieve some of the hostility and tension that's festered in the first half of the workday. "Find a form of exercise that you enjoy and that helps to relieve the everyday stresses, and you'll be less susceptible to letting rage get the best of you," says Aaron R. Kipnis, Ph.D.

If you're a couch potato, take note: Research shows the intensity of exercise isn't a key factor in reducing anxiety. In one study, people reported their emotions after either a brisk 10-minute walk or a 45-minute workout. Both groups reported feeling less tense and more energetic. So even a quick trip around the block can change your mind, literally.

■ **TAKE AN EXTRA 10.** Once a week, treat yourself to a 70-minute lunch break—without your beeper and cell phone—and don't be in a hurry to get back to the grind. Chances are you're working 50-plus hours a week, and that extra 600 seconds without any communiqués from your boss, coworkers, or spouse won't get you canned and will do you wonders, says anger-management expert John Lee, M.A.

If finding "me time" during a workday isn't practical, make time for yourself after hours. Just 10 minutes a day can refresh your outlook on life, according to the American Psychological Association. Spend some time alone in your bedroom, turn off your phone, or meditate to your favorite soothing music.

■ **BREAK THE CHAIN.** Plan ahead to avoid a layering of minor everyday things that could make you blow your top. For example, if you're taking an airplane trip, take a book or crossword puzzles with you, because chances are you'll have delays, says Lee.

■ **BRAINSTORM.** Reviewing your past behaviors can provide valuable insight and a better chance at changing future behaviors. Make mental notes of things that upset you and caused you to overreact, and think of other ways to respond in the future, suggests Marilyn J. Sorensen, Ph.D. "As you do this, try to remember what you were telling yourself at the time, and whether those statements were based on fact, truth, or history," she says. "If your thoughts seemed distorted or exaggerated, you'll see how your self-talk in those situations led you to overreact." Thinking is the motor that propels feelings, and irrational thinking will cause those emotional juices to flow in a hostile direction. Ask yourself if this is really

---

Are You About to Blow?

The symptoms leading up to full-blown rage are easy to spot, according to Lynne McClure, Ph.D. Here are four signs that you might be about to erupt.

Palpitations. Your heart feels as if it were about to pound its way out of your chest, and your breathing becomes quite shallow.

Overheating. Your body temperature rises, and you start to sweat. "That's where the old saying, 'Boy, did he get hot under the collar' comes from," says Dr. McClure.

Fixation. You're consumed with whatever is making you angry. "If you're in a meeting with 14 people and find that you're completely riveted on that one person that made you angry 2 weeks ago, then you have a problem," she says.

Overreacting. You're letting other everyday things, such as the absence of toner in the office copier, set you off. "When little things get you enraged, that's often a sign that you have unresolved anger," says Dr. McClure.

---

the behavior and image you want to project. If not, consider what you would do or say differently, and in the future try to base your self-talk on fact, truth, and history, she says.

■ **PREPARE FOR HECKLERS.** Stand-up comedians like Chris Rock have deep reservoirs of comebacks to deal with hecklers. You should, too, suggests Karyn Buxman, R.N. "We all work with certain people who push our buttons," she says. Think ahead and develop a humorous and *kind* response or two to keep them off balance. Humor is a great tool to diffuse tense situations.

ANGER DIFFUSION

Despite our best efforts, we all get angry sometimes. Here's how to keep your flash of fury from turning into an ugly incident.

■ **CALL A TIME-OUT.** If you find yourself coming to a boil, remove yourself from the situation to clear your head, suggests Dr. Sorensen. "Call 'time-out' to let the other person know you are not going to continue the interaction at that time," she says. Suggest a later time to readdress the problem.

Once you've given yourself some time and space, evaluate the situation. Consider valid reasons for what is happening and assess your reactions, says Dr. Sorenson. "Focus on creating a win-win outcome, rather than simply having your way or spouting off."

■ **GIVE TIME TRAVEL A TRY.** Take a page from Michael J. Fox in *Back to the Future* and transport yourself 10 months or 10 years into the future—without that cool DeLorean, of course. "Will what's making you angry right now really matter in 10 years, 10 months, or even 10 minutes?" asks Buxman. "For 99 out of 100 things, probably not."

■ **KEEP YOUR HANDS BUSY.** When anger strikes, do something constructive with your hands, legs, feet, face, and jaw—anything that will release the tension in your muscles and distract you. For instance, if you're at home, take a bath towel in both hands and twist it as tightly as you can, suggests Lee. As you twist it, let out sighs, moans, or grunts. After 10 to 15 minutes, imagine that the knots that used to be in you are now in the towel.

If rage visits you in the office, grab a toy. "To ease the potential anger-producing incidents at work, people should have toys or things to amuse them in their desk, whether that's wind-up toys or cushy balls," says Buxman.

■ **DIVERT YOUR ATTENTION.** If, for example, the person in front of you in the "10 items or less" supermarket line has 36 items and you're Yosemite Sam–angry about it, Buxman recommends distracting yourself until the counting-challenged shopper has made it through the checkout line. Flip through a supermarket tabloid article, check out what's on TV tonight, or chat with the more rule-abiding person in line behind you.

■ **DON'T DRINK ALONE.** When you're angry, a can—or 12—of beer may seem like your best friend. But drowning your anger with alcohol, especially alone, can make the problem worse. It's when you're drunk that you're most likely to leave the boss a threatening voice mail. Instead, call your best friends and invite them out for a gripe-session happy hour. Sure, enjoy a few drinks, but use the time to vent your anger and get it out of your system. Before you know it, you'll be laughing and will be over whatever had you steamed in the first place.

■ **SCREAM UP A STORM.** If you've had a bad day at work, Lee suggests pulling into the nearest parking lot and, with the windows rolled up, screaming as loud as you possibly can. Swear. Name names. If you're at home, take a pillow and holler into it. The pillow will muffle the noise so that the nosy neighbor can't hear you. How long should you scream? "As long as you have the energy to yell," says Lee. "It might seem simple, but you're releasing that anger right away."

PANEL OF ADVISORS

KARYN BUXMAN, R.N., IS A PUBLIC SPEAKER WHO SPE-CIALIZES IN THERAPEUTIC HUMOR AND IS THE PRESIDENT OF HUMORLAB, A COMPANY THAT HELPS PEOPLE MANAGE THEIR STRESS AND ORGANIZATIONS IMPROVE THEIR BOTTOM LINE THROUGH HUMOR, BASED IN SAN DIEGO.

AARON R. KIPNIS, PH.D., IS A PSYCHOTHERAPIST IN SANTA MONICA, A PROFESSOR OF PSYCHOLOGY AT PACI-FICA GRADUATE INSTITUTE IN SANTA BARBARA, CALI-FORNIA, AND THE AUTHOR OF *ANGRY YOUNG MEN*.

JOHN LEE, M.A., IS THE FOUNDER AND DIRECTOR OF SEV-ERAL MENTAL HEALTH PROGRAMS RELATED TO ANGER MANAGEMENT, AUTHOR OF *FACING THE FIRE*, AND A LIFE COACH IN MENTONE, ALABAMA.

LYNNE MCCLURE, PH.D., IS A LEADING EXPERT IN HIGH-RISK EMPLOYEE BEHAVIORS IN MESA, ARIZONA, AND THE AUTHOR OF *ANGER AND CONFLICT IN THE WORKPLACE* AND *RISKY BUSINESS: MANAGING EMPLOYEE VIOLENCE IN THE WORKPLACE*.

MARILYN J. SORENSEN, PH.D., IS A CLINICAL PSYCHOLO-GIST IN SHERWOOD, OREGON, AND AUTHOR OF *BREAKING THE CHAIN OF LOW SELF-ESTEEM*, *LOW SELF-ESTEEM: MIS-UNDERSTOOD AND MISDIAGNOSED*, AND *LOW SELF-ESTEEM IN THE BEDROOM*.

Hot Flashes

13 Ways to Put Out the Fire

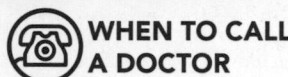
WHEN TO CALL A DOCTOR

Hot flashes and night sweats are rarely serious enough to demand medical attention. Still, if you are just feeling lousy or haven't slept well in weeks, you shouldn't put up with them, says Mary Jane Minkin, M.D. "Your doctor can make it better."

Perhaps the most common complaints about menopause revolve around the dreaded hot flashes—waves of heat that start in the chest and spread to the neck and head, leaving women sweaty, hot, flushed, and irritable.

According to Mary Jane Minkin, M.D., about 75 percent of women experience hot flashes. A single hot flash can last anywhere from 30 seconds to 30 minutes, but 2 to 3 minutes is the norm. Women typically experience them for 3 to 5 years.

As if hot flashes weren't bad enough, they turn into an even more annoying beast in the twilight hours. Nocturnal flashes, or night sweats, wake women at all hours of the night, soaking them in pools of perspiration. Because night sweats disrupt sleep cycles, they may be even more difficult to deal with than daytime hot flashes. They can leave a woman fatigued, exhausted, and begging for one good night of sleep.

Hot flashes and night sweats are the result of the drop in estrogen that women experience during perimenopause (the 2 to 8 years before menopause) and menopause, which technically occurs after 12 months with no periods. This estrogen deficiency, as well as other hormonal changes, interferes with the way your body regulates heat.

If the heat is too much to bear, the following tips can help you get a handle on both daytime and nighttime hot flashes.

■ **WEAN YOURSELF OFF THE BEAN.** Hot caffeinated beverages are a common hot flash aggravator. "You can drink soda or hot herbal tea if you'd like," says Dr. Minkin. "It's not the heat or the caffeine alone that seems to cause hot flashes. But the combination of the two really bring them on strong."

■ **LOSE WEIGHT.** Fat acts as insulation that prevents heat from spreading throughout the body. Too much fat can cause the body to overheat. Hot flashes may just be the body's way of trying to dissipate heat, according to researchers. They found that women with higher body weight had more hot flashes and night sweats than their slimmer counterparts.

■ **RELY ON EXERCISE.** Not only does it give strength to your heart and bones, but regular exercise also reduces the occurrence of hot flashes and night sweats. "I'm a big believer in exercise," says Dr. Minkin. Exercise reduces menopausal symptoms, helps you sleep, keeps bones strong, and maintains heart health. Dr. Minkin recommends exercising three to five times a week for 30 to 45 minutes at a time.

■ **FIND LOW-SWEAT EXERCISE.** There's just one problem with recommending exercise for menopausal women. "When women have hormonal problems, the last thing they want to do is sweat," points out Larrian Gillespie, M.D. However, moderate exercise can actually keep you cool. A study by the University of Illinois found that women in their forties and fifties who walked or did yoga for 3 hours a week reported fewer hot flashes and night sweats.

Dr. Gillespie recommends a low-sweat exercise such as swimming, yoga, and Pilates, which improves flexibility and strength without building bulk.

■ **KNOW THE TRUTH ABOUT HORMONE REPLACEMENT.** There's a myth that it's dangerous to go on and off hormone replacement therapy (HRT). "I don't know how it got started," says Dr. Minkin. The truth is, HRT is a very flexible thing. So if hot flashes and night sweats make both your days and your nights miserable, Dr. Minkin recommends at least trying HRT for a couple of months. If you don't like it, you can always go off the medicine whenever you want. If you decide you want to go back on it again, you can do that, too.

■ **CONSULT YOUR CALENDAR.** "One thing I encourage women to do if they're going to stop taking estrogen is to stop in a cool month," says Dr. Minkin. If you quit in July, you'll discover that a 90°F summer afternoon is a really bad time to get hot flashes.

■ **TRY SOME BLACK COHOSH.** "Black cohosh is mysterious," says Dr. Minkin. The herb is not a plantlike estrogen, like the phytoestrogens

---

What the Doctor Does

To keep cool and get in her daily dose of exercise all at the same time, Larrian Gillespie, M.D., walks on a treadmill situated directly under a ceiling fan.

found in soy and flax, and nobody is really sure why it works so well. Still, Dr. Minkin admits, dozens of studies and her own patients have convinced her that black cohosh is a legitimate herb for relieving hot flashes. The most commonly available brand is Remifemin, which you can find in drugstores. Follow label directions.

■ **DOUSE THE HEAT WITH FLAXSEED.** In a preliminary study at the Mayo Clinic, researchers found that flaxseed may reduce hot flashes. Twenty-nine women who reported 14 hot flashes a week or more had a 50 percent reduction of hot flashes after eating about 4 tablespoons of flaxseed a day for 6 weeks. Larger studies, however, are needed to confirm these effects.

In the meantime, let your doctor know if you'd like to treat hot flashes with flaxseed. If you want to give flaxseed a trial run, the researchers suggest sprinkling 2 tablespoons of flaxseed meal on your cereal, yogurt, or fruit once a day for 3 weeks. Then increase the flaxseed to 2 tablespoons once a day. Be sure to drink plenty of water throughout the day. Increasing the amount gradually may prevent some of the gastrointestinal upsets that flaxseed can cause.

■ **STUDY YOUR SOY OPTIONS.** Adding more soy foods into your diet may be quite helpful for overcoming hot flashes and other menopausal symptoms, says Dr. Gillespie.

Researchers have noted that women living in Asian countries where soy is commonly consumed have fewer hot flashes than women in the United States. In a study at Beth Israel Deaconess Medical Center in Boston, women who took a soy supplement had 52 percent fewer hot flashes after 12 weeks than those who took a placebo. The researchers say that the degree of improvement is similar to that of taking a prescribed medication but without any side effects.

Another advantage of soy, which is bursting with phytoestrogens, is its wide availability. Your best bet is to shoot for one to two servings a day (the amounts found in a typical Asian diet). You're likely to find an array of soy foods at your grocery store, including edamame, tofu, and miso. You also may want to ask your doctor about soy-based forms of hormone replacement therapy.

■ **TRY DEEP BELLY BREATHING.** In some women, belly breathing alone can help reduce the severity of a hot flash. To give it a try, lie on your back with your hands on your abdomen. Imagine that your abdomen is a balloon that you fill with air as you inhale and deflate as you exhale, says Dr. Gillespie. Repeat this six to eight times a minute whenever you experience hot flashes.

■ **RELY ON COTTON.** If night sweats are a persistent problem, all-cotton sheets and pillowcases will "breathe" and wick moisture away from your skin, says Dr. Minkin. Avoid flannel, satin, or cotton/polyester blends, which trap wetness around your body. It may also help to keep a light cotton quilt at the foot of your bed. If you get the chills following a nocturnal flash, pull this over you for comfort. Other cottony items to have on hand while fighting night sweats include an all-cotton, short-sleeved, knee-length nightgown; all-cotton underwear; and a small cotton towel to wipe off the sweat. Avoid full-length nightgowns and other blends of underwear. They'll only trap heat and make you uncomfortable.

■ **IMAGINE YOURSELF NAKED.** Sometimes, the power of positive thinking can overcome all other forms of intervention. Take a few long, deep breaths and imagine yourself naked, rolling gently through cold mountain snow. If all else fails, it's worth a shot.

PANEL OF ADVISORS

LARRIAN GILLESPIE, M.D., IS A RETIRED ASSISTANT CLINICAL PROFESSOR OF UROLOGY AND UROGYNECOLOGY IN LOS ANGELES AND PRESIDENT OF HEALTHY LIFE PUBLICATIONS. SHE IS AUTHOR OF *THE MENOPAUSE DIET* AND *THE GODDESS DIET.*

MARY JANE MINKIN, M.D., IS A CLINICAL PROFESSOR OF OBSTETRICS AND GYNECOLOGY AT YALE UNIVERSITY SCHOOL OF MEDICINE AND AN OBSTETRICIAN-GYNECOLOGIST IN NEW HAVEN, CONNECTICUT. SHE IS COAUTHOR OF *WHAT EVERY WOMAN NEEDS TO KNOW ABOUT MENOPAUSE* AND *A WOMAN'S GUIDE TO MENOPAUSE AND PERIMENOPAUSE.*

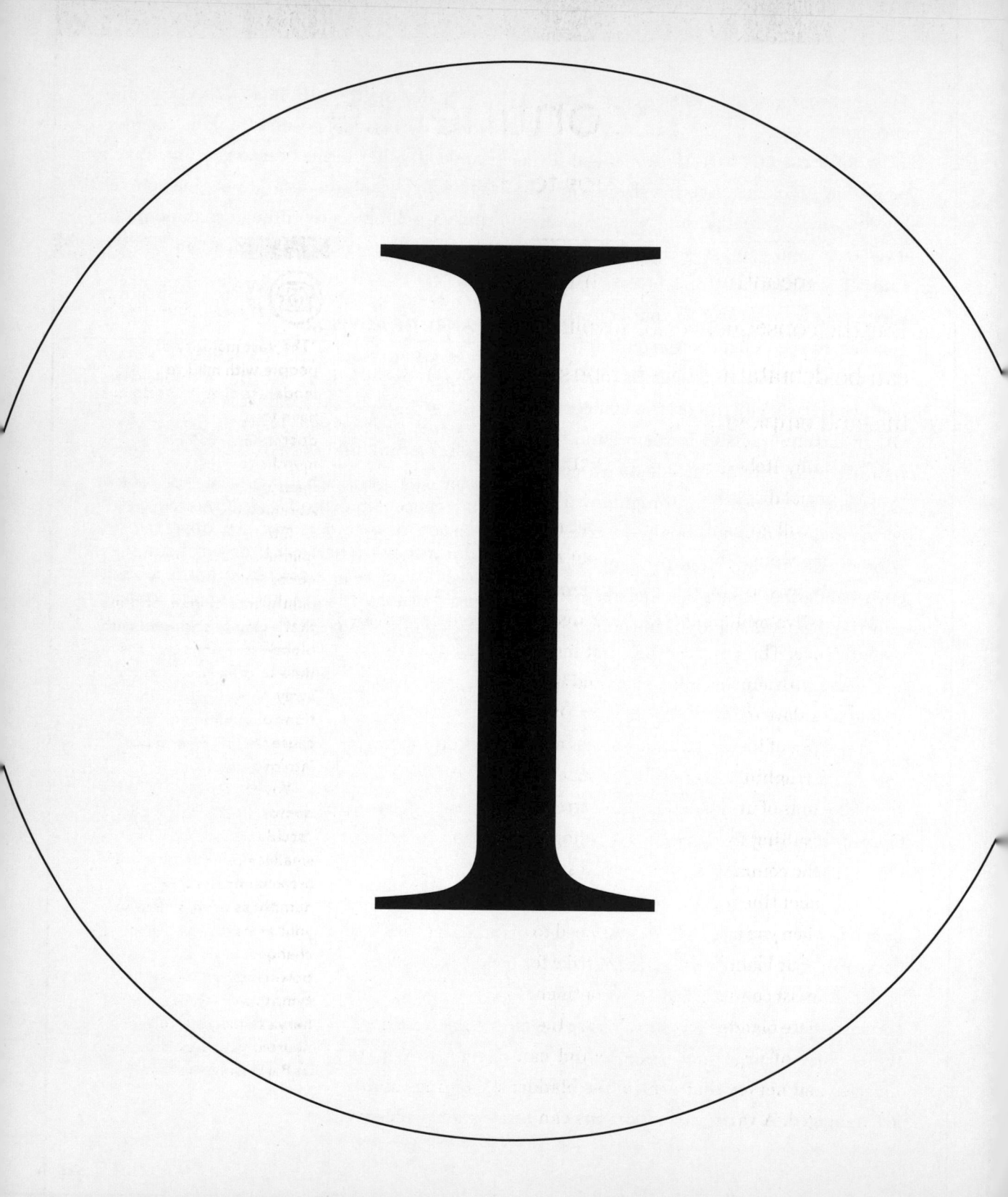

Incontinence

18 Tips to Gain Control

Urinary incontinence is a symptom, not a disease. But the consequences of involuntary loss of urine can be debilitating to a person's self-esteem, social life, and employment.

That's why Robert Schlesinger, M.D., prefers to call incontinence a "social disease."

"People will go to almost any extent to adjust their lives to it. We had one woman who didn't go out of her house for 3 years because she was so ashamed," Dr. Schlesinger says.

Twenty-five million adult Americans are affected by urinary incontinence. The great news is that incontinence can often be controlled with simple medications and lifestyle changes. "No one should be a slave to their bladder," says Dr. Schlesinger.

Two types of incontinence are stress and urge incontinence. If coughing, laughing, exercising, or sneezing causes you to leak small amounts of urine, you may have stress incontinence. Physical changes resulting from pregnancy, aging, childbirth, and menopause are the common culprits behind stress incontinence.

Urge incontinence (otherwise known as overactive bladder) happens when you suddenly feel the need to urinate and then lose control of your bladder. It seems to strike for no apparent reason, and is the most common form of incontinence in men and women. Inappropriate bladder contractions are the most common underlying cause of urge incontinence and can develop when the muscles and nerves that control the bladder's "holding" ability are damaged. A variety of conditions can cause such problems,

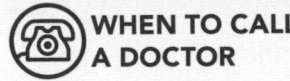

WHEN TO CALL A DOCTOR

"The vast majority of people with mild to moderate symptoms do not have to rush off to see a doctor. Give yourself 3 months to see if lifestyle measures work," says Abraham N. Morse, M.D.

Other symptoms—painful urination, incontinence that accompanies painful intercourse, or urine that's cloudy or tinged with blood—are signs that it's time to call a doctor right away. Urinary tract infections or even tumors can cause the bladder to go into overdrive.

You should also call a doctor if you're having large "accidents" rather than small leaks. Or if accidents are accompanied by numbness or weakness in your arms or legs, vision changes, or a change in bowel habits. These symptoms may be a sign of nerve damage or other neurological problems, such as Parkinson's disease.

including an enlarged prostate, a stroke, or a pinched nerve.

In most cases, incontinence is a matter of degree. But it's not a normal part of aging, says Neil M. Resnick, M.D. "It's not inevitable, and it's not irreversible." Because so many medical conditions can cause or contribute to it, it's important to let your doctor know if you're experiencing incontinence. But there are also some ways to help yourself.

■ **KEEP A BLADDER DIARY.** Keep track of the times you've had a urinary leak. Record the time, what you were drinking, when you went to the bathroom, and what you were doing at the time, such as coughing, laughing, sneezing, or exercising. The diary will help you and your doctor track down the cause.

■ **GO EASY ON FLUIDS.** Your bladder diary may reveal that you've been drinking gallons of water. If you're on a diet that requires taking in a lot of liquids, try drinking a little less and your incontinence problems may ease up.

People have come to believe that a large intake of fluid is healthy. "There is nothing magic about drinking eight glasses of water a day," says Dr Schlesinger. The more you drink, the more you'll have to void. "People should drink as they are thirsty," he says.

When you do drink, sip it throughout the day instead of downing large amounts at once.

■ **AVOID ALCOHOL.** Alcohol is a great stimulant for trotting to the bathroom. It also impairs your ability to know when to go.

■ **AVOID CAFFEINE.** Caffeine is another well-known diuretic. It also irritates the bladder and stimulates muscle contractions, which can aggravate the symptoms of urge incontinence, says Abraham N. Morse, M.D.

Caffeine is found in beverages, but also in foods such as chocolate and in medications such as Excedrin. Doctors advise limiting caffeine intake to no more than 200 milligrams daily, about the amount in 12 ounces of coffee. Your diary will help you track whether you're getting too much.

Switching to decaffeinated coffee or to tea will help, but it may not eliminate the problem, Dr. Morse says. There are other substances in coffee and tea that act as bladder irritants.

■ **AVOID CITRUS JUICES.** The acids in grapefruit, orange, tomato, and other fruit juices can cause bladder woes for many people. The only way to know for sure if these acids are part of the problem is to cut them out of your diet to see if your condition improves.

■ **SKIP THE OXALIC ACIDS.** Some people find relief when they stop eating foods containing oxalic acid, says Meg Gotelli, C.N. Oxalic acid is a natural compound that in high amounts can cause kidney and stomach problems. Cooked spinach, rhubarb, chocolate, and even cigarettes all have oxalic acid (which gives you yet another reason to quit smoking).

■ **DRINK "FLAT" WATER.** The carbon dioxide bubbles in fizzy water and soft drinks make the urine more acidic, which can trigger the urge to urinate, says Dr. Morse.

■ **BUILD UP YOUR BUGS.** The healthy bacteria, *Lactobacillus acidophilus*, provide protective bacteria in the urethra and the digestive tract, says Gotelli. Take a 1 billion strength lactobacillus acidophilus capsule once a day with a meal. These supplements are especially helpful if you're on a course of antibiotics, she says. Antibiotics strip away all bacteria, good and bad, which can result in recurrent bladder infections. You should see improvements after 2 to 4 weeks. Once you've finished the supplements, eat 6 ounces of plain yogurt a day to help with urinary health.

■ **TRY "DOUBLE VOIDING."** When you urinate, stay on the toilet until you feel your bladder is empty. Then, stand up and sit down again, lean forward slightly at the knees, and try again.

■ **KNOW WHEN YOU SHOULD GO.** It's a good idea to empty your bladder on a regular basis, Dr. Schlesinger says. For example, don't sit at the dinner table and hold it until dinner's over. This practice may lead to a bladder infection and an overstretched bladder. Also, if your bladder is too full and your sphincter muscle weak, he says, you're likely to leak when you cough, sneeze, or laugh. Your best bet is to empty your bladder before and after meals, and at bedtime.

■ **DO KEGEL EXERCISES.** This exercise was developed in the late 1940s by Arnold Kegel, M.D., to help women with stress incontinence during and after pregnancy. The experts say that doing this exercise reduces and may even prevent some forms of incontinence in both genders and at all ages. Here are the guidelines from the National Association for Continence.

1. Without tensing the muscles of your legs, buttocks, or abdomen, imagine that you're trying to hold back gas by tightening the ring of muscles (the sphincter) around the anus, and for women also around the vaginal area. This exercise identifies the pelvic muscles.

2. When you're urinating, try to stop the flow, and then restart it. This identifies the correct pelvic muscles. This exercise won't build the pelvic muscles, but you can use it as a bimonthly test of how strong your muscles have become after a few weeks of Kegels. Every 2 weeks you should be able to hold your urine longer.

3. Once you've isolated and identified the correct muscles, you're ready for the complete exercise. Slowly tighten, lift, and draw in those muscles, and hold them for 5 seconds. Then rest for 10 seconds. Practice this exercise over several weeks to try to build your holding time to 10 seconds.

■ **OUTSMART THE URGE.** If you have urge incontinence, you have almost no warning of the need to go. Don't panic. Instead, at first notice, relax. The same muscles you use to clench your buttocks can also be used to short-circuit those "gotta go" sensations. Clench the muscles as tightly as you can, and hold the tension for a few seconds. Doing this several times in a row often makes the urge to urinate disappear. "It's like biting your lip when you have to sneeze," says Dr. Morse.

When the urge sensation passes, walk slowly, without panic, to the nearest restroom.

■ **QUIET YOUR MIND.** Another strategy for sudden urges is to "breathe deeply, calm yourself down, and have confidence that you're not going to make a mess," says Dr. Morse. If you can calm yourself for 30 to 60 seconds, there's a good chance the urge will go away, he says.

■ **BE READY FOR EMERGENCIES.** If incontinence at night is a problem, and your doctor has ruled out fluid retention, keep a bedpan within reach of your bed. Remove any furniture or rugs that you could trip on during a quick nocturnal visit to the bathroom. Add nightlights to help you find your path without delays.

■ **COMPENSATE FOR YOUR AGE.** As you age, it takes longer to get places—including the bathroom. So make sure you always know bathroom's location, and position yourself as close to it as possible.

■ **REVIEW YOUR MEDS.** Any drugs that relax the nerves or muscles can cause incontinence. If you're on medications to calm anxieties so you can sleep or relax, your bladder may not be sending the "I'm full" message to your brain quick enough, according to the National Kidney and Urologic Diseases Information Clearinghouse. Talk to your doctor if you suspect that your medications may be causing or contributing to your incontinence.

■ **BUY SPECIAL SUPPLIES.** There are several brands of absorbent underpants, pads, and shields. The products absorb 50 to 500 times their weight in water, neutralize odor, and congeal fluid to prevent leakage. The type you need depends on your individual anatomy and the kind and degree of your incontinence.

■ **REDUCE THE TENSION IN YOUR LIFE.** "Whenever you're anxious or depressed, your body sensations are magnified in a negative way," says Dr. Morse. "If you're anxious to begin with, feeling as though you have to rush to the bathroom is one more thing that can put you over the edge."

Take a hint from your bladder and unwind. Give yourself an hour each day to do something that's just for you, like taking a long walk, watching some TV, or going to a movie or visiting museum.

PANEL OF ADVISORS

Infertility

16 Ways to Get a Baby on Board

Few experiences can compare to the joy of bringing a child into the world. And virtually nothing is as distressing as trying to make a baby—and failing.

Infertility is the inability to conceive a child after 6 to 12 months of having sexual intercourse without using birth control. A variety of factors contribute to infertility, including genetics, health conditions, and lifestyle choices. And while infertility may be traced to a single cause in either you or your partner, it can also be caused by a combination of factors, from infection to stress to medication.

If you and your partner have been unable to get pregnant, you're far from alone. Overall, 2.1 million married couples face infertility. About one-third of infertility problems are linked to the man's reproductive system, another third is caused by the woman's reproductive system—which has more tasks to perform in the baby-making process—and the last third is a combination of the couples' reproductive systems.

But take heart, especially if you're an older mommy wannabe. While you and your partner will need to see a doctor to determine the cause of your infertility, there's a lot that you can do on your own to increase your odds of conceiving. Try one or all of these expert-recommended tips.

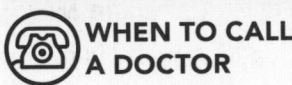

WHEN TO CALL A DOCTOR

If you're younger than 35, and you and your partner have not conceived after a year of unprotected sex, see your gynecologist. If you're age 35 or older, see your doctor if you haven't conceived after 6 months.

REMEDIES FOR WOMEN

■ **PLAN AHEAD, IF YOU CAN.** Unfair as it is, it's a biological fact: A woman's age dramatically impacts her fertility, says Robert Stillman,

M.D. A healthy 30-year-old woman has about a 20 percent chance of getting pregnant every month. By age 40, however, a woman's chance of pregnancy drops to 5 percent every month.

That's *not* to say that if you're in your twenties or early thirties, you should have children if you're not emotionally or financially prepared, says Dr. Stillman. But knowing up front that your odds of conceiving dwindle with age can help you make an informed decision about when to get pregnant.

■ **PRACTICE THINK-AHEAD BIRTH CONTROL.** If you're older than 35, it may be better to avoid two birth-control methods: Depo-Provera ("the Shot") and Norplant, says Dr. Stillman. Both can linger in a woman's body long after she stops taking them—sometimes, up to several years. If you prefer a hormonal method of birth control (rather than, say, condoms or diaphragms), use the Pill, says Dr. Stillman. "When you're ready to conceive, there will be less chance of a long delay."

If you're under 35, Depo-Provera and Norplant are probably quite safe, says Dr. Stillman. "There will be enough time for them to leave your system, even at the end of the spectrum."

■ **GET TO YOUR "FERTILITY WEIGHT."** Twelve percent of all infertility cases stem from weighing too much or too little. If you're overweight, losing just 5 to 10 percent of your weight may dramatically improve your chances of ovulating and conceiving. If you're drastically underweight, try your best to gain. "Women biologically need a certain amount of body fat

to carry and bear a child," says Dr. Stillman.

■ **KEEP UP WITH YOUR WORKOUTS.** It's a myth that women should stop working out while they're trying to conceive, says John Jarrett, M.D. In fact, regular exercise can help you cope with the emotional stress that you might be feeling as you try to get pregnant.

■ **LIMIT CAFFEINE.** Some studies show a connection between high caffeine intake and decreased fertility in women. Even though the jury is still out, if you're trying to conceive it's a good idea to keep your daily caffeine below 250 milligrams a day, or 1 or 2 cups of coffee, says the Mayo Clinic.

■ **DON'T WORRY, BE FERTILE.** Researchers at Harvard studying women who had been trying to conceive for an average of 3 years found that after a stress-reduction program, 42 percent had successful pregnancies within 6 months. In another study, women having trouble getting pregnant were randomly assigned to either a stress-reduction group or a support group, or received no psychological intervention. Within 1 year, 55 percent of the women in the stress-reduction group and 54 percent of the women in the support group had given birth. By comparison, only 20 percent of those who had no treatment conceived.

If you're feeling defeated by infertility, try to set those worries aside by regularly engaging in activities that you find relaxing, whether it's doing yoga, reading a book, or taking a walk.

■ **TIME YOUR OVULATION.** Sperm has a small window of opportunity to fertilize a willing egg near ovulation, and monitoring body temperature may help identify that time. Most women's basal body temperature, or temperature at rest, increases slightly after ovulation. Take your temperaturee every morning before getting out of bed and record it on a graph that also documents the days of your menstruation. After a few months, you should be able to spot a pattern that indicates when you usually ovulate and are most fertile

Many women find that using an ovulation detection kit is easier. These kits, which you can buy over-the-counter, measure your levels of urinary luteinizing hormone (LH), a hormone that stimulates release of the egg.

■ **OR THROW TIMING OUT THE WINDOW.** If a woman is on a reliable 28-day cycle, she ovulates around day 14, says Dr. Jarrett. "So having sex on days 10, 12, 14, 16, and 18 will pretty much cover your bases."

■ **LIE STILL.** Lying still for 5 to 10 minutes after intercourse may improve your chances of conceiving, because it helps keep your partner's semen where it needs to be, says Dr. Stillman. (It's not necessary to do something drastic to keep semen inside you, he adds. So forget about standing on your head.)

REMEDIES FOR MEN

■ **LOSE THE LOVE HANDLES.** What's good for the goose is good for the gander. Women aren't the only ones who should watch their weight. Men who are obese have lower volumes of seminal fluid and a higher proportion of abnormal sperm, according to Scottish researchers. The scientists studied over 5,300 men at the Aberdeen Fertility Centre. Those who had a healthy body mass index (BMI), between 20 and 25, had better levels of semen and normal sperm than those who had a higher BMI. While these findings need more scientific support, the researchers advise that "men who are trying for a baby with their partners should first try to achieve an ideal body weigh."

■ **STAY OUT OF HOT TUBS.** Hot tubs can be detrimental to a man's fertility because the intense heat can kill the sperm in his testes,

Cures from the Kitchen

Daddy wannabes should consider filling their plates with fresh fruits and vegetables. The nutrients they contain may help "grow" healthy sperm.

Here's why. Studies conducted at the Cleveland Clinic Urological Institute's Center for Reproductive Medicine suggest that abnormally high levels of free radicals may cause infertility in some men. Free radicals are "crippled" oxygen molecules that are generated naturally by our body processes. They damage healthy cells—and spermatozoa.

"Sperm require small amounts of free radicals to fertilize an egg," says study author Ashok Agarwal, Ph.D. "But too many free radicals can damage the sperm's cell membrane and DNA, compromising the sperm's ability to fertilize."

The researchers theorize that antioxidant vitamins, such as beta-carotene, vitamin C, and vitamin E, may benefit the sperm of men under high oxidative stress—for example, smokers and avid exercisers—because these vitamins may help neutralize free radicals.

says Dr. Stillman. Spending more than 30 minutes in water 102°F and above can lower your sperm count.

■ **EAT TOMATOES.** Lycopene, a powerful antioxidant found in tomatoes and other foods, may protect sperm from oxidative damage. Scientists at McGill University induced DNA damage in sperm bathed in a lycopene solution and untreated sperm. The solution-treated sperm showed less damage than the untreated sperm.

Researchers need to do more exploring before recommending lycopene for infertility in men. However, most experts agree that food plays a vital role in fertility, so incorporate more antioxidant-rich fruits and veggies into your diet whenever possible.

REMEDIES FOR MEN AND WOMEN

■ **BREAK OUT THE CONDOMS.** If you're not currently in a monogamous relationship and want to have children someday, use a condom— every time. Sexually transmitted diseases such as chlamydia and gonorrhea, which often cause no symptoms, can cause infertility in both men and women.

■ **SAY *SAYONARA* TO SOY FOODS.** Women who are trying to conceive should avoid soy foods, such as tofu and soymilk, advises Dr. Stillman. "They contain plant estrogens, called phytoestrogens, that compete with a woman's natural estrogen, and they can throw off a woman's ovulation cycle," he says. "We've seen women who have stopped ovulating completely."

Men should heed the same advice. In the largest human study of phytoestrogens and semen quality, researchers at the Harvard School of Public Health found that men who ate the most soy had less sperm than men who didn't consume soy at all.

■ **DON'T OVERDO THE DEED.** Having sex until you're ready to drop will *not* increase your chances of conceiving, says Dr. Stillman. "In fact, having sex four or five times a day is counterproductive." That's because a man's sperm count drops dramatically right after ejaculation, and it typically takes 48 hours to regain a normal level.

■ **DRINK LIGHTLY OR NOT AT ALL.** Research shows that women who consume as few as five drinks a week may hinder conception. Men who consume large amounts of alcohol can impair their fertility as well. Alcohol can damage the liver, and estrogen levels rise in men with liver damage, which can impair sperm production.

PANEL OF ADVISORS

ASHOK AGARWAL, PH.D., IS HEAD OF THE ANDROLOGY LABORATORY AND DIRECTOR OF THE CENTER FOR REPRODUCTIVE MEDICINE AT THE CLEVELAND CLINIC FOUNDATION IN OHIO.

JOHN JARRETT, M.D., IS A REPRODUCTIVE ENDOCRINOLOGIST IN INDIANAPOLIS.

ROBERT STILLMAN, M.D., IS A CLINICAL PROFESSOR IN THE DEPARTMENT OF OBSTETRICS AND GYNECOLOGY AT GEORGETOWN UNIVERSITY SCHOOL OF MEDICINE IN WASHINGTON, D.C., AND MEDICAL DIRECTOR AT THE SHADY GROVE FERTILITY REPRODUCTIVE SCIENCE CENTER IN ROCKVILLE, MARYLAND.

Ingrown Hair

11 Ways to Get a Clean Shave

An ingrown hair lives up to its name, for instead of growing outward, it grows back into the skin. When the tip of the hair punctures the skin, it can cause inflammation and pain. Naturally curly hairs, especially beard hairs in African-American men, commonly become ingrown.

If inflammation is also a problem, many experts recommend letting the hair grow, if feasible. When hairs are longer, they don't twist and puncture the skin.

Dermatologists say that tweezers are the only way to get rid of an ingrown hair, but there are other methods to make sure ingrown hairs don't return. Follow these tips to ease your discomfort.

■ **SEND TWEEZERS TO THE RESCUE.** If you can see an ingrown hair beneath the skin, apply a warm, damp compress for a couple of minutes to soften the skin, says Rodney Basler, M.D. Then sterilize a needle or tweezers and pluck the hair. Follow with an antiseptic such as hydrogen peroxide or rubbing alcohol.

■ **BRING THE HAIR TO THE SURFACE.** If you can't see the ingrown hair, don't go fishing for it, Dr. Basler says, "because it might not be an ingrown hair at all." Instead, treat it with a warm compress until you can see a hair lurking there. Then use a sterilized needle or tweezers to pull it, and follow with an antiseptic.

■ **THINK ABOUT GROWING A BEARD.** "The curlier your hair is, the more likely you are to get ingrown hairs," says Dr. Basler. If it's a real problem, seriously consider growing a beard.

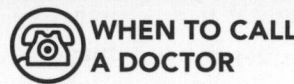

WHEN TO CALL A DOCTOR

Left untreated, most ingrown hairs resolve on their own. If you seem especially prone to ingrown hairs or if the pain from a hair continues for more than a few days, see a dermatologist. You may have an infection that should be treated with antibiotics.

■ **SOFTEN YOUR WHISKERS.** If there's no way you can have a beard, properly preparing your whiskers for shaving helps prevent ingrown hairs. Wash your face thoroughly with soap and water for 2 minutes, says Jerome Z. Litt, M.D. That softens the hair. Rinse well, apply shaving cream or gel, and leave it on for 2 minutes to further soften the hair.

■ **DON'T PULL YOUR SKIN.** Many men tend to pull their skin taut to get a closer shave. Once the skin is released, the short hairs pull back below the surface of the skin. Their sharp tips can reenter the skin and this can cause an ingrown hair, says Dr. Litt.

■ **HIDE BEHIND YOUR SHADOW.** Reconcile yourself to having a constant five o'clock shadow, Dr. Basler says. Don't shave close. The best way to do this, he says, is to use an electric razor.

■ **KEEP A ONE-TRACK MIND.** Those 3-, 4-, and 5-track razors are double trouble. The first blade cuts and sharpens the hair; the second blade cuts below the skin level, Dr. Litt says. The result: The sharpened hair curls around and slips back into the skin. Instead, use a single-track razor and settle for a shave that isn't as close.

■ **TRAIN YOUR WHISKERS.** Does your beard grow in several directions? Dr. Litt advises you to train it to grow out straight. Do this by shaving in two directions: down on the face, and up on the neck (to prevent neck nicks). Don't shave in all kinds of different directions or back and forth. "You won't get as great a shave at first," he says, "but if you keep shaving down on the face and up on the neck, your beard should start growing out straight in a matter of months."

■ **TRY THE AFTERSHAVE SPECIAL.** Put a damp towel on your face for a few minutes after shaving, Dr. Basler says. "It softens the whiskers so they're less able to repenetrate the skin." Use a creamy aftershave lotion, not the typical alcohol-loaded aftershave splash. "It's soothing and keeps the hair moisturized," he says.

■ **FIGHT INFECTION.** If a whisker burrows inside your skin despite your best efforts, you can cut down on the amount of bacteria it carries with it. A 10 percent benzoyl peroxide solution has some antibiotic effect, Dr. Basler says, and probably will help if used as an aftershave. Typical aftershaves contain lots of alcohol and may also help decrease the bacterial load.

■ **LADIES, SHAVE DOWN INSTEAD OF UP.** "Women typically shave their legs from ankle to knee," Dr. Litt says. This is against the grain and can cause ingrown hairs. Instead, shave down, from knee to ankle.

PANEL OF ADVISORS

RODNEY BASLER, M.D., IS A DERMATOLOGIST AND ASSOCIATE PROFESSOR OF INTERNAL MEDICINE AT THE UNIVERSITY OF NEBRASKA COLLEGE OF MEDICINE IN LINCOLN.

JEROME Z. LITT, M.D., IS A DERMATOLOGIST AND ASSISTANT CLINICAL PROFESSOR OF DERMATOLOGY AT CASE WESTERN RESERVE UNIVERSITY SCHOOL OF MEDICINE IN CLEVELAND AND AUTHOR OF *YOUR SKIN: FROM ACNE TO ZITS* AND *CURIOUS, ODD, RARE AND ABNORMAL REACTIONS TO MEDICATIONS.*

Ingrown Nails

7 Feet-Treating Methods

Few things so small drive a man or woman to distraction more than an ingrown nail. The pain can bedevil even the most placid people. How can a minor problem hurt so much?

Ingrown nails typically start when a nail—usually on the big toe—grows or is pushed into the soft, tender tissue alongside it. People whose toenails are somewhat convex are more susceptible, but anyone can get one. The result: a red, painful, tender toe.

Although the long-term goal is to prevent future ingrown nails, the overriding immediate need of most folks is to soothe the pain. Here's how to accomplish both.

■ **TRY AN OVER-THE-COUNTER PRODUCT.** There are a variety of nonprescription products that may soften the nail and the skin around it. Many of them include anti-inflammatory agents, such as tea tree oil, menthol, and other botanicals, says Wilma Bergfeld, M.D. Other over-the-counter products contain chemicals, such as salicylic acid, to soften the nail plate and relieve the pain. Dr. Scholl's Ingrown Toenail Relief Strips and Outgro Solution are two products that may help. Make sure you read and follow all of the directions to the letter. *Don't* use them if you have diabetes, impaired circulation, or an infection.

■ **GET A WISP OF RELIEF.** Your mission is to help that embedded toenail grow out over the skin folds at its side. Start by soaking your foot in warm water to soften the nail (add 1 teaspoon of table salt for every pint of water). Dry carefully, then gently insert a *wisp* (not a wad) of sterile cotton beneath the

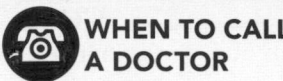

WHEN TO CALL A DOCTOR

If your toe becomes infected, you need to see a doctor. Signs to look for include swelling, redness, pain, and warmth when touched. Pus-filled blisters may also form. The doctor will most likely treat your infection with soaks, removal of infected skin, and antibiotics, says Wilma Bergfeld, M.D.

Letting an ingrown nail get out of control spells serious trouble. If you have poor circulation, a nail infection can ultimately lead to gangrene.

Sometimes a bloody growth, called proud flesh, builds up on the side of the nail. This inflamed soft tissue can become quite sensitive when it extends into the nail groove. Doctors may cut away a small portion of the ingrown nail during a minor operation and prescribe antibiotics to fight infection.

Protect Those Toes from Accidents

While ingrown nails come mostly from improper cutting, they can also result from any number of accidents. Stubbing your toe is one cause. Dropping a heavy object on your toe is yet another.

Wear stout, comfortable shoes for housework. If you constantly handle heavy objects, such as machinery and crates at work, protect your toes with work shoes that have steel toeboxes.

burrowing edge of the nail. The cotton will slightly lift the nail so that it can grow past the sore skin. Apply an antiseptic as a safeguard against infection. Be sure to change the cotton insert daily until the nail has grown past the trouble spot.

■ **REMEMBER: V IS *NOT* FOR VICTORY.** Whatever you do, don't fall for that old wives' tale about cutting a V-shaped wedge out of the center of the nail. People think that an ingrown nail is too big and that if you take a wedge from the middle, the sides will grow toward the center and away from the ingrown edge. However, that's simply not true. All nails grow from back to front.

■ **LET YOUR TOES BREATHE.** Simply put, ill-fitting footwear can cause an ingrown nail, especially if your nails tend to curve. This is why you should avoid pointed or tight shoes that press on toenails. Opt instead for sandals, where appropriate, or wide-toed shoes. If necessary, modify offending shoes by cutting out the portion that presses on your toe. That may seem a little drastic, but a badly ingrown nail will put you in a drastic mood. Likewise, stay away from tight socks and panty hose.

■ **STAY ON YOUR TOES WHEN SHOE SHOP-PING.** Buying properly fitted shoes can spare you from toenail woes. Keep these feet-friendly guidelines in mind:

1. Shop in the p.m. hours when feet are at their largest. Shoes that are purchased in the morning when your feet aren't swollen may be too tight later in the day.

2. Wear soft absorbent socks to allow for a roomy, comfortable fit.

3. Opt for shoes made of breathable material, such as canvas or leather.

4. Choose a shock-absorbent sole to reduce pressure on the toes.

■ **CUT NAILS WITH PRECISION.** Never cut your nails too short. Soften them first in warm water to reduce possible splitting, then cut straight across with a substantial, sharp, straight-edged clipper. Never cut a nail in an oval shape, which causes the leading edge to curve down into the skin at the sides. Always leave the outside edges parallel to the skin. And don't trim the nail any deeper than the tip of the toe; you want it toenail long enough to protect the toe from pressure and friction.

If your nails are thick and difficult to cut properly, apply a cream that contains urea or lactic acid. (Your pharmacist can recommend one.) These ingredients make the nail softer and easier to trim.

■ **FIX MISTAKES PROPERLY.** If you accidentally cut or break a nail too short, carefully smooth it with an emery board or nail file at the edges so that no sharp points are left to penetrate the skin. Don't be tempted to use scissors, no matter how small. There is simply not enough space for you to work them properly, and they often leave a sharp edge.

PANEL OF ADVISORS

WILMA BERGFELD, M.D., IS A SENIOR DERMATOLOGIST IN THE DEPARTMENTS OF DERMATOLOGY AND PATHOLOGY AT THE CLEVELAND CLINIC IN OHIO.

Insomnia

23 Steps to a Good Night's Sleep

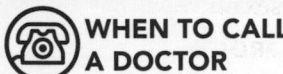
WHEN TO CALL A DOCTOR

Serious sleeping troubles sometimes can result in what experts call chronic insomnia, which could be caused by psychiatric disturbances, breathing problems, or unexplained leg movements during the middle of the night. Experts agree that if you can't easily fall asleep or stay asleep throughout the night for a month or so, it may be time to consult an expert.

According to the American Sleep Disorders Association, a doctor will diagnosis insomnia based on your medical history, sleep history, and possibly a sleep study. If your doctor can't offer any advice, have her recommend a sleep-disorders specialist.

Insomnia ranks right behind the common cold, stomach disorders, and headaches as the reasons people seek a doctor's help. The Centers for Disease Control and Prevention report that more than 25 percent of Americans say they don't get an adequate amount of sleep, and 10 percent experience chronic insomnia.

At one time, doctors might have automatically prescribed a pill or two to ease you into dreamland, but that isn't always the case today. Researchers and doctors are learning more about sleep each year, broadening their knowledge of how to deal with its related problems.

Indeed, behavioral treatments are often most effective. There are also quite a few commonsense approaches that you can use to try to correct the problem yourself. It may take just one therapy, or it may take a combination. In any case, the key to success is discipline. As Michael Stevenson, Ph.D., says, "Sleep is a natural physiological phenomenon, but it's also a learned behavior."

■ **SET A RIGID SLEEP SCHEDULE 7 DAYS A WEEK.** Sleep medicine experts insist on people trying to be as regular with their habits as possible. Be sure to wake up at the same time every morning. And don't sleep in, trying to make up for "lost" sleep, says Mortimer Mamelak, M.D. This goes for the weekends as well. Don't sleep late on Saturday and Sunday mornings. If you do, you may have trouble falling asleep Sunday night, which can leave you feeling washed out on Monday morning.

■ **DON'T WASTE YOUR TIME IN BED.** Don't stay in bed if you can't sleep. Get out of bed, relax, and sit quietly for a while before returning to the bedroom. By spending too much time in bed awake you prolong the cycle of insomnia. You need to learn to associate your bedroom with sleep, not with lying awake for hours, says Dr. Stevenson.

■ **SET ASIDE SOME "QUIET TIME" BEFORE BED.** "Some people are so busy that when they lie down to go to sleep, it's the first time all day that they've had to think about what happened that day," says David Neubauer, M.D.

An hour or two before bedtime, sit down for at least 10 minutes. Reflect on the day's activities and try to put them into some perspective. Review your stresses and strains, as well as your problems. Try to work out solutions. Plan tomorrow's activities.

This exercise may help clear your mind of the annoyances and problems that might keep you awake once you pull up the covers. With all that mental detritus out of the way, it's easier to fill your mind with pleasant thoughts and images as you try to drift off to sleep. If, for some reason, cold reality begins to seep into your conscience, shut it out by saying, "Oh, I've already dealt with that, and I know what I'm going to do about it."

■ **DON'T TURN YOUR BED INTO AN OFFICE OR A DEN.** "If you want to go to bed, you should be prepared to sleep," says Magdi Soliman, Ph.D. "If there's something else to do, you won't be able to concentrate on sleep."

Don't watch TV, talk on the phone, argue with your spouse, read anything, eat anything, or perform mundane tasks in bed. Use your bedroom for sleep and sex only.

■ **KEEP YOUR BEDROOM AS DARK AS POSSIBLE.** "Darkness helps our brain understand that it's time to sleep," says Sonia Ancoli-Israel, Ph.D. Black-out curtains can help block the sunlight. Install a night-light to help guide you to the bathroom, she says.

■ **DON'T WATCH THE CLOCK.** Looking at the clock puts a time pressure on you and, in the middle of the night, actually wakes you up more and makes it harder to fall back to sleep, says Dr. Ancoli-Israel. Turn the clock face away from you so you aren't tempted to look at it, but you can still hear the alarm, she says. Also, cover the clock on the TV.

■ **AVOID "PICK-ME-UPS" AFTER TWILIGHT.** Coffee, colas, and even chocolate contain caffeine, the powerful stimulant that can keep you up, says Dr. Neubauer. Try not to consume them after 4:00 p.m. Don't smoke either; nicotine is a stimulant.

Other foods can cause acid reflux or heartburn, which occurs when stomach acids back up into the esophagus. Avoid foods most likely to cause reflux when you lie down, such as citrus fruits, fatty and fried foods, garlic, onions, mint, and tomato-based foods. (For more anti-heartburn strategies, see page 313.)

■ **SAY NO TO A NIGHTCAP.** Avoid excessive alcohol at dinner and throughout the rest of the evening, suggests Dr. Stevenson. And don't fix a nightcap to relax you before bed. Alcohol may help you fall asleep, but it later disrupts your sleep by causing you to awaken.

■ **QUESTION YOUR MEDICATION.** Certain medications, such as asthma sprays, can disturb sleep. If you take prescription medication routinely, ask your doctor about the side effects. If your doctor suspects that a drug could be interfering with your sleep, she may change the time of day you take it, or replace it with another medication.

■ **BYPASS SEDATIVES.** If you are in pain before bedtime, resist the urge to take a sedative or hypnotic medication. Although they increase your sleep time, they also decrease the quality of your sleep. You should take a non-narcotic analgesic such as acetaminophen instead, says Dr. Soliman.

■ **EXAMINE YOUR WORK SCHEDULE.** Research has shown that people who work on "swing" shifts—irregular schedules that frequently alternate from day to night—have problems sleeping, says Dr. Mamelak. The stress of an up-and-down schedule may create jet lag–like tiredness all the time, and sleep mechanisms can break down altogether. The solution: Try to get consistent shift hours, even if it's at night.

■ **CREATE A COMFORTABLE SETTING.** "Insomnia can often be caused by stress," says Dr. Stevenson. "When you get into bed, and you're nervous and anxious, your nervous system is aroused, impairing your ability to sleep. Soon, your bedroom becomes associated with sleeplessness, so when you go to bed an arousal is triggered instead of sleepiness." Wind down before bed, and then go to bed when you are sleepy.

Make your bedroom comfortable. Redecorate with your favorite colors. Make it as soundproof as possible, and hang dark curtains to keep out the sunlight.

Buy a comfortable bed. It doesn't matter whether it's a coiled-spring mattress, a waterbed, a vibrating bed, or a mat on the floor. If it feels good, use it. Wear loose-fitting sleep clothes. Make sure the bedroom's temperature is just right—not too hot, not too cold—and that it's not stuffy, says Dr. Soliman. Adequate oxygen promotes restorative sleep. Be sure there's no clock within view that can distract you throughout the night.

■ **TURN OFF YOUR MIND.** Keep yourself from rehashing a stressful day of worries by focusing your thoughts on something peaceful and nonthreatening, says Dr. Stevenson. Play some soft, soothing music as you drift off or some environmental noise, such as the sound of a waterfall, waves crashing on a beach, or the sound of rain in a jungle. The only rule: Be sure it's not intrusive and distracting.

■ **USE MECHANICAL AIDS.** Earplugs can help block out unwanted noise, especially if you live on a busy street or near an airport,

Light Up Your Life

Researchers at the National Institute of Mental Health (NIMH) found that bright lights in the morning could help chronically poor sleepers set their circadian rhythms, or "body clocks," on a more regular pattern.

According to Jean R. Joseph-Vanderpool, M.D., who conducted sleep research there for many years, some people find they just can't get started in the morning.

This is why when his research subjects awoke, say, around 8:00 a.m., they were placed in front of high-intensity, full-spectrum fluorescent lights for 2 hours—strong light that resembles what you might encounter on a summer morning in Washington, D.C. Those lights, in turn, told the body it's morning and time to get moving. Then, in the evening, they would wear dark glasses so that their bodies would know it was time to begin to wind down.

After several weeks of the therapy, Dr. Joseph-Vanderpool's patients reported more alertness in the morning and better sleep at night. In addition, their moods improved and they had fewer cravings for sweets.

At home, he says, you can accomplish the same effect by walking around the neighborhood, sitting in the sun, or doing some yard work as soon as you arise. During the winter, consult your doctor about the best type of artificial light to use.

says Dr. Ancoli-Israel. Eyeshades screen out unwanted light. An electric blanket warms you, especially if you're a person who always seems to be on the brink of a chill.

■ **LEARN AND PRACTICE RELAXATION TECHNIQUES.** The harder you try to sleep, the greater the chances that you'll end up gnashing your teeth all night rather than stacking some Zzzs. That's why it's so important to relax once you're in bed.

"People often concentrate too much on their sleep and try too hard," Dr. Stevenson says. "The key to successfully falling asleep is to focus on becoming more relaxed and *let* sleep happen to you instead of trying to *make* it happen to you."

Biofeedback exercises, deep breathing, muscle stretches, or yoga may help. Special audiotapes can teach you how to progressively relax your muscles.

Here are two techniques that doctors have found particularly successful.

■ Slow down your breathing and imagine the air moving in and out of your lungs as you breathe from your belly. Practice this during the day so it's second nature once you're in bed.

■ Program yourself to turn off unpleasant thoughts as they creep into your mind. To do this, think about enjoyable

The Herbal Approach

Help for insomnia may be as close as the herbal aisle of your grocery store. Here are a few herbs to try.

Valerian. This herb has been used for centuries to combat insomnia. Valerian is the most studied herbal remedy for insomnia, says David Neubauer, M.D. Research shows that extracts of the root are an effective treatment for mild to moderately severe insomnia. It not only helps you fall asleep faster but also improves sleep quality. Try taking one or two 350- to 450-milligram capsules about 30 minutes before bedtime.

Lemon balm. The lemony-smelling leaves and pretty white flowers appear to produce relaxing effects. In one small preliminary study, extracts of lemon balm and valerian improved the quality of sleep in much the same way as a sleeping drug called triazolam (Halcion) does. Steep ⅓ to 1 teaspoon of the dried herb for 10 to 15 minutes in 5 ounces of boiling water, and then drink the tea about an hour before bedtime.

Chamomile. A bright, daisylike flower, chamomile has an age-old reputation for calming nerves and gently aiding sleep. Drinking one or two cups of tea before bed will help soothe you into sleep.

Lavender oil. The essential oil of lavender contains linalool, which helps give lavender its distinct smell. The oil's odor is thought to be calming, and so may be helpful in cases of insomnia. One study of elderly people with sleeping troubles found that inhaling lavender oil was as effective as some commonly prescribed sleep medications. Similar results were seen in another trial that included young and middle-aged people with insomnia. Sprinkle a few drops of pure essential oil onto a piece of tissue and tuck it under your pillow, or use an aromatherapy diffuser.

experiences. Reminisce about good times, fantasize, or play some mental games. Try counting sheep or counting backward from 1,000—by 7s.

■ **TAKE A WARM BATH.** One theory suggests that normal body temperatures play off the body's circadian rhythm. Those temperatures are low during sleep and at their highest point during the day.

Along these lines, it's thought that the body begins to get drowsy as temperature drops. So taking a warm bath just a few hours before bedtime raises that temperature, says Dr. Neubauer. Then, when it begins to drop, you'll feel more tired, which makes it easier for you to fall asleep.

■ **MAKE SOME NOISE.** White noise, that is. Listening to a TV or radio when trying to sleep usually isn't helpful, but many people find that they sleep better when there is some white noise from a sound-generating device or from a bedside fan. White noise can be soothing and help block out extraneous sounds, such as neighborhood noise and traffic, says Dr. Neubauer.

■ **TAKE A HIKE.** Get some exercise late in the afternoon or early in the evening, says Dr. Neubauer and Dr. Soliman. It shouldn't be too strenuous—a walk around the block is just fine. Not only will it fatigue your muscles but it will also raise your body temperature, and it may help induce sleepiness as a warm bath would. Exercise may help trigger the deep, nourishing sleep that your body craves most for replenishment. An evening stroll about 2 hours before bedtime also decreases and can even prevent "restless leg syndrome," which is the reason many people to lose sleep to begin with, especially the elderly, says Dr. Soliman.

PANEL OF ADVISORS

SONIA ANCOLI-ISRAEL, PH.D., IS A PSYCHOLOGIST, A PROFESSOR IN THE DEPARTMENT OF PSYCHIATRY AT THE UNIVERSITY OF CALIFORNIA AT SAN DIEGO, SCHOOL OF MEDICINE, AND THE DIRECTOR OF THE UNIVERSITY OF CALIFORNIA AT SAN DIEGO GILLIN LABORATORY OF SLEEP AND CHRONOBIOLOGY.

JEAN R. JOSEPH-VANDERPOOL, M.D., IS CHIEF MEDICAL OFFICER OF SUNWEST BEHAVIORAL HEALTH ORGANIZATION IN EL PASO, TEXAS.

MORTIMER MAMELAK, M.D., IS DIRECTOR OF THE SLEEP DISORDERS CLINIC AT BAYCREST HOSPITAL AT THE UNIVERSITY OF TORONTO.

DAVID NEUBAUER, M.D., IS ASSOCIATE DIRECTOR AT THE JOHNS HOPKINS SLEEP DISORDERS CENTER IN BALTIMORE. HE IS ALSO A GENERAL PSYCHIATRIST IN THE DEPARTMENT OF PSYCHIATRY AT THE JOHNS HOPKINS UNIVERSITY, ALSO IN BALTIMORE.

MAGDI SOLIMAN, PH.D., IS A PROFESSOR OF NEUROPHARMACOLOGY AT FLORIDA A&M UNIVERSITY COLLEGE OF PHARMACY IN TALLAHASSEE, FLORIDA.

MICHAEL STEVENSON, PH.D., IS A PSYCHOLOGIST AND CLINICAL DIRECTOR OF THE NORTH VALLEY SLEEP DISORDERS CENTER IN MISSION HILLS, CALIFORNIA.

Irritable Bowel Syndrome

19 Coping Suggestions

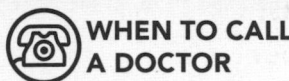 **WHEN TO CALL A DOCTOR**

Diarrhea, constipation, and bloating, especially when accompanied by abdominal pain that seems aggravated in stressful situations and relieved by passing stools, are the cardinal signs of irritable bowel syndrome.

While these symptoms can occur commonly in many individuals, when you find that they are limiting your activities or making you feel depressed or anxious, it's time to see your doctor for proper treatment. Other symptoms may indicate a more serious condition. See your doctor if you have:

- Blood in your stool
- Unexplained weight loss
- Diarrhea or urinary incontinence that causes you to wake up at night
- Diarrhea or urinary incontinence that cause you to have "accidents"
- Constipation, diarrhea, abdominal pain, or any combination of the three so severe that you can't work for several days or engage in social activities

Many people with irritable bowel syndrome, or IBS, develop a sixth sense about public restrooms. They know where to find one in a hurry and are used to leaving a table of friends at dinner or a sale at Bloomingdale's to dash to the bathroom.

Doctors aren't sure what causes IBS, but many believe it's a combination of factors, including muscle contraction or "motility" disturbance, and increased sensitivity of nerves in the digestive tract. The walls of the intestines are lined with layers of muscles that contract and relax as they move food from the stomach through the intestinal tract. In people who don't have IBS, the muscles contract and relax in regular rhythm. In people with IBS, the muscle contractions in the intestines can be stronger, producing diarrhea or constipation, and, in addition, the nerves fire more strongly, producing pain.

Another theory blames an overgrowth of intestinal bacteria. Some IBS patients were thought to have a condition known as "small intestine bacterial overgrowth," in which the bacteria that normally live in the colon somehow find their way into the relatively sterile small intestine. Now we know that there may not necessarily be an overgrowth of bacteria as much as replacement of "good" bacteria with "bad" bacteria, which can affect the motility and sensitivity of the nerves.

The upshot of coping with IBS means identifying the food,

drinks, or stressful events that trigger alternating bouts of diarrhea, constipation, and abdominal pain. Sometimes people with IBS get all three at the same time. A sense of bloating or fullness and mucus in the stool are some of the other complaints.

Some doctors think that IBS may be second only to the common cold as America's most widespread medical complaint. Yet there's plenty of good news: For one, IBS does not appear to raise your risk for colorectal cancer. And IBS doesn't trigger changes in the bowel tissue or cause inflammation. After a diagnosis of IBS, the following tips can ease symptoms and discomfort.

■ **TAKE THE NEWS IN STRIDE.** "There's a very good connection between stress and an irritable bowel," says Douglas A. Drossman, M.D. Overly anxious and driven people are prone to IBS, according to a study published in the *British Medical Journal*. Researchers studied more than 600 people who had gastroenteritis (a condition that can lead to IBS). Six months later the people who had developed IBS were significantly more likely to report high levels of stress and a more pessimistic view of illness than those who didn't develop IBS.

What you don't want to do to yourself is get stressed *because* you have an irritable bowel, which then just creates a vicious cycle. Especially during flare-ups of abdominal pain, it's important to take a deep breath.

"Think about what's happening. Recognize that it's happened before and it will pass. Once you've had an evaluation and are given a diagnosis of IBS by your physician, give up your fears of cancer or other serious diseases. People don't die from an irritable bowel, and these symptoms are far more typical of IBS than anything else," he says.

■ **BECOME A MORE RELAXED PERSON.** Anything you can do to help yourself unwind should help to alleviate your symptoms, says Dr. Drossman. You may benefit from relaxation techniques, such as meditation, self-hypnosis, or biofeedback. If the stress in your life is particularly problematic, consider psychological counseling. The key is to find what best works for *you*.

■ **KEEP A STRESS DIARY.** People with an irritable bowel have an intestinal system that overreacts to food, stress, and hormonal changes. "Think of your irritable bowel as a built-in barometer, and use it to help you determine what things in your life are most stressful," says Dr. Drossman. If, for instance, you have stomach pain every time you talk to your boss, see it as a sign that you need to work on that relationship (perhaps by talking it over with your boss, a friend, a family member, or a therapist). Keep a written record of your symptoms for a week or two, taking note of what was happening just before the pain began and see if any patterns emerge.

■ **LOG IN YOUR FOOD AND BEVERAGE INTAKE, TOO.** Certain foods and beverages, just like stress, can activate an irritable bowel, so also record in your diary the foods and beverages that give you the most trouble, says Dr. Drossman.

Make note of what you eat during the day, the symptoms you have, when these symptoms occur, and what foods cause you to feel ill. Tracking your diet will help you identify foods that trigger your IBS.

■ **ADD FIBER TO YOUR DIET.** Many people with IBS do much better simply by adding fiber to their diets. Fiber is more effective with those who tend to have constipation. A diet that's high in fiber keeps the colon mildly distended, which may prevent spasms. Some types of fiber draw water into the stool, so passing stools is easier. Experts recommend a diet that will keep bowel movements soft and painless to pass. The best fiber to add to your diet is the insoluble type—found in bran, whole grains, fruit, and vegetables. High-fiber foods can cause bloating and gas, but for some people those symptoms go away after a few weeks. Increasing your fiber intake by 2 to 3 grams should make those problems less likely, according to the National Digestive Diseases Information Clearinghouse.

■ **SEND PSYLLIUM SEED TO THE RESCUE.** If you need to treat symptoms of constipation with your IBS, you can increase your fiber intake with crushed psyllium seed, says Dr. Drossman. It's a natural laxative sold in drugstores, supermarkets, and health food stores. Unlike chemical laxatives often found on the same shelves, psyllium-based laxatives such as Metamucil and Konsyl are nonaddictive and generally safe, even when taken over long periods. Keep in mind that laxatives only treat the constipation, not the pain, which is usually manageable. In some cases you may need to see your doctor for medication to treat the pain, advises Dr. Drossman.

■ **DRINK LOTS OF FLUIDS.** To keep your bowels moving smoothly, you need not only fiber but also fluids, especially if you have diarrhea. You'll need more on August days when you play tennis than on December days that you spend at the movies, but in general, you should drink between six and eight glasses of fluid a day.

■ **TURN TO YOGURT.** Scientists have long known that bacteria play an important role in maintaining your health. Probiotics, or foods that contain beneficial bacteria, will someday be recognized as "a new essential food group," predicts Gary Huffnagle, Ph.D. "I believe we'll eventually have research-based minimum daily requirements for probiotics," he says, "just as we do for many vitamins and minerals." Adding a probiotic, such as yogurt, to your diet may help alleviate some of the symptoms of IBS. Research

Visualize Yourself Pain-Free

It's normal to panic during an attack of abdominal pain. But ironically, stress makes the pain worse by tensing the bowel.

How can you break this nasty cycle?

With visualization, says Donna Copeland, Ph.D. It's a very effective tool for dealing with pain and anxiety, she says. Learning visualization techniques with a professional is probably the best route. But there's nothing wrong with trying on your own.

Dr. Copeland suggests the following: If you feel pain, stop what you're doing, find a comfortable place to sit or lie down, close your eyes, and—instead of focusing on your pain—see yourself:

- Diving expertly into the warm ocean surf off a beautiful, white-sand tropical beach

- Standing atop a tall, snow-crested mountain, breathing the cool air, and listening to the crunch of snow under your feet

- Sitting in a large hot tub, chatting idly with several of your closest friends

- Walking through a lush garden in a far-off, exotic land

shows that the bacteria in many types of yogurt can lessen the gas, pain, and bloating that IBS causes. Lactobacilli and bifidobacteria hold the most promise, so look for yogurts containing these bacteria. If you have a lactose or milk intolerance, then try a probiotic supplement, says Dr. Huffnagle. Although probiotics are generally considered safe, discuss them with your doctor before using them to treat IBS.

■ **RECONSIDER DAIRY PRODUCTS.** One fluid you may be better off without is milk. "A large number of people who say they have IBS are really lactose intolerant," says William J. Snape Jr., M.D. It means that your body has difficulty absorbing lactose, an enzyme found in milk. Your doctor can test you for lactose intolerance, or you can give up dairy products for a couple of days and see how you do. In either case, you may find that this one dietary change can clear up all your problems. (For more information on lactose intolerance, see page 391.)

■ **CUT OUT THE FAT.** Here's one more good reason to eat a low-fat diet. "Fat is a major stimulus to colonic contractions," says Dr. Snape. In other words, it can worsen your IBS. A good place to begin to cut the fat out of your diet is by eliminating heavy sauces, fried foods, and salad oils, he says.

■ **BEWARE OF SPICY FOODS.** Some people with IBS are sensitive to foods laden with peppers and other spices. In fact, preliminary research shows that the nerve fibers in people with IBS send more pain signals to the brain when they eat chile peppers and other spicy foods than people without IBS.

■ **DON'T BREW TROUBLE.** Coffee is a major cause of woe among people with IBS, says Dr. Snape. To some extent, the culprit may be caffeine, but it may also be the resins in the coffee bean itself. You may get some relief if you switch to decaffeinated. If you don't, try cutting down on all coffee.

■ **RECONSIDER ALCOHOL.** Alcoholic beverages can exacerbate your problems, but it's probably not the alcohol itself, says Dr. Snape. Rather, it's the complex carbohydrates in beer and the tannins in red wine that probably cause the most grief. People with IBS should avoid these two drinks, he says.

■ **PUT OUT THAT CIGARETTE.** "A large number of people experience IBS problems with smoking," says Dr. Snape. The most probable culprit is the nicotine of your cigarettes, so if you're trying to quit with the help of nicotine gum, you may not see any difference in your tummy problems.

■ **SPIT OUT THE GUM.** Gums and candies artificially sweetened with sorbitol are not easily digested and can worsen your IBS, says Dr. Drossman. While the amount of sorbitol found in one stick of gum or one hard candy isn't likely to affect you greatly, if you gobble up 10 or more pieces a day, it's time to cut back.

■ **EAT REGULAR MEALS.** It's not only *what* you eat, but *how* you eat that can vex an irritable bowel, says Dr. Snape. Digesting a lot of food eaten all at once overstimulates the digestive system. That is why it's much better to eat frequent small meals rather than to ingest infrequent large ones.

■ **GO FOR A JOG.** Exercise strengthens the entire body, including the bowel. It helps relieve stress, and it releases endorphins that help you control pain. All in all, regular exercise will more than likely calm your irritable bowel. Be careful, however, not to overdo it. Oddly enough, too much exercise can lead to diarrhea.

■ **CALL A HOT-WATER BOTTLE TO THE RESCUE.** If you experience abdominal pain, the best thing to do is to sit or lie down, take a deep breath, and try to relax. Some people have discovered that putting a hot-water bottle or a heating pad directly on their tummy helps, says Dr. Snape.

PANEL OF ADVISORS

DONNA COPELAND, PH.D., IS A RETIRED PROFESSOR OF PEDIATRICS (PSYCHOLOGY) AND CHIEF OF THE BEHAVIORAL MEDICINE SECTION AT THE UNIVERSITY OF TEXAS M. D. ANDERSON CANCER CENTER IN HOUSTON. SHE IS ALSO A CLINICAL PSYCHOLOGIST AND PAST PRESIDENT OF THE AMERICAN PSYCHOLOGICAL ASSOCIATION'S DIVISION OF PSYCHOLOGICAL HYPNOSIS.

DOUGLAS A. DROSSMAN, M.D., IS A PROFESSOR OF MEDICINE AND PSYCHIATRY, AND CODIRECTOR OF THE UNIVERSITY OF NORTH CAROLINA CENTER FOR FUNCTIONAL GI AND MOTILITY DISORDERS AT CHAPEL HILL.

GARY HUFFNAGLE, PH.D., IS A PROFESSOR OF INTERNAL MEDICINE AT THE UNIVERSITY OF MICHIGAN MEDICAL SCHOOL IN ANN ARBOR AND A PROMINENT PROBIOTICS RESEARCHER.

WILLIAM J. SNAPE JR., M.D., IS THE DIRECTOR OF NEUROGASTROENTEROLOGY AND MOTILITY AT CALIFORNIA PACIFIC MEDICAL CENTER IN SAN FRANCISCO.

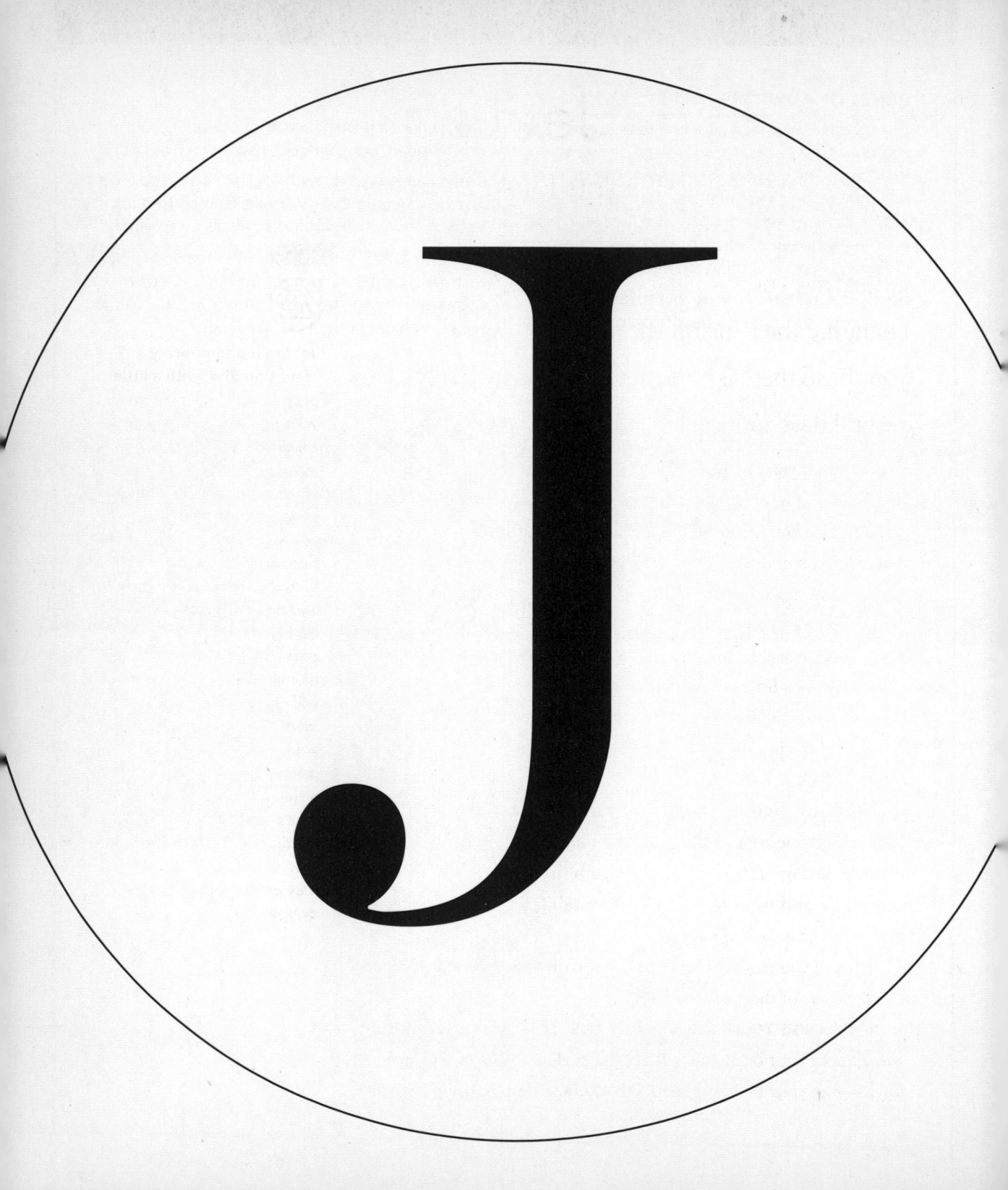

Jet Lag

17 Hints for Arriving Alert

Adjusting your inner body clock isn't as easy as changing the time on the clock on the wall. Inside your head there is a master clock that actually takes several days to reset.

Yet when you fly across several time zones, you ask your body to adjust to a new time and a new place. Your body takes about 1 day per time zone crossed to reset itself, and adjusts slightly faster when you travel west. This difference between clock time and your body's time is why you get jet lag. And the more time zones you cross, the more you suffer.

Although we often speak of a single inner clock, your body really has a whole set of clocks controlled by a main clock. "Every cell in the body is like a clock and they all set themselves according to signals they receive from the brain," says Timothy Monk, Ph.D.

Normally, your body clock cycles on the 24-hour rotation of your home time zone. But rapid time changes disrupt all that. The result is jet lag—fatigue, lethargy, inability to sleep, trouble concentrating and making decisions, irritability, and perhaps even diarrhea and a lack of appetite.

Though you can't make time stand still, there's a lot you *can* do to take some of the zap out of jet lag.

■ **CHANGE YOUR SLEEP PATTERNS.** If you're traveling eastward, move your bedtime up and rise earlier in the morning a few days before your trip, suggests Dr. Monk. If you're traveling west,

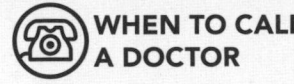
WHEN TO CALL A DOCTOR

Jet lag is a temporary condition that, with a little preparation and changes in your pre- and post-travel routine, is fairly easily for most people to overcome. Some travelers, however, have a harder time adjusting to time zone shifts than others.

If you travel frequently and have difficulty establishing a routine sleep pattern, go see your doctor or a sleep specialist. Either will likely review your medical history, analyze your medications, and perhaps ask you to keep a sleep diary. In a few cases, people are asked to participate in a sleep study test. A doctor or specialist may prescribe medications or light therapy.

Send Travel Stress Packing

That frustrating sleeplessness that travelers experience isn't always caused by out-of-sync body rhythms. Experts say that two types of travel-related stress, called "first-night effect" and "on-call effect," commonly throw a monkey wrench into the best "lie down" plans. First-night effect occurs when travelers can't adjust to a new or an unfamiliar environment. On-call effect amplifies concerns that sleep will be disturbed by a phone call, hallway noises, or other sounds. Here are some recommendations from the National Sleep Foundation that are designed to help you rest much easier:

Take it with you. Bring along small objects from home to give your room an element of familiarity and ease the transition to a new environment. Pack a coffee mug, family photo, favorite blanket, or something that reminds you of home.

Divert p.m. messages. If your hotel has voice mail services for guests, take advantage of it. Before bedtime, have your phone calls transferred to voice mail.

Check out your room. Foil possible disturbances before they happen. Make sure your curtains are closed to block out morning rays, use your Do Not Disturb sign, and set heating or air conditioning temperatures to avoid a middle-of-the-night adjustment.

delay your bedtime and sleep a little later in the morning. This will help your internal clock adjust to a new time zone.

■ **CONSIDER A SUPPLEMENT.** Melatonin supplements may help overcome symptoms of jet lag in travelers crossing five time zones or more. Melatonin, a natural hormone produced by your body, signals the part of your brain that regulates the sleep-wake cycle. While the effectiveness of melatonin supplements require more study, the Centers for Disease Control and Prevention says that they are generally considered safe. The does you take depends on the severity of sleep problmes and health conditions. Talk to your doctor before using melatonin.

■ **TIME YOUR FLIGHT CAREFULLY.** Try to book a flight that lands in the early evening. "If this isn't possible, after landing try to remain awake until 10 p.m. local time," says Dr. Monk. "If sleep is irresistible, take a short nap in the afternoon, no more than 2 hours, and set an alarm clock."

Doing this gives your body optimal opportunity to adjust to the change in time zones, says Dr. Monk.

■ **RESERVE A SEAT IN THE SUN.** This will depend on the time of day you're flying, as well as the direction. But the extra sun exposure will help get your body's "master clock" in sync with your new time zone.

■ **SET YOUR WATCH.** When your plane takes off, change your wristwatch to the time zone of your destination, says Dr. Monk. Just this one simple move will remind you of your new schedule and help you stick to it.

■ **STAY ACTIVE IN-FLIGHT.** You'll feel more refreshed once you land if you move around a bit while you're en route to your destination. Take a walk to the back of the plane, stop and do a few deep knee bends, then return to your seat. Or stay in your seat and stretch as best you can. You also might try squeezing a ball in the palm of your hand or pressing your hands together in front of your chest.

■ **DRINK PLENTY OF FLUIDS.** Airplane cabins are notoriously dry, Dr. Monk says, and fluids help combat the dehydration that induces fatigue. Dehydration obviously won't help you beat jet lag.

■ **AVOID ALCOHOL.** Alcohol is a diuretic and further dehydrates you. Ask for juice or water instead.

■ **ADOPT GOOD SLEEP HYGIENE.** "It's important to recognize how fragile your sleep will be once you've arrived," says Dr. Monk. There are a few things you can do to ensure better sleep in your temporary digs that first night or two.

How Three Famous Globe-Trotters Tried to Cope

If you need a personal strategy for beating jet lag, check out tips from famous globe-trotters Henry Kissinger, Dwight D. Eisenhower, and Lyndon Johnson.

Take the diplomatic route. Several days before the flight, go to bed 1 hour earlier and get up 1 hour later. This was former secretary of state Henry Kissinger's routine. The problem with this plan, experts say, is the rigidity it demands. Kissinger couldn't always follow it consistently, and most people would probably have the same problem. There's also no proof that this approach measurably reduces jet lag.

Arrive extra early. President Eisenhower tried to arrive several days before a meeting with foreign leaders. The problem with Eisenhower's plan is that often he didn't arrive early enough to compensate for the one-time-zone-crossed-equals-one-day-of-adjustment rule.

Live by your home clock. After arriving at a new destination, President Lyndon Johnson insisted on maintaining his home schedule—eating and sleeping at his usual time. He even arranged meetings at hours that were convenient by Washington, D.C., time but not so convenient for the foreigner leaders with whom he was meeting.

Perhaps you can get away with this if you're the president of the United States, but for the average traveler, it may be hard to get dinner reservations for 2:00 a.m.—even in Paris.

- Remember to pack earplugs, and a night-light or a dim flashlight. You can use the earplugs to block out unfamiliar noises and other nighttime distractions. Use a night-light in place of jarring bright room lights, says Dr. Monk.

- Keep a small pack of (nonchocolate) cookies by the bed, just in case you wake up hungry in the middle of the night.

■ **GET BETTER SLEEPY-BYE TIME.** The quality of your sleep can be affected by things you eat or drink within 5 hours of bedtime. So abstain from caffeine, and eat and drink within moderation during that time period.

■ **DON'T PLAY CATCH-UP.** If you lose sleep because of the change in time zones, don't try to compensate for it by lingering in bed the next morning. You'll only feel worse. Instead, get up at the same hour that you usuallly do, but in your new time zone. So if you usually roll out of bed at 7:00 A.M. when you're at home, then set your alarm for 7:00 A.M. This will help coordinate your body clock with the actual time.

■ **SOAK UP SOME SUNSHINE.** Get out in the sun at your destination as much as possible, says Dr. Monk. This exposure sends a powerful message to your biological clock that it is now in a new time zone.

The eye has special light receptors that are specific for sending signals to the area of the brain in which the master clock resides. The clock then sends messages to other areas of the brain to stimulate wakefulness and activity.

■ **MAKE A DATE WItH THE SUN.** Some experts agree that the time of day you get out in the sunshine is also important. Light earlier in the day appears to shift the body's clock to an earlier hour, while light later in the day seems to shift the body's clock to a later hour, according to Al Lewy, M.D., Ph.D.

So if you've traveled east, Dr. Lewy suggests getting outside in the morning. And if you've traveled west, he recommends getting outside later in the afternoon. But keep in mind that this works only when you've crossed six or fewer time zones.

■ **EXERCISE.** Research suggests that westbound travelers may be able to reset their own circadian rhythms if they establish a workout routine once they arrive at their destination. Scientists at the University of Colorado, Boulder, and Harvard Medical School simulated the jet-lag conditions of a 9-hour time difference for 18 fit men. Half of the men did three 45-minute rounds on a stationary bike, while the other half of them didn't exercise at all. After comparing the hormone levels of the two groups, researchers discovered that the internal body clocks of the exercisers moved $3^1/_2$ hours closer to their new time zone, while the nonexercisers moved only $1^1/_2$ hours closer.

"Exercise can help reset the clock by providing an 'arousal signal,'" says Kenneth P. Wright, Ph.D. If you're traveling west, you might wish to try exercising 2 hours after your usual bedtime, says Dr. Wright.

■ **REVERSE THE PROCESS.** If possible, use these tips to prepare for your return flight home, too. Jet lag is a two-way sky.

PANEL OF ADVISORS

AL LEWY, M.D., PH.D., IS A PSYCHIATRIST AT OREGON HEALTH SCIENCES UNIVERSITY SCHOOL OF MEDICINE IN PORTLAND.

TIMOTHY MONK, PH.D., IS A PROFESSOR OF PSYCHIATRY AND DIRECTOR OF THE HUMAN CHRONOBIOLOGY RESEARCH PROGRAM AT THE UNIVERSITY OF PITTSBURGH SCHOOL OF MEDICINE.

KENNETH P. WRIGHT, PH.D., IS AN ASSISTANT PROFESSOR IN THE DEPARTMENT OF INTEGRATIVE PHYSIOLOGY AT THE UNIVERSITY OF COLORADO, BOULDER.

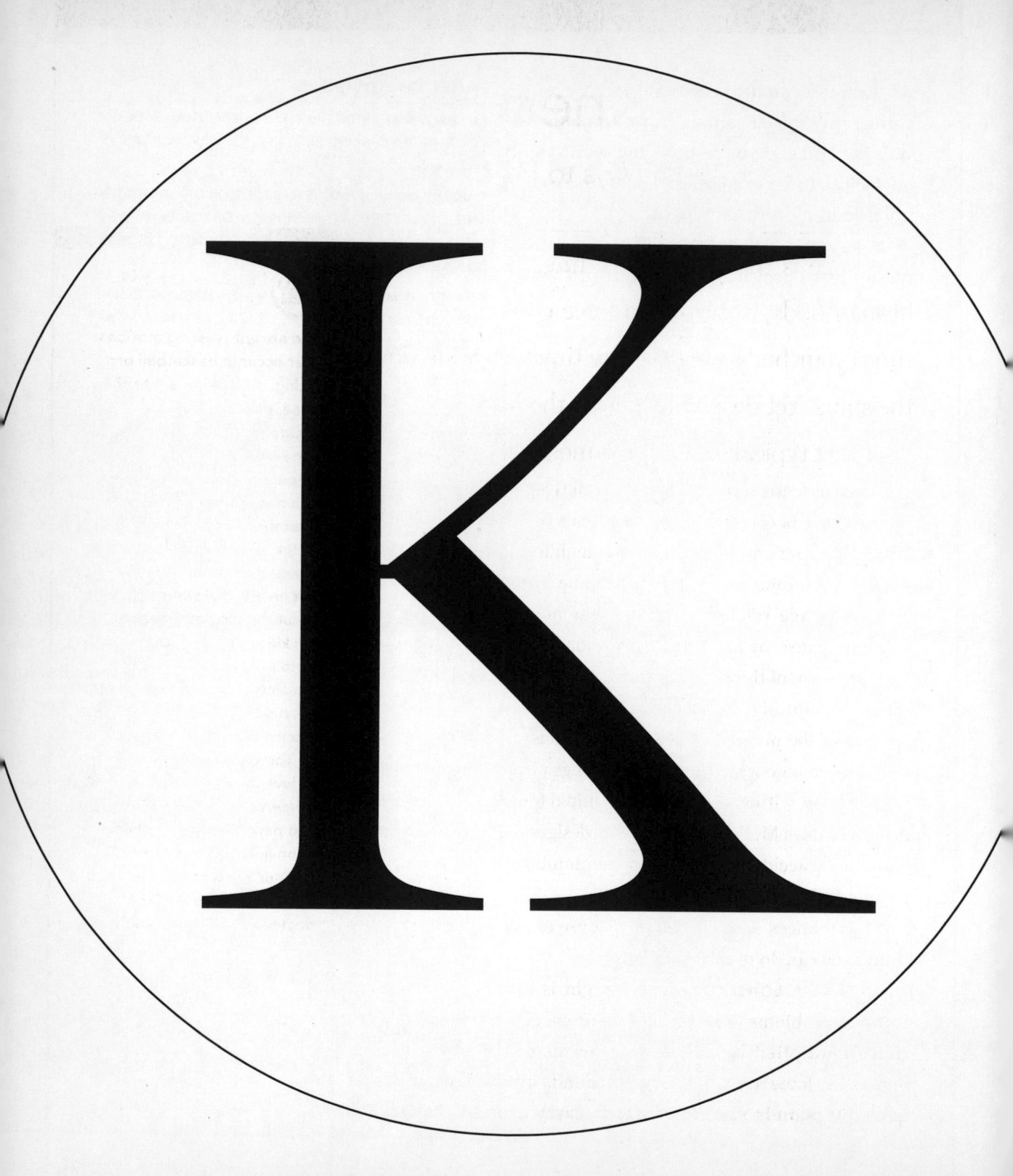

Knee Pain

18 Ways to Handle the Hurt

The knee is the strongest of the 187 joints in the human body, absorbing a force equivalent to $4\frac{1}{2}$ times your body weight every time you walk down the stairs. Yet despite its power, the knee is also the joint that typically causes the most suffering.

As Americans have become more active, sports-related knee injuries have become more common. But you don't have to be an athlete to experience knee pain. Automobile accidents commonly involve knee injuries. So do falls. Some knee pain stems from overuse or age-related wear and tear on the joint. The most common cause of knee pain is osteoarthritis, a degenerative wearing down of the cartilage cushions in the joint, causing bones to scrape painfully against each other.

Part of the problem is design, or rather the inability of knee design to change whenever human beings place new demands on it. "The knee, without question, is ill suited for the jobs we ask it to do," says James M. Fox, M.D. It wasn't designed for football, soccer, automobile accidents, carpentering, plumbing, or squatting and kneeling all day long.

If your knees ache because of overuse or abuse, here are a few things you can do to make amends.

■ **TAKE A LOAD OFF.** Body weight is a major contributor to knee problems, says Dr. Fox. For every pound you weigh, that's multiplied by about six in terms of the stress placed across the knee area. If you're 10 pounds overweight, that's an extra 60 pounds your knee has to carry around. As Dr. Fox

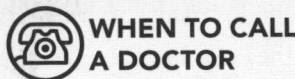

WHEN TO CALL A DOCTOR

The abrupt twisting motions that occur in basketball or skiing, or side impact to the knee, perhaps from a car accident or football tackle, can result in a knee injury. Generally the cruciate ligament or the medial or lateral collateral ligament of the knee is damaged. These injuries may or may not involve pain when they occur, but you may hear a buckle sound or "pop." Tendinitis and ruptured tendons can happen with overuse, or when you attempt to break a fall.

These injuries may be followed by swelling, tenderness, radiating pain, and perhaps some discoloration and loss of motion.

Your knee should be iced, and then seen by a doctor as soon as possible.

observes, "You don't put a Mack truck on Volkswagen tires."

■ **DON'T BOTHER WITH BRACES.** Knee braces can be purchased at just about any sporting goods store, but the experts say to leave them on the shelf. Some braces are meant to unload pressure that's affecting a specific area in the knee, but these are typically cumbersome, expensive, and require a prescription from your physician. "The wraps or braces you buy off the shelf at a sporting goods store shouldn't be used for anything more than to remind you that you have a bad knee," says Dr. Fox.

Some of them can do more harm than good, by pushing your kneecap into the joint, says athletic trainer Marjorie Albohm.

■ **TRY AN INSERT.** Some patients find relief from knee pain with shoe inserts called orthotics, says Dr. Fox. When they are placed in the shoe, they can redistribute pressure and reduce impact on the knee.

There are a variety of orthotics available in drugstores and doctors offices. They can also be custom made just for your knee ailment. Start with the commercially made ones at your local pharmacy. If they don't help, try the orthotics available through your physician or a physical therapist before springing for an expensive custom-made one, suggests Dr. Fox.

■ **GO HOMEOPATHIC.** Arnica, an herb that comes from a European flower, has natural anti-inflammatory properties. German scientists found that it reduces swelling of the knee from surgery. Use homeopathic arnica as an adjunct to ice or conventional medications you may be using for knee pain, suggests Jane Guiltinan, N.D. Rub arnica ointment on bruises or strained muscles, or take it up to six times a day in the form of three pellets placed under the tongue.

■ **REACH FOR A NONPRESCRIPTION MEDICATION.** Ibuprofen is the over-the-counter painkiller of choice recommended by our experts. It reduces inflammation and provides pain relief without causing as many stomach problems as aspirin. Acetaminophen is fine as a painkiller and causes fewer stomach problems, but it does little to reduce inflammation.

Studies have also shown ibuprofen can significantly improve joint mobility in people with acute knee ligament damage.

■ **TRY AN ALTERNATIVE.** Methylsulfonylmethane, more commonly called MSM, is derived from sulfur and may prevent joint and cartilage degeneration, say scientists at the University of California, San Diego. People with osteoarthritis of the knee who took MSM had 25 percent less pain and 30 percent better physical function at the end of a 3-month trial at Southwest College of Naturopathic Medicine.

Start with 1.5 to 3 grams once daily, suggests Leslie Axelrod, N.D. For severe pain, increase the dose to 3 grams twice daily, she says. Studies show that dosages as low as 500 milligrams three times daily helps improve pain and function.

■ **GIVE YOUR KNEE SOME C.** Australian scientists discovered that vitamin C, found in produce like bell peppers, kiwifruit, tomatoes, and oranges, reduces knee pain by protecting your knees against arthritis. Researchers studied 293 middle-aged people who were free of knee pain. Ten years later their knee tissue was assessed with an MRI. Those eating high amounts of vitamin C in their diets were less likely to have bone degeneration that leads to knee pain and the development of knee osteoarthritis. Researchers also found that other antioxidants, including lutein and zeaxanthin found in green veggies (such as spinach), can protect against arthritis and age-related wear and tear.

■ **TRY THE RUB THAT SOOTHES.** Some menthol lotions produce heat, which can relieve symptoms and make you feel more comfortable, says Dr. Fox. By covering the knee in plastic after applying the lotion, you can make the liniment even hotter. Be careful that you don't burn your skin or cause irritation.

■ **FIND A SPICY CURE.** Over-the-counter creams that contain capsaicin, an extract from chile peppers, may tone down knee pain. A study found that nearly 40 percent of arthritis patients reduced their pain by half after using capsaicin cream for a month. These creams, such as Zostrix and Capzasin-P, may be irritating to the skin, so try a small test spot for a few days before applying it to your entire knee, and don't apply it to broken skin.

■ **STRENGTHEN WITH EXERCISE.** The only things holding the knee together are the muscles and the ligaments, says Dr. Fox. Building up the muscles is critical because they are supporting structures. If the muscles don't have enough power or endurance, you're going to be in trouble with your knees.

Stronger muscles provide you with a stronger joint, one that's better able to withstand the considerable strain that even walking or stairclimbing places on the knees. The goal of these exercises is to strengthen your quadriceps, the muscles in front of your legs, and your hamstring muscles, in the back of your thighs. These two muscles must be in balance, says Dr. Fox. If just one or the other is developed, it causes stress on the knee joint.

The following exercises are not hard to do, and they hurt a lot less than aching knees.

■ **Isometric Knee Builder.** Sit on the floor with your sore knee straight out in front of you. Place a rolled towel under the small of the knee, then tighten the muscles in your leg without moving the knee. Hold that contraction and work up to keeping the muscles taut for at least 30 seconds, then relax. Repeat this tightening and relaxing up to 25 times.

■ **Sitting Leg Lifts.** Sit with your back against a wall and place a pillow in the small of your back. (Sitting against a wall ensures that the leg muscles do the lifting. This type of leg lift won't aggravate back pain.) Once you're in that position, do the isometric contraction described above for a count of five, then raise your leg a few inches and hold it to a count of five, then lower it and relax for a count of five. Work up to doing three sets of 10 lifts each, always using the five-count for pacing.

A word of caution: If an exercise causes increasing discomfort or pain, stop, Dr. Fox advises. You have to listen to your body. Don't work through the pain.

■ **TRY TO MODIFY.** Athletes with chronic knee problems have to modify their levels of training or daily activity, says Albohm. "But that doesn't mean turning into a couch potato." If you like racquetball and you have a chronic knee condition that racquetball gradually made worse, you're probably going to have to stop that activity, she says.

Options? Try swimming, cycling, or rowing, all activities that are beneficial to health without placing great strain on the knees. The key phrase is "non-weight-bearing" activity. In fact, by helping to strengthen thigh muscles, non-weight-bearing exercises such as cycling and rowing can give you better knees without sacrificing aerobic capacity or caloric burn.

Whatever you do, don't give up a healthy lifestyle because of knee pain. No one should have to stop being active, Albohm says. Simply avoid anything that causes pain in that knee.

■ **CHANGE TO A SOFTER RUNNING SUR-FACE.** A lot of runners have pain caused by tendinitis that results from poor training habits, says Dr. Fox. These are not significant mechanical problems, he says, and they can often be minimized by a change in running surface.

For starters, run on grass before asphalt and asphalt before concrete. Concrete is the hardest surface of all and should be avoided as much as possible. Don't make a habit of jogging on sidewalks. Try to find a golf course to run on once the golfers have left. "When you run a mile, your foot strikes the ground between 600 and 800 times," Dr. Fox says.

■ **TRY RICE.** Following any activity that causes knee pain, Albohm says to immediately rest the area and apply ice, compression, and elevation for 20 to 30 minutes. That advice is commonly called RICE, short for rest, ice, compression, and elevation.

"Don't underestimate the power of ice," says Albohm. Ice is a tremendous anti-inflammatory and will really help the condition.

Keep your icing routine simple, she says. When you return from working out, just prop the leg up, wrap an elastic bandage around it, and apply an ice pack for 20 to 30 minutes. That should always be your first try at relieving pain.

■ **USE HEAT WITH CAUTION.** When there is *no* swelling present, using a heating pad before an activity may let you exercise with less pain. But, Albohm cautions, if there's any swelling, don't use heat. Also, don't use heat *after* an activity, she says. We're assuming the area is becoming irritated by activity, and heat is only going to increase any irritation that's there.

■ **UPDATE YOUR SHOES.** If your shoes can't absorb the shock anymore, says Gary M. Gordon, D.P.M., that shock has to go someplace. So it goes through your foot, up your shin, and into your knee. Sometimes it keeps on going, up to your hip and back as well.

"I tell runners that they should change their running shoes every 300 miles," Dr. Gordon says. If they run less than that, they need new shoes once a year. Aerobic dancers and basketball and tennis players who work out twice each week can probably get by with new shoes every 4 to 6 months. But if they exercise four times or more each week, they need new shoes every 2 months. Most people don't want to hear that. (Except maybe the shoe manufacturers.)

■ **EXERCISE IN WATER.** The buoyancy of water makes it the perfect place to gently exercise a sore knee joint, says fitness consultant Lisa Dobloug. Try your regular knee exercises slowly underwater. Swimming and specific exercises for strengthening the quadriceps and hamstring muscles will keep you in shape without putting stress on your knees, she says.

■ **LIMBER UP IN THE MORNING.** To keep the knee and hamstring muscles supple, start with an a.m. stretch, suggests Dobloug. Lie on your back with one leg bent and your foot flat on the floor. Lift the other leg slowly toward the ceiling, foot flexed, leading with your heel. Then slowly lower your leg. Repeat 12 times with each leg.

■ **FIRST AND FINALLY, STRETCH AND MOVE SLOWLY.** Many of Dobloug's clients are older and have special needs when it comes to protecting their knees. Her emphasis is on the quality—not quantity—of exercise and the importance of stretching and moving correctly.

It's very important to warm up, she says. Take about 5 minutes and do very light stretching before you begin to exercise. Maybe go through the motions of whatever exercise you'll be doing in a very light manner.

PANEL OF ADVISORS

MARJORIE ALBOHM IS A CERTIFIED ATHLETIC TRAINER AND PRESIDENT OF THE NATIONAL ATHLETIC TRAINERS ASSOCIATION IN DALLAS. SHE SERVED ON THE MEDICAL STAFFS FOR THE 1980 WINTER AND 1996 SUMMER OLYMPICS AND THE 1987 PAN AMERICAN GAMES.

LESLIE AXELROD, N.D., IS PROFESSOR OF CLINICAL SCIENCES AT SOUTHWEST COLLEGE OF NATUROPATHIC MEDICINE AND HEALTH SCIENCES IN PHOENIX.

LISA DOBLOUG IS PRESIDENT OF SAGA FITNESS, A PERSONAL TRAINING AND SPA CONSULTING COMPANY IN WASHINGTON, D.C. MANY OF HER CLIENTS ARE OLDER PEOPLE WHO WISH TO REMAIN ACTIVE AND WHO APPRECIATE HER SOUND AND APPROPRIATE ADVICE ABOUT EXERCISING.

JAMES M. FOX, M.D., SPECIALIZES IN ARTHROSCOPIC SURGERY OF THE KNEE AND SPORTS MEDICINE AT SYNERGY HEALTH MEDICAL GROUP IN LOS ANGELES. HE IS AUTHOR OF *SAVE YOUR KNEES, AGAIN* AND WAS A MEMBER OF THE MEDICAL STAFF FOR THE 1984 SUMMER OLYMPICS.

GARY M. GORDON, D.P.M., IS CHIEF OF PODIATRY AT THE UNIVERSITY OF PENNSYLVANIA SPORTS MEDICINE CENTER AND HAS A PRACTICE IN GLENSIDE, PENNSYLVANIA.

JANE GUILTINAN, N.D., IS A PROFESSOR OF NATUROPATHIC MEDICINE AT BASTYR UNIVERSITY IN KENMORE, WASHINGTON, AND THE FORMER PRESIDENT OF THE AMERICAN ASSOCIATION OF NATUROPATHIC PHYSICIANS.

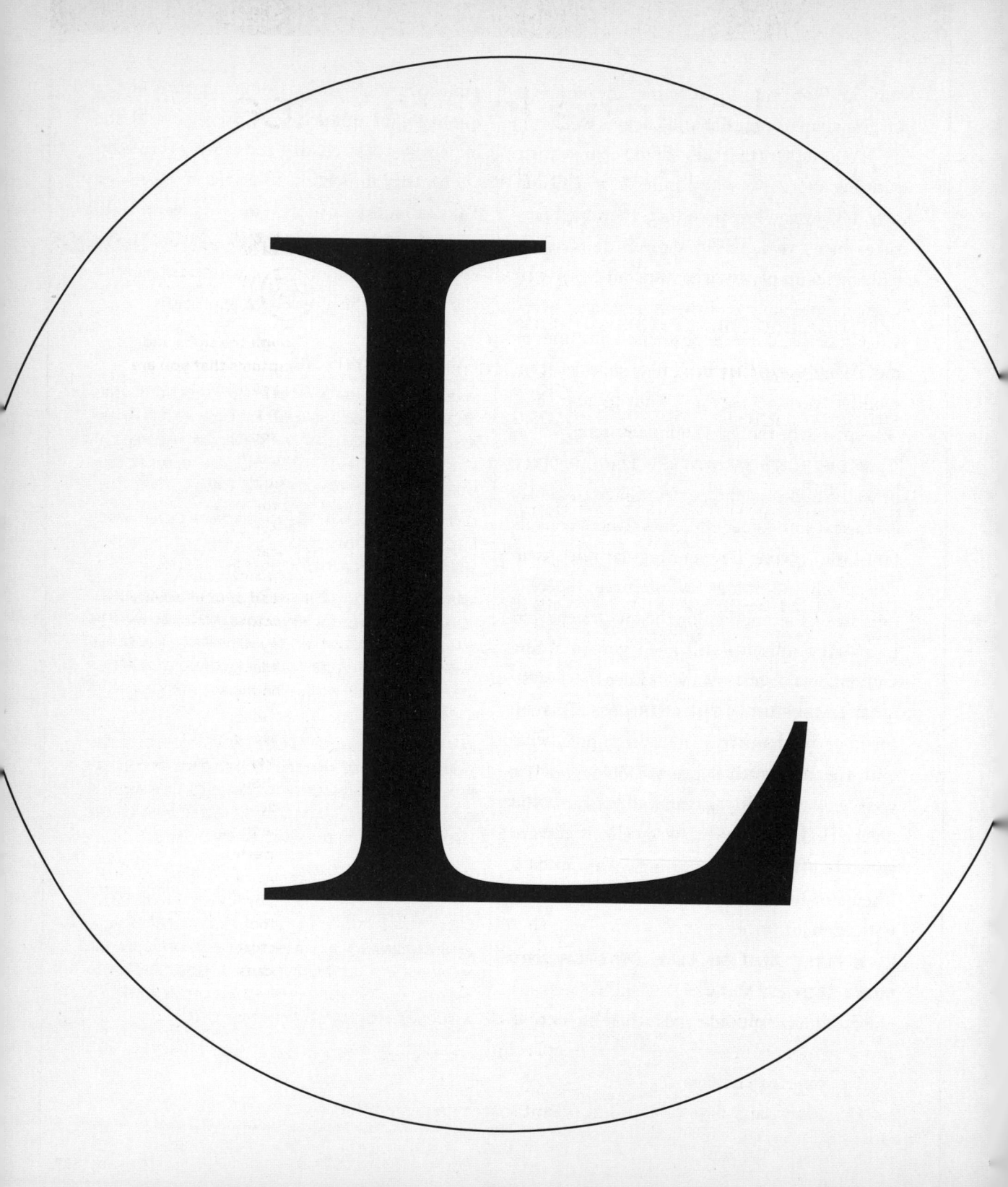

Lactose Intolerance

9 Soothing Ideas

If you feel symptoms such as cramps, bloating, diarrhea, and nausea after eating dairy foods, you're definitely *not* in the minority. It all started thousands of years ago, when humans turned from hunting and gathering, discovered agriculture, and began raising domesticated animals for milk. This was exclusive to certain regions of the world, says nutritional researcher Dennis Savaiano, Ph.D.

As a result, only about 25 percent of the world is genetically equipped to digest properly a sugar found in dairy foods called lactose. The other 75 percent may feel discomfort after eating dairy foods, a problem called lactose intolerance. In nature, most animals that drink milk as babies become lactose intolerant in adulthood, including, ironically, cows. So it's not just you.

Ideally, your small intestine produces enough of an enzyme called lactase, which is the key component that breaks down the lactose in dairy foods. If you don't have enough, the lactose gets to your colon, where your natural bacteria "eat" the lactose and give off clouds of gas, including hydrogen and carbon dioxide, which gives you that bloated feeling.

Up to 50 million Americans are lactose intolerant, and the problem most commonly affects the people of African, Asian, and Native American descent.

However, dairy foods are an important source of calcium for

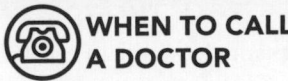 **WHEN TO CALL A DOCTOR**

Though the signs and symptoms that you are lactose intolerant may seem pretty evident, it's not something that you should diagnose and treat without speaking with your doctor first. In many cases, the symptoms could indicate a different or more serious condition instead of or in addition to lactose intolerance.

If you think you might have lactose intolerance, be on the lookout for cramping, gas, bloating, nausea, or diarrhea between 30 minutes and two hours after eating dairy products. If you experience these things, your doctor can perform several tests, such as a lactose tolerance test, hydrogen breath test, or stool acidity test, to see if lactose intolerance is truly the cause of your problems.

Americans, providing three-fourths of our intake of the mineral, says Dr. Savaiano, an expert on lactose intolerance. Even if you think you have lactose intolerance, you can still enjoy milk, cheese, and other dairy foods without discomfort. Here's how.

■ **TAKE THE TOLERANCE TEST.** Since everyone's degree of tolerance is different, find out how much of a good thing you can have before you stop enjoying it, says Theodore Bayless, M.D. Try drinking two glasses of skim milk on an empty stomach, he suggests. If you notice excessive gas or a "laxative effect" in the next 2 to 4 hours, lactose intolerance may be playing a role.

However, even if you do have lactose intolerance, odds are good that you can handle 8 ounces or less at a time, Dr. Savaiano says.

■ **DON'T FORGET YOUR CALCIUM.** "Milk products are a major source of calcium," Dr. Bayless says. "Most people should get the calcium equivalent of two glasses of milk daily." If milk is your main source of calcium and you cut back on it, then you should supplement your diet with substitutes like Tums, sardines with bones, spinach, and broccoli, he says. Calcium-fortified juices and cereals, calcium supplements, and lactase enzymes, pills, or lactase-treated milk can also help you maintain a healthy calcium intake.

■ **NEVER DRINK MILK ALONE.** "Some people find that their symptoms disappear if they consume their dairy products with meals," Dr. Bayless says. Dr. Savaiano agrees, suggesting instead of drinking just a glass of milk, have it with food.

■ **EAT YOGURT.** The fermentation process that produces yogurt depends on organisms that also produce lactase, the enzyme in short supply in lactose-intolerant people, says Naresh Jain, M.D. The bacteria themselves also probably break down the lactose in the milk.

Here are some other tips on yogurt.

■ **Choose Regular Yogurt.** Try to find yogurt that has not been repasteurized. Look for the National Yogurt Association's Live and Active Culture (LAC) seal on the label to make sure that the product you purchase meets the association's minimum standard of 10 million organisms per gram. In addition, frozen yogurt is not the same as yogurt—it's more of an ice milk, Dr. Savaiano says. So stick with regular yogurt.

■ **Choose Fat-Free.** "Fat slows gastric emptying," Dr. Jain says. Yogurt with fat in it sits in the stomach for a longer time. This means stomach acid may have more of a chance to kill the beneficial organisms. Since lactose digestion takes place in the small intestine, you want your organisms to get there as soon as possible, even if your stomach acid doesn't kill them. Although this is still only a theory, Dr. Jain says, it's probably best to stick with fat-free yogurt.

■ **Consume It Regularly.** Even if you don't have enough enzymes in your small intestine to deal with the lactose, "the bacteria in your large intestine are very adaptable, and if they regularly see lactose coming into their diet, they will adapt to using it very effectively," Dr. Savaiano says, and they'll then create less gas. In one study, Dr. Savaiano and his colleagues found that lactose-intolerant teen girls who ate dairy foods for 21 days were able to tolerate it, and their natural intestinal bacteria adapted to the diet.

■ **ADD YOUR OWN LACTASE.** Several companies make lactase enzyme and add it to milk. Or you can buy it in liquid form and add it yourself. Lact-Aid, resulting from research done by Dr. Bayless and David Paige, M.D., at Johns Hopkins University Hospital in Baltimore, comes in tablets you can take when you eat lactose-containing foods. Also, a few drops of the lactase liquid in a quart of milk will render the milk flatulence-free and give it a slightly sweeter taste.

The tablets and drops are available over the counter in drugstores. Supermarkets nationwide carry Lact-Aid milk, which is free of lactose.

■ **TRY BUTTERMILK.** "Buttermilk should be pretty much tolerable," Dr. Jain says. This is because it contains less lactose per 1-cup serving than whole, fat-free, and all types of milk in between. Despite its name, buttermilk has less fat and less cholesterol than even 2 percent milk.

■ **SAY "CHEESE."** When eating cheese, stick with harder varieties, says Dr. Savaiano. Lactose is water-soluble and is found in the whey, which is runny, rather than the curds, during the cheese-making process. Hard cheeses are made with curds while, for example, cottage cheese contains the whey.

■ **BEWARE OF FILLERS.** Lactose is a common filler in many kinds of medication and nutritional supplements. In some pills and for some people, Dr. Jain says, there's enough lactose to cause the symptoms of lactose intolerance. Read labels carefully. Ask your pharmacist if your medication has a lactose filler.

■ **CALL A HOTLINE.** Lact-Aid has a toll-free phone number for questions about lactose intolerance. Call 800-LACTAID.

PANEL OF ADVISORS

THEODORE BAYLESS, M.D., IS A GASTROENTEROLOGY PROFESSOR IN THE JOHNS HOPKINS UNIVERSITY SCHOOL OF MEDICINE IN BALTIMORE.

NARESH JAIN, M.D., IS A GASTROENTEROLOGIST IN NIAGARA FALLS, NEW YORK.

DENNIS SAVAIANO, PH.D., IS A PROFESSOR AND DEAN OF THE COLLEGE OF CONSUMER AND FAMILY SCIENCES AT PURDUE UNIVERSITY IN WEST LAFAYETTE, INDIANA.

Laryngitis

13 Ways to Make It Easier to Swallow

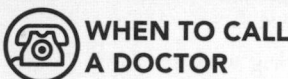
WHEN TO CALL A DOCTOR

If your voice loss is accompanied by pain so severe that you have trouble swallowing your own saliva, see a physician immediately, says George T. Simpson II, M.D. Swelling in the upper part of your larynx may be blocking your airway.

You should also contact your doctor if you cough up blood, hear noises in your throat when you breathe, or find that voice rest doesn't help your hoarseness.

If your laryngitis lasts more than 2 weeks, see a doctor who specializes in throat problems such as an otolaryngologist, says Adam Klein, M.D. These specialists have the experience and equipment to inspect your vocal cords—not merely the back of your throat—and quickly diagnose the problem, which can be caused by such issues as growths on the cords.

Housed in your larynx, your vocal cords—or vocal folds, which doctors might sometimes call them—are little bands of stretchy tissue that come together and move apart like a pair of lips. When you speak or sing, air passes through them while they vibrate just like you're blowing someone "the raspberry," says Adam Klein, M.D. Each time you speak or sing, your vocal cords move hundreds of times each second, possibly even 1,000 times.

Sometimes your vocal cords grow irritated or inflamed, a condition called laryngitis. Your throat may feel sore, but the most common symptom is that your voice sounds different. The vocal cords swell; imagine having two fat lips and trying to buzz them together, Dr. Klein says. They may not vibrate at all, and in that case, you can't make a peep. Or they may vibrate, but because they're heavier, they vibrate more slowly, so the result is that the pitch of your voice drops.

The common cold and other viral infections of the upper airways are frequent causes of laryngitis. It often accompanies the flu, bronchitis, pneumonia, measles, whooping cough, or any infection of the upper airways. Acid juices from the stomach that escape into the throat can wreak havoc with your vocal cords. And any opera singer or campaigning politician can tell you, straining the voice is a common cause of hoarseness, as are exposure to tobacco smoke and allergies.

If your timbre is now as deep and croaky as Clint Eastwood's, follow our experts' tips to recover your true voice.

■ **GIVE IT A REST.** For run-of-the-mill laryngitis, "the best thing you can do is rest your voice," Dr. Klein suggests. When your vocal cords are swollen, those persistent vibrations you create while speaking inflict trauma on them. It's especially bad if you try to maintain your usual speaking or singing performance, since you have to push harder to make your vocal cords vibrate at the usual frequencies.

■ **AVOID EVEN WHISPERING.** Although you may think that whispering is softer and gentler on your tender tissues, it's not. "Whispering causes you to bang your vocal cords together as strongly as if you were shouting," explains George T. Simpson II, M.D.

■ **PRIORITIZE YOUR NOISEMAKING.** If you just have to speak, preserve your words for the times that are absolutely necessary, and the rest of the time "zip it," Dr. Klein says. Avoid speaking in noisy environments—if you must speak, head somewhere quieter. Send text messages with your cell phone, stick to e-mail, or carry a pad of paper and pen with you to jot down your thoughts.

■ **GIVE THEM SOME STEAM.** "Singers swear by steam showers," Dr. Klein says. This helps keep your tissues moist and lubricated, helping them vibrate better. So give yourself some relaxation and step into a hot shower on a regular basis while you're coping with laryngitis.

If you're a professional singer who doesn't currently have laryngitis and you want to keep it that way, do your vocal warmups in a hot, steamy shower to reduce strain, he says.

■ **DRINK UP.** Staying well hydrated helps your vocal folds when you have laryngitis, Dr. Klein says. And it's the perfect time to remember to drink those eight 8-ounce glasses daily that health experts recommend. Avoid caffeinated and carbonated drinks—caffeine can worsen acid reflux. A hot cup of caffeine-free herbal tea can be helpful.

■ **USE A COLD-AIR HUMIDIFIER.** The layer of mucosa that blankets your vocal cords needs to be kept moist. When it's not, mucus can become sticky and adherent, a virtual flypaper for irritants. Fight back with a cold-air humidifier, says Scott Kessler, M.D.

■ **AVOID BREATHING THROUGH YOUR MOUTH.** "Breathing through your nose is a natural humidifier," says Dr. Kessler. "People who have a deviated nasal septum breathe through the mouth while asleep. That exposes the voice to dry and cold air. Evaluating how you breathe is critical to understanding the nature of hoarseness."

■ **NIX THE CIGARETTES.** Smoking is a prime cause of throat dryness, says Dr. Kessler. It also relaxes your upper stomach muscles, which allows your harsh stomach juices to contact the larynx.

■ **WATCH FOR REFLUX.** So-called laryngeal reflux can be worsened by sleeping on a full stomach; drinking caffeine or alcohol; eating mints, citrus fruits, spicy foods, and tomato sauce; taking aspirin or excessive vitamin C; and doing exercises such as abdominal crunches and the "downward facing dog" yoga pose, Dr. Kessler says. Avoiding these may help reduce episodes of laryngitis.

■ **BEWARE OF AIRPLANE AIR.** Talking on an airplane can sabotage your voice. This is because the pressurized air inside the cabin is so dry. To keep your cords moist, breathe through your nose, says Dr. Kessler. Chew gum or suck on lozenges so that you'll have no choice but to keep your mouth closed.

■ **CHECK YOUR MEDICATION.** Certain prescription and over-the-counter drugs, such as antihistamines for allergies, can be very drying, Dr. Kessler says. When your vocal cords are dry, "speaking or singing is like running a car engine without oil," he says. Use these with caution or avoid when you're hoarse—though talk to your doctor before changing your medication regimen. Some other culprits can include blood pressure and thyroid medications.

■ **RESPECT YOUR VOICE.** If you have a presentation to do and you find yourself hoarse, it's better to cancel than risk doing long-term damage to your voice, says Dr. Kessler.

■ **CONSIDER VOICE TRAINING.** If you're a professional speaker or singer—or you're required to communicate with your voice a lot—it's a good idea to get some voice training. A professional can advise you how to get the muscles around your larynx to work together as a team so you can use them more effectively.

PANEL OF ADVISORS

SCOTT KESSLER, M.D., IS AN OTOLARYNGOLOGIST SPECIALIZING IN THE CARE OF VOICE PROFESSIONALS AND IS ON THE ATTENDING STAFF AT THE MOUNT SINAI MEDICAL CENTER IN NEW YORK CITY. HE IS THE PHYSICIAN FOR METROPOLITAN OPERA AND BROADWAY PERFORMERS, RECORDING ARTISTS, TV, RADIO, AND MOVIE PERSONALITIES, AND CLERGY.

ADAM KLEIN, M.D., IS AN ASSISTANT PROFESSOR OF OTOLARYNGOLOGY AND A SURGEON AT EMORY HEALTHCARE IN ATLANTA, GEORGIA, WHOSE SPECIALTIES INCLUDE THROAT AND VOICE PROBLEMS. HIS CLIENTS INCLUDE MANY PROFESSIONAL SINGERS AND SPEAKERS.

GEORGE T. SIMPSON II, M.D., IS A PROFESSOR OF OTOLARYNGOLOGY AND SURGERY AT THE UNIVERSITY OF BUFFALO.

Leg Pain

8 Tips to Ease the Pain

A variety of problems can lead to aching legs, including back problems, varicose veins, and nerve damage. Overuse, from an extra-vigorous workout, or an injury like that from a fall, can also cause leg pain. However, a certain type of pain in the leg can point to potentially life-threatening problems in your cardiovascular system.

Intermittent claudication is a chronic pain experienced in the leg while walking. It most often affects the calf, but sometimes the buttock and thigh. It's estimated to affect 3 to 10 percent of the American population, with nearly one-fifth of the population older than 65 having the problem. Though a painful and serious condition in its own right, intermittent claudication is really the *symptom* of a larger, more serious problem—peripheral arterial disease.

Arterial disease is caused by a buildup of plaque in the arteries that run along the "periphery" of your body, such as those carrying blood to your legs and feet. The plaque limits the amount of oxygen-rich blood that can reach your muscles, and the pain is your legs' way of alerting you that they're not getting enough blood during physical activity. Once you stop the activity, the discomfort stops too. Although cramps, aching, and tiredness are the most frequent symptoms of mild to moderate peripheral arterial disease, less than 20 percent of people with the condition have these signs.

If you have leg pain from arterial disease, you may also have

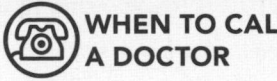 **WHEN TO CALL A DOCTOR**

Leg pain is a symptom of many conditions, some very serious. If your pain is severe, worsens rapidly, or lasts for more than a week, see your doctor as soon as possible. In addition to recommending lifestyle changes, your doctor can prescribe medicines that can improve your walking endurance. In some cases, a surgical procedure is necessary to "bypass" the blocked part of your artery by attaching another blood vessel, or performing a procedure to create more space through the narrowed artery.

Chronic foot problems that get infected are a leading cause of amputation in people who have intermittent claudication. If you have a cut, scrape, blister, or other foot problem that develops the redness, swelling, heat, and pain of infection, seek immediate medical help.

plaque limiting the flow of blood to your heart and brain, which puts you at higher risk of heart attack and stroke, says Wilbert Aronow, M.D. Research found that every year, roughly 6 percent of those who have intermittent claudication, the first phase of arterial disease, will have a heart attack or stroke, or die of cardiovascular causes.

For this reason, intermittent claudication should not be taken lightly. Not only is it important to treat the pain from walking, but it is also vital to reduce any underlying cardiovascular risk. It's important to see your doctor regularly to monitor its progress. The pain in your legs, after all, is only a symptom. The real disease is a killer. On the upside, there are a number of things that you can do at home to rid yourself of claudication's pain and help slow the progression of peripheral arterial disease.

■ **STOP SMOKING.** "Smoking is a powerful risk factor for intermittent claudication," says Nieca Goldberg, M.D. Research has found that more than 80 percent of those people with peripheral arterial disease, or PAD, currently smoke or previously smoked.

Quitting smoking isn't usually easy, but consider the following: Cigarette smoking increases the damage the disease can do by substituting carbon monoxide for oxygen in the already oxygen-starved muscles of your legs. Nicotine also causes constriction of the arteries, which further restricts bloodflow, possibly damaging the arteries themselves and leading to blood clots. In extreme cases, these clots can result in gangrene and may require amputation of a limb.

■ **KEEP YOUR BLOOD SUGAR UNDER CONTROL.** Diabetes raises your risk of peripheral arterial disease and intermittent claudication, Dr. Goldberg says. Because your goal is to keep the problem from growing worse, staying on top of diabetes is an important self-care method. Your doctor can measure your hemoglobin level to assess your long-term blood sugar control, says Dr. Aronow.

Important steps for controlling your diabetes, according to the National Institutes of Health, include taking prescribed medications, checking your blood sugar regularly, eating a healthy diet, and getting at least 30 minutes of physical activity on most days. If the thought of exercise sounds too painful to your already-aching calves, keep reading.

■ **START WALKING.** Both Dr. Goldberg and Dr. Aronow stress the importance of regular exercise, as do other experts on peripheral arterial disease. Patients are often surprised when their doctors recommend that they walk regularly, Dr. Goldberg says, but after doing it for a while, you'll likely find that you can go farther without pain. Experts aren't entirely sure why exercise helps treat claudication, but it may be from the increased muscle strength and improved delivery of oxygen to your leg muscles.

Try to walk 30 to 45 minutes at least three times a week, ideally in a supervised setting in which a trained professional can get you started, encourage you to go far enough, and make sure you're exercising safely. You know the term "no pain, no gain"? Well, that's the goal to keep in mind. You should walk until your legs are in "near-maximal" pain, says Dr. Aronow, then rest by standing or sitting briefly until your symptoms subside. Keep repeating the cycle of walking and resting until your session is finished.

If you're exercising on your own, consider walking in a shopping mall, Dr. Aronow says. You're protected from bad weather, and malls offer plenty of places to sit and rest.

Be warned that improvement won't happen overnight. It might take at least a month or two before you see any change.

When researchers reviewed the results of three studies on physical activity and claudication, they found that exercise increased people's maximum walking distance by 150 percent over a period of 3 to 12 months.

■ **TAKE A LOAD OFF.** Obesity can be a major problem for those with claudication, not only because of the strain it places on circulation but also because of the damage it inflicts on the feet. Change your diet and get more physical activity so you can shed unnecessary pounds. Losing as little as 5 pounds can help.

■ **AVOID HEATING PADS.** Because of the restricted bloodflow in the legs, people who have intermittent claudication often experience cold feet, too. But regardless of how cold your feet may be, never warm them with a heating pad or a hot-water bottle. Because bloodflow is restricted, the heat can't be dissipated and could actually burn your feet. Try loose wool socks to warm your feet instead.

■ **TAKE CARE OF YOUR FEET.** People with diabetes have to be particularly careful with the health of their feet because poor circulation can turn minor injuries into serious problems. The same goes for people with peripheral arterial disease. Be sure to wash and dry your feet daily, check for injuries, and wear properly fitting shoes—with inserts if necessary—to prevent injuries to your feet, Dr. Aronow says.

■ **KNOW YOUR BLOOD PRESSURE AND CHOLESTEROL LEVEL.** If you have intermittent claudication, it's important that your doctor check you for high cholesterol and high blood pressure, and, if necessary, get these risk factors under control, say Dr. Aronow and Dr. Goldberg.

■ **TRY FOLATE.** Homocysteine is an amino acid that's linked to a higher risk of heart disease. By increasing your intake of folate, a B vitamin also known as folic acid, you can help lower your levels of homocysteine. Foods that are good sources of folate include fortified cereals, beans, broccoli, spinach, and orange juice.

PANEL OF ADVISORS

WILBERT S. ARONOW, M.D., IS A CARDIOLOGIST AND CLINICAL PROFESSOR OF MEDICINE AT NEW YORK MEDICAL COLLEGE IN VALHALLA.

NIECA GOLDBERG, M.D., IS A CARDIOLOGIST IN NEW YORK CITY FOCUSING ON WOMEN'S HEALTH AND IS AUTHOR OF *NIECA GOLDBERG'S COMPLETE GUIDE TO WOMEN'S HEALTH.*

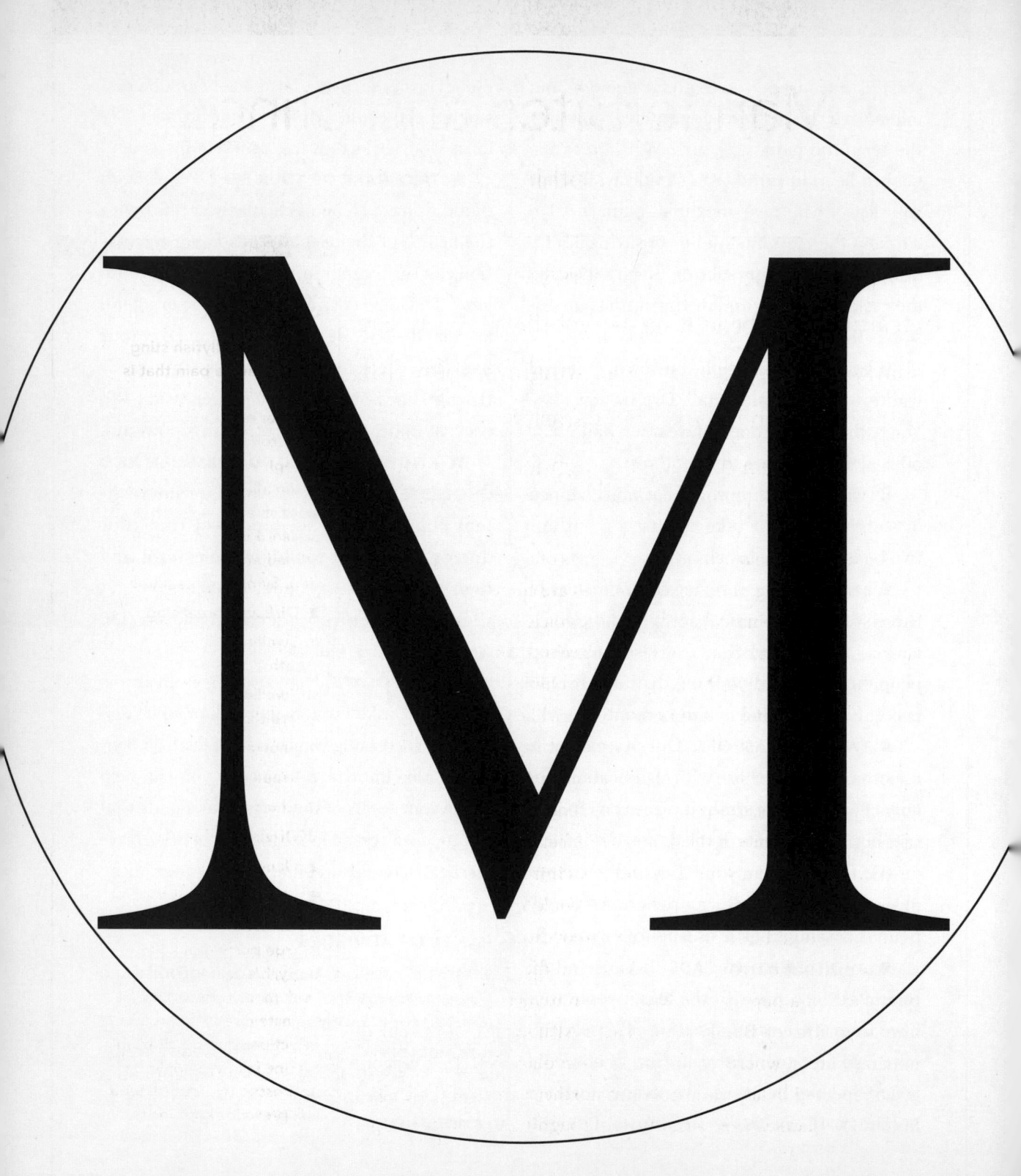

Marine Bites and Stings

11 Soothing Strategies

Where unsuspecting swimmers swim, dangerous creatures may be lurking. Forget the relatively rare sharks. Jellyfish, sea urchins, stingrays, spiny fish, coral, and even microscopic parasites are far more likely to make a day at the beach feel like, well, no day at the beach.

Jellyfish are the most common culprits of ocean vacations gone awry. Their flowing, translucent tentacles are covered with stinging capsules called nematocysts. When a tentacle brushes up against your skin, the nematocysts are ejected, piercing the skin and injecting stinging venom. The result: a burning, throbbing, itching sensation that can feel as minor as a paper cut or more like a bee sting.

Unfortunately, jellyfish aren't the only stinging creatures in the sea. Stingrays, scorpion fish, and even catfish all have venomous spines. Sea urchins, though not usually venomous, have protruding spines that can pierce beach-goers' bare feet.

All this might make fresh water swimming seem less hazardous. Not necessarily. A dip in a lake could impart an annoying itch. That would be swimmer's itch—a condition caused by larval flatworms that burrow into the skin and die. Each one leaves a bump, called a papule, that can be even itchier than a mosquito bite, says Harvey Blankespoor, Ph.D. Although it can occur in marine waters, where it's known as clam digger's itch, it is more often reported in lakes and ponds in northern areas of the United States. Dr. Blankespoor estimates that roughly 250,000 people get

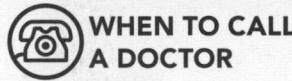

WHEN TO CALL A DOCTOR

Any time a jellyfish sting causes severe pain that is not alleviated by over-the-counter medications, get to a doctor, recommends Joseph W. Burnett, M.D.

An allergic reaction to a jellyfish sting is rare but not unheard of, and it requires immediate medical attention. Symptoms include:

- Difficulty breathing
- Swelling around the mouth
- Swelling of the limb where the sting occurred
- Shortness of breath
- Wheezing
- Chest pain
- Dizziness
- Nausea
- Stomach cramps

If you have a rash over a large portion of your body, it's a good idea to seek medical care, Dr. Bernstein says. In addition, infections that result from marine injuries should be addressed by a doctor who will prescribe antibiotics.

swimmer's itch each year, and the four worst states for the problem are Michigan, Minnesota, Wisconsin, and Washington.

To prevent these painful encounters, avoid swimming in infested waters, especially after stormy weather, and be careful not to step on beached creatures that appear to be dead. Choose a beach with trained lifeguards, who are likely to be familiar with the species you may encounter and can help keep you out of the riskier spots.

Here's how to soothe yourself if one or so sea creatures do attack.

JELLYFISH STINGS

■ **POUR ON THE VINEGAR.** Ordinary vinegar may be your best defense against nematocytes left behind by many, but not all, jellyfish. "The weak acid is useful to stop them from firing," says Joseph W. Burnett, M.D. Pour vinegar directly over the affected area for about 30 seconds, he suggests. Once you've neutralized the nematocysts, you can safely pick off the tentacles. If you don't have any vinegar with you, ask a lifeguard. Some of them keep a bottle in their first-aid kits.

However, if you think you've been stung by a Portuguese man-of-war, don't apply vinegar or anything else. First remove the remaining nematocysts and seek immediate medical attention, particularly if you are in severe pain. These creatures, with tentacles that can reach 40 feet or more, are common in the waters off Hawaii.

Avoid removing any tentacles adhering to the skin with your bare fingers—you could get another sting. "Pick off the big pieces with a gloved hand, tweezers, or scrape them off with the edge of a shell, a sand shovel, or the dull side of a knife blade," says Jeffrey N. Bernstein, M.D.

■ **RINSE IT WITH SALT WATER.** If you don't have anything to neutralize the stingers, flush the area with ocean water. "Salt water is handy and safe," observes Craig Thomas, M.D. Avoid other old wives' remedies like alcohol, ammonia, urine, and bleach. They may be harmful, causing the nematocysts to discharge more venom.

■ **CHARGE IT!** One common method for removing the desensitized nematocysts is to cover the sting with shaving cream to help draw them out and then scrape them off with a credit card, says Dr. Bernstein. Don't have a can of shaving cream in your beach bag? Ask the lifeguard because some of them keep it in their first-aid kits. Do this only after you've treated the area with vinegar, since pressure will otherwise trigger more stinging.

■ **HEAT IT UP.** Dr. Bernstein and his colleagues conducted a study to determine whether heat or ice worked better to relieve the pain of jellyfish stings. In the test, of those treated with ice packs, just over half reported pain relief within an hour. Almost all those treated by immersing the sting in hot water felt no pain an hour later. "Water should be hot to the touch, but obviously not so hot that you burn yourself," explains Dr. Bernstein. After you scrape off the jellyfish nematocysts, stick the stung area in hot water until you feel no pain when you remove it. If hot water is unavailable, apply a heating pad to the area instead.

■ **PUT IT ON ICE.** While heat may be more effective, ice is often handier at the beach. Scrape off the nematocysts and place an ice pack or a bag of ice directly on the sting for some pain relief, says Dr. Bernstein. Keep it on until the pain subsides.

■ **HEAD TO THE DRUGSTORE.** For the pain of a jellyfish sting, take aspirin, acetaminophen, or ibuprofen, says Dr. Burnett.

"Topical preparations don't work in the initial treatment phase. They don't penetrate deeply enough to ease the pain. An over-the-counter hydrocortisone cream or a topical antihistamine may be helpful if symptoms persist beyond 24 hours. Consult a physician if symptoms last more than a few days," Dr. Bernstein says.

OTHER WATER WOES

■ **SPECIAL CARE NEEDED FOR SEA URCHIN INJURIES.** A stroll along coastal waters could prove painful if you step on a hidden sea urchin. These creatures have sharp, brittle spines that penetrate the skin and break off. Surprisingly, small pieces embedded in the skin may be best left untreated. "Big, loosely penetrated spines can be plucked off, but otherwise they have to be dug and cut out, which does more harm than good," says Dr. Thomas. The spines will either work themselves out or they will dissolve within 3 weeks. It's rare for infection to occur, but, just in case, watch for signs of redness and swelling.

■ **TREAT VENOMOUS FISH STINGS.** Stingrays hide just beneath the sand. Surprise one, and you're likely to discover that the end of its tail contains a powerful stinger. Stingray stings are immediately painful, just like a bee sting, says Dr. Thomas. To relieve pain, remove the stinger and any poison tissue remaining on your skin by rinsing with salt or fresh water. Then, pull out any embedded parts with tweezers.

Dr. Bernstein has some firsthand experience with stingray stings . . . make that first-*foot* experience. While on the west coast of Mexico, he stepped on a ray and felt "one of the most painful things I've ever felt in my life," a pain that shot from the bottom of his foot up his spine. His friends knew what to do: They heated up water and he soaked his foot, which provided almost immediate pain relief. You may have to leave your foot in hot water for 20 minutes to an hour, he recommends.

To *prevent* stingray stings, do what he calls the "stingray shuffle" while walking in their territory. Slide your feet along the ocean floor so if you contact a ray, it will scurry away. Their stinging mechanism is a reflexive action that may fire when you step on them: "You feel a squish before you feel the pain," he notes.

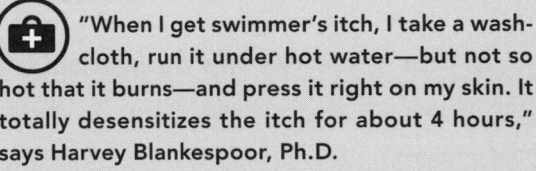

What the Doctor Does

"When I get swimmer's itch, I take a washcloth, run it under hot water—but not so hot that it burns—and press it right on my skin. It totally desensitizes the itch for about 4 hours," says Harvey Blankespoor, Ph.D.

Other fish, like catfish or scorpion fish, have venomous spines that cause a painful reaction if they scrape your skin. Again, immersion in hot water will bring relief. "We recommend hot water for most marine venoms because the heat disables the venom's proteins," says Dr. Bernstein.

■ **QUELL CORAL PAIN.** Coral can give snorkelers or waders a nasty scrape. "These cuts are a combination of a sting, from the nematocysts in the coral, and a dirty cut. They get infected often," says Dr. Thomas. Clean the wound thoroughly, removing any fragments of coral in the skin with tweezers. Then scrub the area with gauze soaked in clean, fresh water, and coat with an antiseptic containing bacitracin. Fresh water, in treating coral cuts, is unlikely to trigger nematocysts and is essential for cleaning the wound.

■ **SOOTHE SEA LICE.** Not really lice at all, sea lice are jellyfish larvae, sometimes encountered in warm ocean waters. Often, they get trapped inside a swimmer's bathing suit or under a T-shirt. Once they sit there for a while, they start stinging. "It causes an almost allergic reaction," says Dr. Bernstein. "You'll get an itchy irritation in the area around the waistband or under the bathing suit." Shower to remove any larvae that might still be on your skin, then treat the itch with an over-the-counter antihistamine, such as Benadryl, or a hydrocortisone cream.

■ **SQUELCH SWIMMER'S ITCH.** Swimmer's itch, which is actually caused by an encounter with a waterborne parasite, can affect every part of the body that's been in the water. The parasite leaves a small, round, itchy bump wherever it has entered. Bumps show up within 15 minutes of contact with the parasite and last for 1 to 2 weeks. Here are a few recommended remedies for soothing that itch.

■ **Try Over-the-Counter Treatments.** Swimmer's itch that covers the entire body or is intensely irritating could require a doctor-prescribed antihistamine, says Dr. Blankespoor. Less-severe cases can be treated with topical anti-itch formulas, such as cortisone creams. Or look for a nonprescription cream or ointment containing benzocaine, such as Boil-Ease, to relieve itching.

■ **Don't Drip Dry.** Toweling off the moment you step out of the lake won't always protect you against swimmer's itch. But some species of the parasite enter only as the water dries on the skin, so it's a good idea to dry yourself immediately after a swim.

PANEL OF ADVISORS

JEFFREY N. BERNSTEIN, M.D., IS MEDICAL DIRECTOR OF THE FLORIDA POISON INFORMATION CENTER IN MIAMI.

HARVEY BLANKESPOOR, PH.D., IS A BIOLOGY PROFESSOR AT HOPE COLLEGE IN HOLLAND, MICHIGAN, WHO STUDIES SWIMMER'S ITCH.

JOSEPH W. BURNETT, M.D., IS A FORMER CHAIRMAN OF DERMATOLOGY AT UNIVERSITY OF MARYLAND IN BALTIMORE, AND PRESIDENT OF THE INTERNATIONAL CONSORTIUM FOR JELLYFISH STINGS.

CRAIG THOMAS, M.D., IS THE PRESIDENT OF HAWAII EMERGENCY PHYSICIANS ASSOCIATED AND THE COAUTHOR OF *ALL STINGS CONSIDERED.*

Memory Problems

21 Ways to Forget Less

Though people may joke about forgetting names or struggling to find a word that's on the tips of their tongues, others seriously fear losing their memory or mental abilities as they age. However, it's worth keeping in mind that there's a huge difference between those occasional "senior moments" and the memory loss caused by conditions such as dementia or Alzheimer's disease.

All sorts of issues that are relatively minor when compared with Alzheimer's can contribute to memory loss. These include high blood pressure, side effects from medications, alcohol use, stress, depression, lack of sleep, nutritional deficiencies, and simply normal aging. Some of the more serious causes include head injury and stroke.

Occasional forgetfulness is rarely a sign of disease. But it's not something you necessarily have to live with, either. A combination of mental exercises and lifestyle changes offer a good chance at improving your memory and keeping it strong for years to come.

■ **GIVE YOUR MIND A WORKOUT.** The brain is like other parts of the body. The more it's exercised and challenged, the stronger it gets over time, says Gunnar Gouras, M.D.

People who are mentally active form additional neural connections, Dr. Gouras explains. In other words, they have a larger "reserve" of brain circuits, so they're more likely to stay mentally

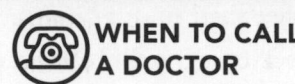 **WHEN TO CALL A DOCTOR**

Because memory declines can be caused by many physical problems, such as depression, thyroid disorders, nutritional deficiencies, or even urinary tract infections, it's important to see a doctor as soon as you notice any changes, says Cynthia R. Green, Ph.D.

Ask yourself if your memory has gotten significantly worse in the past 6 months, says Dr. Green. Are the changes seriously affecting your ability to function? Are your friends or family concerned? The answers to these questions will give you a sense of the seriousness of the changes.

Another thing to consider is whether you're taking a new medication, Dr. Green says. Many drugs, including antihistamines and medications for heartburn, anxiety, and high blood pressure, have memory impairment as a side effect. In many cases, switching to a new drug or changing the dosage may be all that's needed to reverse the problem.

sharp. A study of 678 nuns, for example, found that those with the most education and language abilities were less likely to develop Alzheimer's later in life.

In a 2007 study, volunteers who believed they had mild memory problems followed either their normal routines for 2 weeks or a special program involving mental stimulation, a healthy diet rich in omega-3 fats and antioxidants, stress reduction, and exercise. At the end of the study, those following the program showed positive changes through brain imaging that suggested their brains were working more effectively.

So keep your mind busy. Do crossword and Sudoku puzzles. Read challenging books. Play Scrabble. Virtually any activity that keeps the mind active could help reduce the risk of age-related memory decline.

■ **KEEP YOUR LIFE INTERESTING.** Your body tends to invest resources in the body parts that you're using, says Keith Lyle, Ph.D. "If you're not exercising your brain, it's like when you're not using a muscle very much—your body doesn't put resources into that organ. It says, 'I don't need to. I can get by with a relatively low level of resources here.'" As we get older, many of us tend to steer toward the things we've always done. We stick to the familiar routines, particularly if we develop physical limitations that reduce our ability to get around, he says.

That's why it's important to expose ourselves to novel situations. When you do, you help maintain a higher level of brain functioning. Read books about topics you don't know much about. Listen to new kinds of music. Take a different route home instead of the one that's so familiar you barely have to pay attention to it. Learn new skills, even if it's something nonacademic such as quilting.

■ **PUT INFORMATION INTO SMALLER BITE-SIZE CHUNKS.** It's easy to forget—or fail to learn—information that comes in large chunks. It's much easier to remember things when you break them down into smaller chunks, says Cynthia R. Green, Ph.D.

Phone numbers are a good example. They're customarily divided into three units—the area code, the first three numbers, and the final four numbers. They're fairly easy to remember because they're broken into small, manageable pieces of information.

You can use this same technique to manage all kinds of information. When you shop, for example, divide the shopping list into logical pieces: produce, freezer, and dairy foods.

■ **MAKE YOURSELF REMEMBER.** Researchers have found that people who read information several times, like a chapter in a book, don't remember it better than people who only read it once, Dr. Lyle says. The key to remembering a certain fact is to keep retrieving the information. Dredge it up from your memory, set it aside, and bring it up again later.

When he was interviewing for a job, Dr. Lyle was meeting dozens of new people every day, and so he wanted to remember their names so he could make a good impression. "When I'd go back to the hotel that night, I'd think about those names," he says. "If you do it enough, you'll retain the information for a long time to come."

■ **FORM MENTAL PICTURES.** It's easier to remember things when you have a visual image in your mind to go along with them. Suppose you've just been introduced to someone named Bill at a party. Repeat the name a few times in your mind, and also form a mental picture of a $1 bill. The combination of mental repetition and a visual image will help you remember his name in the future.

■ **MAKE MENTAL CONNECTIONS.** When you were in school, you may have learned to spell "principal" by thinking of the word "pal." It was an effective way to link the new information with something you already knew. It's a quick and easy way of giving information meaning, says Dr. Green.

"I was at a conference and I met a woman named Regina," says Dr. Green. "As soon as she said her name, I connected it to a friend of mine who's also named Regina, which made the name easier to remember."

You can form connections with almost anything. Suppose the number on your spot in the huge airport parking lot is R88. Link it to something that you already know, like the fact that Ronald Reagan was president in 1988. Thus, R88.

■ **TRY THE STORYTELLING TECHNIQUE.** Another way to remember names or other information is to weave them into little mental stories, says Dr. Green. If you meet someone named Frank Hill, for example, you might think something like, "Frankly, he's getting over the hill."

■ **WRITE IT DOWN.** While attending Yale, Dr. Lyle recalls a sign hanging in a laboratory that said "A short note is better than a long memory." Jotting down notes is an "underappreciated" aspect of memory enhancement, but when older people are more successful at remembering to do things, it may not be because they have better memories—it may be because they're more organized and make more notes for themselves. So make sure you have appointment books, calendars, and notepads available, and use them frequently.

■ **CREATE "FORGET-ME-NOT" SPOTS.** Some things are always getting lost or forgotten—car keys and reading glasses, for example. One of the best memory aids is simply to put these and other commonly lost items in the same places all the time.

The minute you walk in the door, put your keys on a table by the door, Dr. Green suggests. Keep your reading glasses next to the couch or bed. As long as you're consistent, you'll never have to worry about losing these or other items again.

■ **PRACTICE AHEAD OF TIME.** Memory isn't just a matter of retrieving information from the *past*—it also involves remembering things you need to do in the future. If you're out to lunch and recall that you need to send

Pay Attention

If you find that your memory isn't as good as you'd like it to be, make a special effort to focus your attention on the things you want to remember.

"The number one reason we forget things is that we weren't paying attention in the first place," says Cynthia R. Green, Ph.D.

One way the brain sorts information is by routing it to short-term or long-term memory. Long-term memories tend to stay with us, while short-term memories tend to be fleeting. If you don't focus your attention on remembering new things, they'll never make the all-important transition into your long-term memory.

"My favorite technique for remembering names is repetition, in which I say the name back to the person," says Dr. Green.

You can use the same technique for anything. When you put the car keys down, for example, simply repeat to yourself where you're putting them. When you meet someone new, repeat the name in your mind a few times. Making the effort to remember things will help ensure that you do.

---

an important e-mail when you get back to your office, picture yourself doing it, Dr. Lyle says. Imagine sitting at the computer, filling in the subject line, typing out the message, then hitting Send. "It takes only a second or two to picture, yet it enhances the likelihood that we'll remember to do it," he says.

■ **GET PLENTY OF SLEEP.** Being sleep deprived impairs your ability to retrieve memories you've stashed away. A 2008 study found that being sleepy might make you remember things that didn't even happen! Volunteers memorized lists of related words, and in testing later, those who were sleep deprived were more likely to recall words that hadn't been on the list.

Aim for at least 8 hours of sleep each night—

if you're having memory problems, you might need even more sleep to function at your best.

■ **TAKE A MULTIVITAMIN.** The B vitamins, especially vitamin B_{12}, play key roles in memory and mental functions. "As people get older, it becomes harder to absorb B vitamins from the diet," says Dr. Green. "A vitamin B_{12} deficiency can cause significant memory loss."

She recommends a multivitamin that provides 100 percent of the Daily Value for vitamins B_6 and B_{12} and folic acid. Supplements in gel, liquid, or powder forms may be better absorbed than solid supplements, she adds.

■ **GET EXTRA VITAMIN E.** This is an antioxidant nutrient that helps block the harmful effects of free radicals, which are unstable oxygen molecules in the blood. It may reduce buildups of cholesterol and other fatty substances in blood vessels in the brain, and it also appears to reduce inflammation.

Vitamin E is mainly found in nuts, wheat germ, and cooking oils, so it's difficult to get enough in your diet without taking supplements. The optimal dose has not been established, but up to 400 IU of vitamin E daily is probably sufficient, Dr. Gouras says.

■ **EAT LIKE THE MEDITERRANEANS DO.** A 2008 study, in which researchers combined studies that included more than 1.5 million people, found that eating a Mediterranean diet may help protect your memory. The researchers found that people who ate more of the foods common in the diet of Mediterraneans—lots of fruits and vegetables, fish, legumes, and a moderate amount of red wine, but less dairy foods and red and processed meats—had a 13 percent lower incidence of Alzheimer's and Parkinson's disease.

■ **GIVE GINKGO A TRY.** Researchers at the Medical Research Centre at the University of Surrey in Guildford, England, found that taking 120 milligrams of ginkgo three times daily improved memory, concentration, and alertness in test subjects. An herb, ginkgo appears to improve circulation that helps enrich brain cells with the nutrients that they need to stay healthy.

■ **EXERCISE REGULARLY.** Walking, hiking, biking, and other avenues of exercise are among the best ways to increase bloodflow throughout the body, including in the brain. "Regular aerobic exercise also protects us from other illnesses such as stroke, diabetes, and high blood pressure, which contribute to memory problems," Dr. Green says.

■ **KEEP STRESS AT MANAGEABLE LEVELS.** People who are frequently tense or anxious tend to have high levels of cortisol and other stress hormones. Over time, elevated levels of these hormones can affect the hippocampus, which is the part of the brain that controls memory, Dr. Green says.

Stress and anxiety also affect memory indirectly, she adds. If you're tense all the time, you're more likely to have sleep problems—and the resulting fatigue can make it harder to remember things.

"You can't avoid stress entirely, but you can balance it with activities that help you relax," says Dr. Green. "It might be taking the time to do some coloring with your kids. Take a bath or have a massage. Anything that shifts your attention away from what's stressing you out can be helpful."

■ **KEEP CHOLESTEROL LOW.** Laboratory studies have shown that mice given a high-cholesterol and high-fat diet are more likely to develop Alzheimer's disease at an earlier age, Dr. Gouras says. In addition, research suggests that adults who take statins—prescription medications that lower cholesterol—might have a significantly lower risk of developing Alzheimer's disease.

More research is needed to conclusively

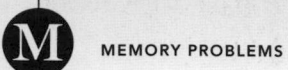

show that lowering cholesterol—either with drugs or with dietary changes—will protect against Alzheimer's disease or memory loss, Dr. Gouras says. But because a diet lower in saturated fat and sugars (which can be converted to fat) has so many other benefits, such as reducing the risk of stroke or heart disease, it's worth the extra effort.

■ **DRINK MORE WATER.** About 85 percent of the brain consists of water. People who don't drink enough can get dehydrated, which leads to fatigue and makes it harder to remember things. Try to drink at least eight 8-ounce glasses of water daily.

■ **DON'T GIVE IN TO DEPRESSION.** It makes it hard to concentrate, and it also causes people to feel tired and sluggish. Among elderly adults, in fact, depression is often mistaken for Alzheimer's disease or other forms of dementia, Dr. Gouras says.

"Depression can be caused by Alzheimer's disease, and it has been found that older patients who get depressed have a higher risk of developing Alzheimer's disease," says Dr. Gouras.

PANEL OF ADVISORS

GUNNAR GOURAS, M.D., IS A PROFESSOR OF NEUROLOGY AND NEUROSCIENCE AT THE WEILL MEDICAL COLLEGE OF CORNELL UNIVERSITY AND ADJUNCT PROFESSOR AT THE FISHER CENTER FOR ALZHEIMER'S RESEARCH AT ROCKEFELLER UNIVERSITY, BOTH IN NEW YORK CITY.

CYNTHIA R. GREEN, PH.D., IS AN ASSISTANT CLINICAL PROFESSOR OF PSYCHIATRY AT MOUNT SINAI SCHOOL OF MEDICINE IN NEW YORK CITY, WHERE SHE FOUNDED THE MEMORY ENHANCEMENT PROGRAM. SHE IS ALSO PRESIDENT OF MEMORY ARTS, A CONSULTING FIRM THAT PROVIDES MEMORY FITNESS TRAINING TO CLIENTS, AND AUTHOR OF *TOTAL MEMORY WORKOUT*.

KEITH LYLE, PH.D., IS A PROFESSOR AT THE UNIVERSITY OF LOUISVILLE, WHERE HE RESEARCHES MEMORY ISSUES, INCLUDING MEMORY ENHANCEMENT, AND AGING AND BRAIN FUNCTION.

Menopause

16 Ways to Embrace the Change

Throughout history, menopause didn't create problems for a lot of women, because most women didn't live long enough to experience it. The average age of menopause in the Western world is 51, and experts confident that the usual onset of menopause has remained the same for centuries. But in the United States, females born even in 1900 lived an average of 48 years.

So if you're approaching menopausal age, perhaps you can find cheer in the fact that at least you get the opportunity to experience a new phase in your life.

And here's another positive news flash about menopause: It's not a disease, nor does it have to present life-altering changes. Many women cruise through menopause with minimal symptoms, and many of the symptoms that women do experience can often be controlled naturally.

Doctors commonly define menopause as the absence of periods for 1 year without other obvious causes. According to the North American Menopause Society, American women enter menopause between the ages of 40 and 58.

The symptoms of menopause vary widely from woman to woman. There may be few for some women, and others may be hit like a gale-force wind. As women age, their estrogen levels drop, which triggers menopause and also increases the risk of

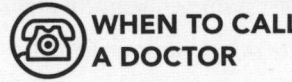 **WHEN TO CALL A DOCTOR**

Mary Jane Minkin, M.D., has a few rules for when you should see your doctor about menopause-related symptoms. First, she recommends an annual exam no matter what. Also, if you have irregular spotting or strange bleeding for any reason, see your doctor, she says. Finally, if menopause leaves you feeling unwell in general, see your doctor.

cardiovascular disease and osteoporosis. The most common symptoms are weight gain, vaginal changes (including dryness and loss of tissue elasticity), sleep disturbances, emotional changes, and hot flashes.

But that doesn't mean *you* have to have these symptoms. Eat right, exercise, and talk to your doctor about the possibility of hormone replacement therapy (HRT), other medications, or herbal remedies. They all can help smooth your transition, enabling you to enjoy the benefits of menopause: no more periods, no more PMS, and no more pregnancy worries.

■ **STAMP OUT THE BUTTS.** Your chances of developing heart disease and osteoporosis jump during menopause. Smoking makes these odds even higher. That's not the only reason to quit. "Smokers have a 2-year-earlier menopause on average than nonsmokers," says Mary Jane Minkin, M.D. Quitting smoking at an early age is critical both for your reproductive health and for a healthy transition into menopause. Granted, if you quit at 48, it won't stop early menopause, but if you're 22 or 23, it might help, she says.

Here's another good reason to quit smoking: When there's smoke, there's more likelihood of hot flashes. (For more on Hot Flashes, see page 348) Research has found that 50 percent of smokers have troublesome hot flashes, compared with 33 percent of women who have never smoked, Dr. Minkin says.

■ **REFRAIN FROM BINGE DRINKING.** Too much booze is another no-no for both bone

and heart health as you transition into menopause. "Drinking a glass of wine a day is fine," says Dr. Minkin. But drinking a bottle a day is definitely not good for either your heart or your bones. Drinking alcohol excessively inhibits bone formation, according to the National Osteoporosis Society, and this is the time of your life when fragile bones become a bigger health concern. (For more on Osteoporosis, see page 468.) And alcohol brings on hot flashes, one of menopause's greatest discomforts, says Dr. Minkin.

■ **BONE UP ON CALCIUM.** You can get a healthy dose of daily calcium from dairy products. "The reality, however, is that most women don't drink a lot of milk and eat a lot of cheese because they're legitimately worried about saturated fat and calories," says Dr. Minkin. To ensure adequate calcium intake, Dr. Minkin recommends taking 1,000 milligrams of supplemental calcium a day.

■ **DON'T FORGET VITAMIN D.** This is the other nutrient that Dr. Minkin pinpoints as crucial to good menopausal health. Although the standard minimum vitamin D recommendation is 400 to 800 IU per day, experts recommend no less than 800 IU daily for women older than 60, Dr. Minkin says.

■ **KNOW THE TRUTH ABOUT HRT.** A persistent myth exists that it's dangerous to go on and off HRT. "It's not," says Dr. Minkin. In fact, she adds, women should feel free to experiment with HRT until they find the combination that works best for them—or decide they don't need it at all.

Dr. Minkin also addresses the other major concern surrounding HRT—the risk of breast cancer. "Taking estrogen for 2 months will not give you breast cancer," she says. Most providers are comfortable with patients continuing estrogen therapy for up to 5 years, she says. After that, you face a small rise in the risk of breast cancer. She doesn't stop HRT for those women taking it for 5 years. Instead, she reviews their dosage at every visit. The North American Menopause Society suggests that estrogen and progesterone are more beneficial if you use them for short-term symptom relief at a younger age.

HRT consistently turns up as one of the best remedies for one of the most troublesome symptoms of menopause: hot flashes, says Dr. Minkin.

■ **KNOW THE TRUTH ABOUT YOUR DIET.** "Women metabolize foods differently than men," says Larrian Gillespie, M.D. "Where men use carbohydrates for energy, women use carbohydrates to store as fat so we're able to procreate in the face of starvation." Plus, she notes, alterations in estrogen levels make these diet differences even more pronounced as we progressively age

To counteract the weight gain typical of menopausal women, Dr. Gillespie recommends eating five or six smaller meals interspersed throughout the day rather than three large meals. "These meals should each be around 250 to 300 calories," she adds.

■ **TRY A LUBRICANT.** Another typical complaint of menopause is decreased sexual desire, sometimes caused by low estrogen–induced physical changes in the vagina. "If the lack of interest in sex is caused by physical discomfort, there are a number of over-the-counter lubricants you can try. You can also ask your doctor about estrogen creams, tablets, or rings," says Dr. Minkin. You can safely use vaginal estrogens "forever," she says, since only a minimal amount is absorbed in your body. "If there are emotional issues involved, however, the couple really needs to focus on matters in their relationship."

■ **TRY THE OLD-FASHIONED SLEEP AIDS.** If sleep is a problem, Dr. Minkin advises some of the old tricks that your grandmother might have taught to you. "Drinking a warm glass of milk, taking a warm bath, or not focusing on the day's events can help you sleep more restfully," she says.

■ **SHARE YOUR TROUBLES WITH FRIENDS.** Much of the stress of menopause for women is

Cures from the Kitchen

As a natural phytoestrogen, soy has proven useful for helping women overcome the symptoms of menopause in numerous studies. You can choose from a variety of soy food products readily available at your grocery store. Mary Jane Minkin, M.D., recommends 45 to 60 milligrams of isoflavones per day. A ½ cup of tofu or a glass of soymilk each day is a good source of isoflavones.

from other life changes that may be occurring at the same time. "Kids are finishing college and moving back home, parents are aging and developing health problems, and husbands are going through their second childhoods. These are all issues I hear from my patients," says Dr. Minkin. Friendships can help you overcome these emotional land mines. "Volunteer your time for a charitable organization, or join a menopause support group," she says. "These are great ways to meet friends, share life's stresses, or just get together and share experiences."

■ **BREATHE DEEPLY.** In one study, 33 women with frequent hot flashes were given lessons in deep breathing, muscle relaxation, or a placebo treatment. Those in the deep breathing group saw their hot flashes cut in half. Practice by sitting comfortably and inhaling deeply through your nose so your belly expands, then exhale through your mouth. Repeat for 15 minutes, taking 5 seconds to breathe in and 5 seconds to exhale. Do this for 5 minutes whenever you have a hot flash.

■ **GIVE YOUR PARTNER A BOOK.** You might feel comfortable with your understanding of your physical and emotional transitions at this point in life. But your partner may be totally oblivious to the changes going on in your body and doesn't understand why things get tough for you from time to time. "Have your partner read up on it to understand the changes your body is going through and then hopefully react with patience and encouragement," says Dr. Minkin.

■ **BUY BLACK COHOSH.** "This is my favorite herb to use for menopausal symptoms. It really does make a big difference," says Connie Catellani, M.D. Studies in menopausal women show that black cohosh may be helpful in treating mild to moderate hot flashes. Research focusing on a standardized black cohosh extract called Remifemin has found it performs on par with estrogen replacement treatment.

Scientists have yet to determine precisely how black cohosh works, but it may help control the effects of estrogen. Some doctors say it shouldn't be used daily for more than 6 months because its long-term effects have not been studied. But women appear to tolerate it well, and adverse events seem to be rare when women take it for 6 months at a time.

To prevent menopausal symptoms, take one or two 40-milligram capsules or tablets of extract (standardized to 2.5 percent triterpene glycosides) twice a day. The dosage for standardized extract is $\frac{1}{2}$ to 1 teaspoon (60 to 120 drops) twice a day, says Dr. Catellani. If you are currently taking HRT and would like to switch to black cohosh, talk to a health care practitioner. You may need guidance to make the transition. Otherwise, you'll have a flare-up of menopausal symptoms.

■ **GET MILK THISTLE.** If you've been taking synthetic hormones and having symptoms related to excess hormone levels—such as breast tenderness, headaches, or bloating—it may mean that your liver isn't "clearing" the breakdown products of these drugs well, says

Serafina Corsello, M.D. To help it out, she recommends milk thistle, or silymarin, an herb that protects the liver against harmful substances and even helps repair and regenerate injured liver cells. Milk thistle is best taken as a standardized extract.

The usual dose for milk thistle is 420 milligrams, divided into two or three doses a day for 6 to 8 weeks, then a reduction to 280 milligrams daily, Dr. Corsello says.

■ **SEEK OUT ST. JOHN'S WORT.** Hormone-related depression, if experienced at an earlier stage in life, may return during menopause, Dr. Catellani says. St. John's wort, long recognized for its ability to fight "melancholy," has been shown to be effective for mild to moderate depression. "It's less likely than prescription antidepressants to cause side effects, such as fatigue, loss of sexual interest, or dry mouth," she explains.

The dosage used in most clinical trials was 300 milligrams in capsule form, three times a day, of an extract containing 0.3 percent hypericin, one of the active ingredients in St. John's wort. And you may need to use it regularly for 2 to 3 weeks before you see an effect. If symptoms persist, seek immediate help from a qualified mental health professional.

■ **CONSIDER KAVA.** Kava is emerging as the herb of choice for women who want to mellow out when life puts them on edge. A 2007 article in the journal *American Family Physician* recommended kava for short-term use in people with mild to moderate anxiety, based on the results of a number of studies. Kava has few side effects compared with prescription antianxiety drugs, is not addictive, and in therapeutic doses does not affect concentration or alertness.

The standard dosage is 70 milligrams of standardized kava extract, taken two or three times a day. "It does work, and it does have a sedating effect, so I might recommend it for short-term situational anxiety," Dr. Catellani says. "But personally, I prefer that women look at and change the things that are causing them anxiety rather than take a pill, whether it's herbal or not."

PANEL OF ADVISORS

CONNIE CATELLANI, M.D., IS A PHYSICIAN IN SKOKIE, ILLINOIS, WHO USES ALTERNATIVE THERAPIES AS PART OF HER PRACTICE.

SERAFINA CORSELLO, M.D., WAS THE MEDICAL DIRECTOR OF THE CORSELLO CENTERS FOR COMPLEMENTARY-ALTERNATIVE MEDICINE IN NEW YORK CITY, AND CURRENTLY FOCUSES ON LIFESTYLE AND NUTRITIONAL COUNSELING. SHE IS AUTHOR OF *THE AGELESS WOMAN*.

LARRIAN GILLESPIE, M.D., IS A RETIRED ASSISTANT CLINICAL PROFESSOR OF UROLOGY AND UROGYNECOLOGY IN LOS ANGELES AND PRESIDENT OF HEALTHY LIFE PUBLICATIONS. SHE IS AUTHOR OF THE BOOKS *THE MENOPAUSE DIET* AND *THE GODDESS DIET*.

MARY JANE MINKIN, M.D., IS A CLINICAL PROFESSOR OF OBSTETRICS AND GYNECOLOGY AT YALE UNIVERSITY SCHOOL OF MEDICINE AND AN OBSTETRICIAN-GYNECOLOGIST IN NEW HAVEN, CONNECTICUT. SHE IS COAUTHOR OF *WHAT EVERY WOMAN NEEDS TO KNOW ABOUT MENOPAUSE* AND *A WOMAN'S GUIDE TO MENOPAUSE AND PERIMENOPAUSE*.

Morning Sickness

13 Ways to Counteract Queasiness

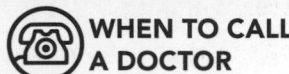 **WHEN TO CALL A DOCTOR**

Consult your physician about your morning sickness if:

■ You notice you've lost a pound or two. Normally, weight gain during pregnancy continues even if you can't keep all your meals down.

■ You feel dehydrated or are not urinating.

■ You find that you can't keep anything down—no water, no juice, nothing—over a period of 4 to 6 hours.

At its most severe, morning sickness can spiral into a condition doctors call hyperemesis gravidarum. Left untreated, it can disturb the essential electrolyte balance in your body, cause pulse irregularities, and, in its severest form, damage the kidneys and liver.

Women with hyperemesis gravidarum are usually hospitalized overnight and treated with an intravenous solution of glucose, water, and vitamins, as well as some medications.

Doctors aren't entirely sure why so-called "morning sickness" occurs during pregnancy. It may have developed as a way to keep mothers-to-be from eating foods that could be possibly harmful to the baby. It may also be from hormonal changes during pregnancy.

But what you're probably more interested in when you have it is how to make it *stop*! Though some women with the condition merely feel mild nausea, others have such severe symptoms they have trouble getting through the day.

Morning sickness is really a misnomer for the vomiting and nausea that affects more than 75 percent of pregnant women. It usually stops after the first 3 months after conception, but sometimes it continues throughout the pregnancy. Some women find that nausea hits at any time of the day or night. Others report feeling worse in the evening, after a long day at work. Some say that certain smells trigger it.

Typically, morning sickness begins around the sixth week of pregnancy—about the same time the placenta begins serious production of human chorionic gonadotropin (HCG), a pregnancy hormone. In most women, symptoms peak during the 8th or 9th week and usually subside after the 13th week.

Knowing that it's temporary isn't a complete source of comfort, though. Research has found that 25 percent of pregnant women have such extreme nausea and vomiting that they take time off from work. More than half become depressed or have difficulties with their relationships because of morning sickness.

The good news about this upsetting condition: Nausea and vomiting are associated with a greater chance of successful pregnancy, according to Tekoa King, C.N.M., M.P.H, a certified nurse-midwife. In one study of 411 women, those *without* morning sickness had more miscarriages and low-birth-weight babies. Another study that combined the results of extensive previous research found a significantly lower risk of miscarriage in women with nausea and vomiting.

With that good news in mind, try these remedies below so that you can say, "I've lost that queasy feeling."

■ **EXPERIMENT.** What worked for your sister, your best friend, or the woman down the street may not do it for you. "There are as many remedies as there are women," says certified nurse-midwife Deborah Gowen, C.N.M. You may need to try a couple of strategies before you find one right for you.

■ **EAT THE WAY YOUR BABY EATS.** The child growing inside you nourishes itself by raiding your bloodstream for glucose 24 hours a day. If you don't take care how you replenish the supply, your blood sugar levels can drop sharply.

Your best tactic, King says, is to switch the way you eat to match how the baby eats: a little bit at a time. Put glucose into your system quickly and easily by eating simple sugars, such as those in fruit. Grapes and orange juice are excellent choices.

■ **AVOID FRIED, FATTY FOODS.** That grilled cheeseburger with onion rings may have looked great to you last week, but you might not want to chance it now.

"Anything fried often seems to make pregnant women more nauseated," King says. The body takes longer to digest such foods, she says, which means they sit in the stomach longer.

■ **CARRY RAW ALMONDS WITH YOU.** Snacking on them fulfills the requirement of small, frequent meals. They contain some fat and some protein, and are high in calcium and potassium. They're portable, too, and tastier than crackers, Gowen says.

■ **KEEP NIBBLES ON YOUR NIGHT TABLE.** If almonds don't appeal to you, or if nausea strikes in the morning, keep crackers by your bed. Moving around on an empty stomach can

Cures from the Kitchen

Although the kitchen may be the last room a nauseated, pregnant woman wants to visit, she'll find several helpful beverages there. Gregory J. Radio, M.D., FACOG, recommends drinking small amounts of clear fluids frequently. Clear broth, fruit juice, and herbal teas such as ginger, raspberry leaf, and chamomile fill the bill. Ginger tea is especially known as a superior remedy for morning sickness. "I don't mean to endorse a product," he says, but Gatorade is usually superb because it can help maintain your electrolytes—substances that regulate the body's electrochemical balance.

Massage to the Rescue

The next time your mate expresses sympathy about your morning sickness, tell him he can do something to help—acupressure massage. Daily allover massage is ideal as a preventive strategy, says Wataru Ohashi, an ohashiatsu teacher.

But if your partner won't go for that, show him the instructions for this quickie technique. It can help in a pinch. Go ahead and hand the book over now.

Have the woman recline on her right side. Sit behind her, supporting her back with your left leg. Slip your left arm under hers and grasp her left shoulder.

With your right hand, massage her entire neck three times. Then place your palm against the base of her skull and stretch her head away from her shoulders.

Next, use your thumb to press down her back in the grooves between the left shoulder blade and the spine and then around the perimeter of her shoulder blade out toward her side. Keep the pressure on for 5 to 7 seconds per point. If you find a sore spot, gently give it extra attention. Slip your thumb as far under her shoulder blade as is comfortable for her.

Begin with gentle pressure and let your partner tell you if she wants more pressure. Always use your body weight, not your muscle power. "The feeling is totally different," says Ohashi.

"If you stimulate the external, you can eliminate the internal discomfort," says Ohashi. The trigger points you use in this exercise affect the stomach and the hormonal system, he says.

make you feel worse, says King, who considers morning sickness "one of my many areas of expertise. I'm the 'vomiting woman' at work." So eat something to bring your blood sugar up before you get out of bed in the morning or in the middle of the night.

■ **TRY GINGER.** This herbal remedy is one of the first methods King recommends "when women are having nausea but they're not throwing up and they're not dehydrated, and they don't want to use medication." She's seen that it can provide women some relief. Although you can get ginger in tea or cookies, the smell may be a turnoff when you're nauseous. Instead, try it in capsule form. Take 500 milligrams twice a day or 250 milligrams four times a day, she advises. However, if you're at risk of hemorrhage, avoid ginger.

■ **PRESS THE RIGHT SPOT.** Another natural remedy that some women find helpful is pressing a particular acupressure point on your wrist called the P6 point, King suggests. This may simply work as a placebo ... but if it works, you're not likely going to care why.

To find the spot, place your fingertip in the center of your wrist—between two tendons—the width of two fingers away from the crease where your palm starts. Press and await relief. As an alternative, you can wear a motion sickness device called Sea Band that puts pressure on the inside of your wrist.

■ **CONSIDER A ONE-TWO PUNCH.** Another solution for nausea is to take half a 25-milligram tablet of Unisom, an over-the-counter sleep aid, in the morning along with 10 milligrams of vitamin B_6. In the evening, again take one tablet along with another 10 milligrams of B_6, King suggests. This combination recreates a medicine called Benectin, which is no longer available in the United States, she says. Before trying this, ask your doctor if this might be helpful for you.

■ **IF YOU'RE TAKING PRENATAL VITAMINS, CHECK WITH YOUR DOCTOR.** In some instances, they can make you sick to your stomach, Gowen says. Your doctor or midwife may be able to switch you to a different brand or a chewable vitamin that won't upset your stomach.

■ **TRUST YOUR BODY'S WISDOM.** "Eat whatever appeals to you, as long as you're not eating junk," Gowen says. "Avoid caffeine, artificial sweeteners, and all drugs. But if you crave pasta, then eat it. It really does work when women listen to their bodies."

■ **KEEP CALM.** If you continue to put on weight, and dehydration isn't a problem for you, you're probably doing just fine.

"Women don't tend to lose beyond what their body stores can handle," says King. "I think we just don't know the magic of what goes on inside the mother. My belief is that you can really be fairly ill with morning sickness, yet you can continue nourishing your baby very well."

PANEL OF ADVISORS

DEBORAH GOWEN, C.N.M., IS A CERTIFIED NURSE-MIDWIFE IN ARLINGTON, MASSACHUSETTS.

TEKOA KING, C.N.M., M.P.H., IS A NURSE-MIDWIFE AND DEPUTY EDITOR OF THE *JOURNAL OF MIDWIFERY & WOMEN'S HEALTH.*

WATARU OHASHI IS AN INTERNATIONALLY KNOWN TEACHER OF OHASHIATSU AND FOUNDER OF THE OHASHI INSTITUTE, A NONPROFIT ORGANIZATION IN NEW YORK CITY.

GREGORY J. RADIO, M.D., FACOG, IS CHAIR OF PRIMARY CARE IN THE DEPARTMENT OF OBSTETRICS AND GYNECOLOGY AT LEHIGH VALLEY HOSPITAL IN ALLENTOWN, PENNSYLVANIA, AND ASSISTANT CLINICAL PROFESSOR OF OBSTETRICS AND GYNECOLOGY AT MILTON S. HERSHEY MEDICAL SCHOOL OF PENNSYLVANIA STATE UNIVERSITY.

Motion Sickness

19 Quick-Action Cures

Cures from the Kitchen

Folk remedies for motion sickness have probably been around since before the first buggy ride. Here are some that are worth trying.

GINGER. Although the remedy is tried and true, ginger passed scientific scrutiny when an experiment showed that two powdered gingerroot capsules were more effective than a dose of Dramamine in preventing motion sickness.

OLIVES AND LEMONS. Motion sickness causes you to produce excess saliva, which can make you nauseated, some doctors say. Olives produce chemicals called tannins, which make your mouth dry. Hence, the theory goes, eating a couple of olives at the first hint of nausea can help diminish it, as can sucking on a mouth-puckering lemon.

SODA CRACKERS. They won't stop salivation, but dry soda crackers may help absorb the excess fluid when it reaches your stomach. Their "secret ingredients" are bicarbonate of soda and cream of tartar.

The French call seasickness *mal de mer*, and even the most seasoned sailors can suffer from it. When travelling by air, it's called airsickness. On land, it's car sickness. At amusement parks, it's ride sickness. At least one visitor a day turns green on Disney World's Space Mountain or the Big Thunder Mountain roller coaster. Regardless of what you call it, it's all the same thing: that queasy, uneasy feeling collectively known as motion sickness.

Your body relies on several systems to keep you operating properly when you're in motion, says Tim Hain, M.D. These include structures in your inner ears; your eyes; so-called somatosensors around your body that take in information such as touch; and an internal mental sense of motion, in which your mind anticipates the motions that you'll soon be making.

"In general, when a mismatch occurs between one or more of these, there's potential for motion sickness," Dr. Hain says. For example, if you're in the backseat of a car reading a book as you travel over bumpy, curvy roads, your inner ears are reporting that you're bouncing all around, but your eyes are fixed on the book in front of you. This is a common recipe for motion sickness.

Although not everyone gets motion sickness, the signals are

pretty clear when it does occur. Dizziness. Sweating. Pale skin and feelings of nausea. If things don't improve, you throw up.

Once you feel the symptoms coming on, motion sickness can be very difficult to stop, especially if you've reached your particular point of no return—usually once nausea sets in. But the following remedies can help nurse the symptoms, perhaps even cutting them short. Better yet, they may keep them from starting in the first place the next time you're bobbing and rolling, rolling and bobbing along on a choppy sea's waves.

■ **THINK ABOUT MOTION WELLNESS.** "Motion sickness is partly psychological," says Horst Konrad, M.D. "If you think you're going to throw up, you're probably going to." Instead, turn your thoughts to something more pleasant than your surroundings.

■ **LEAVE NURSING THE SICK TO SOMEONE ELSE.** It's a common occurrence. You're on a fishing boat. Everything's going along fine until someone gets sick. You watch in sympathy, maybe even offer a comforting shoulder. Before long, you're the next body down. Then another hits the deck. It's the domino theory in action. As cruel as it may sound, do your best to ignore others who are sick, says Dr. Konrad. Otherwise, you're liable to end up in the same proverbial boat.

■ **GET YOUR NOSE OUT OF THE JOINT.** Bad odors such as engine fumes, the dead fish on ice in the back of the boat, or the airline food passing by on the flight attendant's cart can contribute to nausea, says Dr. Konrad. Aim your nose elsewhere.

■ **BUTT OUT.** If you're a smoker, you may think that lighting up can calm you, deterring motion sickness. Wrong. Cigarette smoke contributes to impending nausea, says Dr. Konrad. If you're a nonsmoker, you should hightail it to the nonsmoking section when you feel queasiness coming on.

■ **TRAVEL AT NIGHT.** Your chances of getting sick diminish when you travel at night because you can't see the motion as well as you can during daylight, says Roderic W. Gillilan, O.D.

■ **THINK BEFORE YOU DRINK.** "Too much alcohol can interfere with the way the brain handles information about the environment, setting off motion sickness symptoms," says Dr. Konrad. What's more, alcohol can dissolve into the fluids in your inner ear, which can send your head spinning, he says. Drink in moderation, if at all, during plane and ship travel.

■ **EAT BEFORE YOU GO.** Oftentimes people won't eat before they begin an activity that's likely to cause motion sickness, says Max Levine, Ph.D. This seems reasonable, but it's not a good idea. "Having an empty stomach is one of the worst things you can do. It seems that if you get your stomach into its normal rhythm of contraction, it's more likely to stay that way than if it's sitting there with nothing to do in the first place."

In one of Dr. Levine's studies, participants sat with their head inside a rotating drum painted with black and white stripes for several minutes, which, not surprisingly, can induce nausea. Those who drank a high-protein shake first reported fewer symptoms than those who'd eaten nothing, and measurements of their stomach activity found less excess churning. So eat a snack containing protein before you head off on your potentially stomach-churning activity. Just make sure it's low in fat—a high-fat food such as a cheeseburger wouldn't help.

■ **GET ENOUGH SLEEP.** "Your chance of getting motion sickness increases with fatigue," says Dr. Gillilan. So be sure to get your usual quota of sleep before taking off on a trip. If you're a passenger in a car or plane, catching a few Zzzs while en route can help, too, if only to temporarily ward off potentially sickening stimuli.

■ **GET BEHIND THE WHEEL.** Being in control of your situation—or even *feeling* like you're in control—can help reduce nausea, Dr. Levine says. In other research involving the striped rotating nausea machine, when participants were given a button to push that they thought controlled the rotation, they had less-severe symptoms, even though they were exposed to as much spinning as the people without the button.

So when you're traveling, you may be less likely to feel sick if you're the driver rather than the passenger. It's also a good idea to stick with familiar routes so you can get to your destination more effectively and better anticipate the types of movements that are coming up, Dr. Hain says.

■ **GET CAUGHT UP ON YOUR READING SOME OTHER TIME.** Obviously, if reading in a moving vehicle tends to trigger motion sickness, save your reading material for later. Sure, skimming the pages may make the time go by faster, but the nausea and vomiting that ensues will make the trip feel *much* longer.

If you absolutely must read, there are ways to do it without getting sick, says Dr. Gillilan. Among them:

■ Slouch in the seat and hold the reading material close to eye level. "It's not the reading itself that makes you sick," he says, "but the angle at which you're doing it. When you look down while traveling in a car, the visible motion from the side windows strikes the eyes at an unusual angle, and that triggers the symptoms. This method brings your eyes into the same position as if you were looking down the road."

■ Hold your hands next to your temples to block out the action, or turn your back to the window nearest you.

■ **SCAN THE HORIZON.** In a car, move up to the front seat and focus on the road ahead or the horizon. This can help bring signals from your body and your eyes into balance. The same goes for travel on a ship or boat: Don't stare down at the water, where you'll see the craft rise and fall and the waves crash around you. Instead, fix your eyes on a point

A Space-Age Cure That Goes to Extremes

"...Four, three, two, one—liftoff!" With an earth-shaking roar, white-hot jets propel Spacelab 3 and its four-member crew into the stratosphere, where it turns its back on a world still tremulously shivering. But the folks in ground control aren't the only ones shaken up by the blast. A mere 7 minutes into the flight, one of the crew members has his first "vomiting episode," an incident that is rerun numerous times during the mission.

Being motion sick in space is a serious problem for astronauts. "At any one time, the whole crew could be incapacitated," says Patricia Cowings, Ph.D. "Potentially, it could be disastrous. Throwing up while wearing a helmet could be fatal." And there's no easy solution, since motion sickness medications can have dangerous side effects.

But new horizons are opening up, thanks to a biofeedback training program. For decades, Dr. Cowings and her colleagues have been making people sick in order to help astronauts feel better.

"Essentially, our routine involves bringing a person up to our lab and making him throw up," says Dr. Cowings, known to her colleagues as the "Baroness of Barf." A devious device aids this process: a chair that rotates while moving volunteers' heads at various angles, a process that throws off the inner ear's sense of balance in a few minutes. "It works on virtually everyone," she says.

While rotating, the subject is monitored for physiological responses such as heart rate, breathing rate, sweating, and muscle contractions. "No two people have exactly the same response," Dr. Cowings says. "Motion sickness is actually a kind of fingerprint that's unique to each person." Once the fingerprint is revealed, it's a map for each person to learn to control his particular responses through a combination of deep relaxation and exercise of muscles—muscles we don't realize we can exercise, like those in blood vessels.

If you can learn to successfully control your early responses, you may prevent more violent ones from coming up. The success rate is so great that Dr. Cowings and her colleagues patented the technique. "About 60 percent can completely eliminate their symptoms when we retest them in the chair. Another 25 percent can significantly decrease their responses. And the training remains effective for up to 3 years," she says.

The results are promising enough to suggest that an actual cure for motion sickness is on the horizon, says Dr. Cowings.

on the horizon, preferably an unmoving object like the shoreline.

■ **WEAR ACUPRESSURE WRISTBANDS.** Sold in many marine and travel shops, these lightweight wristbands have a plastic button that is supposed to be worn over what Eastern doctors call the Nei-Kuan acupressure point inside each wrist. Pressing the button for a few

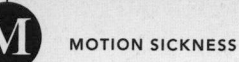

minutes should protect you against nausea.

■ **GET OVER-THE-COUNTER RELIEF.** Non-prescription remedies such as Dramamine and Bonine can be helpful, but you need to take them *before* you get sick, Dr. Hain says. If you're susceptible to motion sickness, take the remedy 30 minutes before you start moving. Also, beware that these medications cause drowsiness, so they may not be a good choice if you need to be alert.

■ **REMEMBER, TIME HEALS ALL WOUNDS.** This includes motion sickness. You may feel like you're going to die, but motion sickness doesn't kill. Your body should eventually adjust to the environment in a ship or boat—although it might take a few days.

So be patient. Things will get better.

PANEL OF ADVISORS

PATRICIA COWINGS, PH.D., IS THE PRINCIPAL INVESTIGATOR OF PSYCHOPHYSIOLOGICAL RESEARCH LABORATORIES AT NASA'S AMES RESEARCH CENTER IN MOFFETT FIELD, CALIFORNIA. SHE'S ALSO A PROFESSOR OF PSYCHIATRY AT THE UNIVERSITY OF CALIFORNIA, LOS ANGELES.

RODERIC W. GILLILAN, O.D., IS A RETIRED OPTOMETRIST IN EUGENE, OREGON, WHERE HE STILL WORKS IN EDUCATION REGARDING MOTION SICKNESS.

TIM HAIN, M.D., IS A PROFESSOR OF NEUROLOGY, OTOLARYNGOLOGY, AND PHYSICAL THERAPY-HUMAN MOVEMENT SCIENCE AT THE NORTHWESTERN UNIVERSITY MEDICAL SCHOOL IN CHICAGO.

HORST KONRAD, M.D., IS A PROFESSOR OF OTOLARYNGOLOGY AT THE SOUTHERN ILLINOIS UNIVERSITY SCHOOL OF MEDICINE IN SPRINGFIELD.

MAX LEVINE, PH.D., IS AN ASSISTANT PROFESSOR OF PSYCHOLOGY AT SIENA COLLEGE IN LOUDONVILLE, NEW YORK, WHERE HE FOCUSES ON MIND-BODY ISSUES RELATED TO NAUSEA.

Muscle Pain

37 Ways to Relief

You have more than 600 muscles in your body, and pain can strike any of them. Perhaps you've developed a painfully strained muscle or tendon—typically in your lower back or in the back of your upper leg. Maybe you have delayed onset muscle soreness after a workout. Perhaps you're sound asleep not challenging your muscles at all and you're awakened by a piercing calf cramp.

No matter the source of the pain, you may feel like your body has turned against you. But fear not—you can regain control of the muscle that's hurting and possibly prevent the pain from happening in the future.

■ **CEASE WHAT YOU'RE DOING.** "Rule number one is to stop the activity," says Martin Z. Kanner, M.D. He jokingly says his medical practice has two kinds of patients: "People who should exercise and won't, and people who shouldn't exercise and do." People who are working toward a goal such as a marathon, or teenage athletes who can't see beyond their next game, often have a hard time giving their bodies a break. But if you have muscle pain that's bad enough to be consulting this chapter, now is the time to stop pushing yourself.

A cramp may require only minutes of rest, but a severe strain may need days or weeks.

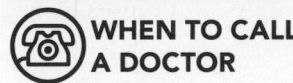 **WHEN TO CALL A DOCTOR**

Most of the time, the pain of a sudden muscle cramp, strain, or even extreme soreness is a lot worse than the injury. But not always.

Cramping, for example, could be the result of a nerve injury. Or, in rare cases, it could be the result of phlebitis—inflammation of a vein. Phlebitis can become serious if a deep vein is involved, but is typically not serious when the inflammation is located in a superficial vein. (For more information, see Phlebitis on page 475.

Muscle problems that take on abnormal characteristics and linger *may* be more serious. Consult your doctor.

425

Stretch to Strengthen

Give muscles the attention they need, and they tend to do their jobs quietly. Ignore them, and they'll scream for attention by cramping or becoming strained when moved the wrong way.

When that happens, you may be able to quiet them again with some simple stretching exercises. But if you want them to remain quiet, you probably will have to incorporate stretching into the daily activities in regular life.

Here are a few suggestions from doctors, athletic trainers, and physical therapists to help you keep your attention on work and play, not on muscle pain.

Toe the towel. To stretch and strengthen ankle muscles, sit on the floor and loop a towel around the ball of your foot while holding the ends of the towel in each hand. Alternately point your toes up and down while pulling the ends of the towel toward you and keeping your legs straight. Repeat several times with both feet.

Toe the towel again. This time don't move your toes. Lean back with the towel looped around your foot until you feel the stretch in the calf muscle. Hold for 15 seconds and repeat several times.

Use the steps. To stretch your calves, stand on the bottom step of a staircase and hold the railing for balance. Move one foot back so that the ball of the foot is at the edge of the step and your heel hangs off the back. Then, with both knees slightly bent, drop your heel below the step and feel a stretch in the back of your lower leg. Hold for 30 seconds, then switch legs.

■ **SERVE YOURSELF A BIG HELPING OF RICE.** This stands for rest, ice, compression, and elevation, Dr. Kanner says. Hopefully, you're already resting: Refrain from athletic activity, and avoid putting any weight on the injured area if you're really in pain.

The remaining steps in the formula help reduce inflammation and swelling in the injured muscle.

To ice an injured muscle, wrap a bag of ice cubes in a cloth and apply it to the sore spot for no more than 20 minutes at a time, Dr. Kanner says. A good alternative is a cloth-wrapped bag of frozen veggies, which you can mold around the body part—he knows one woman who's been using the same bag of peas for years.

You can get compression from wrapping the injury snugly with an elastic bandage—but not so tight that your body tingles or turns a darker color on the other end of the bandage. Leave on for no more than 4 hours at a time. Elevate your arm or leg above the level of your heart to help reduce swelling. You may need to prop up your arm or leg on a pillow.

■ **GET WARM.** About 48 hours after the injury, you can begin stretching the sore muscle a little and heating it—preferably at the same time. This will help avoid "contractures,"

Get into bed. Actually, sit with one leg stretched out on the bed and hang the other leg over the side. Then lean forward until you feel the stretch in your hamstring (the back of the thigh) and hold for 10 to 15 seconds. Repeat several times, then switch positions and stretch the other hamstring.

Stand on one leg. To stretch your quadriceps (the front of the thigh) muscles, stand on one leg and hold your opposite foot so that the ankle is touching your buttocks and your knee points toward the floor. Hold for 10 seconds. Repeat five times with each leg.

Reach back. For a good shoulder stretch, place one arm, with elbow bent, behind your head, and using the opposite hand, gently pull your elbow behind your head.

Reach around. Another good shoulder stretch is to hold one arm, with elbow bent, across your midriff and use the opposite hand to gently pull the arm across the front of your body.

Stretch your wrists. Make a fist, then span or spread your fingers as far as possible. Relax. Repeat three or four times.

Stretch your forearms. Hold your arms straight out in front of your body with your palms facing down. Bend your hands up, so that your palms face away from you. Hold that stretch for 5 seconds. Then bend your hands down, so that your palms are facing toward you. Hold that stretch for 5 seconds. Repeat three or four times.

muscle tightness that won't loosen back up. Your natural tendency is not to move the part of your body that hurts, Dr. Kanner says, but it's important that you do. Step into a hot shower and slowly start circling the achy part. Go just to the point of pain, and don't push further. Whirlpools and heat wraps offer other good methods of warming yourself.

■ **LOOK FOR ARNICA ON THE INGREDIENT LIST.** Old-time folk remedies for sore muscles contained arnica, a yellow-orange flower found in Europe and North America. Arnica-containing lotions are available at many health food stores and some supermar-

kets. You should test a small patch of skin before applying it liberally. Note: Some people are allergic to a chemical in the flower.

■ **STRETCH FOR PREVENTION—IF YOU'D LIKE.** Although you may have memories of a high-school gym teacher urging you to reach further toward your toes, research has gone "back and forth" on whether stretching is beneficial for your muscles during physical activity, says Gregory Snow, D.C., C.C.S.P.

A 2004 review of studies didn't find enough evidence to support stretching before or after exercise among serious or recreational athletes—or discourage it, either. A 2007 study in the journal *Sports Medicine,* however, suggested warming up first with low-intensity movements that create slight sweating, then stretching. This is all done within 15 minutes before your workout or event.

Warm up for at least 5 minutes (stretching cold muscles may raise your risk of injury), then stretch if you'd like, Dr. Snow suggests. Once you're finished with your exercise, stretch again. That final stretching session "is helpful for recovery and feeling good the next day and keeping the muscles lengthened after the activity, when they're most fatigued," he says. See "Stretch to Strengthen" on pages 426–427 for more ideas.

■ **TRY SOME CAFFEINE BEFOREHAND.** One study found that women who had the amount of caffeine equivalent to that in 2½ cups of coffee an hour before a 30-minute bike ride had roughly half the leg muscle pain as riders who didn't have caffeine.

Caffeine may block an inflammatory chemical from attaching to areas in your brain or muscles that are associated with pain, according to the lead researcher. Even one preexercise cup of coffee may help.

■ **DRINK SOME CHERRY JUICE.** It may not often be considered a sports drink, but cherry juice contains natural anti-inflammatory chemicals that can reduce pain and swelling. Participants in one study who drank 16 ounces daily for 3 days before a hard workout felt less muscle soreness two days later.

■ **ACCEPT YOUR LIMITATIONS.** "Those of us older than 40 think we can do everything we did 20 years ago, and we can't," Dr. Kanner says. He compares muscles with rubber bands: At 20, they're like a fresh rubber band that springs back after you stretch it. At 40, they're more like a rubber band that's fallen behind the couch for several years. It's stiffer and will snap more quickly when you overstretch it.

Although it's important to stay active as you get older, make sure your pace and activities change to accommodate your body's evolving limits.

■ **WEAR WARM CLOTHING.** If you're exercising in cold weather and feel you're getting stiff and sore, warm up with more clothes. You may be able to halt muscle problems right there.

In cold weather, former New York Jets head trainer Bob Reese had players wear running tights under their uniforms to retain the heat. "The players like the compressive feeling it gives them, and the tights support the muscles a little bit," he says.

■ **CHANGE POSITIONS.** Whether you're bent over a keyboard typing or bent over a bicycle pedaling, your wrists and forearms are vulnerable to cramping and soreness, says Scott Donkin, D.C. But there's one important difference between cyclists and office workers—when cyclists buy bikes, a salesperson is usually there to make sure they select the bike that best fits them. Yet office workers, who have fingers and hands of all different sizes,

Banish Nighttime Leg Cramps

Few things hurt worse than a charley horse—the searing pain of a calf muscle cramp that can wake you from the dead of sleep.

What happened? Basically, your calf muscle got stuck. Leg muscles contract when you turn or stretch during sleep. When a muscle stays contracted, a sudden cramp can result.

Here's how to stop night cramps and, hopefully, head off a recurrence later in the night.

Lean into the wall. Stand 3 to 5 feet away from a wall, keeping your heels flat and your legs straight. Lean into the wall in front of you as you support yourself with your hands. Hold for 10 seconds and repeat several times.

Massage the cramp. Massage the calf by rubbing upward from the ankle. If night cramps are a constant problem, you may want to do this before you go to bed.

Loosen the covers. The pressure of heavy blankets on your legs could be partly to blame.

Wear loose, flowing roomy PJs. Snug-fitting pajamas will only exacerbate nighttime leg cramps if you're prone to them.

Use an electric blanket. The electric blanket on your bed can do more than keep you warm all over on cold winter nights; it can also keep your calf muscles warm and pain-free.

Sleep on your side. Sleeping on your stomach with your legs straight out and your calves flexed invites cramping, says Scott Donkin, D.C. "Try sleeping on your side with your knees bent upward and a pillow between them."

Consider more calcium. "A calcium deficiency can make the muscles trigger-happy; the contractions in the muscles are stronger," Dr. Donkin says. The Daily Value for calcium is 1,000 milligrams a day (1,200 if you're older than age 50).

---

typically use the same office equipment. With the selection of ergonomic accessories out there for desk jockeys, all it takes is a little research and testing to find a setup that puts you in a comfortable, ergonomically correct position.

"The wrist and hands should be used in what is known as the neutral position," according to Dr. Donkin. "In this position, the wrist is bent neither forward, backward, inward, nor outward."

If you have long hands and fingers, you can reduce the strain on the wrist by adjusting the keyboard to a more horizontal position (flat with the work surface) as long as it does not put your arms or shoulders in a strained position. For those who have short hands and fingers, a higher incline on the keyboard will make the keys easier to reach.

■ **REPEAT THE ACTIVITY THAT MADE YOU SORE.** It sounds counterintuitive, but it helps.

"Do the activity again the very next day," Reese says, "but with much less intensity. It will help work out some of the soreness."

Moderate exercise has been shown to release brain chemicals called endorphins that act as natural painkillers. Also, the movement can stimulate bloodflow to the achy muscles, which may help remove inflammatory substances that are contributing to the pain.

■ **TRY THE CURCUMIN CURE.** The spice turmeric contains curcumin, which has an anti-inflammatory property that may work like nonsteroidal anti-inflammatory drugs. Look for curcumin supplements containing 95 percent curcumin; the typical dosage is 400 milligrams three times daily.

■ **GET ROLLING.** Exercisers have been flocking to foam rollers—firm foam tubes that you use to massage your muscles by resting your body weight on them. For example, for sore thighs, lie on your left side with your weight resting on the roller under your left thigh. Extend your left leg and cross your right leg over it, and rest your weight on your left forearm and right foot. Push up slightly from the floor with your right foot and work your left thigh across the roller for 2 minutes, stopping briefly at sore points. Switch sides and repeat on your right side.

■ **BRANCH OUT.** When one set of muscles hurt, use some others. For example, walkers experiencing sore lower leg muscles should mix in some swimming or bicycling (which works the upper legs) in order to continue exercising while healing.

■ **LOSE WEIGHT.** If sore muscles and muscle strains have become a chronic problem, the extra weight you're asking them to move may be at least partially to blame. Get rid of those unwanted pounds by changing your diet and exercise habits.

■ **BE REALISTIC.** If running always makes you hurt, for example, then you may have to find another exercise. "Running is one of the most dangerous sports for injuries," says Gabe Mirkin, M.D. When you run, both feet leave the ground, creating repeated impact when you land. None of his athletic friends from mid-century are still running, he says, and though he claims that "I can't run across the street," he's doing 100-mile bike rides at a fast pace even in his seventies.

■ **BALANCE OUT YOUR STATIN DRUG.** People taking statins to lower their cholesterol may run into a common side effect: muscle pain. Research has found that taking 100 milligrams of the supplement coenzyme Q10 (CoQ10) daily helped reduce soreness in a small group of people on statins. Taking the drugs may lower your body's natural production of CoQ10, contributing to pain. If you're taking a statin, ask your doctor if this remedy may help.

■ **CHANGE YOUR SHOES.** Wearing the wrong kind of shoes or shoes that don't fit well could explain the foot, leg, and even back pains you feel while exercising, says sports medicine expert Mike McCormick.

■ **DON'T JUST SIT THERE—MOVE!** Whenever you're sitting down for long periods of time—whether at work in front of the computer or at home in front of the TV—get up and move at least once an hour, Dr. Snow says. This keeps your blood flowing and your muscles loosened.

■ **LOOSEN YOUR CLOTHING.** If you feel a leg cramp coming on, you may want to shed tights or other snug clothing to give your muscles a little more room.

■ **DRINK UP.** Dehydration is often a big contributor to cramping, McCormick says. "We overstress the need to force liquids, especially before, during, and after physical activity. And for good reason."

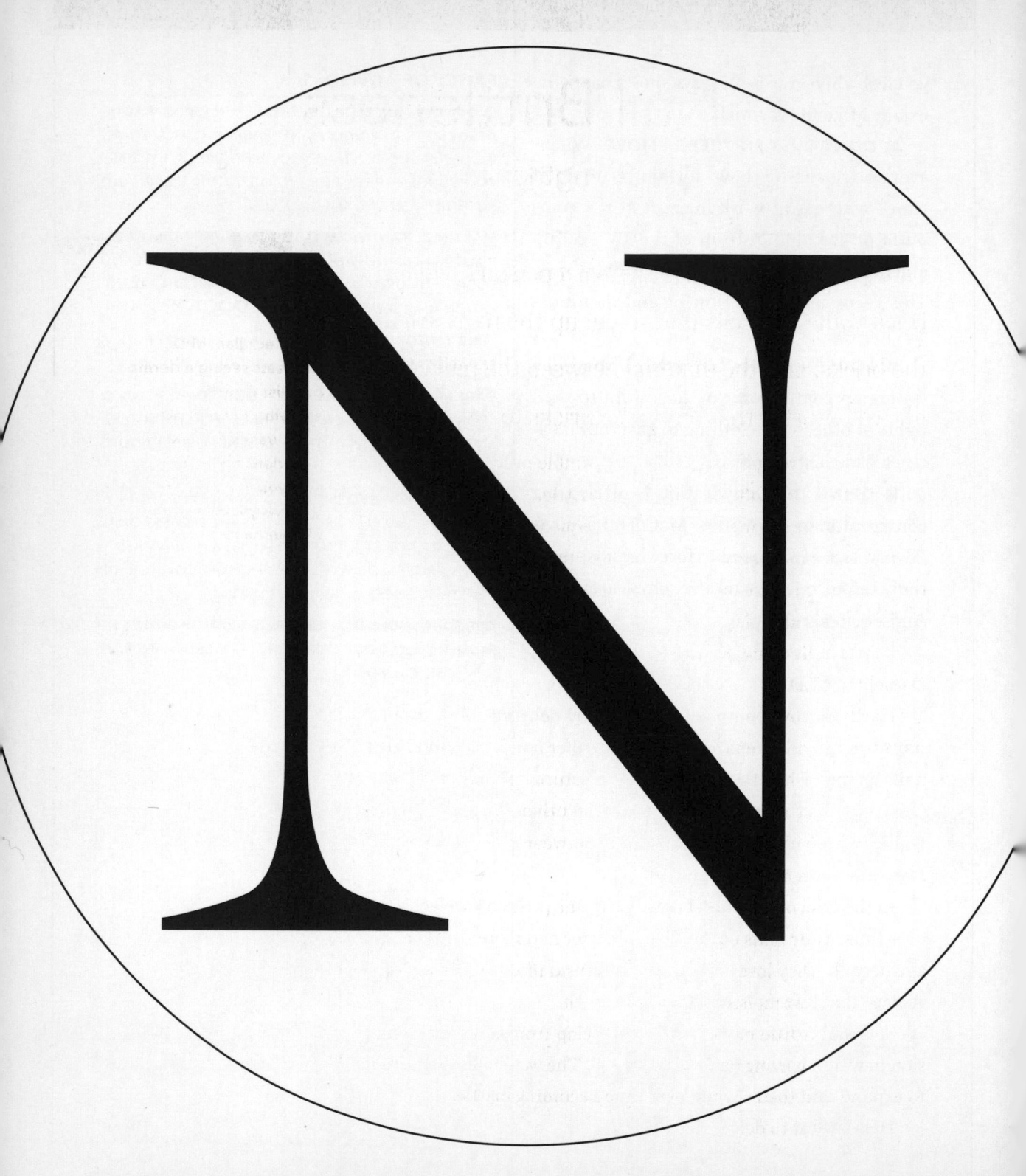

Nail Brittleness

14 Strengthening Secrets

Paul Kechijian, M.D., compares a person's nails to a brick wall. The cells that make up the nails are like the bricks, and the material between the nail cells is like the mortar that binds the bricks together.

But even strong brick walls can crumble over time, and your nails can also become damaged and brittle. The main causes of brittle nails are aging, followed by frequent hand washing and drying, and exposure to household cleaning products, he says. All of these lead to decreased moisture in the hands. Exposure to nail cosmetics can also play a role.

Brittle nails come in two varieties: hard and soft, says C. Ralph Daniel III, M.D.

Hard and brittle nails are caused by dehydration—too *little* moisture in and around nails. On the other hand, soft and brittle nails happen when there's too *much* moisture in and around nails. One type isn't more common than the other, according to Dr. Daniel. "I see about a fifty-fifty split between the two types," he says. "But both are treatable."

In the case of hard and brittle nails, the problem can get worse over time. Your nails naturally get harder and more brittle as you age because they lose some of their natural moisture. If you don't replace that lost moisture, they may crack.

Soft and brittle nails, however, develop from constant immersion in water, leaving nails waterlogged. The water causes the nails to expand and then shrink, over time becoming brittle.

Here's what to do.

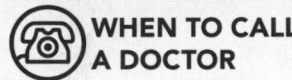

WHEN TO CALL A DOCTOR

Paul Kechijian, M.D., suggests seeing a dermatologist if you've been applying a moisturizer for 2 weeks and are still experiencing brittle nails, or if your nails hurt or affect the everyday function of your hands.

No Thumbs-Up for Nail Strengtheners

The corner drugstore is often the first stop for people with brittle nails. They turn to nail strengtheners in the hope of transforming their brittle nails into unbreakable ones. Our experts say that these nail strengtheners aren't all that they're cracked up to be.

Nail strengtheners purportedly contain an ingredient that binds to damaged nails to make them thicker. But you can't change the quality of the nail simply by applying something to the surface, says Paul Kechijian, M.D. Instead of fixing the problem of brittle nails, he says, they merely camouflage the brittleness.

■ **REACH FOR SOME HAND CREAM.** After washing and drying your hands apply a moisturizing hand cream to your hands and nails each time. The hand cream traps moisture, keeping your hands and nails from drying out, says Dr. Kechijian.

Because your nails expand like an accordion when they absorb water and then contract when the water evaporates, products that attract and bind moisture to your nails, both morning and night, are the most effective. Over-the-counter creams with 5 percent lactic acid, such as Lac-Hydrin Five, best fit this description. "You might also try any glycolic acid preparation (Total Skin Care Glycolic Gel is one) or any good moisturizer available at your neighborhood drugstore. Ask your pharmacist to recommend one, or try a few until you find one you like," Dr. Kechijian says.

■ **SHOP AROUND.** Over-the-counter moisturizers are sold in many different scents and textures. Dee Anna Glaser, M.D., suggests finding your favorite aroma and feel.

The reason? You're more apt to use a product you enjoy.

Dr. Glaser also encourages people with brittle nails to keep small tubes of moisturizer on hand so that they can apply it after every washing. Stash tubes by all the sinks at home as well as in your car glove compartment and desk drawer at work.

■ **AVOID ALCOHOL.** Some perfumed hand lotions contain alcohol. Avoid these types if your nails are brittle. The alcohol only makes your brittle nails worse because of its drying effect, says Dr. Daniel.

■ **KEEP NAILS SHORT AND SWEET.** Longer nails are more subject to trauma and are more likely to crack or get caught on something and tear. Dr. Kechijian also proposes cutting your nails after showering, when they're softer and less likely to break.

■ **EAT A WELL-BALANCED DIET.** Brittle nails can be the result of something you are—or aren't—eating, says Dr. Glaser. "Eating a well-balanced diet and taking a daily multivitamin and mineral supplement to get your recommended daily allowance are important. Any trendy diet that includes only a few foods or excludes certain food groups can produce nail problems," she adds.

■ **DOUBLE GLOVE.** If washing dishes is on your daily "to-do" list, Dr. Kechijian suggests investing in several pairs of cotton gloves to use under your rubber dishwashing gloves. The vinyl exterior of the dishwashing gloves keeps water and detergent off your nails, and the cotton gloves absorb sweat so that your nails and hands don't get soggy inside the glove.

■ **DISH OFF SOME CHORES.** While agreeing wholeheartedly that people with brittle nails should wear gloves while doing household chores, Audrey Kunin, M.D., has an even better way to limit your water exposure: Get someone else to wash the dishes.

Cures from the Kitchen

Rub oil or thick hand cream into your nails while applying your hand moisturizer for better results, says Audrey Kunin, M.D. You can use expensive store-bought creams or look in your kitchen for vegetable oil or shortening.

Dee Anna Glaser, M.D., recommends this extra-soothing nighttime treatment. Before you go to bed, apply vegetable oil to your hands, then put on vinyl gloves or wrap your hands in plastic wrap to keep the oil off bedspreads and pillowcases. The hand coverings force the oil to penetrate your skin, preventing your hands from getting too dry.

■ **GO WITH ACETATE, NOT ACETONE.** Be sure to use nail polish removers that contain acetate. "Acetone nail polish removers are stronger, but they can take much-needed moisture out of your nails and make them brittle," says Dr. Daniel.

■ **DON'T PICK.** Avoid picking or peeling polish—this removes the protective top layer from the nails.

■ **ADD SOME CALCIUM.** A lack of calcium in the diet is another cause of brittle nails, says Dr. Kunin. Calcium supplements can work wonders for strengthening nails. If you don't get three servings of milk, cheese, or yogurt every day, take a 500-milligram calcium supplement daily if you are under age 50, or 1,000 milligrams of calcium if you are older than 50.

■ **GIVE SOY A TRY.** Boni Elewski, M.D., says that just 5 grams of soy protein a day will help toughen up your brittle nails. You can try tofu, tempeh, soymilk, or edamame; all are available in most grocery stores. Each 8-ounce serving of soymilk provides 6 grams of soy protein and is cholesterol-free.

■ **HORSE AROUND WITH BIOTIN.** Years ago, Swiss researchers proved that the B vitamin biotin increased the toughness of horse hooves, says Dr. Daniel. Today, doctors recommend the vitamin for toughening human nails.

"Biotin doesn't work in every case, but I've found it to be effective in anywhere from one-third to one-half of the cases I've seen," says Dr. Daniel.

Cauliflower is a rich source of biotin, as are legumes such as peanuts and lentils; however, you'd have to eat a lot of them to get enough biotin. Instead, take 3 milligrams of biotin in supplement form daily, Dr. Elewski says. Biotin typically comes in 600-microgram doses, which would require five tablets. If you don't want to take that many, a type called Biotin Forte comes in 3-milligram doses. This dosage could increase your nail thickness within 6 months.

■ **MANAGE YOUR MEDS.** Some common drugs, such as diuretics, can cause dehydration and could worsen a preexisting case of brittle nails. Check with your doctor if you think your medications are contributing to your brittle nails.

Nail Discoloration

12 Nail Remedies

Your eyes may be the windows to your soul, but your nails can reveal a lot about your body.

"Nail discoloration can be caused by a variety of conditions, such as reactions to medications (blue discoloration), bacterial infection (green-black), fungal infection (yellow), or even melanoma (black or brown discoloration)," says Audrey Kunin, M.D. Smoking can stain nails a very unattractive brown, while the wrong nail polish can leave them tinged an unnatural orange-yellow.

According to Coyle S. Connolly, D.O., the most common cause of discolored nails is a condition called onychomycosis. This nail fungus occurs when organisms known as dermatophytes move in under your nails. According to the National Onychomycosis Society, 11 million new cases are diagnosed each year.

Why so common? Toenails and fingernails and surrounding skin are prone to everyday wear and tear, which invites dirt, germs, and infection-causing fungi to take up residence there.

The first sign of a fungal infection is a change in color. The nail often becomes yellow to brown, and then it gets thicker and may develop a bad odor. Debris may collect beneath the nail, and a white area on the nail edge may form as the nail begins to lift from the nail bed. The infection can spread to other nails and even the skin. Toenails are affected more frequently than fingernails. This whole process often happens more frequently with age, Dr. Connolly says. In addition, age alone—without fungal infection—can also cause your nails to become yellow, but in this case, the nails are just discolored, but not thick and misshapen.

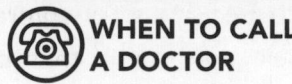

WHEN TO CALL A DOCTOR

According to Coyle S. Connolly, D.O., onychomycosis is not a problem to be ignored. "In fact, if left untreated, it can spread to other nails and make everyday activities, such as walking or writing, painful and difficult," he says.

See your doctor if:

■ You notice unexplained changes in the color of your nail.

■ Your nails appear to be abnormally thick.

■ The area surrounding your nails are painful or tender.

■ You have swelling on the skin surrounding the nail.

■ You have a nail that appears to have separated from the nail bed.

"If it's a fungus, it's best to catch it in its earlier stages. If the discoloration is a symptom of something more serious, early detection is even more important," Dr. Connolly says.

Here's how to treat off-colored nails, or keep these changes from happening to you.

■ **KEEP CLEAN.** Because fungi are everywhere, including the skin, they can be present months before they find opportunities to strike. By following proper hygiene and regularly inspecting your feet and toes, you can reduce your chances of the problem, or even stop the chain of events once it starts, says Paul Kechijian, M.D.

"Clean, dry feet resist disease. A strict regimen of washing the feet with antibacterial soap and water every night before bedtime, and remembering to dry thoroughly, is the best way to prevent an infection," says Dr. Kechijian. This habit helps rid the feet of excess bacteria from shoes and gives them a full night of cleanliness before they are back into shoes.

■ **WEAR YOUR SHOES IN YUCKY SURROUNDINGS.** If you're prone to developing fungal infections, walking barefoot in public facilities can expose your feet to the troublesome fungi, Dr. Kechijian says. So slip your feet into shoes or sandals rather than placing your bare feet in harm's way.

■ **SNIP NAILS SHORT.** "Longer nails can get caught on things or rub against tight shoes, which can cause the nail to lift from its bed," says Dr. Connolly. "That opening can invite fungus inside." Clip toenails straight across so that the nail doesn't extend beyond the nail bed, he suggests.

■ **KEEP THEM COOL.** Use a quality foot powder—talcum, not cornstarch—and wear shoes that fit well and are made of materials that breathe, says C. Ralph Daniel III, M.D. The reason? "Sweating makes matters worse, since it creates a warm, moist environment—perfect for spreading nail fungus," he says. The fungus digests the nail keratin, the protein that makes up the nail, causing the discoloration, which ranges from white to yellow and less often green to black.

■ **WASH YOUR HANDS.** Fungal infection can spread from your feet to your hands. So wash your hands after inspecting your feet, says Dr. Connolly. Also, smooth away dead skin by gently scrubbing it with soap and water, because fungus often attaches itself to dead, dry skin and moves on to other areas. "Watch for any rash or nail involvement of any new rash," he advises.

■ **WATCH THOSE NAIL PRODUCTS.** Ordinarily, any moisture that collects underneath the surface of the nail passes through the porous structure of the nail and evaporates. Acrylic nails applied to the tops of the nails may impede that, however. The moisture trapped below can become stagnant and unhealthy, ideal conditions for fungi and similar organisms to thrive, says Dr. Daniel.

■ **TRY VINEGAR.** Sometimes nails can develop a greenish hue caused by a bacterial infection, Dr. Connolly says. Pour some white vinegar in a bowl and soak your nails in it a few times a day. Vinegar is actually a mild acid, and it can be helpful in these cases.

■ **OR TRY LEMON JUICE.** To remove run-of-the mill stains from your fingernails, soak them in lemon juice, suggests Gina Morgan, a nail care instructor.

■ **PREVENT POLISH STAINS WITH A BASE COAT.** A base coat is typically a clear nail polish that goes onto your fingernails first, keeping the colored fingernail polish—and its potential lingering stain—off your nails, Morgan says. It also helps keep the polish on your nails.

■ **COVER THEM UP.** If you have staining that's not linked to fungus or any other growth on your fingernails, and you don't have pain or other symptoms of a true health problem, then feel free to just cover it up with nail polish, Dr. Connolly suggests.

■ **BE CAREFUL WHEN GETTING YOUR NAILS DONE.** When getting a manicure or pedicure, ask the nail technician not to be overly aggressive with your cuticles, Dr. Connolly says. This thin seal of skin around the edges of your nail acts like a sort of "weather strip," keeping out the elements. Oftentimes when people visit the nail salon, their cuticles are overly trimmed and pushed back, providing an opening for invisible attackers to enter.

■ **DON'T EXPECT TOO MUCH FROM NON-PRESCRIPTION TREATMENTS.** Over-the-counter treatments for nail fungus typically don't work well, if at all, Dr. Connolly says. Nails are so thick, and made of such strong material, that these treatments penetrate poorly. Your doctor can prescribe medications that you take orally, which attack the fungal infection from the inside out. Even these take many months to work.

PANEL OF ADVISORS

COYLE S. CONNOLLY, D.O., IS A DERMATOLOGIST AND ASSISTANT CLINICAL PROFESSOR AT THE PHILADELPHIA COLLEGE OF OSTEOPATHIC MEDICINE AND THE PRESIDENT OF CONNOLLY DERMATOLOGY IN LINWOOD, NEW JERSEY.

C. RALPH DANIEL III, M.D., IS A CLINICAL PROFESSOR OF DERMATOLOGY AT THE UNIVERSITY OF MISSISSIPPI MEDICAL CENTER AND A CLINICAL ASSOCIATE PROFESSOR OF DERMATOLOGY AT THE UNIVERSITY OF ALABAMA AT BIRMINGHAM.

PAUL KECHIJIAN, M.D., IS A FORMER CLINICAL ASSOCIATE PROFESSOR OF DERMATOLOGY AND CHIEF OF THE NAIL SECTION AT THE NEW YORK UNIVERSITY MEDICAL CENTER IN GREAT NECK. HE'S NOW IN PRIVATE PRACTICE IN GREAT NECK.

AUDREY KUNIN, M.D., IS A COSMETIC DERMATOLOGIST IN KANSAS CITY, MISSOURI, THE FOUNDER OF THE DERMATOLOGY EDUCATIONAL WEB SITE WWW.DERMADOCTOR.COM, AND AUTHOR OF *THE DERMADOCTOR SKINSTRUCTION MANUAL*.

GINA MORGAN IS AN INSTRUCTOR AT THE INTERNATIONAL SCHOOL OF SKIN AND NAIL CARE IN ATLANTA.

Nail Ridges

7 Ridge Reducers

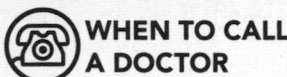

WHEN TO CALL A DOCTOR

Report any nail irregularities to your doctor or dermatologist immediately. Sudden nail changes (such as nail ridges) or swelling and pain could signal a serious problem, says Dee Anna Glaser, M.D.

Palm readers carefully inspect your hands to try to figure out what life may someday offer you. The only trouble is they could be looking at the wrong side of your hands. For predicting your future health, you may be better off consulting your fingernails, not your palms.

The ridges that appear in your nails, either vertically or horizontally, can indicate several serious medical conditions, says Dee Anna Glaser, M.D.

Vertical, or longitudinal, ridges, which run from the base of the nail to the tip, are most typical. They are usually normal and are related to aging or genetics. "Anyone over age 50 can expect to see more ridging in their nails as they age," says Paul Kechijian, M.D.

Severe ridging and cracking or sudden onset of vertical ridges serve as an alert to see a doctor, since they could be a sign of poor general health, poor nutrient absorption, or iron deficiency, Dr. Glaser says. They may also indicate rheumatoid arthritis or a circulatory or kidney disorder.

Horizontal, or transverse, ridges, which run from left to right, may occur as a result of severe psychological or physical stress, such as from infection or disease, Dr. Glaser says. Often called Beau's lines, they can occur after illness or trauma to the nail and with malnutrition. They can also be the result of habitually picking at or chewing your nail and cuticle, a nervous tic in some people.

Hormonal changes, genetics, and the way your body uses cal-

The ABCs of Nail Care

Because many nail disorders result from poor nail care, developing good nail habits today will help keep them healthy. Remember the following tips:

Keep them short. Shorter nails are less likely to crack or get caught on something and tear, says Paul Kechijian, M.D. He also suggests cutting your nails after bathing, when they're softer and less likely to break.

Stay on the straight and narrow. Nails should be cut straight across and rounded slightly at the tip for maximum strength, says C. Ralph Daniel III, M.D.

Avoid biting your fingernails. Your five-finger feeding frenzy worsens the condition of your nails, says Coyle S. Connolly, D.O.

cium are all factors that contribute to the rise of nail ridges. Nail ridges don't always signal a larger problem, though. "Remember, vertical ridges are like gray hair. You can expect to see more of them as you grow older," Dr. Kechijian stresses.

Here are some ways to reduce the ridges.

■ **BUFF 'EM.** You can gently buff your nails with a buffing block to minimize the ridges, Dr. Glaser says.

■ **BE GENTLE.** Don't try to completely buff out the nail ridges—overzealous buffing can weaken the nail plate, Dr. Kechijian says.

■ **EAT A WELL-BALANCED DIET.** Ridged nails can be the result of something lacking in your diet, Dr. Glaser says. "When people come into my office with severe nail changes, I immediately ask them for a dietary history to make sure that they aren't on some fad diet keeping them from getting their recommended daily allowance of vitamins and minerals," she says. "If they're not eating a well-balanced diet,

then a proper diet and a vitamin supplement might help the health of their nails."

■ **DON'T OVERDO IT WITH THE EMERY BOARD.** "Filing your nails is actually sanding your nails," says Dr. Kechijian. "If you oversand them, it will thin the nail and cause damage, which invites infection. So avoid overdoing it."

PANEL OF ADVISORS

COYLE S. CONNOLLY, D.O., IS A DERMATOLOGIST AND ASSISTANT CLINICAL PROFESSOR AT THE PHILADELPHIA COLLEGE OF OSTEOPATHIC MEDICINE AND PRESIDENT OF CONNOLLY DERMATOLOGY IN LINWOOD, NEW JERSEY.

C. RALPH DANIEL III, M.D., IS A CLINICAL PROFESSOR OF DERMATOLOGY AT THE UNIVERSITY OF MISSISSIPPI AND AN ASSOCIATE PROFESSOR OF DERMATOLOGY AT THE UNIVERSITY OF ALABAMA AT BIRMINGHAM.

DEE ANNA GLASER, M.D., IS A PROFESSOR OF DERMATOLOGY AT SAINT LOUIS UNIVERSITY SCHOOL OF MEDICINE IN MISSOURI.

PAUL KECHIJIAN, M.D., IS A FORMER CLINICAL ASSOCIATE PROFESSOR OF DERMATOLOGY AND CHIEF OF THE NAIL SECTION AT THE NEW YORK UNIVERSITY MEDICAL CENTER IN GREAT NECK. HE'S NOW IN PRIVATE PRACTICE IN GREAT NECK.

Nausea and Vomiting

15 Stomach-Soothing Solutions

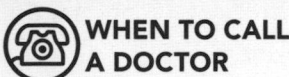 **WHEN TO CALL A DOCTOR**

"There are at least 25 different diseases that could cause chronic nausea," says Kenneth Koch, M.D. If your nausea doesn't go away in a day or two, it's a good idea to see your doctor.

Vomiting, on the other hand, can be a sign of something serious, and if it's persistent or contains blood, seek medical attention. Also see a doctor if you've gone 24 hours without being able to keep any food down and nothing seems to help, Dr. Koch says.

"If your thirst is severe and you notice you're not urinating very much—especially if you're light-headed when you stand up, a sign of dehydration—see a doctor," he adds. "If you know it's the flu, or it's something you've eaten, you might try to go a bit longer."

Nausea can also be a sign of a heart attack. If that may be the problem, get to a hospital right away.

The world is full of things that make our stomachs turn. Depending on the situation, everything from eating egg salad to giving blood to reading credit card bills can make you clutch your belly in agony.

Normally, your stomach contracts three times a minute, which is the ideal speed for grinding up food and passing it along the digestive system, says Max Levine, Ph.D., a psychologist who studies mental and emotional issues related to nausea. If your stomach contracts faster than that, it can make a kind of quivering motion, he says—it's a bit like what happens to your heart when it develops an irregular heartbeat.

And what happens when that twisting, turning tummy becomes too much to bear? You guessed it—you vomit. "If the stomach's not contracting, it makes it easier for things to move back up in the other direction," he says. Below are tips to help you keep nausea in check before you reach the point of no return and lose your lunch. If it's too late, you can also take steps to nurse your stomach—and the rest of yourself—back to good health.

■ **TRY OVER-THE-COUNTER REMEDIES.** A product called cola syrup—which contains corn syrup, caffeine, and flavorings—is helpful for treating nausea and upset stomach. Adults should take 1 to 2 tablespoons as needed. Another treatment available without a prescription is Emetrol, which contains the sugars dextrose and fructose, and the dosage for adults is also 1 to 2 tablespoons every 15 minutes for up to an hour or until you have relief.

An alternative to these treatments is a glass of 7UP or cola. Pour a glass and let it stand until it becomes flat and lukewarm, then drink it. If your "countdown clock" until you get sick is ticking fast, you can pour the drink back and forth between two glasses to help it lose its fizz faster.

■ **CHOOSE CLEAR LIQUIDS.** Even if you're craving food, stick with clear liquids such as tea and juice, says nausea researcher Kenneth Koch, M.D. Drink the liquids warm or at room temperature, not cold, to avoid further shock to your stomach. Drink no more than 1 to 2 ounces at a time.

■ **GET MINTY FRESH.** Mint makes your mouth a more pleasant place . . . and it may help your stomach, too. Peppermint leaves contain menthol, which is a digestive aid, and peppermint tea can ease nausea and vomiting. Steep a tablespoon of peppermint leaves in a cup of hot water, let it steep, strain, and drink.

■ **EAT CARBS FIRST.** If you need something to eat, and your nausea isn't too bad, eat light carbohydrates in small amounts—such as toast or crackers, Dr. Koch says. As your stomach starts to settle, graduate to light protein, like chicken breast or fish. Fatty foods are the last thing to add to your diet. If your problem is not nausea but vomiting, start with Jell-O. Then follow the progression mentioned previously to introduce other foods back into your diet.

■ **GET OUT OF THE PINK.** The stomach soother Pepto-Bismol—as well as Mylanta and Maalox—is for disease-provoked stomach upsets, not for a queasy stomach. If your nausea is caused by inflammation or irritation, however, Dr. Koch says it's reasonable to start with them. But none of our experts wholeheartedly recommend them. As Samuel Klein, M.D., says, none is specifically designed for nausea. You should probably avoid these products altogether if you're already vomiting. By then, it's usually too late.

■ **PLAN AHEAD.** A lot of medical research is devoted to the problem of dealing with nausea after chemotherapy. A problem that arises with nausea is that people may associate the foods they've eaten recently with their queasy stomach, and after a few times, whenever they eat that food—or think about eating it—they start to feel sick, Dr. Levine says. This

Cures from the Kitchen

Hawaiian Punch may be a great remedy to try for nausea or an upset stomach (although it may not be advisable if you have diabetes). The sweet drink contains fructose, the same active ingredient as in the nausea reliever cola syrup. Plus, Hawaiian Punch is caffeine-free and just a quick convenience-store run away. Just as with other liquids that can be used to relieve nausea, make sure you sip small amounts of Hawaiian Punch slowly.

association is called "scapegoating," and it's especially a problem for people with cancer who are trying to keep their weight from dropping. If you're undergoing chemotherapy, it's best to avoid eating your favorite foods or those you're tolerating before you go for a treatment. That way you won't become averse to eating them.

■ **FIND RELIEF IN THE MEADOW.** Meadowsweet, a pleasant-tasting wildflower, can be quite effective in reducing nausea, says Lois Johnson, M.D. To make a soothing cup of meadowsweet tea, mix 1 tablespoon of dried herb per cup of boiling water, and steep for 5 to 10 minutes, then strain. Then sip the concoction slowly. Rosemary is another ideal herb to add to the mixture.

■ **RUB YOUR WRIST.** A potentially helpful idea that showed up in the pages of the journal *American Family Physician* in 2007 is to use acupressure on a spot on your inner wrist. Researchers found that stimulating the P6 point on the underside of the wrist using a variety of techniques, including acupressure, successfully relieved nausea and vomiting. Rubbing the point also compared well against antinausea drugs.

To find the P6, run your fingertip about 2 inches up your inner wrist away from the crease at the edge of your palm. The spot is found between two tendons.

■ **SETTLE YOUR MIND.** Anxiety can trigger nausea and vomiting, because your body's fight-or-flight impulse makes it easier for your stomach to kick into those out-of-rhythm contractions, Dr. Levine says. When you're in a high-stress situation and feel your stomach start to churn, practice muscle relaxation, deep breathing exercises, or other steps to calm yourself down.

Cooling your face can spur your parasympathetic nervous system into action, Dr. Levine says, which slows your heart rate and spurs digestion. It may be helpful to soak a washcloth in cold water and apply it to your face when stress has you feeling nauseous.

■ **FIND OUT IF NAUSEA IS APPROACHING.** If you're going to undergo a medical treatment that could cause nausea—such as chemotherapy or surgery—ask your doctor if you're likely to feel sick to your stomach afterward. Although health care providers are often hesitant to tell people to expect nausea, it doesn't feel as severe when you're not surprised by it, Dr. Levine says.

■ **END IT ALL.** One of the most effective ways to stop nausea is to allow yourself to vomit, Dr. Koch says. At the very least, you'll have a temporary respite from that queasy feeling. Although it's okay to just let it go, he doesn't recommend *making* yourself vomit, however.

■ **REPLACE IMPORTANT FLUIDS AND NUTRIENTS.** "The ultimate goals for someone who's got a lot of vomiting are not to get dehydrated and not to lose weight," Dr. Koch says. You lose a lot of fluid in vomiting, so the best thing you can do is drink water, tea, and weak juices to replace them. Gatorade, Pedialyte, and juices such as apple and cranberry also help replace nutrients flushed out while vomiting.

■ **SIP—DON'T SLURP.** Sipping your fluids in tiny swallows lets your irritated stomach adjust, Dr. Koch says. Sip no more than 1 to 2 ounces at a time. In addition, sipping small amounts enables you to determine how much fluid you can handle at one time.

■ **USE THE COLOR CODE.** If your urine is deep yellow, you're not getting enough fluid. The paler it gets, the better you're doing at rehydrating.

PANEL OF ADVISORS

LOIS JOHNSON, M.D., IS A PHYSICIAN IN SEBASTOPOL, CALIFORNIA, AND A PROFESSIONAL MEMBER OF THE AMERICAN HERBALISTS GUILD.

SAMUEL KLEIN, M.D., IS A WILLIAM H. DANFORTH PROFESSOR OF MEDICINE AND NUTRITIONAL SCIENCE AND DIRECTOR OF THE CENTER FOR HUMAN NUTRITION AT WASHINGTON UNIVERSITY SCHOOL OF MEDICINE IN ST. LOUIS.

KENNETH KOCH, M.D., IS A PROFESSOR AND MEDICAL DIRECTOR OF THE DIGESTIVE HEALTH CENTER AT THE WAKE FOREST UNIVERSITY BAPTIST MEDICAL CENTER IN WINSTON-SALEM, NORTH CAROLINA.

MAX LEVINE, PH.D., IS AN ASSISTANT PROFESSOR OF PSYCHOLOGY AT SIENA COLLEGE IN LOUDONVILLE, NEW YORK, WHERE HE FOCUSES ON MIND-BODY ISSUES RELATED TO NAUSEA.

Neck Pain

29 Ways to Get the Kinks Out

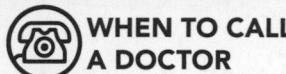
WHEN TO CALL A DOCTOR

Severe or lasting neck pain may require a doctor's care. If, for example, you've been in an auto accident and have severe neck pain afterward, you may have whiplash and should see a doctor, says Mitchell A. Price, D.C.

In general, persistent neck pain warrants professional medical evaluation.

When undue strain isn't placed on your neck, its seven vertebrae and 32 muscles do a pretty good job of holding up your 10- to 12-pound head. Still, that's a heavy load resting on a relatively small structure, leaving your neck vulnerable to a variety of stresses that can result in acute or chronic pain.

Naturally, some people—because of their occupations—are more at risk than others. Hairstylists, for example, work in a bent-over position all day long, notes Robert Kunkel, M.D. Office workers, machine operators, and carpenters also have been found to have more neck problems from the repetitive arm movements they make throughout the day.

Regardless of your job or lifestyle, neck pain can be eased and prevented by applying a few time-tested methods, replacing bad habits with good ones, and giving your neck regular exercise. Help is on the way.

■ **USE ICE, THEN HEAT.** If you've had a neck injury, apply an ice pack wrapped in a thin cloth—such as a T-shirt—to the injury for 15 minutes at a time. After ice has reduced inflammation, use heat later on as a wonderful soother. Or you can try a heating pad or a hot shower.

■ **KEEP LIVING YOUR LIFE.** If you've hurt your neck, "Try not to get caught up in your pain. Try to resume your normal activities or do as much as you can do," says Gregory Snow, D.C.,

C.C.S.P. It can be a little uncomfortable—you certainly don't want to create pain—but the sooner you can get back to your activities, the better you'll be. People with this kind of injury may fear developing more pain and reduce their physical activity, then start losing their physical abilities and mental well-being, he says. If your neck does hurt, you should try to focus on what you *can* do rather than your limitations.

■ **STOP SMOKING.** If you smoke, your neck would like to make a request: Please stop. Smoking reduces the amount of oxygen that travels around your body, thus impairing your ability to heal and recover from injuries, Dr. Snow says.

■ **PRESS ON THE PAINFUL SPOT.** Relieve muscle tension by applying moderate pressure to the area for 3 minutes. Don't press as hard as you can, but use your fingertips to exert steady, constant pressure on the affected point. At the end of 3 minutes, your pain may improve dramatically.

■ **TAKE A PAIN RELIEVER.** Over-the-counter anti-inflammatories such as aspirin or ibuprofen will help reduce pain and inflammation. Follow label instructions.

■ **TURN TO HERBS.** Turmeric and ginger help reduce production of leukotrienes, substances that can trigger inflammation. Take 1 to 2 grams of each herb a day until your pain is relieved, advises Mark Gostine, M.D.

■ **EAT A HEALTHY DIET.** Cut down on foods high in saturated fats such as red meat and full-fat dairy; they promote pain. Dr. Snow recommends that you limit these foods—and fast food, while you're at it—and focus more on foods that can help reduce inflammation and contain omega-3 fatty acids, found in salmon and sardines.

■ **ADD FLAX OIL TO YOUR JUICE.** Flaxseed contains alpha linolenic acid, a substance similar to the omega-3 fatty acids found in fish that can prevent joint swelling. Take 2 teaspoons a day, Dr. Gostine recommends. Refrigerate your flax oil—it spoils quickly.

■ **GIVE GLUCOSAMINE A TRY.** Evidence suggests that this supplement may help repair joints. Dr. Gostine recommends taking 1,500 milligrams a day to ease neck pain, but be patient; you may go several weeks before you feel an effect.

■ **TAKE YOUR VITAMINS.** Antioxidant vitamins such as vitamins C and E, taken on a regular basis, can help to prevent the painful deterioration of joints in your neck and elsewhere in your body. Take 1,000 milligrams of vitamin C and 400 IU of vitamin E daily.

■ **SIT IN A FIRM CHAIR.** Sitting in a chair without good back support can create havoc further up your spine, making neck problems worse and even causing new ones, says Mitchell A. Price, D.C.

■ **POSITION YOUR HEADREST AT THE PROPER HEIGHT.** Keep the headrest in your

Exercise Away Neck Pain

Even your neck muscles need to be stretched and strengthened. Here are some exercises to combat stiffness and prevent problems in the future. Do each exercise five times twice a day. Do the first three exercises for 2 weeks before starting the rest.

■ Slowly tilt your head forward as far as possible. Then move your head backward as far as possible.

■ Tilt your head toward one of your shoulders, while keeping your shoulder stationary. Straighten, then tilt toward the other shoulder.

■ Slowly turn your head from side to side as far as possible.

■ Place your hand on one side of your head while you push toward it with your head. Hold for 5 seconds, then relax. Repeat three times. Then do the same exercise on the other side.

■ Place your hand on the front of your head while you push your head forward. Then provide slight resistance to the back of your head while you push your head backward. Hold for 5 seconds, then relax. Repeat three times.

■ Hold light weights—say, 3 to 5 pounds—in your hands while shrugging your shoulders. Keep your arms straight.

vehicle elevated so it's even with the crown of your head. If it's too low and you're rear-ended by a vehicle, your head could possibly jerk back over the headrest, which is an invitation for neck injuries, Dr. Snow says.

■ **STAY FIT.** Regular exercise is important for treating and preventing all types of pain. Staying fit helps your body cope with injuries better and recover from them faster, Dr. Snow says. Even if you're not overweight, you should still stay physically active.

■ **WATCH YOUR BODY.** While doing chores around the house and yard, keep your body in a neutral posture, Dr. Snow advises. This means your head is upright on your shoulders, your shoulders are back, your chest is out, and your shoulders are above your hips and parallel to them. "Basically, it's what your mom told you about good posture," he says.

■ **BE CAUTIOUS WITH CAR SEATS.** If you're putting a baby or young child into a car seat, it's a bad idea to hold the child, lean deep into the car, and put the child into the seat with your arms extended, Dr. Snow says. It's much safer to sit on the seat while holding the child, move your legs into the car, then place the child into the seat.

■ **CAREFUL WITH YOGA.** Although exercise is good, yoga isn't necessarily a good idea if you have neck or back problems, Dr. Snow says. If you do practice yoga, be sure to work with a well-trained instructor who can help you avoid positions that might aggravate your problem.

■ **IMPROVE YOUR MENTAL HEALTH.** People with depression, anxiety, and stress have been found to be more likely to have back and neck pain, and more likely to experience it for longer periods of time, Dr. Snow says. If you're having depression or anxiety that may be playing a role in your neck pain, consider seeing a mental health professional for treatment and advice. Learning stress-reduction practices such as meditation or progressive muscle relaxation may also be beneficial.

■ **SEE EYE TO SCREEN.** If you stare at a computer monitor all day, you might need to position it at eye level. If you force yourself to look up or down hour after hour, your neck may spasm, says Dr. Price.

While we're on the subject of good ergonomics, keep your elbows, hips, and knees bent at 90 degrees, Dr. Snow says. Sit up straight and avoid leaning back in your chair.

■ **KEEP MOVING.** Set an alarm at work that alerts you to get up and move around every hour, Dr. Price says. This can reduce your neck strain and get your blood circulation moving. In addition, regularly do the following exercise while seated in your chair: Lift your shoulders all the way up, bring them back as far as you can; lower them as far as you can; and then bring them as far forward as possible. Repeat this 10 times in both directions, he advises.

When you're at home using your computer or watching TV for long periods of time, remember to get up and move on a regular basis.

■ **GET A TELEPHONE HEADSET.** If you talk on the phone a lot while you're doing other activities, either at work or home, ask your employer for a headset or buy one for home, Dr. Snow says. Holding the phone between your neck and shoulder while you use your hands can lead to stiffness and pain.

■ **SLEEP ON A FIRM MATTRESS.** A lot of neck problems begin, as well as worsen, with poor sleeping habits that wrench the spine out of alignment. A firm mattress is important, Dr. Price says.

■ **AVOID SLEEPING ON YOUR STOMACH.** This is bad not only for your back but also for your neck, says Dr. Price. Instead, sleep in the fetal position—on your side with your knees pulled up toward your chest. Oftentimes sleeping with a pillow between your knees can help prevent you from rolling back onto your stomach, Dr. Snow says.

■ **WRAP UP.** When it's cold and damp outside, cover your neck well. The weather can aggravate neck stiffness and pain, Dr. Kunkel says.

PANEL OF ADVISORS

MARK GOSTINE, M.D., IS AN ANESTHESIOLOGIST AND PAIN MANAGEMENT SPECIALIST AND A COFOUNDER OF MICHIGAN PAIN CONSULTANTS, BASED IN GRAND RAPIDS.

ROBERT KUNKEL, M.D., IS ON THE CONSULTANT STAFF OF THE NEUROLOGICAL CENTER FOR PAIN AT THE CLEVELAND CLINIC IN OHIO. HE SPECIALIZES IN HEADACHE.

MITCHELL A. PRICE, D.C., IS A CHIROPRACTOR IN READING, PENNSYLVANIA.

GREGORY SNOW, D.C., C.C.S.P., IS DEAN OF CLINICS AT PALMER COLLEGE OF CHIROPRACTIC, WEST CAMPUS, IN SAN JOSE, CALIFORNIA.

Night Blindness

10 Ways to Deal with the Dark

We all have more trouble seeing when the lights go out, which means that night blindness affects everyone to some degree, because it usually takes a moment for the retina to adjust to changes in light, explains Alan Laties, M.D.

But for some people, night blindness is more than momentary.

"Nearsighted people can at times be slower to adapt to the dark," Dr. Laties says. But some other people simply *can't* see in the dark. These people have a rare condition called congenital stationary night blindness.

Unfortunately, doctors don't have a bag of ready-to-issue cures for night blindness. But if you don't see well at night and your doctor has ruled out an eye disorder, our experts offer the following practical advice for driving safely at night, when night blindness poses the biggest problem.

■ **GET A PAIR OF NIGHT GLASSES.** Millions of people take advantage of glasses to improve their vision. Glasses can improve night myopia, which is defective night vision, especially of distant objects, says Creig Hoyt, M.D.

Pilots will tell you that they have more trouble seeing runways at night. To combat this problem, at night they often wear glasses with stronger prescriptions, Dr. Hoyt says. What works for a pilot trying to land a plane on a narrow strip of pavement ought to help you keep your car on the driveway and out of the front yard.

Consider wearing a stronger prescription at night or getting

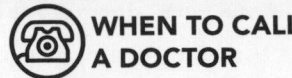 **WHEN TO CALL A DOCTOR**

If you're having problems with night vision, you should have your eyes examined by an ophthalmologist, says Alan Laties, M.D. It's the best way to protect your vision.

Occasionally, night blindness can be an early symptom of a progressive eye disease.

glasses for night driving, even if you currently don't wear glasses during the day, Dr. Hoyt says.

■ **KEEP YOUR HEADLIGHTS CLEAN.** Dirty headlights can greatly reduce your visibility and will only make an already bad problem worse, says safety researcher Charles Zegeer.

Auto-parts stores carry headlight-cleaning kits that can repair the age-related haze that can form on the shields over your headlights. The kit may include a foam pad and a polishing compound.

■ **PLAN AHEAD.** Careful route planning can make night driving easier and safer. When possible, select roads that are divided or have very little traffic.

■ **SLOW DOWN.** By getting your foot off the gas pedal, you give yourself more time to react to unexpected hazards. Increase your regular following distance by 3 to 4 seconds to allow for extra stopping time.

■ **EXPECT THE UNEXPECTED.** The roads don't belong just to cars, but also to walkers, runners, cyclists, and wayward deer. It's your responsibility to watch for others sharing the road. It's even more important if you have trouble seeing at night to keep your eyes on the road and off your cell phone, radio, iPod, and other distractions.

■ **RESPECT THE RAIN AND FOG.** These two conditions make night driving especially dangerous, Zegeer says. He recommends keeping your headlights on low beam in fog for better visibility.

■ **DON'T TAKE CHANCES.** If fog or travel conditions become too bad, says Zegeer, pull off at a rest area, service station, or parking lot. Avoid stopping on the shoulder of the road.

■ **LOOK TO THE RIGHT.** Try to direct your gaze to the right edge of the road—this will keep your eyes from looking directly into oncoming headlights.

■ **LEAVE THE DRIVING TILL TOMORROW.** If night blindness is really a problem, drive only during the day. Even good lighting conditions at night, such as those in a big city, can be troublesome to someone with night blindness.

■ **THINK ABOUT VITAMIN A.** Researchers have found that people who've had gastric bypass surgery for weight loss may develop night blindness from a deficiency of vitamin A, a nutrient essential for eye health. This type of surgery bypasses part of the small intestine that helps absorb vitamin A. If you've had bariatric surgery and are having vision trouble, ask your doctor to check you for vitamin A deficiency.

PANEL OF ADVISORS

CREIG HOYT, M.D., IS FORMER CHAIRMAN OF THE DEPARTMENT OF OPHTHALMOLOGY AT THE UNIVERSITY OF CALIFORNIA IN SAN FRANCISCO.

ALAN LATIES, M.D., IS A PROFESSOR OF OPHTHALMOLOGY AT THE SCHEIE EYE INSTITUTE OF THE UNIVERSITY OF PENNSYLVANIA SCHOOL OF MEDICINE IN PHILADELPHIA.

CHARLES ZEGEER IS DIRECTOR OF THE PEDESTRIAN AND BICYCLE INFORMATION CENTER AT THE UNIVERSITY OF NORTH CAROLINA IN CHAPEL HILL.

Nosebleed

15 Hints to Stop the Flow

Whether it's a boxer in the ring, a kid who took a ball to the nose, or an office worker who collided with a door, nosebleeds are always alarming and often very painful.

Vast amounts of blood circulate through capillaries in the nose, so bleeding can be copious when blood vessels break. Nosebleeds can also occur when your mucous membranes become irritated by a cold or winter's dry indoor heat. People with high blood pressure or atherosclerosis (hardening of the arteries) are especially vulnerable to nosebleeds, as are those taking certain medications, such as anticoagulants, anti-inflammatories, and aspirin. Nose blowing, nose picking, excessive sneezing, allergies, and foreign objects in the nose can also prompt bleeding.

Nosebleeds seem to be the most common among children, largely from their sometimes aggressive style of playing, says Sally Robinson, M.D. "Most nosebleeds in children are the result of too-vigorous blowing, an accidental smack in the nose during rough-and-tumble play, or reckless picking with a sharp fingernail," she says.

Whatever the cause, most nosebleeds are no cause for alarm, and you can do many things to stop them. Here's what the experts say.

■ **REASSURE YOUR CHILD.** If a child gets a bloody nose, step one is to stay calm. This will help your child remain calm, which makes the bloody nose much easier to manage. "Explain to your child in a calm tone that the nosebleed isn't serious and that you can stop it quickly with your child's help," says Dr. Robinson.

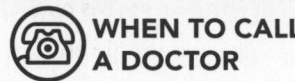

WHEN TO CALL A DOCTOR

Nosebleeds are rarely serious, but there are instances that demand immediate medical attention. Head for the emergency room if:

■ You've applied pressure for 10 to 15 minutes, but your nose still bleeds.

■ Your nosebleed results from a head injury.

■ You've been diagnosed with atherosclerosis or high blood pressure, and your nose has bled for more than 10 minutes.

■ You have blood pulsating from the nose or coming from both nostrils.

■ You have difficulty breathing.

■ You bruise easily, or there is a history of clotting problems in your family.

Finally, if your nosebleeds become too frequent and don't seem to be associated with a cold or an irritation of the mucous membranes, schedule an appointment with your physician.

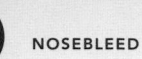

■ **BLOW THE CLOT OUT.** Before you try to stop your nosebleed, give your nose one good, vigorous blow, says Alvin Katz, M.D. That should remove any clots that are keeping the blood vessel open. A clot acts like a "wedge in the door," he explains. Blood vessels have elastic fibers. If you can get the clot out, you can get the elastic fibers to contract around that tiny opening.

■ **FILL THE VOID WITH COTTON.** Once the clot is removed, Dr. Katz advises putting a small amount of nasal decongestant on a ball of cotton and inserting it about a ½ inch into the bleeding nostril. This will soak up any additional blood and help stop the bleeding.

■ **PINCH THE FLESHY PART OF YOUR NOSE.** Once the cotton is in place, use your thumb and forefinger to squeeze shut the soft part of the nose with a tissue or clean washcloth. Apply continuous pressure for 10 minutes, and then remove the cotton. If the bleeding doesn't stop, pinch again for another 5 to 7 minutes. The bleeding should stop by the time you're through.

■ **WATCH THE CLOCK.** Ten minutes may seem like an awfully long time while you're sitting there pinching a child's nose, but Dr. Robinson says it's important not to let up. "Don't give up too soon," she says. "If you don't hold the nose long enough, the bleeding will start again shortly after you let go."

■ **SIT UP STRAIGHT.** This is important, as leaning back while a nose is bleeding can cause blood to run down the back of the throat, says Keith Bly, M.D. "This not only tastes bad and can initiate a coughing fit, but also the blood can irritate the stomach and cause vomiting," he says.

■ **CHILL OUT.** While you're pinching the nose shut, place a cold washcloth or towel against the back of the neck or the bridge of the nose to provide additional relief and slow bleeding. "This can constrict blood vessels and help stem the flow," says Dr. Bly.

■ **RUN INTERFERENCE.** Sitting still for 10 minutes is usually no problem if you're an adult, but it can be maddening for a child. That's why Dr. Robinson recommends talking to your child to keep him or her calm during that time. Explain exactly what you're doing, and why you're doing it.

■ **REACH FOR THE SPRAY.** In almost all cases, going through the steps listed above is sufficient to stop a nosebleed. If it doesn't, however, a last resort is an over-the-counter nasal spray such as Afrin, which can shrink blood vessels and help a scab form.

■ **KEEP IT FROM COMING BACK.** Once it's gone, there are still a few steps you can take to prevent new bleeding, says Dr. Robinson. "After a nosebleed has stopped, moisturizing the inside of the nostrils with petroleum jelly and keeping a humidifier in the room can keep the delicate tissue from drying and cracking," she says. "And the Afrin may be useful at this point to help prevent further bleeding."

■ **DON'T PICK.** It takes 7 to 10 days to heal the rupture in the blood vessel that caused your nose to bleed. Bleeding stops after the clot forms, but the clot becomes a scab as healing continues. If you pick your nose during the next week and knock the scab off, you'll give yourself another nosebleed, says Jerold Principato, M.D.

■ **HUMIDIFY THE AIR.** When you breathe, that moist lining in your nose works to make sure that the air that reaches your lungs is well humidified. So it follows that when your surroundings are dry, your nose has to work harder. A cold-mist humidifier, operating when the air is dry, helps moisturize airways and tissue linings. "Moist tissue has better resistance and less reactivity than dry tissue," says Dr. Katz.

Dr. Katz recommends filling the humidifier with distilled water to protect against impurities in tap water. Also, be sure to clean the unit properly, according to the manufacturer's instructions, at least once a week.

■ **WATCH YOUR ASPIRIN INTAKE.** Aspirin can interfere with clotting. If you're prone to nosebleeds, don't take unnecessary aspirin.

■ **BE CAREFUL IN CHOOSING ORAL CONTRACEPTIVES.** Estrogen influences blood supply and mucus production. Anything that changes the estrogen balance in your body—including menstruation—can make you more prone to nosebleeds. Certain oral contraceptives also alter the balance. If nosebleeds are a problem and estrogen hormone is a suspect, discuss this with your doctor when you choose your birth control pill.

■ **DON'T SMOKE.** Along with the 2,001 other bad things it does to the body, smoking really dries out the nasal cavity, says Mark Baldree, M.D. It can make you more prone to nosebleeds.

PANEL OF ADVISORS

MARK BALDREE, M.D., IS A STAFF MEMBER IN THE DIVISION OF OTOLARYNGOLOGY IN THE DEPARTMENT OF SURGERY AT GOOD SAMARITAN MEDICAL CENTER IN PHOENIX.

KEITH BLY, M.D., IS AN ASSISTANT PROFESSOR OF PEDIATRICS IN THE UNIVERSITY OF TEXAS MEDICAL BRANCH CHILDREN'S EMERGENCY ROOM IN GALVESTON.

ALVIN KATZ, M.D., IS AN OTOLARYNGOLOGIST AT THE MANHATTAN EYE, EAR, NOSE, AND THROAT HOSPITAL, LENOX HILL HOSPITAL, AND PRESBYTERIAN HOSPITAL IN NEW YORK CITY. HE IS PAST PRESIDENT OF THE AMERICAN RHINOLOGIC SOCIETY.

JEROLD PRINCIPATO, M.D., IS AN OTOLARYNGOLOGIST IN BETHESDA, MARYLAND.

SALLY ROBINSON, M.D., IS A CLINICAL PROFESSOR OF PEDIATRICS AT THE UNIVERSITY OF TEXAS MEDICAL BRANCH CHILDREN'S HOSPITAL IN GALVESTON.

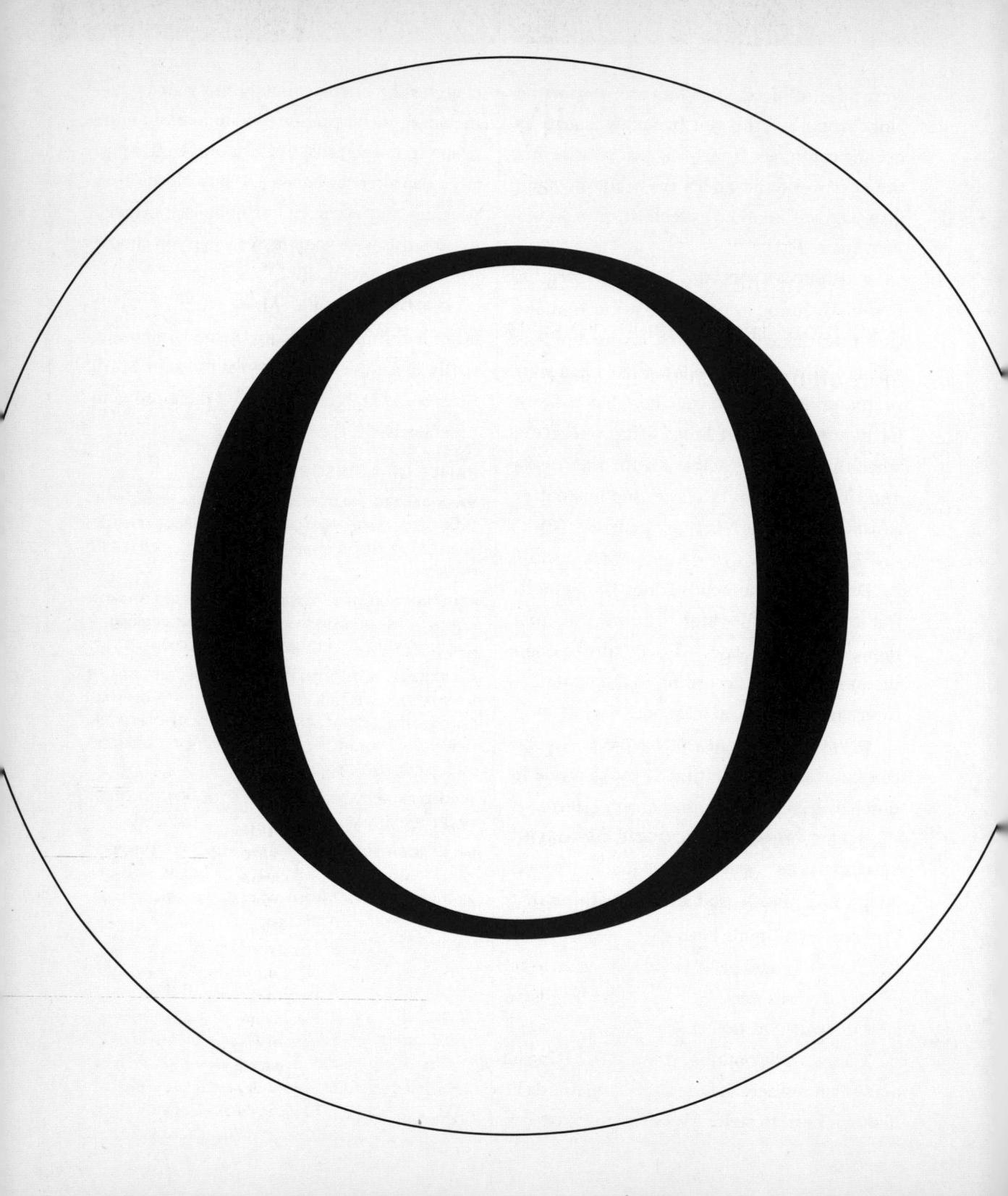

Oily Hair

15 Neutralizing Solutions

If you're in the group that believes that blondes have more fun, consider this: They also have more oil in their hair. And those with silky, baby-fine hair tend to have the worst problem of all with oiliness. "Fine textured hair is more prone to oiliness because there is space for more hairs per square inch," says hair care specialist Philip Kingsley. "As each hair has its own oil glands, there are more glands covering a smaller circumference of hair."

Blondes with fine hair have as many as 140,000 oil glands on their scalps, says Kingsley. Compare that with redheads, who average 80,000 to 90,000 hairs per head. They rarely have oily hair, he says. Brunettes typically fall somewhere in the middle.

Hair color isn't the only factor that affects oiliness, though. "Androgens, or male hormones, control oil flow, too," says Kingsley. "Oily-skinned people have oilier hair, as oily skin can be a sign of androgen response." Stress boosts bloodstream levels of androgens in women as well as in men.

There's really nothing wrong with having oily hair, but it can be a bit of a nuisance. "It leaves the hair looking limp and lifeless, and makes it hard to style," says dermatologist Jason R. Lupton, M.D.

Cures from the Kitchen

Your mother told you to never brush your hair near food, but that doesn't mean the kitchen can't provide some home remedies for oily hair. Try these hair-care pro tips.

TRY AN APPLE CIDER VINEGAR RINSE. Put a teaspoon of apple cider vinegar in a pint of water and use as your final rinse. This solution removes soap residue that can weigh down oily hair. And don't worry about smelling like a salad; the vinegar's aroma subsides quickly.

FRESHEN UP WITH LEMON. Squeeze the juice of two lemons into a quart of the best water you can find, says hairstylist David Daines. Distilled water is a great choice.

SWITCH TO BEER. Daines recommends fresh beer as a setting lotion for oily hair. "Beer gives the hair lots of body, and the alcohol is a drying ingredient," he says. Store it in a closed plastic container in your shower; otherwise, it will keep for only a couple of days. Then blow-dry from underneath, and style as desired.

"People with oily hair and scalps are more likely to be prone to dandruff and acne."

Because you're stuck with the *type* of hair Mother Nature gave you (if not the color), here's what our experts advise.

■ **SHAMPOO FREQUENTLY.** The most important thing you can do to combat an excessively oily scalp is to shampoo at least once a day. This seems like a no-brainer, but many people with oily hair don't do it because of a common misconception. "Some people are afraid that shampooing too much causes dry scalp and dandruff, but in reality, it's oil buildup that causes dandruff, so washing your hair often is the best thing you can do," says Judith Hellman, M.D.

■ **GO WITH THE HERBAL VARIETIES.** Professional hairstylist David Daines suggests going the natural route. "I tell my clients to look for more natural or herbal shampoos, and to check the labels," he says. "Ingredients such as chamomile and yarrow seem to have drying qualities."

■ **LOOK FOR A SPECIAL SHAMPOO.** If that doesn't work, the next line of defense is to try a shampoo made specifically for oily hair. "Over-the-counter varieties include the ones that contain selenium, zinc, salicylic acid, or even tar," says Dr. Hellman. "Medicated shampoos can be prescribed by a dermatologist."

■ **SHAMPOO THE RIGHT WAY.** One common mistake that people with oily hair make is scrubbing too hard while shampooing. This only irritates the scalp and makes things worse, says Daines. "Oily hair should be shampooed only once, not rubbing or scrubbing the scalp too much but concentrating on the hair shaft."

■ **GET OUT OF CONDITION.** If you have oily hair that tends to flatten out as the day goes on, the last thing you want to do is coat it with more oil. "The natural oils in the scalp will act as a conditioner," says Dr. Lupton. "Adding conditioner will just leave the hair with an oilier, limp appearance."

■ **KNOW WHEN TO USE IT.** If you have longer hair and are prone to split ends, you'll want to condition just the ends of your hairs, says Daines. "Short hair shouldn't need it, as it's usually trimmed more often," he says. But apply conditioner if you dye your hair or go swimming, says Dr. Hellman.

■ **APPLY ASTRINGENT.** You can help slow oil secretion by applying a homemade astringent directly to your scalp. Kingsley suggests mixing up equal parts witch hazel and mouthwash, and using cotton pads to dab on to the scalp. The witch hazel acts to cut oil, and the mouthwash has antiseptic properties, he says. If your scalp is very oily, use this first before each shampoo.

■ **DRY HAIR IN THE OPPOSITE DIRECTION FROM WHICH IT GROWS.** Left on its own, oily hair tends to be limp and lank. To coax more fullness into it, be creative with your blow-drying technique, says Kingsley. Use a brush to lift the hair up at the roots, or bend forward at the waist and gently brush your hair up over the top of your head.

■ **DON'T OVERBRUSH.** "Be careful not to brush your hair too much," says Dr. Lupton. "This will drag the oil from the scalp throughout your full head of hair."

■ **DON'T GO HAIR CARE CRAZY.** Dr. Lupton also recommends not going overboard on the amount of "product" you put in your hair, because it can be difficult to get it all out when shampooing.

■ **GET THE RIGHT CUT.** Beat the straight, matted-down hair blues by asking your stylist to cut body into your hair. "Today's fashions are leaning toward a 'bob' length just around the chin or a little longer. If you have oily hair, you might have to keep it shorter. It's trial and error," says Daines. "It's up to you and your stylist to try different looks and styles. Hair styles should change as you would change clothing styles. If your stylist doesn't want to change, change stylists."

■ **LEARN TO RELAX.** When you're under stress, your body produces more androgens. And androgens help boost oil production. Kingsley's advice? Relax. Experiment with different relaxation techniques, such as meditation, tai chi, and yoga, and practice the one that works best for you.

PANEL OF ADVISORS

DAVID DAINES IS A PROFESSIONAL HAIRSTYLIST AT GIL FERRER IN NEW YORK CITY.

JUDITH HELLMAN, M.D., IS A PROFESSOR OF DERMATOLOGY AT MOUNT SINAI HOSPITAL IN NEW YORK CITY.

PHILIP KINGSLEY IS THE FOUNDER OF TRICHOLOGICAL CLINICS IN LONDON AND NEW YORK CITY. HE IS FELLOW AND PAST CHAIRMAN OF THE INSTITUTE OF TRICHOLOGISTS AND HAS BEEN A TRICHOLOGIST (HAIR-CARE SPECIALIST) FOR MORE THAN 50 YEARS.

JASON R. LUPTON, M.D., IS A BOARD-CERTIFIED DERMATOLOGIST IN PRIVATE PRACTICE IN DEL MAR, CALIFORNIA.

Oily Skin

7 Restoratives for a Shine-Free Face

When you think about "oily skin," it usually brings to mind squeaky-voiced, pimply-faced teenagers who are in the midst of that awkward phase. But if you're an adult with oily skin, you know the condition can be just as frustrating for older people as it is for teenagers.

"Oily skin is common in teenagers because of the hormonal changes brought on by puberty. Surging levels of sex hormones can stimulate increased oil production," says Steven Jepson, M.D. "But many adults are affected by oily skin, as well. This is usually from hormonal factors, too. In the twenties, there's an ongoing high production of testosterone and estrogen. In the thirties and forties, it's usually caused by decreasing levels of progesterone and is much more common in women than men."

Heredity can also play a role, as well as pregnancy, stress, and even the type of birth control you use. The wrong cosmetics can easily aggravate an otherwise mild case of oily skin. Some of these causes are within your ability to control, but others you'll have to learn to live with.

Look on the bright side. Skin experts believe that there are some advantages to having oily skin. In the long run, they say that oily skin tends to age better and wrinkle less than dry or normal skin. Meanwhile, here are some tips for a cleaner, drier face.

■ **MAKE MINE MUD.** "Clay masks or mud masks are worthwhile," says Howard Donsky, M.D. Masks cleanse the skin of sur-

Forget the Food Connection

Although some magazines and skin-care books recommend special diets for reducing oily skin problems (usually by cutting out fried and fatty foods), our experts dismiss such things as pure fantasy and wasted effort.

"There are not really any foods that you need to avoid," says Judith Hellman, M.D. "It is a common myth that foods cause oily skin and acne, but it has no roots in reality."

Kenneth Neldner, M.D., agrees. "I don't think diet has any effect. If it does, there's nothing about it that's known to the medical community. If you have dry skin, there's nothing you can eat that will make your skin oily, so there's no reason to think it would work the opposite way for oily skin."

face greasiness and tone the skin—for a while anyway. Realize, however, that their effects are temporary.

Generally, the darker brown the clay or mud, the more oil it can absorb. White or rose-colored clays, though, are gentler and work best on sensitive skin.

■ **CLEAN YOUR FACE TWICE A DAY.** Thankfully, cleaning oily skin doesn't have to be complicated, says Dr. Jepson. He recommends finding a nonsoap cleanser that's designed specifically for the face, and washing with it twice a day, in the morning and at night.

Don't feel the need to wash more than twice, says dermatologist Judith Hellman, M.D. "Oily skin is not a result of inadequate washing or bad hygiene, so overly aggressive washing of the skin is not a good idea," she says. "Generally, washing twice a day is enough."

■ **FOLLOW WITH EXFOLIATION.** For some people, an additional cleansing step might be a good idea, says Dr. Jepson. "I recommend daily exfoliation with a product with beta-hydroxy or alpha-hydroxy acid such as salicylic acid, glycolic acid, and lactic acid," he says. "View exfoliation as the second cleansing step. It removes dirt and oils missed by the cleanser and gets down deep into the pores to remove hidden oil and debris."

This step isn't for everyone, however. "Some cleansers will contain an exfoliating agent and are adequate for people with mildly oily skin," says Dr. Jepson. "But for people with moderate to severe oily skin, I recommend exfoliating with a stronger acid solution as part of a second individual skin care step once or twice daily."

■ **MAKE THE RIGHT MAKEUP DECISION.** "Cosmetics come in two major categories: oil-based and water-based. If you have oily skin, Dr. Donsky recommends choosing only water-based products.

Another possibility, adds Dr. Jepson, is trying mineral-based makeup. "A good mineral makeup will actually help absorb some of the oils and will not clog the pores," he says. "I recommend the Colorescience brand."

■ **TAKE A POWDER.** Baby powder, that is. For additional shine-free protection, some women find that simple products such as Johnson's Baby Powder make a superb face powder when fluffed lightly over makeup. Another handy way to blot the shine is to use rice paper facial tissues. They're coated with a light layer of cornstarch and are easy to stow in your purse for midafternoon touch-ups.

■ **TRY SAW PALMETTO.** Saw palmetto is usually viewed as an herbal treatment for men, but Dr. Jepson says it can help all adults with oily skin. "Saw palmetto can help decrease oil production in the skin in both men and women by blocking the effects of the oil-producing hormones on the sebaceous glands," he says. Be sure to speak with your doctor before taking saw palmetto or any other herb.

■ **BE SMART ABOUT SUNSCREEN.** Sunscreens have oils, but, as Dr. Hellman points out, the risks of skin cancer from sun exposure are much greater than the risks posed by oily skin. "If you use sunscreen, which you should, do wash it off as soon as you go inside and no longer need it," she says.

PANEL OF ADVISORS

Osteoarthritis
25 Ways to End the Ache

The stiffness, pain, and joint deterioration that accompany osteoarthritis have undoubtedly stood the test of time: Researchers have found evidence of the condition in the fossilized remains of 85-million-year-old dinosaurs. And if you're one of the 70 million Americans afflicted with the painful condition, you know all too well how that dinosaur felt.

Some of the osteoarthritis common in America is part of the inevitable wear and tear on your joints. As you get older, the cartilage that cushions your bones wears down over time, and stiffness and pain may result. Other factors are at work besides aging, however. Genetics seems to predispose some people to arthritis more than others. And traumatic injuries can speed up the development of arthritis.

Whatever is behind your arthritis pain, home remedies can play a significant role in reducing it, or even preventing it from occurring in the first place. Read on to see how they can help.

■ **GET TO YOUR IDEAL WEIGHT.** "Being overweight is like carrying around heavy luggage," says Neal Barnard, M.D. "It hurts the knees, hips—literally every joint in the body. The basic rule of thumb is that every extra 10 pounds increases the risk of osteoarthritis in the knees by 30 percent."

Another way to look at it, explains Kevin Stone, M.D., is that

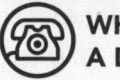

WHEN TO CALL A DOCTOR

If arthritis pain is persistent or if you have 5 to 10 minutes or more of significant morning stiffness, see your doctor, advises Theodore R. Fields, M.D. Also see your doctor if you have loss of motion or swelling in a joint or if the pain stops you from doing activities you find important.

Talk to your doctor if acetaminophen or another over-the-counter pain reliever doesn't help with the pain, says Justus Fiechtner, M.D.

it's not just extra weight, but also extra pressure. "Whatever your body weight is, a force of three to five times that weight is bearing down on your knee joints," he says.

However, it's more than just your knees and hips that are at risk. "It turns out that thinner people are also less likely to develop arthritis in their hands," says Dr. Barnard. That just gives you one more reason to keep that weight off.

■ **EAT FOR THE LONG HAUL.** While specific foods seem to play a role in rheumatoid arthritis, the relationship is less clear when it comes to osteoarthritis. That's why the general dietary advice here is to focus on foods that will help you maintain a healthy weight. "Low-fat, high-fiber foods can help," says Dr. Barnard. "That means vegetables, fruits, beans, and whole grains. These foods typically cause weight loss, which takes the weight off your knees and hips."

The Arthritis Foundation's suggestions for a proper diet are simple: Strive for balance and eat plenty of vegetables, fruits, and grains; take in only moderate amounts of sugar, salt, and alcohol; and limit your consumption of fat and cholesterol. The foundation also advises taking a multivitamin and mineral supplement to get your daily requirements, especially of calcium.

■ **DRINK LOTS OF WATER.** "Hydration helps prevent arthritis," says Michael Loes, M.D. Your joints need lubrication to move smoothly, just like a well-oiled machine. Dr. Loes recommends drinking 9 to 12 eight-ounce glasses of water every day to prevent osteoarthritis pain. If you drink lots of coffee or other caffeinated beverages, which act as diuretics and flush water out of your body, down even more water.

■ **EXERCISE AEROBICALLY.** Whether it's walking, riding a stationary bike, or swimming, daily aerobic exercise can help reduce stiffness and pain, preserving or improving the health of your bones and joints. If you're just getting started, Dr. Barnard recommends a half-hour walk three times a week.

■ **WORK IN SOME WEIGHT, OR RESISTANCE, TRAINING.** Just as aerobic exercise is important, a weekly weight-training regimen is key to building strength in your muscles, bones, and joints. If your muscles aren't strong, joints tend to slip out of alignment, causing more pain for you. If you have osteoarthritis, talk to a physical therapist before beginning a weight-training regimen.

■ **STRETCH.** The third critical aspect of your workout routine is stretching. It's important for maintaining the strength and agility of your joints. "Stretching may not prevent the arthritis, but it will likely help to reduce its impact on your function by keeping you looser and less subject to muscle spasm," says Theodore R. Fields, M.D.

Start with gentle exercises. These include simply rotating your arms, legs, and trunk slowly in as full a range of motion as possible without pain. Dr. Loes recommends a Thera-Band stretcher, a small piece of elastic band that offers resistance as you stretch various body parts. Similar products are available online and in sporting goods stores.

■ **START SLOWLY AND GENTLY.** Overexertion can make osteoarthritis pain worse. "If your exercise causes pain that lasts for more than a half hour after you are finished, you probably did too much. Cut back, then work up to an increased amount," says Dr. Loes.

If you're unsure of your limitations, rely on the trusted guidance of your doctor, who can diagnose your physical limitations, and your physical therapist, who can create a special routine to keep you sufficiently challenged within those limits.

■ **EXERCISE AFTER A HOT SHOWER.** The hot water loosens you up, says Dr. Fields, so you're less likely to experience pain while or after exercising.

■ **BUY GOOD SHOES.** Walking is a great aerobic exercise to reduce your arthritis pain. If you make walking a routine, Dr. Loes recommends investing in a good pair of walking shoes. Look for lightweight shoes made of breathable material, comfortable at the ball of your foot, and that have good arch support and a padded heel.

■ **EXERCISE ON A SOFT, FLAT SURFACE.** A surface that gives under each step minimizes jarring to your joints and hurtful steps that could irritate your arthritis. A smooth, grassy field or a vulcanized rubber running track, like the one at your local high school, are excellent choices.

■ **MAKE FRIENDS WITH WATER.** "In retirement communities, it's not the golfers who are the healthiest," says Dr. Loes, "it's the swimmers." Our experts agree that swimming is the top low-impact, aerobic exercises for arthritis. Dr. Loes recommends the backstroke and sidestroke to condition the paraspinal muscles, those tiny nerve-rich muscles surrounding the spine. Strengthening these muscles will help ease back pain and improve mobility. Water aerobics is also a good choice to relieve and reduce arthritis pain.

■ **BE CAREFUL ABOUT RUNNING.** The good news is that studies show running doesn't cause osteoarthritis, says Dr. Fields. The bad news is that, "in people predisposed to getting osteoarthritis, or in those with knees or ankles that are not well aligned, running can contribute to osteoarthritis," he says. "If a joint such as the knee is injured, then subsequent running, especially on a hard surface, can cause it to progress."

■ **USE EPSOM SALTS.** Added to bathwater, these magnesium sulfate crystals provide extra-soothing comfort for arthritis pain because they help draw out carbon—one of the waste products of your body—through your skin.

■ **STAND UP STRAIGHT.** Bad posture puts a lot of pressure on your joints, causing wear and tear on your bones and cartilage—just as poor alignment in your car causes tires to wear unevenly. It also can cause a lot of extra pain for people with arthritis, says Alan

Lichtbroun, M.D. So stand up straight now; it could save your knees and hips in the long run.

■ **GET HOT OR COLD.** If you feel arthritis pain flaring, Dr. Fields recommends heat or ice to quell the burning. Use ice for sudden flare-ups, chronic pain, or when your joints are inflamed. And reserve the heat treatment—like a hot bath, heating pad, or a hot pack wrapped in a towel—for when you feel sore and achy.

■ **RELY ON ACETAMINOPHEN.** Safe and effective, acetaminophen taken on a daily basis is the standard recommendation for minor arthritis pain. "Tylenol is the main-stay of operation," says Justus Fiechtner, M.D. "It doesn't work for everybody, obviously, but it seems to work well if you don't take too much of it."

"The problem with taking many over-the-counter pain relievers every day is that they increase your risk of developing stomach ulcers," says Dr. Fiechtner. He recommends acetaminophen because, unlike aspirin, ibuprofen, and naproxen (Aleve), which can all cause ulcers, acetaminophen is not associated with stomach problems.

■ **EXPERIMENT WITH GLUCOSAMINE AND CHONDROITIN SULFATE.** You often see the medical community turn a skeptical eye when it comes to supplements. But glucosamine and chondroitin sulfate have worked so well in the treatment of arthritis time and again that critics have now accepted them as a pain treatment for arthritis. "There are enough positive studies and evidence for the safety of glucosamine and chondroitin that someone with osteoarthritis should give it a try," says Dr. Fields.

For those who want to test out glucosamine and chondroitin sulfate, Dr. Fields recommends the dosage in the guidelines of the National Institutes of Health: 500 milligrams of glucosamine and 400 milligrams of chondroitin sulfate tablets three times daily for 2 months, and then twice daily after that. "After 3 months, this supplement can be stopped if no benefit is seen," says Dr. Fields.

■ **LOVE YOUR JOINTS WITH GINGER.** Some studies indicate that this amazing root blocks inflammation as well as anti-inflammatory drugs do (and without side effects). Steep a few slivers of fresh ginger in a tea ball in 1 cup of freshly boiled water for 10 minutes. Let it cool to sipping temperature and drink up.

■ **TAKE A DAILY C SUPPLEMENT.** Try a daily dose of vitamin C to preserve the health of your collagen and connective tissue. Take at least 100 milligrams a day.

■ **ADD IN VITAMIN E.** Though vitamin E has gotten some bad press lately, Dr. Barnard stands behind it as a good treatment for alleviating osteoarthritis pain. "A typical dosage regimen is 200 IU each day, or 100 IU if you have high blood pressure," he says.

■ **MIX IN MAGNESIUM.** In addition to these other nutrients, Dr. Loes recommends 60 milligrams of magnesium a day. "Aside from just helping bones, magnesium helps to ward off cramps and improves sleep," he says.

■ **DON'T FORGET VITAMIN D.** A deficiency of vitamin D was once thought to lead directly to osteoarthritis. While additional studies have not shown this to be the case, the vitamin is still critical for preserving overall muscle strength, which is why Dr. Fields recommends 800 IU daily.

■ **ADD OMEGA-3S TO YOUR REGIME.** The anti-inflammatory effects of omega-3 fatty acids seem to play a role in reducing arthritis pain, explains Dr. Barnard. Add flaxseeds or flax oil to your diet. Try to get 2 teaspoons every day for a healthy dose of omega-3s.

■ **MIX THEM WITH OMEGA-6S.** "The most recent research seems to indicate that combining omega-3s with an omega-6 fat like borage oil, black currant oil, or evening primrose oil makes it even more effective," says Dr. Barnard. Try to get 1.4 grams of gamma linolenic acid (GLA), the most helpful omega-6.

■ **FIND A CAPSAICIN CREAM.** Capsaicin, the active constituent of hot peppers, is available over the counter in a topical cream. (The most commonly available brand is Zostrix.)

Smearing capsaicin cream over your joints inhibits your nerve cells' ability to transmit pain impulses, effectively wiping out arthritis pain. You can find capsaicin cream over the counter at drugstores.

PANEL OF ADVISORS

NEAL BARNARD, M.D., IS THE PRESIDENT OF THE PHYSICIAN'S COMMITTEE FOR RESPONSIBLE MEDICINE IN WASHINGTON, D.C., AND AUTHOR OF *FOODS THAT FIGHT PAIN.*

JUSTUS FIECHTNER, M.D., IS A CLINICAL PROFESSOR OF OSTEOPATHIC MANIPULATIVE MEDICINE AT MICHIGAN STATE UNIVERSITY COLLEGE OF HUMAN MEDICINE IN EAST LANSING.

THEODORE R. FIELDS, M.D., IS A RHEUMATOLOGIST AT THE HOSPITAL FOR SPECIAL SURGERY IN NEW YORK CITY, AN ASSOCIATE PROFESSOR OF CLINICAL MEDICINE AT THE WEILL COLLEGE OF MEDICINE OF CORNELL UNIVERSITY, AND CLINICAL DIRECTOR OF THE H.S.S. GOSDEN ROBINSON EARLY ARTHRITIS CENTER.

ALAN LICHTBROUN, M.D., SPECIALIZES IN RHEUMATOLOGY AND CONNECTIVE TISSUE RESEARCH AT THE ROBERT WOOD JOHNSON UNIVERSITY HOSPITAL IN EAST BRUNSWICK, NEW JERSEY.

MICHAEL LOES, M.D., IS DIRECTOR OF THE ARIZONA PAIN INSTITUTE IN PHOENIX AND AUTHOR OF *THE HEALING RESPONSE.*

KEVIN STONE, M.D., IS AN ORTHOPEDIC SURGEON AT THE STONE CLINIC IN SAN FRANCISCO.

Osteoporosis

19 Ways to Preserve Bone Strength

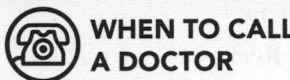

WHEN TO CALL A DOCTOR

All people age 65 or older should have a bone-density test to determine if they're at risk for osteoporosis—or if they already have it, says Robert R. Recker, M.D.

Those with one or more risk factors for osteoporosis—such as a family history of the disease, a history of alcohol or tobacco use, the use of bone-weakening medications (such as steroids or antiseizure drugs), or early menopause—should get the test as early as age 50, Dr. Recker says.

Your doctor will probably advise you to have a test called DEXA, which measures bone density of the hip and spine. If the density is lower than it should be, your doctor may advise you to take estrogen or other medications to prevent further bone loss and add bone density.

The word *osteoporosis* means "porous bones." Comparing two sets of x-rays—one from someone with healthy bones and the other from someone with osteoporosis—makes it immediately clear why the name is appropriate.

Healthy bones on an x-ray appear as a lot of white shapes because the x-rays bounce right off the bone and are not captured on film. On an x-ray revealing osteoporosis, however, you'd see a lot of dark shadows because the bones are so porous that x-rays pass right through them.

In the United States, about 10 million people have osteoporosis—8 million are women, for whom the overall risk of osteoporosis is much greater. The National Osteoporosis Foundation estimates that 44 million Americans, or 55 percent of those age 50 or older, are at risk of developing osteoporosis.

The reason women are at a greater risk of osteoporosis than men is because men's bones are actually a bit stronger to begin with, explains Theodore R. Fields, M.D. Estrogen works to keep women's bones strong, but "after menopause, women lose the protective effect of estrogen, which causes as much as a 5 percent loss of bone density," says Dr. Fields.

The scary thing about osteoporosis is that it's a "silent" disease. It develops over decades without causing pain or other symptoms. "There are no symptoms until you fracture a bone or a vertebra collapses," says James Hubbard, M.D., M.P.H. "The bone mass is slowly and silently lost without you knowing it."

The good news is that bone is constantly regenerated—new cells are created while older cells are taken away. There are many ways to enhance this process and restore bone while also reducing the rate at which bone is removed, including prescription medication. Whether you have osteoporosis already or you want to be sure you never get it, here are some bone-banking strategies to keep your skeleton strong.

■ **EAT A CALCIUM-RICH DIET.** Think of calcium as the cement that makes bones strong. Even though bones are loaded with calcium, cells called osteoclasts constantly break down bone and "steal" calcium for use in other parts of the body. If you don't get enough calcium in your diet, your bones will give up the calcium for other functions in your body.

Your peak bone-building years end at age 30. After that, bones can get perilously weak, especially after menopause, when declines in estrogen levels cause women's bones to lose calcium at an accelerated rate. Get a bone-density test at the first signs of menopause. And men aren't immune to bone loss. They go through a similar process as women, although not as dramatic. "Testosterone is protective of the bones in men, and the drop-off is generally slower and more delayed than the drop-off of estrogen in women," says Dr. Fields. So men are also susceptible to bone loss, and screenings should begin at 50 to 60 years of age.

If you're 30 years or younger, you need 1,200 milligrams of calcium daily. From ages 30 to 50, it increases to 1,200 to 1,500 milligrams daily, and after age 50, you need 1,500 to 2,000 milligrams of calcium each day.

Calcium is among the easiest nutrients to get in your diet, especially if you eat dairy foods, says Robert R. Recker, M.D. A glass of low-fat milk, for example, has about 300 milligrams of calcium. Yogurt and cheese also provide ample amounts. Three or four servings daily of low-fat milk or other dairy foods will provide all or most of the calcium that your bones need to be healthy.

■ **CHOOSE FORTIFIED FOODS.** If you don't enjoy the taste of dairy foods, or if you find you have trouble digesting them, there are plenty of dairy-free calcium sources to choose from. "If you don't eat dairy, the best thing is to eat a lot of fortified foods," says Dr. Recker.

Many fortified juices and breakfast cereals contain as much calcium as a glass of milk. A number of breads, cereals, and snack bars are available with calcium added.

■ **LOAD UP ON PRODUCE.** If you don't eat dairy, load up on fruits and vegetables rich in dietary calcium. Dr. Hubbard recommends dark, leafy green vegetables such as spinach and dark lettuce varieties. And Steven Jepson, M.D., says broccoli, brussels sprouts, and kale are also good choices.

■ **FIND IT IN FISH.** In addition to their other benefits, fish like sardines and salmon contain calcium, says Dr. Hubbard.

■ **EAT SOY FOODS.** Some brands of soy foods are calcium fortified, but that's not the only reason that soy protects the bones. Soy contains phytoestrogens, chemical compounds that act like a weaker form of the bone-protecting estrogen that women can incorporate into their diet.

Soy products, such as tofu and soymilk, are especially helpful for vegetarians, as those two foods often replace the meat and dairy in the diet, say our experts. Of course, everybody can benefit from eating more soy.

■ **SUPPLEMENT YOUR DIET.** The average American does not consume enough calcium every day to prevent osteoporosis. Even women who have healthy diets may still fall short on calcium because so little of this mineral is absorbed. It makes sense to make up the difference with supplements, says Susan Kaib, M.D. "I can't tell you how many patients I've counseled who are taking a medication for osteoporosis but not obtaining enough calcium," she says. "I explain it's like putting the mortar on a fence, but not laying any bricks: You need the supplemental calcium to build the bones along with the medications, too."

Because your body can absorb only 500 to 600 milligrams of calcium at a time efficiently, it's a good idea to take one supplement in the morning and another in the evening, says Dr. Recker. Look for supplements containing 500 milligrams of calcium, and take them two or three times daily. Another, less expensive option is to buy a big bottle of Tums, a calcium-based antacid. If you're getting your calcium from an antacid, choose tablets that are aluminum-free. Aluminum can hinder the body's ability to get enough calcium into the bones.

■ **TAKE SUPPLEMENTS WITH MEALS.** Calcium is absorbed most efficiently in an acidic environment, such as when your stomach is digesting a meal. That's why Dr. Fields recommends taking your calcium supplements after you've eaten.

■ **GET ENOUGH VITAMIN D.** This nutrient is vital for bone health because it helps transport calcium from the blood into your skeleton. Vitamin D is plentiful—right from the sun. But still, most people don't get nearly enough of it, says Dr. Fields. "Most everyone needs a supplement to keep their vitamin D in the normal range, and vitamin D deficiency is very common," he says.

About 800 IU of vitamin D are recommended daily. "There is generally a 400-IU dose of vitamin D in a multivitamin, so you only need an additional 400 IU," says Dr. Fields. "Many people get the bulk of their daily vitamin D combined with their calcium tablet, often with 200 IU of each."

If you're already taking a multivitamin or a calcium supplement, check the amount of vitamin D in it, and adjust your dosage to get to the 800 IU recommended daily.

■ **ENJOY THE SUN.** Millions of people avoid the sun to protect their skin, but they may be harming their bones. Every time sunshine strikes your skin, your body produces bone-protecting vitamin D. If you're outside without sunscreen, approximately 20 minutes of sun exposure will give you about 200 IU of vitamin D. Sunscreen blocks vitamin D production almost completely.

However, Dr. Fields cautions against too much time in the sun. "There are risks to sun exposure such as skin cancer," he says. "Plus, the weather varies from location to location, and it's hard to get enough sun every day. For all these reasons, most people need a supplement."

■ **MAKE SOUP.** Here's an easy and unique way to get more calcium in your diet. Make a homemade soup stock from bones. Add a little vinegar when preparing the stock. The vinegar dissolves the calcium out of the bones. One pint of this soup offers as much calcium as about 1 quart of milk.

■ **EAT LESS SALT.** Americans get tremendous amounts of sodium, and it's our bones that may be paying the price. Salt depletes the body's calcium stores in two ways. It reduces the amount that's absorbed from foods or supplements, and it increases the amount that's then excreted. "The greater your intake of sodium, the greater the loss of calcium," says Dr. Recker.

The upper limit for sodium is 2,300 milligrams daily, but less is better. It's okay to sprinkle a little salt on your food, but try to avoid processed and packaged foods, which

tend to be very high in sodium. Better yet, check food labels at the grocery store, and only buy foods that are labeled low-sodium or sodium-free.

■ **DRINK ALCOHOL IN MODERATION.** For men, that means no more than two drinks daily; for women, one drink is the upper limit. Excessive alcohol consumption decreases bone formation and reduces your body's ability to absorb calcium.

Alcohol can hurt in yet another way. People who drink heavily tend to have poor diets, which results in lower calcium intake and a greater risk of osteoporosis and fractures.

■ **DRINK FEWER SOFT DRINKS AND COFFEE.** Soft drinks give your bones a one-two punch of phosphorus and caffeine. Some studies have suggested that the phosphorus in soft drinks may lead to decreased bone density, especially in the hips. And caffeine intake may lead to decreased calcium absorption.

Though both of these links are not definitively proven, there's enough evidence that it's advisable to limit the soda and caffeine that you intake if you're worried about osteoporosis, says Dr. Fields. "It's reasonable to keep cola intake to one to two cans a day," he says. "Instead of soda, drink some milk. That would also help with your vitamin D and calcium intake."

■ **IF YOU SMOKE, TRY TO QUIT.** On top of all the other health benefits of not smoking, here's another one: Lifelong smokers are 10 to

20 times more likely to develop osteoporosis than nonsmokers, says Dr. Recker.

■ **GET PLENTY OF EXERCISE.** It slows the rate of bone loss and can lead to an increase in bone density. Virtually any type of exercise is helpful, but the best for bone health are weight-bearing exercises, such as walking—in which you move your body against gravity—and resistance exercises, such as lifting weights, says Dr. Recker.

Exercise has other benefits as well. Because it improves muscle tone, coordination, and balance, it can dramatically reduce the risk of falls, which is the leading cause of fractures in the elderly.

You don't have to be a hard-core athlete to build stronger bones with exercise. You don't even have to join a gym. Any activity that gets you on your feet and moving against gravity for 30 minutes four or five times a week adds significant amounts of bone to your skeleton. Add a 15-minute weight-lifting session, and your bones get even stronger.

"Bone is living tissue. Weight-bearing, resistance, and flexibility exercises help combat the potentially crippling effects of osteoporosis," says Dr. Kaib. "Exercises like swimming, however, are not as helpful because the body is floating in the water, which doesn't put as much strain on the bones. If you are hiking, wearing a backpack with even 5 pounds of added weight can help improve your spinal bone density."

What exercises are best for bones? Here are some of your options.

- Walking is a weight-bearing exercise that increases stress on bones in the legs and hips. The stress stimulates bone-building cells to create new bone, which is why women who walk regularly have greater bone density and get fewer fractures than those who are sedentary.

- Running, dancing, aerobics, and other high-impact activities are even better for bone growth than walking is. If you already have osteoporosis, ask your doctor if your bones are strong enough for high-impact exercises.

- Flexing your wrists—by holding a soup can in each hand and bending your wrist toward your forearm, for example—strengthens not only your wrist bones but also reduces the risk of fractures or other injuries.

- Doing household activities can strengthen the bones just as much as "formal" workouts, as long as you do them vigorously. Yard work is a good choice because it involves a lot of pushing and pulling. Even cleaning the house—sweeping, vacuuming, and walking up and down stairs—helps keep bones strong.

PANEL OF ADVISORS

THEODORE R. FIELDS, M.D., IS A RHEUMATOLOGIST AT THE HOSPITAL FOR SPECIAL SURGERY IN NEW YORK CITY, AN ASSOCIATE PROFESSOR OF CLINICAL MEDICINE AT THE WEILL COLLEGE OF MEDICINE OF CORNELL UNIVERSITY, AND CLINICAL DIRECTOR OF THE H.S.S. GOSDEN ROBINSON EARLY ARTHRITIS CENTER.

JAMES HUBBARD, M.D., M.P.H., WAS A FAMILY PRACTITIONER IN MISSISSIPPI FOR OVER 25 YEARS AND IS THE PUBLISHER OF *JAMES HUBBARD'S MY FAMILY DOCTOR*, A MAGAZINE WRITTEN BY HEALTH CARE PROVIDERS FOR THE GENERAL PUBLIC.

STEVEN JEPSON, M.D., IS MEDICAL DIRECTOR OF THE UTAH DERMATOLOGIC AND MEDICAL PROCEDURES CLINIC IN MURRAY, UTAH, AND AUTHOR OF *7 WAYS TO LOOK YOUNGER WITHOUT UNDERGOING THE KNIFE.*

SUSAN KAIB, M.D., IS THE MEDICAL DIRECTOR OF KRONOS OPTIMAL HEALTH COMPANY IN PHOENIX, ARIZONA.

ROBERT R. RECKER, M.D., IS DIRECTOR OF THE OSTEOPOROSIS RESEARCH CENTER AT CREIGHTON UNIVERSITY SCHOOL OF MEDICINE IN OMAHA, NEBRASKA.

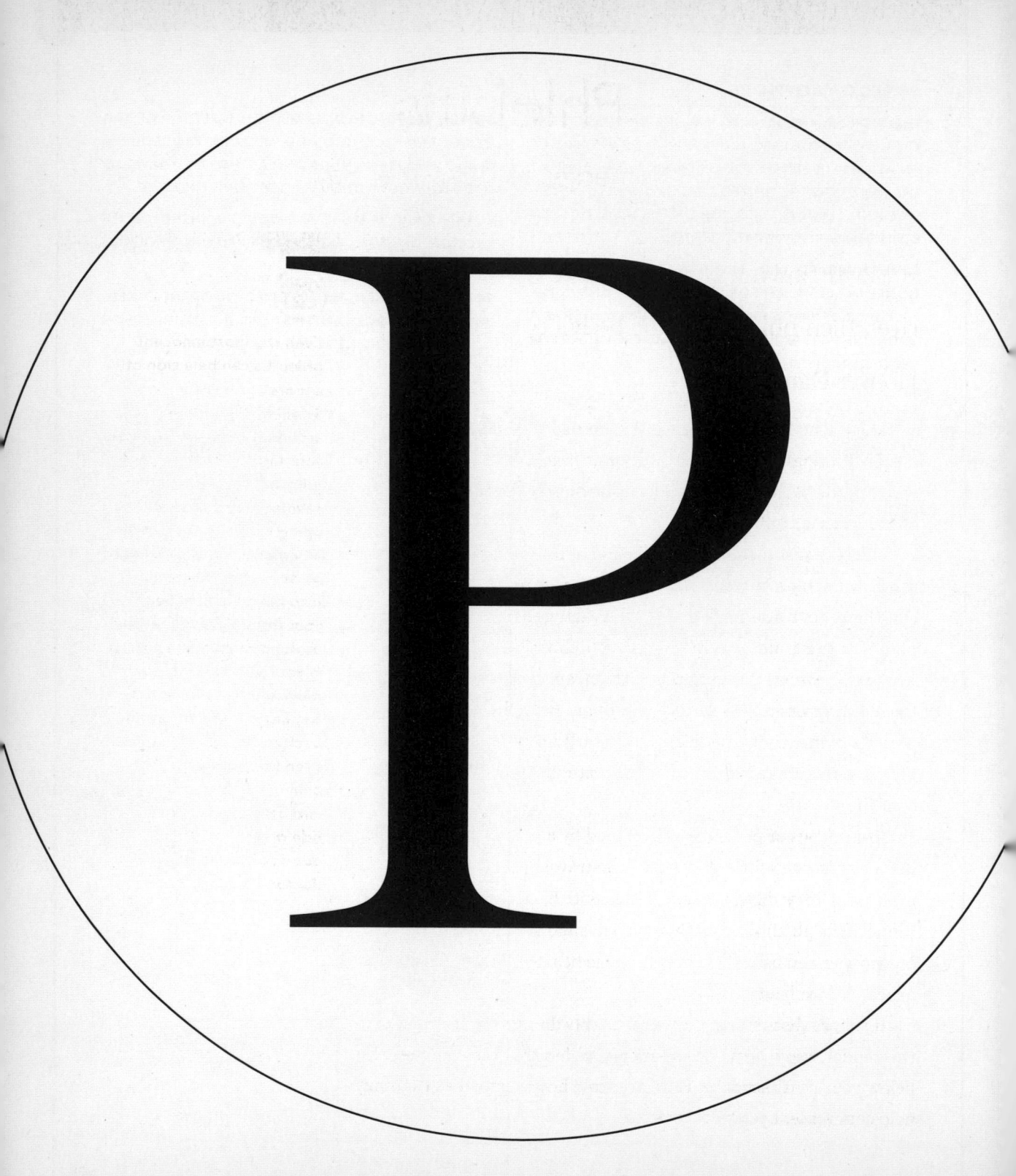

Phlebitis

14 Remedies to Keep It at Bay

If blood flowing through the veins is a peaceful river, then phlebitis is the body's equivalent of the Hoover Dam.

Those who have experienced phlebitis know it as much more: a painful, frightening affliction that can claim a life without warning via a blood clot that surreptitiously lodges in the veins of the heart or lungs.

Phlebitis just means inflammation of the veins. It is more correctly known as thrombophlebitis. "Thrombo" is for the blood clot that is its trademark and primary danger. Two basic types of phlebitis exist: deep vein thrombophlebitis, or DVT for short, which is the more dangerous condition, and superficial phlebitis, the more common, less serious condition. Both are caused by long periods of inactivity, such as a long car trip or lengthy bed rest. Your genes might also put you at a greater risk for developing this condition.

"Both types of phlebitis are defined by a clot in a blood vessel, but a clot in one of the deep veins can travel to the heart or lungs, making it very dangerous," says David L. Katz, M.D., M.P.H. "Superficial phlebitis usually occurs in smaller vessels, so the clots are smaller and usually won't reach the heart or lungs. It's more of a localized problem."

It sounds disturbing, but you probably don't need to stress over the tender, ropy veins of superficial phlebitis you may feel just below your skin's surface. Here are some home remedies that may help complement your doctor's care.

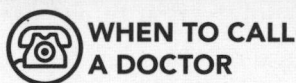

WHEN TO CALL A DOCTOR

Even the most innocent phlebitis can be a sign of a more serious ailment. Swelling or tenderness around a reddened area on your leg is something to tell your physician. If you have a history of developing superficial phlebitis or varicose veins, you might be at risk for deep vein thrombophlebitis. See your doctor if you feel any prolonged pain or swelling in your calf or thigh, and particularly if the pain is coming primarily from the back of the calf. If you feel even the least bit of leg pain or swelling a day or two after a long plane ride or car trip, it's a good reason to pay your doctor a visit.

■ **AVOID INJURY.** While DVT usually has more to do with your overall heart health, superficial phlebitis often occurs after an injury to the leg, says Dr. Katz.

■ **GIVE IT REST AND WARMTH.** If you experience the pain or swelling of phlebitis, one of the first things you can do for immediate relief is elevate your legs and apply a warm compress to the area, says Dr. Katz. "Warm compresses increase bloodflow and help to dissolve the clot," he says. "And elevating the limbs will help to get the blood moving again."

■ **GET SOME EXERCISE.** Exercise is a good way to prevent phlebitis in the first place, as well as keep it from coming back. "If your muscles are stronger and more toned, that means the blood is flowing through them more efficiently," says Dr. Katz. "And that greatly reduces your risk of developing a blood clot."

■ **WALK WHEN YOU HAVE TO RIDE.** Planning a long trip by car? If you've had phlebitis in the past, then make sure your wheels aren't the only things in motion. The main thing is to stop frequently and exercise, says Michael D. Dake, M.D. "Don't take just one pit stop during the day and walk a mile, but rather stop four or five times and walk shorter distances." Exercise prevents your circulation from slowing down during long periods of sitting.

■ **BEWARE THE FRIENDLY SKIES.** Scientific literature is littered with reports of people stricken with deep vein thrombophlebitis following long airplane flights. The condition is so common that it's now known as economy class syndrome, because it rarely seems to strike those passengers seated in roomy, first-class seats.

The best way to prevent DVT, says Dr. Katz, is to get up and walk around every hour or so to keep the blood circulating. In fact, you may want to request an aisle seat to make this easier.

Even while sitting you can do exercises to keep blood flowing. "Simply tense and flex your muscles for a few seconds, and then release them," says Dr. Katz. "Also, lift up your feet, and contract the muscles in your calves while you do this. And check out the videos on an intercontinental flight. Usually a few of the options are exercises that you can do in your seat."

■ **KNOW YOUR RISKS.** Once you've had phlebitis, you're at increased risk of getting it again. Long periods of bed rest make you especially vulnerable. While you might not be able to prevent prolonged bed rest following an injury or a serious illness, certain types of risks, such as elective surgery, can be avoided if you're prone to clotting disorders. Consult your doctor for specific risk factors, but keep in mind that getting up and around can help reduce the risks of developing phlebitis after surgery.

■ **WEAR SUPPORT STOCKINGS FOR SOME RELIEF.** These stockings, available in drugstores and department stores, impede the blood's tendency to pool in the small blood vessels closest to the skin. While there's no documented evidence showing that support stockings do any good in *preventing* phlebitis, they do seem to relieve pain and make some people feel better. The best advice for you? Wear support stockings if you're prone to swollen legs and ankles or varicose veins.

■ **FOLLOW A HEALTHY DIET.** While nutrition doesn't have a direct connection to phlebitis, eating a healthy diet and maintaining a healthy weight are both related to a more efficient heart and better bloodflow. And that, in turn, reduces your risk of experiencing phlebitis, especially the more dangerous DVT.

There are some nutrients, such as garlic and certain antioxidants, that have anti-inflammatory properties, but Dr. Katz says the most important thing is to focus on a whole-diet approach of eating plenty of fruits and vegetables, whole grains, and lean sources of protein. "They've never done the study, but I'm willing to bet if you had 2,000 people on airplanes, and 1,000 of them followed a

Cures from the Kitchen

High-fiber foods are important to your vein health for one simple reason—they keep you regular. If you're constipated, you tend to push too much and too frequently when you have a bowel movement, which puts extra pressure on the valves of your legs. Try to eat around 30 grams of fiber a day from foods like bran cereals, oatmeal, and beans. And remember to drink extra water. Without water, adding fiber can make your constipation worse.

healthy diet, that group would experience less DVT than the other group," he says.

■ **TRY AN OVER-THE-COUNTER SOLUTION.** Some studies suggest that the blood-thinning properties of aspirin, Tylenol, and other over-the-counter pain relievers may help reduce phlebitis by preventing rapid clot formation in those prone to the disease. These studies advise that you take aspirin before prolonged periods of bed rest, travel, or surgery, all of which tend to make circulation sluggish and increase the possibility of clotting.

■ **TRY HORSE CHESTNUT.** Available in tincture or capsules, this herb can really improve stressed veins by helping to strengthen and repair blood vessels that have lost their elasticity, says Teresa Koby, a clinical herbalist. Take 300 milligrams twice a day to relieve symptoms.

■ **ADD VITAMIN E.** While the safety of vitamin E has been called into question in some studies recently, Dr. Katz says taking a low dose is safe and effective for treating phlebitis pain and swelling. "I recommend taking 200 IU daily when you experience pain and for 2 weeks after the pain stops," he says. "Some multivitamins will even provide this much vitamin E."

■ **FIND RELIEF FROM FISH OIL.** Dr. Katz is a big believer in the anti-thrombotic properties of fish oil, which is why he recommends that everyone take 2 grams of a fish oil supplement each day.

■ **ADD ANOTHER REASON TO QUIT.** As if you need any more! Dr. Katz pegs smoking as one of the biggest factors in causing phlebitis because it increases your risk of blood clots. If you still smoke, ask your doctor for help in quitting.

■ **BE CAREFUL WITH CONTRACEPTIVES.** Contrary to popular belief, oral contraceptives don't raise everyone's risk of getting phlebitis, says Dr. Katz. But if you have a rare genetic blood disorder known as Factor V, or Leiden, deficiency, then you shouldn't take them. Your doctor can determine if you have a Factor V deficiency with a simple blood test.

PANEL OF ADVISORS

MICHAEL D. DAKE, M.D., IS A PROFESSOR AT THE UNIVERSITY OF VIRGINIA DEPARTMENT OF RADIOLOGY IN CHARLOTTESVILLE.

DAVID L. KATZ, M.D., M.P.H., IS THE DIRECTOR OF THE YALE GRIFFIN PREVENTION RESEARCH CENTER IN DERBY, CONNECTICUT, AND AUTHOR OF *THE WAY TO EAT*.

TERESA KOBY IS A CLINICAL HERBALIST WITH THE HERBAL RESEARCH FOUNDATION IN BOULDER, COLORADO.

Phobias and Fears

11 Coping Measures

Whether it's the neighborhood dog or being alone in the dark, all of us have fears in our lives. And fears are quite normal, says Simon A. Rego, Psy.D. "Fear is healthy. It gives you an evolutionary advantage," he says. "With a fear of heights, for example, your body is trying to tell you that this is dangerous, and you shouldn't be there." When that fear goes beyond a mere feeling and aversely impacts your ability to function, that's when it becomes a phobia, says Dr. Rego.

"There are as many different kinds of phobias as there are different kinds of people," says Jerilyn Ross, M.A., L.I.C.S.W. In the classic sense, a phobia is "an irrational, involuntary, inappropriate fear reaction that generally leads to an avoidance of common everyday places, objects, or situations," she says. In the real sense, though, a phobia is the fear of fear itself. "A phobia is a fear of one's own feelings and impulses. It's a fear of having a panic attack, feeling trapped, of losing control or getting sick."

Phobias are classified into three types: simple or specific phobias, social phobias, and agoraphobia. People with specific phobias experience a dread of certain objects, places, or situations. People with social phobias avoid public situations, like parties, because

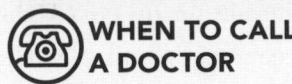

WHEN TO CALL A DOCTOR

If your phobia interferes with your life, seek professional help. Who you seek out is as crucial as seeking help itself. "It's important that you get help from someone who understands phobias," says Jerilyn Ross, M.A., L.I.C.S.W. "Many people with phobias end up going from doctor to doctor before getting a diagnosis and appropriate help."

they're afraid they'll do something to embarrass themselves. Agoraphobics are victims of a complex phenomenon based on a fear of being in public places without a familiar person or an escape plan.

According to Dr. Rego, there are three common pathways to phobias. The first is direct conditioning, in which an experience earlier in life leads to the phobia—for example, being bitten by a dog causing a fear of dogs. The second is vicarious conditioning, in which an experience of someone close to you leads to a phobia. And the final pathway is receiving information or instruction, such as the fear of flight after September 11, or a fear of pit bulls after negative news reports about them.

People with phobias always recognize that their fear is inappropriate to the situation, says Ross. For example, if you're flying on an airplane during a thunderstorm, feeling fearful is a normal reaction. If, however, your boss tells you you'll have to take a business trip in a few weeks and you immediately start worrying about having a panic attack on the plane, that's inappropriate to the situation.

Does this sound like something you've experienced? If so, here's some rational advice for irrational behavior from those who deal with the problem every day.

■ **RELY ON RELAXATION.** If you face a situation in which fear or panic are beginning to take hold, simple relaxation techniques can help, says Cathy Frank, M.D. "Just relax your muscles and mind," she says. "Form images of a place you'd rather be, such as lying on a beach or walking through the woods. This can release tension and bring you back down."

■ **DO SOMETHING DISTRACTING.** Another approach, says Dr. Frank, is to train your attention on something else entirely and focus hard on it. "This usually helps if it's an absorbing activity, such as a crossword, jigsaw puzzle, or computer game," she says. "Other mental exercises that can help are counting backward, playing word games, or thinking about vacation plans. These can work, but they're short-term solutions."

■ **FACE YOUR FEAR HEAD ON.** While these techniques can work, says Dr. Rego, they do nothing to help you face and ultimately overcome your fear. That's why he advocates cognitive behavioral therapy (CBT), which has you face your fear head on to triumph over it. This can be done with the help of a therapist for more severe phobias, or on your own if it's a minor phobia.

■ **ESTABLISH A HIERARCHY.** Of course, there's more to overcoming a phobia than just facing it, says Dr. Frank. One common approach in cognitive behavioral therapy is to create a hierarchy within your phobia of the least anxious aspects of it to the most fearful, and rank them from 1 to 10. "For example, if you're afraid of flying, going to the airport might be a '1,' and going on a very long flight would be a '10,'" she says. "It's best to start by facing the smaller challenges first, overcoming them, and then working your way up to the larger fears."

■ **CHALLENGE IT INTELLECTUALLY.** If you begin to feel panic and anxiety when facing your fear (and you inevitably will), don't let it affect you unchecked, says Dr. Frank. "You need to challenge the thoughts you have about your anxiety," she says. "If you're panicky on elevators, for example, ask yourself, 'What evidence do I have to be afraid of this elevator?' or, 'What's the worst that could happen?' By using Socratic questioning to verify or refute your notions about your phobia, you can gradually begin to overcome it."

■ **BE AWARE.** Even with a gradual approach to facing your fears—and a logical approach to reasoning through them—those with phobias are likely to have panic attacks. David Carbonell, M.D., advocates the "AWARE" technique of facing the attack and allowing it to pass.

The steps involved in "AWARE" are "Acknowledge and Accept," in which you accept the oncoming attack, realize that it's scary, but also accept that it is not dangerous. Once you have accomplished this, you need to "Wait and Watch." Here, you're not trying to run away from the fear, but are instead letting it wash over you. Next are the "Action" steps, in which you bring the panic under control with breathing (see the information

that follows), and resume the fearful activity. Finally, you'll want to "Repeat" the steps if necessary, and then let yourself acknowledge that no matter how it feels now, the attack will come to an "End."

■ **RELY ON BREATHING.** When panic is beginning to take hold, Dr. Carbonell recommends fighting it off with a technique called diaphragmatic breathing, or belly breathing. In the simplest of terms, this is a method for deep breathing, explains Dr. Carbonell. A panic attack often begins a feeling that you can't breathe, but in reality, you're taking rapid breaths, and not exhaling between them.

To combat this, Dr. Carbonell says to breathe by placing one hand on your belt line, and another on your breastbone. Then, exhale forcefully by sighing, as if somebody just told you something very annoying.

Now you can begin the process of inhaling, which you want to do slowly through your nose. As you inhale, push your stomach out. Then hold the breath for as long as it is comfortable, and exhale by opening your mouth, breathing out, and pulling your stomach in. Repeat the process until the panic begins to subside.

■ **PLAY MUSCLE GAMES.** One thing that often occurs during a panic attack is that your muscles tense up. That's why Dr. Frank recommends that people practice muscle control by intentionally tightening their muscles for 10 to

Blame It on Your Ears

Just when you think that your phobia may be all in your mind, along comes Harold Levinson, M.D., who says it's not in your mind at all. It's in your inner ear.

Dr. Levinson has specialized in inner ear–determined disorders since successfully treating his dyslexic and attention-deficit hyperactivity disorder (ADHD) patients with inner ear–enhancing medications. "Not only did the learning, attention, balance, coordination, and rhythmic symptoms improve, but so did their phobia problems," he says.

It was his unique background as both a psychiatrist and a neurologist that led him to this conclusion. "A significant number of my dyslexic and ADHD patients with inner-ear problems also had phobias identical to the patients I was treating in my psychiatric practice. Psycho-therapy neither explained nor helped phobic symptoms, however, whereas these medications often helped dramatically and rapidly."

After 45 years of research on more than 35,000 patients, Dr. Levinson believes that 90 per-cent of all phobic behavior is a result of an underlying malfunction within the inner-ear system and its supercomputer, the cerebellum.

"The sensory and motor mechanisms controlled by the inner ear are not functioning correctly," he explains. For example, balance is controlled in the inner ear. If it is not working correctly and your balance is off, you might be afraid of heights or falling or trip-ping. Similarly, if your eye and hand coordination is impaired, you won't be able to read and write with any accuracy.

Dr. Levinson acknowledges that his was a minority point of view 40 years ago. But thou-sands of success stories are nothing to snicker at, and current independent research is substan-tiating his original concepts. Dr. Levinson is convinced that a trip to an ear specialist is at least worth a try for those who have phobias and related learning, concentration and balance, coor-dination, and rhythmic disturbances.

15 seconds, and then relaxing them. "This gives people a sense of empowerment, that they, and not their emotions, are in charge of their muscles," she says.

■ **BEWARE OF THE EFFECTS OF CAF-FEINE.** While it's not a major factor, Dr. Car-bonell adds that high caffeine intake or caffeine addiction can only heighten your anxiety and increase your reaction to pho-bias. So if you drink a lot of coffee or caffein-ated soda, now might be the time to cut back on your intake.

■ **REWARD YOURSELF.** Overcoming a phobia is nothing to be taken lightly, which is why Dr. Carbonell says it's important to give yourself a pat on the back and congratulate yourself for any breakthroughs that you make. However, it's also important to make sure that the breakthroughs are the type you're after.

"This is good, so long as one defines 'triumph' accurately," says Dr. Carbonell. "A typical triumph in working with a phobia is not to approach the object and then not feel afraid. This motivates a person to fight the fear, which leads nowhere useful. Rather, a triumph is to feel the fear and stay in the situation, working with the fear in an accepting manner."

PANEL OF ADVISORS

DAVID CARBONELL, PH.D., IS THE DIRECTOR OF ANXIETY TREATMENT CENTER, LTD., IN CHICAGO, AUTHOR OF *PANIC ATTACKS WORKBOOK: A GUIDED PROGRAM FOR BEATING THE PANIC TRICK,* AND WEB MASTER OF WWW. ANXIETYCOACH.COM.

CATHY FRANK, M.D., IS A PSYCHIATRIST AT THE HENRY FORD MEDICAL CENTER IN DETROIT, MICHIGAN.

HAROLD LEVINSON, M.D., IS A PSYCHIATRIST AND NEUROLOGIST IN GREAT NECK, NEW YORK. HE DISCOVERED THAT AN INNER-EAR DYSFUNCTION WAS RESPONSIBLE FOR DYSLEXIA AND RELATED LEARNING, CONCENTRATION, AND PHOBIC OR ANXIETY DISORDERS. HE IS COAUTHOR OF *PHOBIA FREE.*

SIMON A. REGO, PSY. D., IS DIRECTOR OF QUALITY MANAGEMENT AND DEVELOPMENT FOR UNIVERSITY BEHAVIORAL ASSOCIATES IN YONKERS, NEW YORK.

JERILYN ROSS, M.A., L.I.C.S.W., IS PRESIDENT AND CHIEF EXECUTIVE OFFICER OF THE ANXIETY DISORDER ASSOCIATION OF AMERICA, DIRECTOR OF THE ROSS CENTER FOR ANXIETY AND RELATED DISORDERS IN WASHINGTON, D.C., AND AUTHOR OF *TRIUMPH OVER FEAR* AND *ONE LESS THING TO WORRY ABOUT.*

Pizza Burn

6 Cooling Treatments

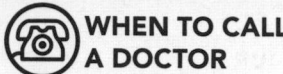

WHEN TO CALL A DOCTOR

A pizza burn usually heals on its own in a week to 10 days. But, if you have a lesion, bump, or scratch, painful or not, that does not disappear within 2 weeks, then it's time to see your dentist.

Richard Antaya, M.D., also advises a trip to the doctor if the burn is so bad that you can't eat or drink. "It's rare for it to get that bad, but it is possible," he says.

We've all been there at one time or another. We know we should let it cool, but that food just looks too good to wait for. Next thing we know, our stomachs get the better of us and . . . ouch! That millimeters-thick tissue on the roof of our mouth is now burned, swollen, and irritated.

Though it's commonly called "pizza burn," that slice is far from the only culprit. "Any hot food can burn your mouth, particularly food in a liquid form or one hard to manipulate in your mouth. Think hot drinks, soups, and melted cheese," says Kimberly Harms, D.D.S.

If the damage is already done, here are some simple ways to help soothe the pain.

■ **KEEP A COOL DRINK ON HAND.** Taking a swig of ice water or other cold drink immediately after the burn can bring temporary and immediate relief, advises Dr. Harms. For more painful burns, put an ice cube in your mouth right away to bring down the temperature, ease the pain, and control swelling, says Dr. Harms, though shortly the cold cube becomes almost equally painful.

■ **BRING ON THE BEN & JERRY'S.** When a doctor advises you to eat ice cream, most people find it hard to argue! And while cool, creamy foods like ice cream and yogurt can help, it's best not to overdo it, says Richard Antaya, M.D. "The cool can bring temporary relief, but be reasonable," he says. "Eating a great big bowl of ice cream is not good for other obvious reasons."

■ **MARCH TO YOUR NEAREST NEIGHBOR-HOOD DRUGSTORE.** Apply an over-the-counter topical anesthetic such as Orabase (other brands that contain benzocaine are just as effective) directly to the burn to help protect the wound, soothe the pain, and speed the healing process, suggests Dr. Harms.

■ **MIX IN A MOUTHWASH.** For another simple remedy, Dr. Antaya recommends dissolving a Maalox antacid tablet in a single dose of Benadryl liquid, swishing it around in your mouth, and spitting it out. "This has a numbing effect that brings immediate relief to the mouth," he says.

■ **AVOID HOT, SALTY, AND CRUNCHY FOODS.** Change your eating habits for a few days, suggests Van B. Haywood, D.M.D. "You'll want to stay away from Tabasco sauce and limit your intake of spicy foods for a few days after suffering a pizza burn," he says. "These types of foods will aggravate the burn and cause you more pain."

Dr. Antaya says the same goes for salty foods, which can bring on the sting and burn, and crunchy foods with sharp edges like potato chips and pretzels, which can aggravate the lesion. And, maybe you should consider striking pizza from your menu for a week or so. Sticking with a bland diet while the thermal irritation heals is a must.

"Most people will eat bland and soft foods for a couple of days after this happens without even thinking about it," says Dr. Haywood.

■ **LEARN FROM YOUR BURN.** To prevent future fires, the best approach, advises Dr. Harms, is to learn some patience. "Make sure your food has had a chance to cool down," she says. "It sometimes helps to take a small taste or sip to minimize damage. If you suspect a drink may be too hot, put an ice cube in it to cool off the liquid."

PANEL OF ADVISORS

RICHARD ANTAYA, M.D., IS A PROFESSOR OF DERMATOLOGY AND DIRECTOR OF PEDIATRICS DERMATOLOGY AT YALE SCHOOL OF MEDICINE IN NEW HAVEN, CONNECTICUT.

KIMBERLY HARMS, D.D.S., IS A DENTIST IN FARMINGTON, MINNESOTA, AND A CONSUMER ADVISOR FOR THE AMERICAN DENTAL ASSOCIATION.

VAN B. HAYWOOD, D.M.D., IS A PROFESSOR AT THE MEDICAL COLLEGE OF THE GEORGIA SCHOOL OF DENTISTRY IN AUGUSTA.

Poison Plant Rashes

15 Itch Relievers

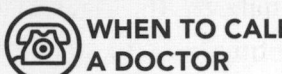

WHEN TO CALL A DOCTOR

In most cases, a poison plant rash isn't serious. You'll just want to stick to the remedies discussed here to relieve the pain and itching until the rash subsides (usually in a couple of weeks). Still, there are a few situations in which the rash may need your doctor's attention, perhaps even immediately. See the list below to find out when you should seek out help.

■ The reaction is severe or widespread, or affects sensitive areas such as your eyes, mouth, or genitals.

■ The rash is still there after 3 weeks.

■ The blisters begin oozing.

■ You develop a fever greater than 100°F.

■ You have any areas of infection that continue to worsen.

■ You have a hard time sleeping at night.

If you've ever had a run-in with poison ivy (or its brethren, poison oak or sumac), chances are you remember the encounter all too well. The red, itchy blisters of the accompanying rash are unpleasant at best and unbearable at worst. The only good news is that you're not alone in this misery: More than 85 percent of people react to this pesky plant the same way.

What most people don't realize is that a poison ivy outbreak is actually an allergy—contact dermatitis, to be precise. And the trigger is an oil secreted by the plants called urushiol. Some people are more sensitive to urushiol oil than others. And a few lucky people are not sensitive to it at all—they can literally roll in the stuff and not get a reaction. But our experts don't advise it. Sensitivity to urushiol can develop at any time. "We're not exactly sure why some people are sensitive to it and some aren't, but it seems to relate to exposure to certain chemicals," explains Richard Antaya, M.D. "If you're not exposed to the oil a lot, your rate of developing an allergy drops dramatically."

Another common misconception about poison plant allergies is that scratching them will actually spread the rash around. In reality, the oil has to make direct contact with the skin to cause the rash. And you can actually get the oil under your fingernails and spread it that way. Still, it's best not to tempt fate by scratching and further irritating your skin.

■ **KNOW YOUR ENEMY.** Ideally, the best approach is to avoid getting a poison plant rash in the first place. You can try to avoid poison ivy, poison oak, and poison sumac simply by steering clear—if you know what the plants look like.

Poison ivy plants have clusters of three shiny leaves, the source of the saying "Leaves of three, let it be." It can grow as a vine or as a shrub, but it always has hair on its trunk. Poison ivy is found throughout most of the country.

The reason that poison ivy claims a lot of victims is that it likes to grow where we like to be: "On the sides of trails, in the rough of a golf course, behind a garage, or at the edge of a forest," says Thomas N. Helm, M.D. "The plants like the transition from forest to open land and are often at the edge of dense tree growth."

Poison oak can be a high-climbing vine or a shrub. Its notched leaves look like those of the common white oak tree. Its berries grow in clusters and are green in summer and off-white in winter. Poison oak grows mostly in the West and Southeast U.S.

Poison sumac stems each have 7 to 13 leaflets. It grows as a tall shrub, sporting green berries in summer that turn yellow-white in winter. The plant can be found in the northern part of the country and sometimes in the Deep South.

■ **BLOCK THAT IVY.** If you know you're going to be around poison ivy, like when you're about to clear it from your yard, prepare your-self first. IvyBlock is a lotion that actually prevents urushiol from penetrating your skin. The lotion leaves a slightly visible film on the skin so that you can see exactly where you're protected. IvyBlock and similar products are available at drugstores.

■ **WASH UP.** If, despite your best efforts, you've been in contact, time is of the essence. "I don't know what the exact breaking point is, but I do know that you can stop an outbreak if you act quickly enough," says Dr. Antaya. If you have access to soap and water, wash any exposed areas as quickly as possible. Or pour rubbing alcohol over your skin immediately. Don't use a washcloth, however, as it just picks up the urushiol oil and spreads it around.

■ **USE WHAT YOU HAVE.** If you don't have water, soap, or rubbing alcohol at your disposal, opt for several premoistened towelettes (like baby wipes) if you have them. If you have a cooler handy, rub ice on the affected area.

If you're *really* roughing it, Dr. Helm has a couple of tips for dealing with the rash. "If you are camping out and not much else is available, I would bathe in a pond or stream every 2 to 3 hours and apply a thin mud layer, which will dry up some of the blisters," he says.

■ **WASH EVERYTHING.** These poison plants have a nasty habit of spreading their oil around, so it's not enough to just wash your skin, says Dr. Antaya. "You'll want to wash everything that may have come in contact with it, including your clothes, your pets, everything," he says. "I have patients that have reacquired poison ivy by wearing the same shirt a few days later."

■ **WATCH OUT IN THE WINTER.** Just because the leaves have left the plant doesn't mean it's any less dangerous. The poison still lurks in the roots and stems, waiting to land. "I had a patient who came in absolutely covered with the rash in the middle of winter," says Dr. Antaya. "It turns out he was cutting trees with a chain saw, and oil from the dormant ivy plant splattered on him."

■ **POP A PILL.** It takes a few hours to a few days after exposure to the plants for the rash to develop, along with its maddening itch. Oral antihistamines are high on Robert Rietschel's, M.D., list of poison plant rash remedies. Two popular over-the-counter brands are Chlor-Trimeton, which contains the active ingredient chlorpheniramine maleate, and Benadryl, which contains the active ingredient diphenhydramine hydrochloride. "You

Cures from the Kitchen

If you don't have an Aveeno oatmeal product readily at your disposal, regular oatmeal can work just as well. Make some soupy oatmeal and allow it to cool. Then scoop the mixture into an old sock and strain out the liquid. You can use this sock as a compress to apply to the rash for 10 minutes every 2 hours.

If you don't want to use your good socks, just strain the oatmeal mixture and smear the liquid over your rash five times a day. Do this until the symptoms subside.

even could take your hay fever medicine if it happens to be an antihistamine," he adds.

■ **USE CALAMINE LOTION.** The time-honored mainstay in poison plant treatment is calamine lotion, a popular skin protectant with a cooling, soothing action that distracts your skin from the itching sensation, says Dr. Rietschel.

With poison ivy, poison oak, and poison sumac, the blood vessels develop gaps that leak fluid through the skin, which then cause blistering and oozing, he explains. "When you cool the skin, the vessels constrict and don't leak as much," he says.

Most calamine lotions contain only about 5 percent calamine, which is actually a form of crystallized zinc. As the lotion dries on your skin, it leaves a powdery residue that absorbs the oozing, develops a crust, and keeps your skin from sticking to your clothes, Dr. Rietschel says. He recommends applying calamine lotion three or four times a day. To keep your rash from getting too dry and making the itch even worse, stop using calamine when the oozing stops, he says.

■ **TRY A COOL DRESSING OR COMPRESS.** Another simple way to bring relief is to moisten a sheet or pillowcase, and lay it over the affected area. "This produces a cooling, calming effect," says Dr. Antaya. "I tell my patients to leave it there until it dries."

Dr. Helm recommends adding a bit of tea to your dressing or compress for additional relief. "Any common black tea contains tannins that are very helpful," he says. "Let it cool, dampen a cloth, and apply it for 10 minutes every 3 to 4 hours."

■ **COUNTERATTACK WITH CORTISONE.** Over-the-counter cortisone creams are too weak and "are absolutely worthless in knocking out a significant rash," Dr. Rietschel says. "But they can relieve minimal itching." Start using them about 2 weeks into the rash, when it's healing, scaling, and itching.

■ **TRY AN OATMEAL ONSLAUGHT.** Colloidal oatmeal dries up oozing blisters. "It works great and is very soothing," says Dr. Helm. Aveeno is the most popular commercial oatmeal preparation for skin care and comes with easy-to-follow instructions. Apply it with a cloth to the blisters, or use it in the bath.

■ **FIND RELIEF WITH JEWELS.** The most popular herbal treatment is jewelweed, also known as impatiens or touch-me-not. James Duke, Ph.D., says he uses jewelweed to stop the rash from developing. "I ball up the whole plant and make sort of a washrag out of it to wipe the poison sap off," he says. Jewelweed is fairly easy to find in the wild, if you know what to look for. The succulent plant has orange and yellow flowers, which bloom from June through September in moist, shaded areas. You may have difficulty finding jewelweed in health food stores, but you can order a bottle from several online suppliers. Slather it on your skin to soothe the itching.

■ **TRY SOME OTHER HERBS.** Herbalists recommend washing the infected area with a grindelia tincture to soothe itching. Also, an echinacea wash helps fight inflammation in the blistered, irritated skin. Mix 1 part echinacea tincture with 3 parts water and rinse the infected areas with the mixture several times a day.

■ **GET MUDDY.** Find a bentonite clay "mud pack" at a health food store, and mix it with water until it forms a thick goo. Spread it over the infected skin to dry up blisters and control the itch, then remove it when it starts to flake off or gets itchy.

For more relief, add $\frac{1}{4}$ to $\frac{1}{2}$ teaspoon of powdered Oregon grape root to the clay poultice to fight infection. If the rash feels hot, add a drop of lavender essential oil to produce a cooling effect.

■ **DON'T GET BURNED.** Don't try to rid your yard of urushiol by burning plants—urushiol takes to the air in a fire. You can inhale droplets of the oil and come down with a serious lung infection, fever, and body-wide rash.

PANEL OF ADVISORS

RICHARD ANTAYA, M.D., IS A PROFESSOR OF DERMATOLOGY AND DIRECTOR OF PEDIATRICS DERMATOLOGY AT THE YALE SCHOOL OF MEDICINE IN NEW HAVEN, CONNECTICUT.

JAMES DUKE, PH.D., HELD SEVERAL POSTS IN HIS MORE THAN THREE DECADES WITH THE USDA, INCLUDING CHIEF OF THE MEDICINAL PLANT RESOURCES LABORATORY. HE IS AUTHOR OF *THE GREEN PHARMACY*.

THOMAS N. HELM, M.D., IS A CLINICAL ASSOCIATE PROFESSOR OF DERMATOLOGY AND PATHOLOGY AT THE STATE UNIVERSITY OF NEW YORK AT BUFFALO.

ROBERT RIETSCHEL, M.D., IS A STAFF DERMATOLOGIST WITH THE SOUTHERN ARIZONA VETERANS AFFAIRS HEALTH CARE SYSTEM IN TUCSON.

Premenstrual Syndrome

26 Ways to Treat the Symptoms

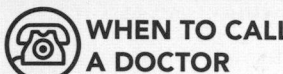

WHEN TO CALL A DOCTOR

The symptoms of premenstrual syndrome rarely call for medical intervention, but drastic circumstances demand drastic measures. If you've tried everything here and nothing seems to help, see your doctor about a prescription medication. In addition, if the symptoms of PMS are seriously affecting your health and other daily activities, see your doctor as soon as possible. You may have premenstrual dysphoric disorder (PMDD), a more serious complication of PMS symptoms.

Think of it as biological warfare, its battles played out on the fields of a woman's body and mind. Once a month, about 2 weeks before she begin to menstruate, the opposing armies—estrogen and progesterone—begin to amass. These female hormones, which regulate the menstrual cycle and affect a woman's central nervous system, normally work in tandem. It's only when one of them tries to outdo the other that trouble looms.

Some women escape the conflict altogether, their hormones striking a peaceful balance before a single sword is drawn. Others are less fortunate. For one woman, estrogen levels may soar, leaving her feeling anxious and irritable. In another, progesterone predominates, dragging her into depression and fatigue.

The battles can rage for days. You may feel bloated and gain weight, or have a headache, backache, acne, allergies, or terrible breast tenderness. You may crave ice cream and potato chips. Your mood may shift without reason, swinging from euphoria to depression. Then, suddenly, the troops clear out and peace of mind returns—just as your period begins.

Though it takes many shapes and sizes, the more than 150 symptoms that can occur during this period are categorized as premenstrual syndrome, or PMS. And though the exact cause is not known, the symptoms are very real and affect most women in one way or another.

"About 85 percent of menstruating women have one or more premenstrual symptoms, but not all of these women have a diagnosis of PMS," says Rallie McAllister, M.D., M.P.H. "When the emotional and physical symptoms interfere with daily life, PMS is typically diagnosed, and PMS affects about 40 percent of American women at some point in their lives. PMS occurs most often in women in their twenties and thirties, but it may occur in teens and older women."

In about 3 to 8 percent of women, the symptoms are so severe that the condition is categorized as PMDD, or premenstrual dysphoric disorder. "It's a severe form of PMS that is characterized by severe mood disturbances, usually irritability but also mood swings, depressed mood, and anxiety that causes functional impairment," says Susan G. Kornstein, M.D.

Regardless of the scope or severity of your PMS symptoms, our experts came up with a number of tips that can help.

■ **EXERCISE.** Many experts agree that exercise may be your best PMS prescription. "Not only does it help reduce the negative effects of any emotional stress, but it also boosts the levels of mood-elevating endorphins, helps regulate fluctuating blood sugar levels, controls appetite, and prevents weight gain," says Dr. McAllister.

The type of exercise you choose really isn't that critical, adds Dr. McAllister. The key is to get yourself moving. "Women should engage in activities that they enjoy," she says. "The main goal is to put your body in motion for at least 30 minutes a day, most days of the week."

■ **RELY ON RELAXATION.** In addition to exercise, Steven Jepson, M.D., says that several other relaxation techniques can help alleviate symptoms as well. "Deep breathing exercises, meditation, and yoga can also help reduce some of the mood symptoms associated with PMS, including mood swings, anxiety, and irritability," he says.

■ **BE PREPARED.** PMS symptoms may not be pleasant, but if you prepare yourself mentally for their arrival every month, you'll have a lot easier time dealing with them, says Dr. Kornstein. "I have found that it helps patients if they are aware of where they are in their menstrual cycle and can anticipate the onset of PMS symptoms, rather than being caught off guard," she says. "Then when the PMS symptoms occur, if they are able to label them as PMS, it may help them not to overreact to situations."

■ **TRACK YOUR SYMPTOMS.** Of course, step one is realizing and accepting the fact that you actually have PMS. And Dr. Kornstein says that the easiest way for a woman to do that is to "chart her symptoms daily over two menstrual cycles to confirm that she has PMS. If she can learn the exact pattern of her particular symptoms, she can try to plan around them."

■ **BE REALISTIC.** Having a positive attitude and getting enough exercise may help, but Dr. McAllister stresses that there's no reason to despair if you still feel bad during this time. "A positive outlook is beneficial to health and healing, but alone, it's rarely a cure," she says. "In many cases, depressed mood and negative emotions are the result of PMS rather than the cause. Fluctuations in serotonin and other mood-elevating neurotransmitters—rather than a bad attitude—are what cause women with PMS to feel down in the dumps or irritable."

■ **AVOID POTENTIAL STRESSORS.** Dr. Kornstein says that one of the easiest things you can do during this time period is also the most practical—simply steer clear of any activities that really stress you out. "Try to avoid stressful events or decisions during the premenstrual time," she says.

■ **DE-STRESS YOUR ENVIRONMENT.** Women with PMS seem to be particularly sensitive to environmental stress, says Susan Lark, M.D. Surrounding yourself with soothing colors and soft music can contribute to greater calm at this and other times of the month.

■ **BREATHE DEEPLY.** Shallow breathing, which many of us do unconsciously, decreases your energy level and leaves you feeling tense, making PMS feel even worse, says Dr. Lark. To ease your discomfort, try practicing inhaling and exhaling slowly and deeply.

■ **SINK INTO A TUB.** Indulge yourself in a mineral bath to relax muscles from head to toe, Dr. Lark suggests. Add 1 cup of sea salt and 1 cup of baking soda to warm bathwater. Soak for 20 minutes.

■ **BE CHASTE.** Consider adding chasteberry to your arsenal of PMS treatments. Most experts recommend it as the top herbal remedy for PMS symptoms. Find it in a tea, tincture, or other preparation at a health food store. Drink a cup of chasteberry tea, or take 5 to 15 drops of tincture, mixed with a few ounces of water, three times a day.

■ **RELY ON ROSEMARY.** According to herbal experts, certain compounds in rosemary may bring hormone levels into balance and reduce symptoms. To make rosemary tea, bring 1 cup of water to a boil and pour it over 1 teaspoon of dried rosemary leaves. Cover and steep for 10 to 15 minutes, then drink warm. During the week you expect your period, drink a cup before lunch and a cup before dinner for 3 days.

■ **TRY SOME OTHER HERBS.** A few other herbal supplements, most notably black cohosh, wild yam, and evening primrose oil, may also be helpful in alleviating the pain, cramping, and mood swings common in PMS, says Dr. McAllister. As with all herbal treatments, you'll want to discuss these options with your doctor before taking them.

■ **GET AN ADVANCE FROM YOUR SLEEP BANK.** If insomnia is part of your PMS, prepare for it by going to bed a few hours earlier for a few days before you expect PMS to set in, says Dr. Lark. It may help alleviate the tiredness and irritability that go hand in hand with insomnia.

Help from the Supplement Aisle

A number of vitamins, minerals, and other supplements may help relieve PMS symptoms, some doctors say. Here's the lowdown on nutritional solutions.

Vitamin B$_6$. Research into vitamin B$_6$ and PMS has shown that increasing your intake of the nutrient can help alleviate symptoms such as mood swings, fluid retention, breast tenderness, bloating, sugar cravings, and fatigue, says Susan Lark, M.D. But, she cautions, don't experiment with the vitamin on your own. B$_6$ is toxic in high doses. Your doctor should supervise any vitamin therapy, including those mentioned below.

Fish oil or flax oil. Inflammation is a major cause of pain and other PMS symptoms, and the omega-3 fatty acids found in fish oil and flax oil are potent anti-inflammatory agents that have been shown in studies to reduce this inflammation, says Rallie McAllister, M.D., M.P.H. Plus, most people just don't get as many of these vital nutrients as they should.

Calcium and vitamin D$_3$. Studies seem to suggest that these two can work in tandem to curb PMS symptoms. "In a 2005 study published in the *Archives of Internal Medicine*, researchers found that women who consumed 1,200 milligrams of calcium and 400 IU of vitamin D had a 40 percent reduction in risk of PMS," says Dr. McAllister. "Vitamin D$_3$ appears to be better absorbed and utilized by the body than Vitamin D$_2$."

Magnesium. Along with calcium comes magnesium, as things just seem to be better when these two minerals are in balance. "When levels of calcium and magnesium are balanced in the body, carbohydrate cravings tend to diminish," says Dr. McAllister. This mineral may also promote restful sleep, reduce muscle cramping, regulate blood sugar levels, and minimize migraines.

The PMS pill. Your best bet for treating PMS with nutritional supplements is to take a balanced supplement every day, says Dr. Lark. Your nearby neighborhood drugstore may even sell products specially formulated for PMS symptoms.

■ **DON'T HIDE THE TRUTH.** Talking about your PMS problems with your spouse, friends, or coworkers does help, says Dr. Lark. You may even find a PMS self-help group where you can share your experiences with others who have PMS. To find one in your area, ask your doctor or call a local women's medical center.

■ **AVOID EMPTY CALORIES.** Many women crave sweets while fighting PMS, but Dr. McAllister says these simple carbohydrates start a vicious cycle. "Sugar cravings lead to eating highly refined carbohydrates, which leads to a rapid spike in your blood glucose level. This leads to overstimulation of the pancreas and a release of insulin, which drives blood sugar levels to below normal, which results in feelings of hunger, fatigue, irritability, and cravings for more sugar.

Ultimately, this ends in weight gain," she says.

■ **FILL UP ON FIBER.** Luckily, there's an easy way to break this cycle, adds Dr. McAllister. Just substitute whole grains and complex carbohydrates with plenty of fiber, found in vegetables, beans, and whole grain bread, in place of nutritionally empty foods. "When women satisfy their carb cravings with complex carbohydrates that are high in fiber, like a bran muffin with a small handful of nuts, they can satisfy their cravings without triggering the destructive cycle."

■ **DECREASE DAIRY.** Dairy has many positive benefits in the American diet—but while you're suffering through PMS, you may want to find those benefits from a different food. "The vast majority of American women have some degree of lactose intolerance, and for these women, eating dairy foods can cause a great deal of bloating and abdominal discomfort," says Dr. McAllister. "In addition, dairy foods may worsen inflammation in the bodies of many women."

■ **RESTRICT SALT.** Dr. McAllister says that salt is another foodstuff you'll want to cut back on. "Salt increases the likelihood of water retention and bloating, and should be eaten in moderation by women with PMS."

■ **GET GOOD PROTEIN AND FATS.** While you're cutting out the dairy and salt, add good proteins and fats, says Dr. McAllister. The essential fatty acids are particularly important, as most women don't get enough, she says. "Good sources of these nutrients include fatty fish such as salmon, tuna, and mackerel, and avocados, nuts, and seeds."

■ **CUT THE CAFFEINE HABIT.** You may want to cut back a bit on the morning coffee while experiencing PMS symptoms, says Dr. McAllister. "Caffeine can stimulate the adrenal glands and trigger production and release of stress hormones, making PMS symptoms worse."

■ **DRINK UP.** While you're cutting out caffeine, you might want to consider replacing it with water and green tea. "Water helps flush toxins from the body and may help control appetite. Drinking sufficient water may actually help reduce bloating," says Dr. McAllister. "Green tea is rich in antioxidants and may help reduce the pain and inflammation associated with PMS."

PANEL OF ADVISORS

STEVEN JEPSON, M.D., IS THE MEDICAL DIRECTOR OF THE UTAH DERMATOLOGIC AND MEDICAL PROCEDURES CLINIC AND AUTHOR OF *7 WAYS TO LOOK YOUNGER WITHOUT UNDERGOING THE KNIFE.*

SUSAN G. KORNSTEIN, M.D., IS A PROFESSOR OF PSYCHIATRY AND OBSTETRICS-GYNECOLOGY AND EXECUTIVE DIRECTOR OF THE INSTITUTE FOR WOMEN'S HEALTH AT VIRGINIA COMMONWEALTH UNIVERSITY IN RICHMOND.

SUSAN LARK, M.D., IS A DISTINGUISHED CLINICIAN, LECTURER, AND WOMEN'S HEALTH EXPERT. SHE MAINTAINS THE WEB SITE WWW.DRLARK.COM AND IS AUTHOR OF SEVERAL BOOKS, INCLUDING *HORMONE REVOLUTION.*

RALLIE MCALLISTER, M.D., M.P.H., IS A BOARD CERTIFIED FAMILY PHYSICIAN IN KINGSPORT, TENNESSEE, AND AUTHOR OF SEVERAL HEALTH-RELATED BOOKS, INCLUDING *HEALTHY LUNCHBOX: THE WORKING MOM'S GUIDE TO KEEPING YOU AND YOUR KIDS TRIM* AND *RIDING FOR LIFE: A HORSEWOMAN'S GUIDE TO LIFETIME HEALTH AND FITNESS.*

Prostate Problems

18 Gland Helpers

Many things start to change as you age, but one of the most frustrating for men is having to get up in the middle of the night to go to the bathroom—and then having to do it all over again a few hours later. It's called frequent nighttime urination, and it's a common complaint among men older than 50. And the usual suspect of this pesky symptom is an enlarged prostate.

Why are so many men plagued by prostate problems? The answer lies in the male anatomy. The prostate—the gland responsible for producing most of the fluids in semen—is situated directly beneath the bladder. Roughly the size of a pea at birth, it begins growing rapidly during puberty, when testosterone levels rise. In adults, it takes on the size and shape of a walnut. When a man hits his mid-forties, his prostate often begins to grow again, probably from changes in hormone levels. The result? A condition called benign prostatic hyperplasia, or BPH, the technical term for enlarged prostate.

About half of men with BPH don't experience any overt symptoms. In others, the prostate presses against the urethra, the tube that passes urine out of the body. This creates a host of urinary difficulties, including frequency, urgency, reduction in flow, difficulty starting urination, discomfort when urinating, and a feeling that the bladder is not completely empty.

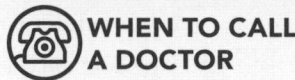 **WHEN TO CALL A DOCTOR**

Two prostate-related problems require immediate treatment: acute prostatitis and urinary retention.

Acute prostatitis occurs when bacteria from the urethra travels to the prostate, creating an infection that must be treated with antibiotics. Unlike other forms of prostatitis, it comes on quickly, producing these severe symptoms:

- Fever, chills, and flulike symptoms
- Pain in the prostate, scrotum, or lower back
- Urinary frequency and blood-tinged urine
- Painful ejaculation

In urinary retention, the prostate enlarges and blocks the flow of urine, potentially damaging the kidneys. If you notice a diminished flow, are unable to completely empty your bladder, or have a continuous urge to urinate but produce only a small trickle of urine, call your doctor immediately.

Time to Test

All men should see their doctors beginning at age 50 for annual exams to screen for prostate cancer risk. The most common screenings used are a blood test to check levels of prostate-specific antigen (PSA) and a digital rectal exam (DRE). Though this test can be slightly uncomfortable, it's a small price to pay for preventing cancer.

BPH isn't the only ailment that strikes the prostate. At one time or another, roughly 50 percent of all men develop prostatitis, a condition in which the prostate gland becomes inflamed. Prostatitis is a term given to three separate conditions. One, acute bacterial prostatitis, is a serious infection. (See "When to Call a Doctor" on page 495.) The second, chronic bacterial prostatitis, is a persistent low-grade infection with intermittent urinary symptoms, similar to those of BPH, along with pain after ejaculation, lower-back pain, and, possibly, semen tinged with blood. Antibiotics are usually needed to treat the infection. The third is a similar condition with identical symptoms, although no bacteria are present. Named chronic nonbacterial prostatitis, it is the most common form, although doctors aren't sure what causes it.

Perhaps the most frightening prospect when it comes to your prostate, though, is prostate cancer, one of the most common cancers among men. Though it affects about one in six men in the United States, the good news is that detection and treatment have improved greatly in recent years. The key is to catch it early, which you can do with the help of your doctor.

The news about your prostate isn't all bad. We'll show you how you can help prevent prostate problems and treat the symptoms if you have them. Follow these tips.

■ **HARVEST THE POWER OF SAW PALMETTO.** One of the most well-known natural remedies for the prostate is saw palmetto, an extract of berries of a tree found in Southeast United States. Though some recent studies, including a 2006 trial in the *New England Journal of Medicine*, have questioned the herb's effectiveness, our experts, including Winston Craig, R.D., Ph.D., Willard Dean, M.D., and Richard C. Sazama, M.D., stand behind saw palmetto as worth trying.

Why does it work? "It's not known yet," says Dr. Craig. Saw palmetto contains phytosterols—compounds similar to cholesterol, found in plants and thought to have health benefits, including aiding urinary difficulties. What's more, it appears to affect dihydrotestosterone, or DHT, found in testosterone. "High levels of DHT are associated with an enlarged prostate," explains Dr. Craig. Compounds in saw palmetto inhibit the production of DHT, and reducing DHT's growth-promoting effects eases urinary symptoms and increases urine flow, he says.

Because saw palmetto is so effective for treating this condition, you should consult your doctor for a proper diagnosis and to establish monitoring before using it. Two or three 500-milligram capsules per day of saw palmetto extract is enough for you to see improvement in 1 to 3 months.

■ **TRY AFRICAN PYGEUM.** Used extensively in Europe for the treatment of BPH, this fruit of an African evergreen tree is effective, possibly because it diminishes inflammation. "The active extract seems to reduce symptoms of frequent nighttime urination and difficulty urinating," says Dr. Craig. African pygeum appears to be a safe herb, but talk to your doctor for proper diagnosis and monitoring before using it to treat enlarged prostate. The standard dosage is usually 100 to 200 milligrams per day in capsule form.

■ **RX WITH NETTLE ROOT.** Nettle root extract has steroidal and anti-inflammatory properties that benefit men with BPH, says Dr. Craig. Take up to six 300-milligram capsules per day, or take it in a combination supplement with saw palmetto.

■ **THINK ABOUT ZINC.** "Zinc is a high priority for natural therapy of the prostate gland," says Dr. Dean. Because zinc is essential to the production of semen, a deficiency can lead to prostate problems. Take 30 milligrams per day. But beware—zinc and copper are linked in the body, so taking zinc for prolonged periods can throw off their balance. To avoid a potential imbalance, take a 2-milligram capsule or tablet of copper as well.

■ **BREAK OPEN THE GREAT PUMPKIN.** Pumpkin seeds contain high levels of phytosterols and zinc—both critical for the prostate's well-being. Dr. Craig recommends taking 1 to 2 teaspoons of ground pumpkin seeds mixed with liquid twice a day. If you'd rather take a combination supplement with saw palmetto and African pygeum, follow the label recommendations for dosage amounts.

■ **LOAD UP ON LYCOPENE.** An overwhelming amount of evidence in recent years has indicated that lycopene, the compound that tints tomatoes red, may reduce your risk of prostate cancer. The evidence is so strong, in fact, that virtually all the experts we spoke with recommended getting more tomato products in your diet. Lycopene is present in much higher concentrations in cooked tomato products than in raw tomatoes, so you'll want to load up on tomato soup, tomato juice, and tomato sauce. "One tomato contains about 3 milligrams of lycopene, but 1 cup of tomato soup contains 24 milligrams!" says William Dunn, M.D.

Though lycopene is usually thought of as a preventer of prostate cancer, Dr. Dunn reports that a recent study showed that lycopene may prevent prostate enlargement as well. Yet another reason to stock up on tomatoes. "Lycopene is also in watermelon, papaya, guava, and red grapefruit," says Dr. Craig.

■ **WATCH WHAT YOU EAT.** When it comes to your diet, the food you eat seems to play a big role in the prevention of everything from an enlarged prostate to prostate cancer. Here, the advice really isn't too much different than what you've been hearing for keeping your heart healthy. "Men approaching middle age should start a diet higher in fruits and vegetables containing vitamin C, lutein, and beta-carotene," says Dr. Dunn. "A study in the *Journal of Clinical Nutrition* supported the finding that BPH could be avoided with this approach."

Another strategy that seems to play a role in prostate cancer prevention is avoiding the saturated fats found in red meat, dairy products, and fried foods.

■ **KEEP ON YOUR TOES.** Men with jobs that require long hours of sitting, especially occupations that constantly put pressure on the prostate area, such as truck driving, are more prone to both prostatitis and BPH. "Periodically throughout the day, take breaks from sitting," recommends Dr. Dean. Getting out of your seat helps prevent circulation from being diminished in that region of the body and helps relieve symptoms.

■ **GET SOME EXERCISE.** Myriad studies point to the fact that increased physical activity

reduces your risk of prostate problems. "A trial at UCLA reported that a high-fiber, low-fat diet coupled with exercise reduced the growth of prostate cells in culture," says Dr. Dunn. "And another recent study showed an association between running and BPH. The greater the distance ran per week correlated with a reduction in BPH risk, regardless of one's weight. Finally, a study from the University of Athens reported that those with more occupational physical activity had less BPH and a trend for less prostate cancer, especially in men over 65," he says.

■ **CYCLE ON A SPLIT SEAT.** If cycling is your preferred form of exercise, beware—it puts pressure on the prostate. This can lead to prostatitis or exacerbate an existing condition, says Martin K. Gelbard, M.D. "Get a split bicycle seat," he recommends. A split seat is cushioned on each side, so your weight rests on the bones of your pelvis, keeping the tension off the prostate.

■ **SOME INTERESTING EFFECTS OF ALCOHOL.** Alcohol provides an interesting conundrum when it comes to prostate health. Studies have shown pretty clearly that moderate consumption seems to help reduce the risk of BPH. "At the same time, I have a hard time advocating alcohol consumption," says Dr. Dean. "The risks of alcoholism are too great, plus it wreaks havoc with your blood sugar, diabetes risk, and obesity, as well as other problems."

The best advice, as with many things, is moderation, advises Dr. Dean. "One or two drinks a night is probably okay," he says. "But any more than that becomes problematic."

■ **SOOTHE IT WITH A SITZ.** A sitz bath, in which the lower half of your body rests in warm water, brings heat to the prostate gland and relaxes lower abdominal muscles. "It reduces inflammation and cuts down on pain and urgency," says Dr. Gelbard. Fill a tub with about a foot of warm water and soak for 15 minutes once a day.

■ **BUY LOOSE COTTON BRIEFS.** Tight, restrictive underclothing also restricts bloodflow to the area surrounding the prostate. "Good bloodflow brings nutrients to the gland and carries out waste products," explains Dr. Dean. And make it cotton. Synthetic undergarments trap sweat, but cotton wicks away moisture, allowing the skin to breathe. This means less accumulation of toxins in the skin directly over the prostate, which affects the underlying organs, he says.

■ **MAKE LOVE MORE.** "Since the prostate is vitally involved in the production of semen, ejaculation can be therapeutic," says Dr. Dean. During ejaculation, muscles surrounding the prostate contract. "Think of it as exercise or gymnastics for the prostate," he says. "It's very good for bloodflow." Most likely to benefit are men who don't have regular sexual relations. Don't worry about passing the bacteria that caused the prostatitis on to your partner—the infection is not transmitted through sexual contact.

■ **RUB IT OUT.** Reflexology is a natural healing therapy that can be effective in promoting health in certain disorders, including prostate ailments, says Dr. Dean. The principle behind reflexology is that the hands and feet contain sensors that connect to all other parts of the body. By massaging the reflex points related to the prostate, you send a signal to the gland that stimulates healing. The point for the prostate is located at the base of the heel on either side. (Charts showing actual points are available at most health food stores.)

Once you find the point, rub it with your thumb, a marble, or a pencil eraser. "Rub for 20 to 30 seconds a couple of times a day," says Dr. Dean. The spot may become sore at first, indicating the gland is, afterall, in need of balance, he explains. With continued rubbing, it becomes less sensitive.

■ **KEEP AWAY FROM COLD MEDICINES.** Decongestants and antihistamines can cause the muscles that control urine flow to contract, making urination more difficult. In some cases, this can completely restrict the flow of urine, leading to a potentially life-threatening condition. If you have allergies, be sure to ask your doctor to prescribe cold and allergy medications that don't contain antihistamines.

■ **DRINK UP.** If you're tempted to drink less because you're tired of so many trips to the bathroom, don't give in to the temptation, warns Dr. Gelbard. "Dehydration creates added stress," he explains. Drinking enough water every day is important for the kidneys to function properly and can prevent urinary infections. You'll want to aim for six 8-ounce glasses a day.

■ **BUT NOT BEFORE BED.** Want to cut back on nightly bathroom visits? Don't drink any liquids after 6:00 p.m., advises Dr. Gelbard. Also be sure to empty your bladder completely before hitting the sack.

PANEL OF ADVISORS

WINSTON CRAIG, R.D., PH.D., IS A PROFESSOR OF NUTRITION AT ANDREWS UNIVERSITY IN BERRIEN SPRINGS, MICHIGAN.

WILLARD DEAN, M.D., IS A HOLISTIC PHYSICIAN IN GLORIETA, NEW MEXICO.

WILLIAM DUNN, M.D., IS A PHYSICIAN IN CANCER CARE AND RADIATION ONCOLOGY AT THE MEDICAL UNIVERSITY OF SOUTH CAROLINA IN CHARLESTON.

MARTIN K. GELBARD, M.D., IS A UROLOGIST IN PRIVATE PRACTICE IN BURBANK, CALIFORNIA, AND THE AUTHOR OF *SOLVING PROSTATE PROBLEMS*.

RICHARD C. SAZAMA, M.D., IS A UROLOGIST AT SACRED HEART HOSPITAL IN EAU CLAIRE, WISCONSIN.

Psoriasis

21 Skin-Soothing Remedies

Our skin is an amazing organ. In addition to being the body's largest, it's constantly renewing itself by replacing the dead skin cells on the top layer (the epidermis) with new cells from below. Though you can't see it, this is happening at the rate of 30,000 to 40,000 cells a minute, or about 9 pounds of dead skin cells a year.

If you have psoriasis, though, it's like someone hit the fast-forward button on your skin. Normally, skin renews itself in about 30 days, but with psoriasis, that process occurs in just 3 days, as if the body has lost its brakes. The result is raised areas of skin called plaques, which are red and often itchy. After the cells reach the surface, they die like normal cells, but there are so many of them that the raised patches turn white with dead cells flaking off.

Psoriasis usually goes through cycles of flare-ups and remission, with flare-ups most often occurring in winter. Sometimes it disappears for months or years. The condition can improve or worsen with age.

Doctors are beginning to understand psoriasis a little better than in years past. Dermatologist D'Anne Kleinsmith, M.D., says that there seems to be a genetic component to the disease. "In one-third of cases, there is a family history of the condition," she says. Other research indicates that it, like diabetes, may be an auto-immune disease.

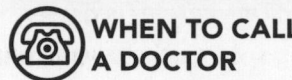

WHEN TO CALL A DOCTOR

The impact of psoriasis on people's lives can range from mildly annoying to completely debilitating. If your condition causes you discomfort and pain, if performing routine tasks has become difficult, or if the appearance of your skin concerns you, go to see your doctor.

While there is no known cure for psoriasis, there are a lot of tips that can help soothe the itching. Here's what can help.

■ **GET SOME SUN.** With regular doses of intense sun, 95 percent of people with psoriasis do improve.

"Dermatologists hate to recommend getting sunlight in most cases, but in the case of psoriasis, this really brings relief," says Richard Antaya, M.D. Ultraviolet waves seem to fight psoriasis, and the UVB rays work the fastest. But a catch-22 does exist. UVB's are also the rays that give you a sunburn and run up the risks of skin cancer. They can also cause people with psoriasis to have a flare-up in previously unaffected areas.

Sunscreen is your weapon of choice for blocking the sun's deadly rays. "The benefits of sunbathing can outweigh the risks of skin cancer and spreading psoriasis if you use sunscreens on the places where you don't have psoriasis and only expose the affected areas to the full force of the sun," says Laurence Miller, M.D. Be sure to talk to your doctor about the amount of sun exposure that's appropriate for you.

■ **TURN ON THE LAMP.** A safer alternative to sun exposure is phototherapy. During this process you expose the skin to ultraviolet rays with the help of a machine. These sessions can take place at a doctor's office, or you can buy a home unit, but talk to your doctor about a proper regimen before using the machine on your own. "People on phototherapy usually start with two or three sessions a week, and then gradually taper down," says Dr. Antaya. "It's not as strong as sunlight, so it helps minimize your risk of skin cancer."

■ **AVOID INFECTIONS AND INJURIES.** When your immune system is compromised, you stand a much greater chance of a psoriasis outbreak, says dermatologist Oanh Lauring, M.D. You often see psoriasis accompany strep throat, cold, flu, and gastrointestinal infections. This means people with psoriasis should be on their guard for preventing illness, particularly in the winter. A flu shot is usually a good precautionary measure.

The other scenario that's likely to bring about psoriasis is trauma, whether it's from surgery or an injury. Just as with avoiding infections, extra vigilance is needed here for those with psoriasis.

■ **DEFEAT DRYNESS.** Speaking of the winter, those cold, dry months are some of the worst for psoriasis. Dr. Lauring says this is when you'll really want to step up your regimen of washing correctly, moisturizing, and using phototherapy.

■ **DE-STRESS YOURSELF.** Stress is another psoriasis trigger, so try to avoid stressful situations, and look into any available relaxation techniques that feel can help you. "Don't minimize the emotions or the level of stress you are under with this diagnosis," says dermatologist Jason R. Lupton, M.D.

■ **USE THE RIGHT SOAP.** Many soaps can be drying, so you'll want to choose a soap with this in mind, says Dr. Lauring. She recommends Dove body wash or Cetaphil.

■ **FEED YOUR SKIN.** Emollients top every dermatologist's list of over-the-counter treatments. Psoriatic skin is dry, and that can mean a worsening of the psoriasis and increased flaking and itching. Emollients help your skin retain water. "Generally, the really thick, greasy emollients work the best because they can actually reduce the appearance of the thick scales," says Dr. Antaya. "Vaseline is a good one to use."

For a natural alternative, you may want to try a soothing herbal cream with calendula and beeswax to seal in moisture. An aloe vera–based cream may also be helpful.

■ **USE TAR.** Over-the-counter coal tar preparations are weaker than the prescription versions but can be effective in treating mild psoriasis, says Dr. Miller. You can apply the tar directly to the plaques or immerse yourself in tar bath oil and treat your scalp with tar shampoo. Because all tars can stain and smell,

Cures from the Kitchen

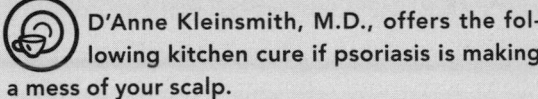

D'Anne Kleinsmith, M.D., offers the following kitchen cure if psoriasis is making a mess of your scalp.

First, heat olive oil until it is warm, but not hot. Massage the oil into your scalp. Leave the oil on for 20 to 30 minutes minimum or overnight, while wearing a shower cap. Wash out the oil with a dandruff shampoo. Do this nightly until your skin clears up, and then continue the treatment once or twice a week as needed.

they're usually washed off after a certain amount of time, but some kinds can be left on the skin to enhance the effect of sunlight or UVB treatments. "Tar makes you more sensitive to the sun, so be careful," he warns.

Dr. Miller says that some new tar products come in gel form. They don't smell like tar pits, and they can be used daily and they wash off easily. "If any tar product causes burning or irritation, stop using it. Never use tar on raw, open skin," he says.

■ **GET WET AND WARM.** If you want to bring relief to psoriasis, few things are easier and more relaxing than a bath. "You want to add Epsom salts to tepid water, and then soak in it for 18 to 20 minutes," says Dr. Antaya. "This will help dissolve some of the scales and exfoliate the skin." Dr. Antaya advises a warm bath, not hot, which increases itchiness. And don't rub the skin—it can make things worse.

Dermatologist Thomas N. Helm, M.D., adds that oatmeal baths may relieve the itchiness of psoriasis.

■ **OR GET WET AND COLD.** A cold-water bath, maybe with a cup or so of apple cider vinegar added, is great for itching. "Another thing that really works is ice," Dr. Miller says. "Just dump some ice cubes into a small plastic bag and hold it against the afflicted skin."

■ **TRY HYDROCORTISONE FOR SMALL AREAS.** "Over-the-counter topical hydrocortisone creams are weaker than their prescription cousins, but they're worth trying, and they're

The Great Cover-Up

Hollywood to the rescue. Cosmetologist and Hollywood makeup artist Maurice Stein helps out clients referred to him by medical doctors across the country, as well as the standard must-be-perfect stars. Here are some of his recommendations.

■ First of all, never try to cover up any open lesion, Stein says, echoing medical advice.

■ "There's a very good over-the-counter cream, applied with a makeup sponge, that can be applied to the scalp to cover up the flaking," Stein says. "Get your doctor's approval first. It's called Couvré, and it comes in black; dark, medium, and light brown; auburn, blond, white, and gray. It works by darkening the scalp to match the color of the hair."

■ For elbows and knees, Stein recommends Indian earth mixed with your favorite emollient and spread over the plaques with a makeup sponge. A rock, ground to face powder consistency, Indian earth can be bought in salons, department stores, health food stores, or online. "A dime-size portion is enough to do your whole body," he says. The emollient will keep the plaques moist, and the Indian earth will disguise their appearance. "If you have to wear clothes over it, pat it dry to remove the excess," Stein advises.

■ If you can't find Indian earth, look for a cosmetic base with a lot of pigment, he says. "The best place to find and test them is at a local cosmetologist's salon."

---

safer on the face and genital areas," Dr. Miller says. "But if you use it all the time in these areas, it will become less effective, and when you give up on it, the psoriasis can rebound. Just use it until you show some improvement, and then gradually wean yourself off."

■ **WRAP IT UP.** Prescription topical steroids is the primary treatment used by many with psoriasis, but there is something you can do at home to increase their effectiveness. "I have patients wrap their feet with plastic wrap after applying the steroids to increase penetration," says Dr. Lauring. "Wearing plastic gloves on the hands has the same effect."

■ **GET A NEW ATTITUDE.** The fact that there's no cure makes psoriasis a particularly frustrating condition for many people. But Dr. Antaya says there are many resources at your disposal. "The National Psoriasis Foundation has a great Web site where you can connect with other people with psoriasis through chat rooms and message boards," he says. "For some people, it just helps them to know they're not the only ones. Others need additional help, such as a psychologist." You can access the National Psoriasis Foundation's Web site at www.psoriasis.org.

Another important point is to realize that

you might not be able to rid yourself of every scale—and that's okay. "I see some of my psoriasis patients maybe twice a year," he says. "There is no law that says every person with psoriasis has to get rid of every flake on the body. I put my hands about a foot apart and say, 'It takes this much effort to get you 80 percent clear.' Then I stretch my arms out as far as I can and say, 'For the final 20 percent, this is what you have to do.' I never say, 'Learn to live with it.' When you think you've run out of treatments, you've gone from A to Z, you start over again at A. Mild psoriasis can be controlled totally by following some of these remedies."

■ **MOVE MORE, DRINK LESS.** "Both alcohol and overweight seem to be associated with psoriasis, but whether the relationship is cause or effect is not entirely clear," says Dr. Helm. "Still, staying fit and active and avoiding excessive alcohol intake is a prudent step toward staying healthy."

■ **GIVE YOURSELF A NUTRITION BOOST.** No specific food seems to be particularly helpful for psoriasis, but decreased immunity seems to increase your chance of an outbreak, so nutrition can still play a vital role, says Dr. Lupton. "Eating a healthy, balanced diet aids in the overall performance of the immune system," he says.

■ **TRY FISH OIL.** Some studies show fish oil may help in treating psoriasis, though results are mixed. Still, the supplement seems to have such positive benefits on other parts of the body that taking fish oil certainly couldn't hurt, says Dr. Lauring.

PANEL OF ADVISORS

RICHARD ANTAYA, M.D., IS A PROFESSOR OF DERMATOLOGY AND DIRECTOR OF PEDIATRICS DERMATOLOGY AT YALE SCHOOL OF MEDICINE IN NEW HAVEN, CONNECTICUT.

THOMAS N. HELM, M.D., IS A CLINICAL ASSOCIATE PROFESSOR OF DERMATOLOGY AND PATHOLOGY AT THE STATE UNIVERSITY OF NEW YORK AT BUFFALO.

D'ANNE KLEINSMITH, M.D., IS A COSMETIC DERMATOLOGIST AT WILLIAM BEAUMONT HOSPITAL IN ROYAL OAK, MICHIGAN.

OANH LAURING, M.D., IS CHIEF OF DERMATOLOGY AT MERCY HOSPITAL IN BALTIMORE, MARYLAND.

JASON R. LUPTON, M.D., IS A BOARD-CERTIFIED DERMATOLOGIST IN PRIVATE PRACTICE IN DEL MAR, CALIFORNIA.

LAURENCE MILLER, M.D., IS A DERMATOLOGIST IN CHEVY CHASE, MARYLAND, A MEMBER OF THE MEDICAL ADVISORY BOARD OF THE NATIONAL PSORIASIS FOUNDATION, AND A SPECIAL ADVISOR TO THE DIRECTOR OF THE NATIONAL INSTITUTE OF ARTHRITIS AND MUSCULOSKELETAL AND SKIN DISEASES OF THE NATIONAL INSTITUTES OF HEALTH.

MAURICE STEIN IS A COSMETOLOGIST AND HOLLYWOOD MAKEUP ARTIST. HE IS THE OWNER OF CINEMA SECRETS, A FULL-SERVICE BEAUTY SUPPLIER FOR THE PUBLIC AND A THEATRICAL BEAUTY SUPPLIER FOR THE ENTERTAINMENT INDUSTRY IN BURBANK, CALIFORNIA.

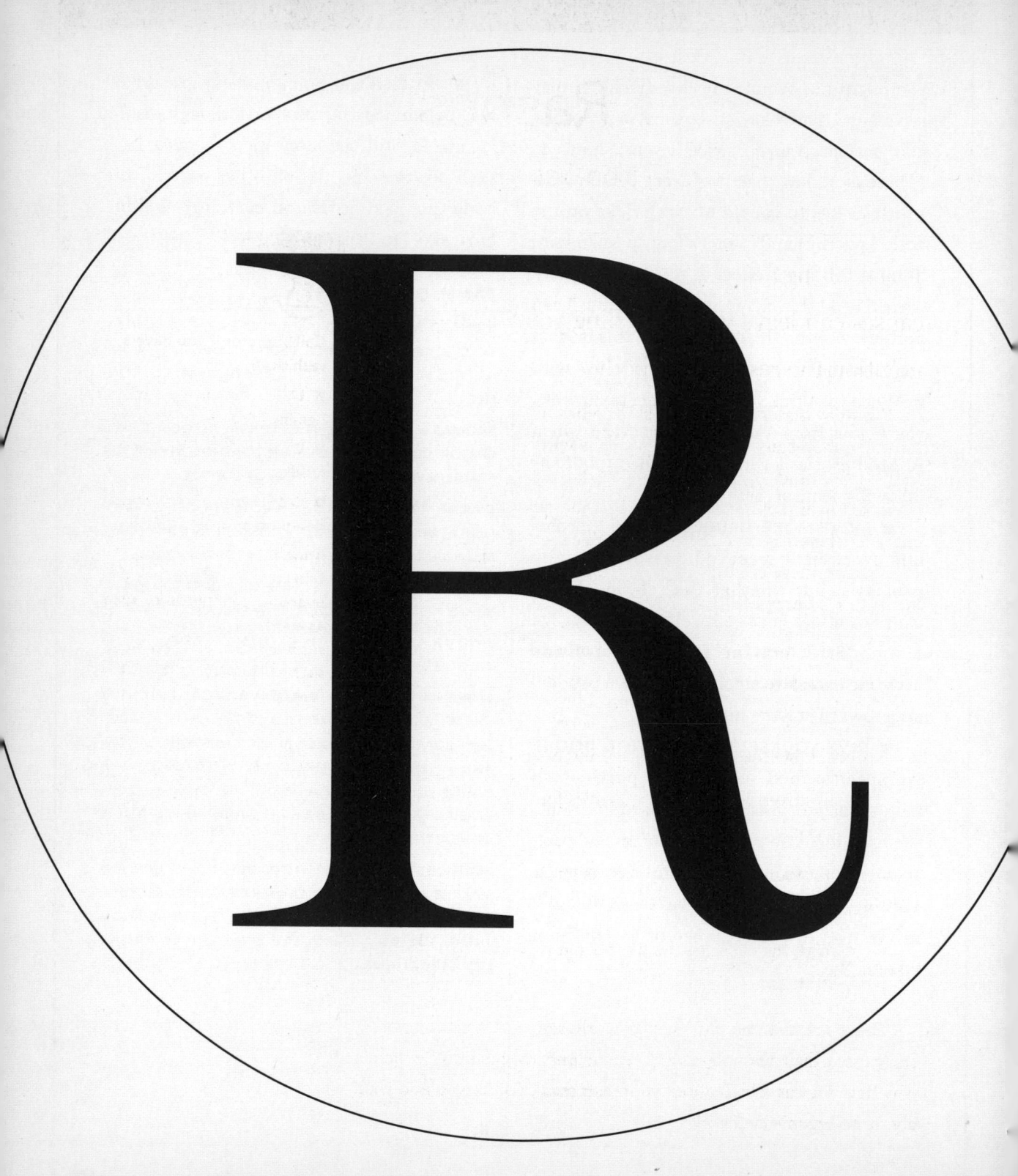

Rashes

15 Skin-Salving Solutions

Rashes sting and burn and come and go. And their causes can leave you scratching your head—not to mention the rest of your body.

Everyday materials that our skin comes in contact with are the most common cause of rashes—which is why dermatologists refer to the appearance of rashes as contact dermatitis. But if your rash is caused by a particular substance, then the phrase is "allergic contact dermatitis" and the triggers are called "allergens."

The five most common rash-producing allergens are the following, says Larry Millikan, M.D.

- Nickel, a metal often mixed with other metals to make costume jewelry

- Chromates, a chemical found in everyday home-improvement products such as cement, paints, and antirust products

- Preservatives or fragrance additives found in hand creams and lotions

- Rubber, found in products such as latex gloves, elastic waistbands, and shoes

- Urushiol, the oil in plants like poison ivy, poison oak, and poison sumac

These are just the most common allergens. Almost anything can cause a rash, though, including food and medications, which is why figuring out what caused your rash may require you and your doctor to become detectives.

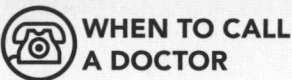 **WHEN TO CALL A DOCTOR**

Call a doctor if you have a rash that:

- Doesn't show signs of healing after 5 to 6 days

- Develops after you take a medication

- Is present on more than one person in a household

Bring all of your medications to the office, even over-the-counter items such as eyedrops, vitamins, supplements, and products such as ibuprofen, says Dee Anna Glaser, M.D.

"The rash is sending a message that your body is not happy about something," says Dee Anna Glaser, M.D. The key is to go to your dermatologist appointment armed with a complete list of substances you've come in contact with that could have caused the rash. Once the doctor determines the cause, he can help you get rid of the rash.

In the meantime, here are some common causes and cures for what itches you.

NICKEL RASH

Nickel is a metal that is often mixed with other metals to make rings, necklaces, and bracelets. Costume jewelry is by far the most common cause of nickel reactions. The good news is that the nickel allergy is easy to diagnose because the rash springs up wherever nickel touches your skin. For example, you may get a rash on your ears if you wear earrings with nickel in them. However, because so many everyday things contain nickel—such as coins, kitchen utensils, paper clips, pens, and keys—you can be exposed to nickel dozens of times a day. Here's what to do.

■ **GO FOR THE GOLD.** Before the next gift-giving event, drop hints to your loved one to spring for a pure gold necklace or bracelet
to replace the costume jewelry that's giving you problems. "I've never heard of anyone who's allergic to pure gold, that's for sure," says Dr. Millikan.

Also, trade in nickel-containing jewelry for pieces made from nickel-free stainless steel, titanium, or surgical-grade stainless steel. If you suspect your watchband is giving you problems, replace it with one made of leather, cloth, or plastic.

■ **CREAM IT.** Try applying an over-the-counter 1 percent hydrocortisone cream, says Jerome Z. Litt, M.D. Prescription brands, such as Cortaid, and generic brands should be identical, according to the FDA.

But be sure that you know what is causing your rash before using hydrocortisone cream on it, Dr. Litt cautions. If the rash is fungal, such as athlete's foot or ringworm, or a yeast infection, then hydrocortisone cream will make the rash much worse.

■ **SOOTHE YOUR SKIN.** A nickel rash can itch like crazy. You might find that a lotion such as calamine can alleviate it. Or mix up a solution of 1 part white vinegar to 16 parts water. Soak a clean soft cloth in the mixture and apply the compress to your rash.

CHROMATE RASH

This is the most common cause of contact dermatitis in the workplace, says Dr. Millikan. This chemical is found in cement, paints, and antirust products. "People with certain blue-collar jobs are exposed to chromate all the time, as are people doing certain home-repair jobs on the weekends," he says.

■ **WEAR GLOVES.** If you can't avoid the chemical, at least avoid getting it on your hands. Wear a sturdy pair of waterproof work gloves to keep the chromate off your skin.

■ **WASH UP.** Make sure to wash your hands often so that any chromate that gets on your skin is not there very long. Because this much washing may dry out your skin, follow with a moisturizing cream or lotion.

■ **USE LIGHTERS.** Some matches contain chromates, so touching unlit matches can contaminate your fingers. Even placing a book of matches in your pants pocket will contaminate it. When you stick your hands in your pockets, bingo! A rash. Rely on a lighter instead.

ADDITIVE RASH

Exposure to preservative and fragrance ingredients used in hand creams, lotions, and other skin-care products causes rashes in many people, says Dr. Millikan.

Common culprits include:

■ Neomycin, an ingredient found in many over-the-counter and prescription antibiotic creams, ointments, lotions, eardrops, and eyedrops

Cures from the Kitchen

To soothe a burning, itching rash, mix together equal parts honey, olive oil, and beeswax. Several studies found this combo heals rashes more quickly than cortisone alone.

You can also speed healing from the inside out by eating more omega-3 fatty acid–rich fish, walnuts, and flaxseed.

■ Preservatives, such as ethylenediamine, which is added to creams to keep them from turning rancid

■ Chemicals that are found in certain laundry detergents and fabric softeners, such as sodium silicate, sodium phosphate, and sodium carbonate

Here's what to do:

■ **PAY ATTENTION.** "Make mental notes of products you were using at the time that the rashes started and report them to your dermatologist," says Dr. Millikan. "That will help your doctor get to the bottom of what's causing them more quickly."

■ **READ LABELS.** Once you realize that an additive causes you problems, scrutinize labels of other products and avoid that additive.

RUBBER RASH

Chemical additives in rubber products, especially latex gloves, can often cause allergic reactions and rashes, including itching, burning, and even welts. They're common among people who wear tightly fitting rubber gloves, such as medical workers. Here are some approaches to try.

■ **TRY A DIFFERENT GLOVE.** Sometimes powder-free rubber gloves may possibly be less allergenic; vinyl (or other synthetic) gloves can be used as a substitute.

■ **HEAD TO VICTORIA'S SECRET.** Undergarments with rubber stretch waistbands are common triggers of rubber rashes. Try lingerie

Rash Relief

Although millions of things can cause rashes, the treatments are pretty much the same. Here's what our experts suggest.

Consider antihistamines. They aren't just for hay fever anymore. Antihistamines will relieve some of your skin irritation, and if you take one of the older forms, it may even help you sleep.

Soothe your skin. Try a cloth compress soaked in water or Domeboro powder, an over-the-counter astringent that you mix with water, to relieve the itch and inflammation. You can also soak in a bath with a special oatmeal bathing product designed to soothe inflamed skin.

Just avoid it. The best thing you can do is to minimize contact with—or better yet, avoid—the allergens and irritants that will trigger an outbreak. If you do get an irritant on you or your clothing, wash it off as soon as possible with soap and warm water.

---

made with spandex instead, and look for items without rubber-backed fasteners or edges.

■ **CHECK YOUR SHOES.** Many cases of allergic contact dermatitis are caused by ingredients used to make shoes, such as leather, certain dyes, adhesives, and, of course, rubber. But because so many parts of your shoe could be causing that foot rash, see your dermatologist for a patch test to determine what exactly you are allergic to before you purchase new shoes. And because hypoallergenic shoes are hard to find and tend to be rather costly, ask your dermatologist for a list of stores or Web sites that sell these shoes so that you can shop around easily.

POISON PLANT RASHES

"If you have a rash that's a perfectly straight line, it's an outside job," says Jacob Teitelbaum, M.D. "The body doesn't work in straight lines. You came into contact with a toxin, such as poison ivy." See Poison Plant Rashes on page 486.

PANEL OF ADVISORS

DEE ANNA GLASER, M.D., IS A PROFESSOR IN THE DEPARTMENT OF DERMATOLOGY AT ST. LOUIS UNIVERSITY SCHOOL OF MEDICINE.

JEROME Z. LITT, M.D., IS A DERMATOLOGIST AND ASSISTANT CLINICAL PROFESSOR OF DERMATOLOGY AT CASE WESTERN RESERVE UNIVERSITY SCHOOL OF MEDICINE IN CLEVELAND AND AUTHOR OF *YOUR SKIN: FROM ACNE TO ZITS* AND *CURIOUS, ODD, RARE AND ABNORMAL REACTIONS TO MEDICATIONS.*

LARRY MILLIKAN, M.D., IS A PROFESSOR EMERITUS IN THE DEPARTMENT OF DERMATOLOGY AT TULANE UNIVERSITY SCHOOL OF MEDICINE IN NEW ORLEANS.

JACOB TEITELBAUM, M.D., IS A BOARD-CERTIFIED INTERNIST AND MEDICAL DIRECTOR OF THE FIBROMYALGIA AND FATIGUE CENTERS, WITH LOCATIONS THROUGHOUT THE COUNTRY.

Raynaud's Phenomenon

26 Toasty Tips

If you have Raynaud's phenomenon, gloves and mittens are just never enough. Your fingers (and sometimes toes) are often so cold, and the reaction to sudden cold as your blood vessels constrict and bloodflow slows can be absolutley excruciatingly painful.

That's because when blood vessels to your extremities constrict, a spasm occurs. Beyond the pain are the color changes. As blood-flow slows to the affected area, the lack of oxygenated blood causes fingers and toes to pale, maybe even take on a bluish tinge.

Yet not everyone experiences Raynaud's in the same way. Some feel numbness from the lack of blood, then their fingers turn red again when the blood returns. In advanced stages of Raynaud's, poor blood supply can weaken the fingers and damage the sense of touch.

Raynaud's is a medical mystery; no one is sure what causes it. Some speculate it has a hormonal connection because women are nine times more likely to have it than men, and 20 percent of all women of childbearing age experience it. Alarmingly, only one in five people with Raynaud's knows it and seeks medical treatment. Because Raynaud's is a conditioned response by the body, it slowly worsens if not properly handled and treated.

Our experts provide some protective suggestions.

■ **TWIRL YOUR ARMS TO GENERATE HEAT.** Force your hands to warm up through a simple exercise devised by Donald McIntyre,

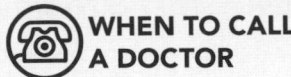

WHEN TO CALL A DOCTOR

Call a doctor if in addition to cold hands and feet:

■ You experience hair or memory loss, which may signal hypothyroidism.

■ You also have numbness and tingling, which could signal a vitamin B_{12} deficiency.

■ Frostiness is paired with pain, burning, or drastic whitening of your fingers or toes, which could indicate peripheral vascular disease.

■ You develop brownish-red ulcers on your hands and feet, which at the extreme can signal permanent damage to your blood vessels.

Although 90 percent of people with Raynaud's have primary Raynaud's, 10 percent have it in tandem with another more serious medical condition or disease, such as sclero-derma, lupus, or rheuma-toid arthritis. Raynaud's might be the first sign, and it could be a decade before the other condition sur-faces.

M.D. Pretend you're a softball pitcher. Swing your arm downward behind your body and then upward in front of you at about 80 twirls per minute. (This isn't as fast as it sounds; give it a try.)

The windmill effect, which Dr. McIntyre modeled after a skier's warmup exercise, forces blood to the fingers through both gravitational and centrifugal force. This warmup works well for chilled hands no matter what the cause.

■ **EAT A HOT, HEARTY MEAL.** The very act of eating causes a rise in core body temperature. This is called thermogenesis. So eat something to stoke your body's furnace before you head outside. And eat something hot to give the stoking a boost. A bowl of hot oatmeal before your morning walk, a soup break, or a hot lunch helps keep your hands and feet toasty even in inclement weather.

■ **DRINK UP.** Dehydration can aggravate chills and frostbite by reducing your blood volume. Ward off a big chill by drinking plenty of warm fluids such as mulled cider, herbal teas, or broth. Plus, drink at least eight glasses of water a day to increase circulation and warmth.

■ **PASS ON THE COFFEE.** Coffee and other caffeinated products constrict blood vessels. The last thing you want when you have Raynaud's phenomenon is to interfere with your circulation.

■ **AVOID ALCOHOL.** Alcohol increases bloodflow to the skin, giving you the immediate perception of warmth. But that heat is soon lost to the air, reducing your core body temperature. In other words, alcohol actually makes you colder. The danger comes from drinking too much and then being subjected to unexpected cold for an extended period, which can lead to severe problems such as frostbite or hypothermia.

■ **DRESS SMART.** To keep warm, you have to dress warmly, says John L. Abruzzo, M.D. Common sense, yes, but many people will slap on gloves and footwear without taking equal precautions to maintain their core temperatures, which is really more important.

■ **CHOOSE FABRICS THAT WICK AWAY PERSPIRATION.** Perspiration is an even bigger cause of cold hands and feet than temperature. Sweat is the body's air conditioner, and your body's air conditioner can operate in cold weather if you're not careful. Your hands and feet are especially susceptible because the palms and heels (along with the armpits) have the largest number of sweat glands in the body. That's why the heavy woolen socks and fleece-lined boots you bought to keep your feet warm may instead make them sweaty and chilly. Try a pair of polypropylene (a synthetic fabric) socks underneath your wool ones.

■ **MAKE SURE GARMENTS ARE LOOSE.** None of your clothing should pinch. Tightly fitting clothes can cut off circulation and eliminate insulating air pockets.

■ **DRESS IN LAYERS.** If you're stepping out into the cold, the best warming measure you can take is to dress in layers. This helps trap

Toasty Tips

The following Raynaud's survival tricks come from Lynn Wunderman, chairman and founder of the Raynaud's Association. Although Wunderman has had Raynaud's for most of her life, she wasn't formally diagnosed until 1990. "I was always freezing as a child," Wunderman says.

"Raynaud's is a very personal experience, so not every solution will work for everyone," Wunderman says. "But because Raynaud's is a conditioned bodily response, the more you expose yourself to cold and the less you protect yourself, the more frequent and severe your attacks will be. The opposite is also true: The more you do things that will help you stay warm and keep you protected, the better you will feel."

■ Drink cold beverages from a glass with a stem instead of out of a tumbler.

■ Put drink cozies on cold containers such as soda cans and yogurt cups to keep the cold away from your hands.

■ Keep a pair of oven mitts close by your refrigerator and wear them when taking things in and out of the fridge and freezer.

■ Run your hands under warm (but not hot) water to warm them up quickly.

■ Wear HeatBands—thin, flat strips that wrap around your wrists (looking sort of like wristbands)—to keep your fingers and hands warm. "Keeping the arteries in your wrist warm keeps your hand warmer, much like wearing a scarf makes your whole body feel warmer," Wunderman says. (Visit the Raynaud's Association's Web site, www.raynauds.org, for more information about HeatBands and the other products mentioned here as well as for links to the manufacturers' Web sites and discount codes.)

■ Try battery-heated gloves, mittens, and socks from companies such as www.bewellshop.com.

■ Try FootHugger brand comfort socks, which are made from extremely thin fleece and keep your feet exceptionally warm.

■ Buy shoes that are a little big so that you can wear thick socks and to minimize discomfort if your feet swell when you're having a Raynaud's attack.

■ Exercise—it helps to increase blood supplies to body tissues.

■ Manage stress any way you can; it's a trigger of Raynaud's attacks. Some people with Raynaud's find biofeedback and tai chi helpful.

■ Find a doctor who listens to you. "A lot of doctors just shrug their shoulders and say, 'Figure out how to stay warm.'" Wunderman says, "Raynaud's is real. Turn the heat up."

heat and allows you to peel off clothes as the temperature changes. Your inner layer should consist of synthetic fabrics, such as polypropylene, which wicks perspiration away from your skin. Silk or wool blends also are acceptable. The next layer should insulate you by trapping your body heat. A wool shirt is one of your best options.

■ **WATERPROOF YOUR BODY.** Choose a breathable, water-repellent jacket or windbreaker. Gore-Tex shoes and boots are the best choices for keeping your feet warm and dry.

■ **WEAR A HAT.** The most body heat is lost from the top of your head. The blood vessels in your head are controlled by cardiac output and won't constrict like those in your hands and feet to keep in heat. So while your head may not feel as cold as those icy fingers and toes, it is important to keep it covered to retain precious body heat.

■ **WEAR MITTENS.** Mittens keep you warmer than gloves because they trap your whole hand's heat, rather than just a finger's worth.

■ **TRY FOOT POWDER.** Clothes aren't the only way to keep dry. "Absorbent foot powders are excellent for helping keep feet dry," says Marc A. Brenner, D.P.M. He cautions people with severe cold-foot problems caused by diabetes and peripheral vascular disease to use a shaker can rather than a spray, because the mist from the spray can actually freeze your feet.

■ **DON'T SMOKE.** Cigarette smoke cools you in two ways. It helps form plaque in your arteries and, more immediately, contains nicotine, which causes vasospasms that narrow the small blood vessels and restrict the amount of blood available to keep your hands and feet warm.

■ **CHILL OUT TO WARM UP.** Stress creates the same reaction in the body as cold. It's the fight-or-flight phenomenon. Blood is pulled from the hands and feet to the brain and internal organs to enable you to think and react more quickly.

Calming techniques abound. Some, such as progressive relaxation, in which you systematically tense and then relax the muscles from your forehead to your hands and toes, can be practiced at any time, in any place.

PANEL OF ADVISORS

JOHN L. ABRUZZO, M.D., IS DIRECTOR OF THE DIVISION OF RHEUMATOLOGY AND A PROFESSOR OF MEDICINE AT THOMAS JEFFERSON UNIVERSITY IN PHILADELPHIA.

MARC A. BRENNER, D.P.M., IS FOUNDER AND DIRECTOR OF THE INSTITUTE OF DIABETIC FOOT RESEARCH IN GLENDALE, NEW YORK. HE IS PAST PRESIDENT OF THE AMERICAN SOCIETY OF PODIATRIC DERMATOLOGY AND AUTHOR AND EDITOR OF VARIOUS BOOKS.

DONALD MCINTYRE, M.D., IS A RETIRED DERMATOLOGIST IN RUTLAND, VERMONT.

LYNN WUNDERMAN IS CHAIRMAN AND FOUNDER OF THE RAYNAUD'S ASSOCIATION IN HARTSDALE, NEW YORK.

Restless Legs Syndrome

20 Calming Techniques

"Restless legs syndrome (RLS) is a very common problem," says Jacob Teitelbaum, M.D. People with daytime RLS have the sensation that they need to keep moving their legs even while they are sitting still, or they get a "creepy crawly" sensation in their legs. Most people, however, have RLS only while sleeping. They may not even be aware of the problem.

"A person with RLS will often extend the big toe while flexing the ankle, the knee, and sometimes the hip. This sensation occurs in the arms as well, and sometimes the whole body," says Dr. Teitelbaum. Other people with RLS feel the need to stretch when still and the sensation is often relieved by movement.

"You may or may not be aware of your movements, but your bed partner probably is," he adds. "You're likely exhausted during the day from not getting good rest. When you have RLS, it's like you're running a marathon in your sleep."

People with RLS say the sensation is like an electrical current flowing through the legs, a "creepy crawly" feeling, aching or itching bones, a sensation "like Coca-Cola bubbling through the veins," "crazy legs," and "the gotta moves." If this sounds all too familiar to you, chances are you have RLS.

The condition, also known as Ekbom syndrome, is usually a chronic annoyance rather than a symptom of a larger disorder.

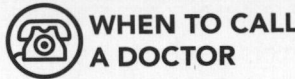

WHEN TO CALL A DOCTOR

If you have restless legs syndrome (RLS), you probably don't have anything to worry about—except the sleep you miss.

But if you're experiencing symptoms for the first time—pronounced sensations in the legs, usually at night—see your doctor. Though rare, these symptoms can be warning signs for serious medical problems such as diabetes, Parkinson's disease, or mineral and electrolyte imbalances.

So for safety—not to mention peace of mind—let your doctor know if you have new leg pains or other symptoms. You can have a sleep study done to look for leg muscle contractions.

Another reason to see a doctor is if crawly legs are keeping you up at night and home remedies just aren't helping. Your doctor may be able to prescribe something to ease discomfort.

"Typically, both lower legs are affected, although the thighs and even the arms can be involved," says Lawrence Z. Stern, M.D. It's not always symmetrical; sometimes it occurs in only one limb.

The origin of the sensations is unknown. Some researchers suspect that an imbalance in the brain's chemistry may be the root cause. A problem with iron metabolism may also be a contributor, and genetics are thought to play a role.

Whatever the cause, RLS can be very frustrating to people who have it, and it can significantly interfere with sleep. Here are a few steps to quiet those jumpy legs.

■ **PUMP UP YOUR IRON LEVELS.** "Although the cause of RLS is not clear, experts suspect it comes from a deficiency of the neurotransmitter dopamine," says Dr. Teitelbaum. Dopamine regulates the smoothness of movement, and your body needs iron to make dopamine. An estimated 25 percent of people with RLS have low iron levels in their blood.

It's a good idea to have your iron levels checked, Dr. Teitelbaum says. But keep in mind that if your levels fall within the "normal" range, that only means you're not in the lowest $2\frac{1}{2}$ percent of the population. (That's like saying if you have an income of $8,100 a year, your income is "normal.") Your ferritin level (the best iron test) should be higher than 50 ng/mL, and your iron percent saturation should be more than 22 percent.

Try taking 20 to 30 milligrams of iron every other day. Be sure to take iron supple-ments on an empty stomach and with vitamin C to help your body absorb it better. Because iron is a little irritating to your stomach, it is absorbed better if you take it every other day instead of every day, giving your stomach the chance to heal. Iron can be toxic if too much builds up in the bloodstream, so it's important to follow dosage instructions very carefully. Stay on the iron until your ferritin blood level is greater than 60 ng/mL (even though anything over 12 is considered "normal").

■ **CALM YOUR LEGS WITH E.** "Vitamin E can be very helpful," says Dr. Teitelbaum. But some patience is in order because it takes 6 to 10 weeks of treatment to help.

Take 400 IU of natural mixed tocopherals a day, says Dr. Teitelbaum. Don't just take alpha tocopheral; you want the whole family of mixed tocopherals.

■ **DON'T EAT A BIG MEAL LATE.** Eating a lot late at night may get the legs really jumping. "It may be the activity of digesting a big meal that triggers something that causes symptoms," says Dr. Stern.

■ **HAVE A PROTEIN SNACK.** "Because RLS may be associated with hypoglycemia, eating a sugar-free, high-protein diet with a protein snack at night may decrease episodes of RLS, and also cramping, at night," says Dr. Teitelbaum.

"I have a very complex diagnostic test for hypoglycemia," he adds. If your hunger is like a light switch that goes off and you feel like you have 3 minutes before you need to eat or else you're going to kill someone, you're hypoglycemic. To avoid that, before you turn in for the night, eat a piece of cheese, some peanut butter, or some turkey.

■ **AVOID SLEEP-INDUCING MEDICATIONS.** They may provide short-term benefits, but many people build up a tolerance to them, and then they have two problems—RLS *and* dependence on the drugs, says Dr. Stern.

■ **DON'T USE ALCOHOL AS A SEDATIVE.** Again, you're only setting yourself up for double trouble, Dr. Stern says.

■ **CUT OUT CAFFEINE.** Avoiding caffeine is important, says Dr. Teitelbaum. Some studies have shown an association between relief of RLS and stopping caffeine. Steer clear of anything with a lot of caffeine for a few weeks, including coffee, tea, soda, energy drinks, and some medications such as Extra-Strength Excedrin.

■ **TRY A TONIC.** Drinking a 6-ounce glass of tonic water each night before bed might calm your restless legs. Tonic water contains quinine, which stops repeated muscle contractions. Some people say even a sip or two before bed helps.

Can't drink tonic water straight? Try this simple, nonalcoholic recipe: Put ½ teaspoon sugar and 2 crushed mint sprigs into a glass. Fill the glass with crushed ice. Add ½ teaspoon lemon juice, 2 tablespoons grapefruit juice, and 4 ounces tonic water. Stir, and drink.

■ **SUPPLEMENT WITH FOLIC ACID.** A small set of people with RLS have the disagreeable leg sensations during the day, instead of when they are at rest or asleep, says Dr. Teitelbaum. These folks also sometimes have numbness

and lightning stabs of pain, which is relieved by massage or movement.

The treatment for this type of RLS is different, he adds. Try supplementing with 800 micrograms of folic acid three times each day. If the problem persists, you may need to see a doctor for a prescription dose of folic acid. It's important to note that folic acid does not help cases of RLS that lack the stabbing pain.

■ **ADD HELPFUL HERBS.** Take theanine (50 to 200 milligrams) and wild lettuce at bedtime, says Dr. Teitelbaum. These both help sleep and may help RLS as well. They can be found in combination (along with four other sleep herbs) in the brand Revitalizing Sleep Formula by Enzymatic Therapy. Theanine raises GABA (gamma amino butyric acid), and wild lettuce raises endorphins, which are two neurotransmitters that have been shown to help settle RLS.

■ **AVOID ALL COLD AND SINUS MEDICATIONS.** These types of medications have been reported to increase the symptoms.

■ **COME IN FROM OUT OF THE COLD.** Several studies have implicated prolonged exposure to cold as a possible cause of RLS.

■ **TAKE TWO ASPIRINS BEFORE BEDTIME.** Doctors can't say why aspirin helps, but apparently it does reduce symptoms in some people.

Other people find that ibuprofen can help to alleviate their symptoms.

■ **LOWER YOUR STRESS LEVEL.** Easier said than done, but it's certainly worth trying. "Stress just worsens the problem," says Dr. Stern. Being organized, giving yourself quiet time, taking deep breaths, and practicing various relaxation techniques are good ways to reduce stress.

Try to relax, especially before going to bed at night. You might try meditation or yoga to help you wind down.

■ **WALK BEFORE GOING TO BED.** In some cases, taking a walk noticeably reduces bedtime bouts, says Dr. Stern. "Exercise changes chemical balances in the brain—endorphins are released—and may promote more restful sleep," he adds.

■ **GET PLENTY OF REST.** Symptoms may be more severe if you allow yourself to become overtired. The following are some tips to try.

■ **Shut off your cell phone.** Researchers at Wayne State University discovered that low-level radiation from cell phones may disrupt production of melatonin, which is a hormone that induces sleep. To make matters worse, cell phones can rev up other areas of your brain. Chatting on your cell for a while before bed can interfere with deep sleep.

■ **Slip on socks.** Who can sleep with freezing cold toes? Plus, when you wear socks, it widens the blood vessels in your feet, allowing your body to transfer heat from its core to its extremities. This cools you slightly, which helps to welcome the sandman.

■ **Set a sleep schedule.** We schedule everything else these days, why not sleep? Scientists at the University of Pittsburgh

Medical Center found that people who follow regular daily routines report fewer sleep problems than do people with more unpredictable lives. Doctors think that recurring time cues synchronize body rhythms and sleep-wake cycles.

■ **Turn down the heat.** Set your thermostat to 60° to 65°F. This will help to nudge your internal temperature down, which is a key ingredient to deep and restful sleep. Plus, you'll save some energy and money.

■ **GET UP AND WALK.** RLS tends to strike at night, when you're at rest. When the urge to move hits, the quickest way to satisfy it is to comply with a stroll around the bedroom.

■ **WIGGLE YOUR FEET.** The idea is to move your feet back and forth when symptoms start.

■ **CHANGE POSITIONS.** "Some people seem to develop symptoms a lot more often when sleeping in one particular position," says Dr. Stern. "Experiment with different sleeping positions. It's harmless and may prove to be worthwhile."

■ **RUB YOUR LEGS WITH AN ELECTRIC VIBRATOR.** Some people say this reduces symptoms; in a few people, however, it could make symptoms worse.

PANEL OF ADVISORS

LAWRENCE Z. STERN, M.D., IS A PROFESSOR IN THE DEPARTMENT OF MEDICINE AT THE UNIVERSITY OF ARIZONA COLLEGE OF MEDICINE IN TUCSON.

JACOB TEITELBAUM, M.D., IS A BOARD-CERTIFIED INTERNIST AND MEDICAL DIRECTOR OF THE FIBROMYALGIA AND FATIGUE CENTERS, WITH LOCATIONS THROUGHOUT THE COUNTRY.

Road Rage

15 Tips for a More Pleasant Drive

The terms *road rage* and *aggressive driving* are often used interchangeably.

But to people who study the ever-increasing vigilante performance of drivers on America's streets and highways, the terms are not synonymous.

Road rage is the deliberate, criminal attempt to hurt or kill a driver or pedestrian, by firing a gun, for example. And although aggressive driving isn't as overtly violent, it can still be deadly.

While most people don't participate in road rage, says Leon James, Ph.D., we all are aggressive drivers.

"We are raised that way from childhood," Dr. James says. We acquire competitive and aggressive attitudes in the car, from parents and TV, for example. By the time we start driving, our attitudes are pretty much set.

Few people, however, consider themselves aggressive behind the wheel, he says. In surveys, 80 percent of drivers say *others* are aggressive on the road, but only about 30 percent admit they're aggressive, too. "There's a 50 percent gap," says Dr. James. In other words, more than half of all aggressive drivers don't realize they're aggressive drivers.

"We define aggressive driving as imposing your own preferred level of risk on others," says Dr. James's wife and coresearcher, Diane Nahl, Ph.D.

People who tailgate, for instance, may be convinced that the other drivers are driving too slowly. "If you get out of their way, they'll consider you to be a good driver," says Dr. Nahl. "If you don't, you're labeled a bad driver."

Cures from the Kitchen

Trade in that pine-scented air freshener for a peppermint candy or cinnamon stick.

In a NASA-funded study, scientists from Wheeling Jesuit University monitored the emotional responses of 25 college students during simulated driving scenarios. The volunteers reported that peppermint lowered their feelings of anxiety and fatigue by 20 percent. Peppermint and cinnamon each decreased their frustration by 25 percent, increased alertness by 30 percent, and made the ride seem 30 percent shorter.

You can buy peppermint and cinnamon oils and aromatherapy diffusers for the car at health food stores.

Some of the "symptoms" of aggressive driving include feeling stressed behind the wheel, cursing, acting hostile, speeding, yelling or honking, making insulting gestures, tailgating, cutting off others, wanting to let the other driver know how you feel, indulging in violent fantasies, or feeling enraged, competitive, or compelled to drive dangerously.

Anonymity is a major contributor to the problem, says Arnold P. Nerenberg, Ph.D. In cars, we tend to dehumanize each other, he says. "We don't think, 'This is a human being like me, with fears, aspirations, love, and vulnerabilities. It's just some jerk that cut me off, and I'm going to teach him a lesson.'"

But there may be a price to pay, Dr. Nerenberg adds. An aggressive driver who contributes to a crash, an injury, or a death is likely to end up in court, or worse.

So here are some tips from the experts on how to relax behind the wheel, as well as some ways to steer clear of aggressive or angry drivers.

■ **LEND SUPPORT.** Learn to accommodate other drivers, says Dr. James. Instead of competing with them, support them. "If they want to enter the lane ahead of you, make space. If they want to pass you, move over and let them. If they want to cut you off, slow down," he says.

"When you're a supportive driver, not only does the stress vanish, but you also begin to enjoy traffic," he says.

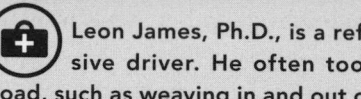

What the Doctor Does

Leon James, Ph.D., is a reformed aggressive driver. He often took risks on the road, such as weaving in and out of lanes.

"I acted like I was in a hurry all the time, even when I wasn't," he says. "It becomes a habit. People who have a habit of getting ahead of everybody else get panicky when they get stuck behind somebody."

Now, Dr. James is much more relaxed in the driver's seat.

It took several years of battling with his wife—who insisted that drivers should consider their passenger's feelings and safety—to realize that she was right.

"I carried a tape recorder in the car and spoke my thoughts out loud, then listened to it later," says Dr. James. From there, it was a matter of "one little skill at a time."

"The one thing that's most helpful is to learn to leave earlier," he says, and he regularly allows an extra 15 to 20 minutes to reach his destination.

"The same events do not stress me out as before," he says. "I am able to be patient."

■ **CUT THEM SOME SLACK.** A driver suddenly slams on his brakes right in front of you, a car makes a left-hand turn from the right-hand lane without the benefit of a turn signal, a car pulls out in front of you, causing you to slam on your brakes—too many cars on the road and too many distractions make for a large margin of error. It's easy to get mad. "Get off the road, idiot," you might think, or worse.

Give other drivers a break, says Dr. James. Think of alternative explanations for a driver's mistake. Maybe she's from out of town. Perhaps he's distracted by a toddler screeching in the backseat. An attitude of latitude is of great benefit, because it counteracts our tendency for hostile judgments and righteous indignation, which are symptoms of road rage. Making mistakes is routine in driving, and for most drivers, a mistake doesn't mean inherent incompetence.

■ **DO IT RIGHT.** "Try life in the right lane," Dr. James suggests. People often avoid the right, or slower, lane because they fear losing time. But if you drive in the slow lane, you'll keep pace with less aggressive drivers and may realize it's not slow after all, he says.

Research shows that the average commute in the United States is 25 minutes. Driving in the fast lane generally saves about 10 percent of that time. So the commuter who rushes arrives at his destination only 2 to 3 minutes ahead of the slower driver. Don't believe it? Time yourself and see.

■ **CONTROL YOURSELF.** Don't let other drivers do it for you, says Dr. Nerenberg. He asks aggressive or angry drivers: "Do you want to turn control over to those people you're calling idiots, or do you want to keep control for yourself?" Losing your cool is turning control over to them. Once you become aware of what they're doing, it's easier to commit to keeping calm on the road.

■ **LISTEN UP.** "Backseat drivers have a bad reputation," says Dr. Nahl. But they may have a point. So listen to the "complaints" of your spouse, your children, and others who ride with you. They are witnesses to your driving.

■ **BE RESPONSIBLE.** To your passengers, that is. "A lot of drivers feel: 'I am the captain of my ship. You just put up with how I drive,'" says Dr. James. The driver controls the air conditioner, radio stations, speed, and just about everything else.

Instead, ask your passengers about their preferences. They'll likely appreciate the respect, and you'll feel better about yourself and calmer while driving.

■ **GET SILLY.** Feeling tense behind the wheel? Try making animal noises, machine sounds, or whatever you find amusing. "Laughter not only interrupts your negative thinking or anger, but also unloads the stress," says Dr. Nahl.

■ **FORGIVE AND FORGET.** If you are the "victim" of an aggressive driver, remind yourself that retaliation isn't worth it. Think about the people waiting for you to arrive at home. "You don't want to do anything that would endanger your life or anyone else's," says Dr. James. "Tell yourself, 'It's just not worth the hassle.'"

■ **HONK WITH CARE.** "Even honking has become a dangerous behavior," says Dr. Nahl. "People often take honking as a great insult, as a sign of disrespect." So you had better be careful about when, where, and why you decide to tap or lay on that horn.

■ **ACKNOWLEDGE YOUR AGGRESSION.** "It's a good first step, but it's a hard thing for people to do," says Dr. Nahl.

People with road rage often focus on other people—those on the outside of the windshield, she says. "We rarely focus on our own behavior."

So one way to tune in: Talk behind the wheel. "The act of speaking your thoughts out loud while you're driving creates awareness," she says.

Better yet, tape-record yourself while driving, and listen later. Research shows people often are surprised by what they've said.

Another option: Carry a notepad in the car. When you arrive at your destination, write down your thoughts and feelings about the drive. Over time, your observations will lend insight that may help you some changes to any aggressive patterns.

■ **DON'T GET ENGAGED.** Avoid confrontations at all costs by never tailgate or making eye contact with any angry drivers. Don't get out of the car or attempt to have a conversation for any reason. Similarly, don't go home or to work if someone is following you. "You don't want that person to know anything about you," Dr. Nerenberg says. If you feel frightened or threatened, go to a safe place, such as a police or fire station.

■ **TALK ABOUT IT.** Meet with your family regularly, especially if you have teenagers, to talk about safe driving, says Dr. Nahl. Ask for feedback on your own driving, allow other family members to openly discuss driving habits or problems, and discuss potential scenarios and actions.

■ **TEACH YOUR CHILDREN.** Babies and toddlers learn a lot in those car seats. "We call this the road-rage nursery," says Dr. Nahl. Before children even learn to speak, they absorb the attitudes of the adults they ride with. They witness firsthand all of the yelling, cursing, and gestures.

So learn to turn around those actions. Say something like: "Mommy just yelled at that other person. I really shouldn't do that." Also ask for your children's help. They might remind you to put on your seat belt, for example. Thank them, and encourage them. "You'll create a whole different culture in the car," Dr. Nahl says. That may pay off in the long run, and your children may be less aggressive when it's *their* turn to drive.

What the Doctor Does

Arnold P. Nerenberg, Ph.D., uses what he calls the "Power Thought System" to keep negative thoughts from arising and overpowering drivers. Remind yourself—hourly, if possible, and never fewer than six times a day—of how you want to be on the road. Think, for example: "I'm going to keep control over myself. I'm not turning control over to you." You'll learn to turn away destructive thoughts.

Test Yourself

Leon James, Ph.D., created the following test for aggressive drivers. The 20 items are arranged along a continuum of escalating degrees of hostility experienced by drivers, beginning with relatively milder forms of aggressiveness (step 1) and going all the way to ultimate violence (step 20). The majority of drivers Dr. James tested go as far as step 13. How far down the uncivilized road do you allow yourself to travel?

1. Mentally condemning other drivers

2. Verbally denigrating other drivers to a passenger in your vehicle

3. Closing ranks to deny someone access to your lane because you're frustrated or upset

4. Giving another driver the "stink eye" to show your disapproval

5. Speeding past another car or revving the engine as a sign of protest

6. Preventing another driver from passing because you're angry

7. Tailgating to pressure a driver to go faster or get out of the way

8. Fantasizing physical violence against another driver

9. Honking or yelling at someone through the window to indicate displeasure

10. Making a visible obscene gesture at another driver

11. Using your car to retaliate by making sudden, threatening maneuvers

12. Pursuing another car in chase because of a provocation or insult

13. Getting out of the car and engaging in a verbal dispute on a street or in a parking lot

14. Carrying a weapon in the car in case you decide to use it in a driving incident

15. Deliberately bumping or ramming another car in anger

16. Trying to run another car off the road to punish the driver

17. Getting out of the car and beating or battering someone as a result of an exchange on the road

18. Trying to run someone down whose actions angered you

19. Shooting at another car

20. Killing someone

What the Doctor Does

Martha Howard, M.D., used to commute a very stressful 16 miles, often twice a day. "I would find myself getting very irritated and annoyed behind the wheel," she says. "'This is bad for my health,' I realized. This is going to kill me. They say hostility is the biggest risk factor for heart attacks, a bigger risk factor even than smoking."

"I started listening to Buddhist lecture tapes while driving. One tape had a car meditation exercise by Thich Nhat Hanh, a famous Buddhist monk. For the exercise, you use the brake light in the car in front of you as a mindfulness wake-up call. When the driver in front of you brakes, instead of cursing and pounding the steering wheel, take it as your cue to breathe and smile and relax. Smiling in itself is huge; just putting your face in a smile changes your body chemistry and helps you relax."

PANEL OF ADVISORS

MARTHA HOWARD, M.D., IS MEDICAL DIRECTOR OF WELLNESS ASSOCIATES OF CHICAGO, AN INTEGRATIVE MEDICINE CENTER.

LEON JAMES, PH.D., IS A PROFESSOR OF PSYCHOLOGY AT THE UNIVERSITY OF HAWAII IN HONOLULU. HE HAS RESEARCHED AGGRESSIVE DRIVING FOR MORE THAN 20 YEARS AND IS COAUTHOR, WITH HIS WIFE, DIANE NAHL, OF *ROAD RAGE AND AGGRESSIVE DRIVING*. DR. JAMES AND DR. NAHL OPERATE THE WEB SITE WWW. DRDRIVING.ORG AND ARE THE CREATORS OF AN ANTI-AGGRESSIVE DRIVING VIDEO SERIES CALLED *ROADRAGEOUS*.

DIANE NAHL, PH.D., IS A PROFESSOR AND INFORMATION SCIENTIST AT THE UNIVERSITY OF HAWAII IN HONOLULU. SHE HAS STUDIED AGGRESSIVE DRIVING FOR MORE THAN 20 YEARS.

ARNOLD P. NERENBERG, PH.D., IS A PSYCHOLOGIST IN WHITTIER, CALIFORNIA, AND A LONGTIME ROAD-RAGE RESEARCHER. HE IS COAUTHOR OF THE AMERICAN INSTITUTE FOR PUBLIC SAFETY'S ROAD RAGE PROGRAM AND AUTHOR OF *A 10-STEP COMPASSION PROGRAM*, FOR LEARNING TO OVERCOME ANGRY DRIVING.

Rosacea

12 Face-Saving Steps

Quick . . . aside from spending lots of time in the public eye, what did former U.S. President Bill Clinton, the late Princess Diana, and the late comedian W. C. Fields all have in common?

They are three of the most famous people in the public eye to have had rosacea (pronounced "rose-AY-shah"), an inflammatory skin condition that often results in redness of the nose, cheeks, forehead, and chin. The skin condition affects more than 14 million Americans, but it is most common in people with fair complexions.

"Rosacea is a common condition, but often the average person confuses it with adult acne or a skin allergy," says Dee Anna Glaser, M.D. It tends to be cyclical. It might be active for a while, then lessen in intensity, and then suddenly flare up again.

Left untreated, the redness becomes more permanent, and tiny blood vessels become visible. Bumps and pimples often develop, and in advanced cases, your nose may become bumpy, red, and swollen. In some cases, your eyes can appear watery or bloodshot, according to Dr. Glaser. That's why it's important to get an early diagnosis and make the life changes necessary to keep the condition under control.

"The key is to know what triggers your flare-ups and to avoid those things as much as possible," says Dr. Glaser.

As a rule, anything that causes a rosacea sufferer's face to get red or flush may trigger a flare-up. Among the most common trip

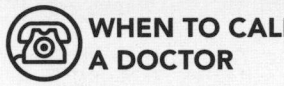

WHEN TO CALL A DOCTOR

When a person starts to show early stages of rosacea, it's wise to see a dermatologist as soon as possible, suggests Dee Anna Glaser, M.D.

"A dermatologist can fully educate the person about rosacea—how to properly wash his or her face, how to deal with the things that trigger flare-ups, what should be avoided, and so forth," says Dr. Glaser. "The sooner the person gets that knowledge, the better."

Plus, many other skin problems, such as sun damage and acne, mimic rosacea, so you could be treating one condition when you really have another.

wires are alcohol, heat, hot drinks, spicy foods, caffeine, stress, and sun exposure. To avoid a flare-up, make the following lifestyle changes.

■ **BE SUN SAVVY.** Sunscreens are helpful in decreasing rosacea. So apply a quality sunscreen to your face each and every time you go outdoors for an extended period of time. A broad-spectrum sunblock with a sun protection factor (SPF) of at least 15 is best for year-round use, says Dr. Glaser. (Broad-spectrum sunblocks protect you from both the ultraviolet A and the ultraviolet B waves of the sun.) Because perspiration and water can wash off your sunscreen, reapply it throughout the day.

■ **COVER YOUR HEAD.** If you're heading to the beach or spending extended time in the midday sun, wear a hat with a 4-inch-wide brim to keep the sun off your face and neck, says Dr. Glaser. Baseball caps, when worn with the bill in front, don't protect your ears, the back of your neck, or even most of your face from the sun.

■ **WATCH THE WEATHER.** Harsh weather, such as cold, blustery wind or blistering hot sunshine, can spike rosacea. Protect your skin year-round.

■ **TURN DOWN THE HEAT OF YOUR BEVERAGES.** A cup of piping hot coffee or hot chocolate may be a trigger for some people with rosacea because hot beverages can make your face flush. Decreasing the temperature of your drink, even slightly, may be all you need to do. "What triggers the rosacea to flare up can be different in different people, so it's up to you to figure out your triggers," says Dr. Glaser. "If it's hot coffee, try drinking it a little cooler. Or if you're a four-cup-a-day coffee drinker, then cut back to one or two cups instead or eliminate coffee entirely."

■ **WATCH WHAT YOU EAT.** Hot, spicy food—seasoned with red and cayenne pepper, for instance—is a common rosacea trip wire. In some cases, other foods cause problems for people with rosacea, including avocados, broad-leafed beans and pods, cheese (especially Brie and hard cheeses because they release histamine, a chemical that turns the skin red), chocolate, citrus fruit, eggplant, liver, sour cream, soy sauce, spinach, vanilla, vinegar, yeast extract, and yogurt.

"Keep a diary or make mental notes of what you eat and how it affects your rosacea," says Dr. Glaser. "Adjust your diet accordingly."

■ **AVOID HIGH-INTENSITY WORKOUTS.** Sure, exercise is essential for a healthy lifestyle, but too much exertion can cause rosacea to flare up, says Dr. Glaser. "You must still get exercise, but make adjustments. Exercise three times a day for 15 minutes rather than 45 minutes straight, to avoid overheating. Or in summer, exercise in an air-conditioned room or gym, or wait until the early evening to exercise outside when the sun is less intense," she says.

■ **STAY OUT OF THE SAUNA OR HOT TUB.** The heat of hot tubs and saunas can bring on flushing and aggravate your condition, according to Larry Millikan, M.D.

■ **BE GENTLE WHEN CLEANSING.** Begin each day with a thorough, but gentle cleansing of your face, says Dr. Millikan. Think "simple." People with rosacea get into trouble when they start using fancy soaps with fragrances, lots of preservatives, or harsh textures, he says.

Spread a gentle cleanser all over your face softly with your fingertips. Then rinse your face with lukewarm tepid, not hot, water to remove all dirt and soap.

Let your face air-dry for a few minutes before applying any topical medication or skin-care products. Then allow the medication to dry for 5 to 10 minutes before applying a moisturizer or makeup.

Repeat the same cleansing process at night.

■ **SELECT SKIN-CARE PRODUCTS WITH DELICATE CARE.** "Steer clear of products that include alcohol or other irritants, which may cause your face to burn, sting, or become red," says Dr. Glaser.

Also avoid products that contain acid and anything that causes a warming sensation on the skin. Favorites include Cetaphil, Dove, and CeraVe. Eucerin's Redness Relief products contain licorice extract, which calms redness.

■ **BATTLE REDNESS WITH RED TEA.** How's this for irony: Red tea, which is brewed from the leaves of a South African shrub, is rich in quercetin, an anti-inflammatory that can help relieve the facial flushing, irritation, and itching associated with rosacea. As a bonus, it also prevents the UV damage that causes fine lines and age spots. You can buy red tea in over-the-counter skin care products such as Jason Red Elements Red Clay Masque ($13.60, www.jason-natural.com).

■ **STRESS LESS.** The National Rosacea Society reports that 79 percent of people with rosacea say mental stress and anxiety aggravate their symptoms. Consider walking, yoga, or tai chi.

■ **BABY YOUR FACE.** People with rosacea who took a low-dose aspirin (81 milligrams) for a month experienced fewer and shorter rosacea flare-ups. The researchers think that aspirin constricts blood vessels, preventing skin from turning red.

PANEL OF ADVISORS

DEE ANNA GLASER, M.D., IS A PROFESSOR IN THE DEPARTMENT OF DERMATOLOGY AT ST. LOUIS UNIVERSITY SCHOOL OF MEDICINE IN MISSOURI.

LARRY MILLIKAN, M.D., IS A PROFESSOR EMERITUS IN THE DEPARTMENT OF DERMATOLOGY AT TULANE UNIVERSITY SCHOOL OF MEDICINE IN NEW ORLEANS.

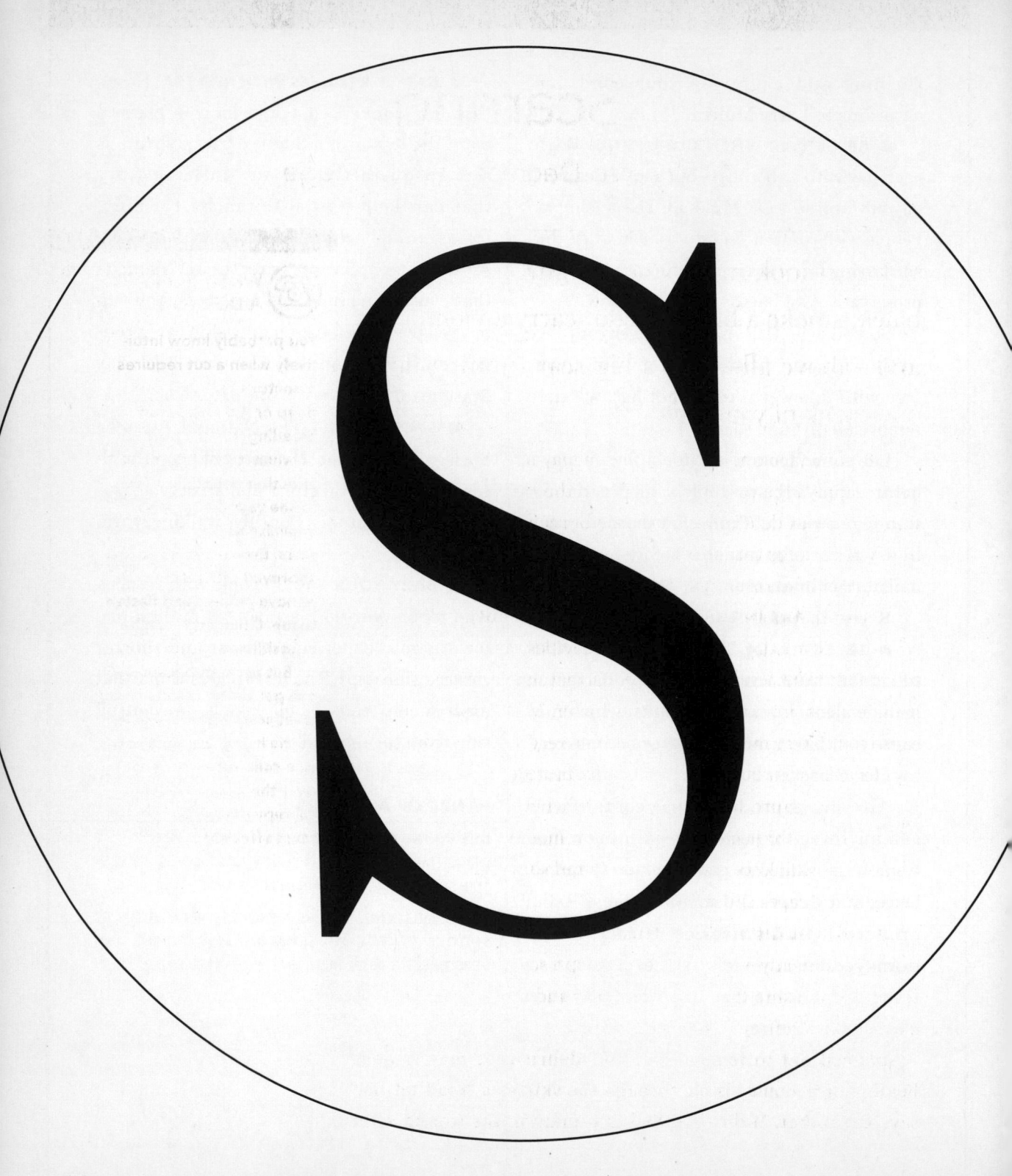

Scarring

14 Ways to Decrease the Damage

Want to look mean and tough? Just dress in black, smoke a big, fat cigar, carry a violin case, and—above all—have a big scar running down one cheek of your face.

Of course, looking mean and tough may not be the look you're after. If that's the case, you've come to the right place. How you treat a cut can determine what kind of scar may develop. Then, how you care for that scar can determine how fast and to what extent it will fade over time. Here's what our experts suggest.

■ **NIP SCARS IN THE BUD.** If you don't want dog hair on your sofa, don't own a dog. If you don't want cavities, don't eat sugar. And if you don't want scars, don't get cut. It's that simple. "Every time the skin gets cut, it scars," says Gerald Imber, M.D. Some people, he says, tend to scar more than others. "It's a very individual thing."

However your body reacts, consider protecting your skin with gloves, long pants, and long sleeves whenever working around thorny, sharp, or jagged objects. If you mountain bike or skate, wear elbow and knee pads, and wrist and shin guards to prevent accidental scrapes and abrasions.

■ **THOROUGHLY CLEAN THE WOUND.** A wound that heals quickly and neatly is less likely to develop a scar than a wound that festers. Make sure that all of your cuts and scrapes are properly cleaned, says Jeffrey H. Binstock, M.D.

It's critical to remove dirt and debris that may impede healing or become visible through the skin as a "road tattoo," says Dr. Imber. If dirt and debris remain in the wound after

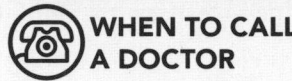 **WHEN TO CALL A DOCTOR**

You probably know intuitively when a cut requires a doctor's call—when it's deep or it doesn't stop bleeding, for example, or when it shows signs of infection. Another reason to see your doctor is to minimize the appearance of scars. Even old scars can be improved with lasers, which remove redness and flatten tissue. Other scars can be repositioned with surgery.

But act fast, because you can get better results if you treat scars within 6 weeks of the injury, the time new skin cells begin forming over the wound. Laser therapy during that time is most effective.

washing, use tweezers cleaned with alcohol to remove particles.

■ **BUT SKIP THE HYDROGEN PEROXIDE.** It destroys white blood cells that help repair wounds, actually slowing healing. Plus, it extends the time that the wound is open and vulnerable. Also not helpful are soap and rubbing alcohol, which can be irritating. Instead, rinse the cut with warm clear water and a gentle soap if necessary, even though it might sting.

■ **KEEP IT MOIST AND COVERED.** Moisture prevents a hard scab from forming, which slows development of new tissue. Plus, cells regenerate faster in a moist environment, so leaving a cut open to the air may promote scarring. Cover your wound with plain petroleum jelly to keep it moist, then slap on an adhesive bandage. Research shows that keeping wounds covered with a bandage speeds healing by as much as 50 percent.

■ **BUT CONSIDER SKIPPING THE OINTMENT.** "Neosporin and other ointments are

Cures from the Kitchen

Keep an aloe plant on your kitchen windowsill, and make the plant your ally for any minor cuts, scrapes, or wounds. Aloe is antibacterial, antifungal, antiviral, and an immune stimulant. Plus, the plant contains vitamins C and E and the mineral zinc, all nutrients shown to speed wound healing.

Studies suggest that commercial aloe preparations lose some of their wound-healing ability, so the plant is your best bet. Just snip off a leaf, slit it open, scoop out the gel, and apply it to your cut.

What the Doctor Does

John F. Romano, M.D., finds that putting a little Mylanta, milk of magnesia, or calamine lotion on a pimple helps to dry it out a bit, possibly preventing a scar.

virtually useless," says Dr. Imber. "They don't penetrate and don't allow the daily washing needed to keep the wound clean."

■ **DON'T PICK AT SCABS.** Mom was right. Picking a scab off a healing wound could increase your chances of leaving behind a scar, says John F. Romano, M.D.

■ **CLOSE GAPS WITH A BUTTERFLY BANDAGE.** If you get a large cut, you should go to a doctor for stitches, particularly if the cut is on the face where a scar would be most visible. But even if a cut is small and you are concerned about scarring, consider using a butterfly bandage, says Dr. Romano. These bandages, available at most drugstores, can help keep the wound closed for better healing and minimal scarring. They should be used only after the wound has been thoroughly cleaned.

■ **EAT A WELL-BALANCED DIET.** Wounds won't heal right unless your body has what it takes to *make* them heal right. What does it take? Protein and vitamins—obtained by eating a good, well-balanced diet—are essential. Of particular importance to wound healing is the mineral zinc. Good sources of zinc include roasted pumpkin and sunflower seeds, Brazil nuts, Swiss and Cheddar cheeses, peanuts, dark-meat turkey, and lean beef.

■ **GET MOVING.** Exercise can speed the healing process by as much as 25 percent. Ohio State University researchers gave 28 sedentary men and women each a small puncture wound. (How'd they get people to volunteer for that?) The researchers then asked half of the people to exercise on a treadmill, ride a stationary bike, or strength-train three times a week, for an hour each time for 3 months, while the other half of the people stayed sedentary. After 3 months, the wounds of the active people healed an average of 10 days faster (in 29 days versus 39 days) than those of the couch potatoes.

The study researchers suggest that exercise increases circulation and helps regulate the immune system and hormones that influence the healing process. They believe that exercise may even help wound healing in people traditionally slow to heal, such as those with diabetes. Is there nothing exercise can't do?

■ **MANAGE YOUR ANGER.** When you have a cut or wound, try to keep your cool. Inability to control strong emotions can slow recovery from an injury. Ohio State University scientists gave 100 volunteers identical blisters on their forearms. The hot-tempered subjects took four times longer to heal than their calmer peers. The researchers think that increased levels of the stress hormone cortisol can suppress your immune system.

■ **COVER YOUR SCARS WITH SUNBLOCK.** Scars have less pigment than the rest of your skin. This means they lack the ability to develop a protective tan, and they are especially vulnerable to sunburn. Cover all scars with a strong sunscreen whenever you head outside.

Also, UV rays slow healing by interfering with new collagen production. Always protect healed wounds with a broad-spectrum SPF 15 or higher sunscreen. It's a myth that scars blend better into surrounding skin after sun exposure. The contrast of a tan actually can make the scar more visible.

■ **LEVEL OUT.** After your scar has healed, an over-the-counter scar treatment, such as ScarGuard Scar Care or Curad Scar Therapy Clear Pads, may help to level raised scars. You can buy them at drugstores.

Cures from the Kitchen

Hasten healing by applying some honey to a cut. Its antibacterial properties help prevent infection and help you to heal faster. Apply a dab of honey to the wound and then cover it with an airtight bandage.

PANEL OF ADVISORS

JEFFREY H. BINSTOCK, M.D., IS A CLINICAL PROFESSOR IN THE DEPARTMENT OF DERMATOLOGY AT THE UNIVERSITY OF CALIFORNIA, SAN FRANCISCO, SCHOOL OF MEDICINE.

GERALD IMBER, M.D., IS AN ATTENDING PLASTIC SURGEON AT NEW YORK–PRESBYTERIAN HOSPITAL IN NEW YORK CITY.

JOHN F. ROMANO, M.D., IS AN ASSISTANT PROFESSOR OF DERMATOLOGY AT THE WEIL MEDICAL COLLEGE OF CORNELL UNIVERSITY AND AN ATTENDING PHYSICIAN AT NEW YORK PRESBYTERIAN HOSPITAL AND ST. VINCENT'S HOSPITAL, ALL IN NEW YORK CITY. HE HAS A PRACTICE IN MANHATTAN.

Sciatica

17 Strategies to Knock Out Nerve Pain

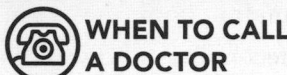 **WHEN TO CALL A DOCTOR**

About the only good thing concerning sciatica is that the pain is usually temporary. It often begins to feel better within 4 to 5 days, and most people will be well on the way to recovery within 6 weeks.

"There's no need to panic if you get sciatica, but it can be extraordinarily painful," says John G. Heller, M.D.

Still, it's important to see a doctor, he adds. For one thing, you'll probably need medication to control the pain. You'll also want to be sure that you aren't risking permanent nerve damage.

One of the most serious warning signs is a loss of muscle function—your foot is dragging, for example. Even more serious is a loss of bowel or bladder control. If you have any one of these symptoms, don't wait to see your regular doctor, Dr. Heller advises. Go straight to an emergency room.

Nearly everyone experiences back pain on occasion, but only an unlucky few ever have to endure the agonizing pain of sciatica.

The sciatic nerve stretches down the lower back region, down the back of the legs to the ankles and feet. Anything that puts pressure on the nerve—a herniated spinal disk, a bone spur, or spinal malalignment—can result in sharp, shooting pains in the buttocks or legs.

A herniated disk is the most common cause of sciatica among young, active adults. This condition occurs when the outer wall of the disk, which normally functions as a shock absorber between the vertebrae, becomes torn, and the inner cushioning material pushes into the spinal canal, where it compresses a nerve root.

Sciatica tends to be short-lived, but sometimes it persists for years. Even simple daily activities—like bending over, sneezing, or having a bowel movement—can trigger attacks. Once the nerve has been irritated or damaged, the pain can persist even when you're lying still.

Because so many things can cause sciatica, and because the nerve can be permanently damaged without prompt treatment, it's essential to see a doctor at the first sign of symptoms. Surgery is sometimes required, but sciatica can usually be controlled with a combination of medications and home care. Here are a few ways to stop the pain and protect the nerve from additional harm.

■ **ICE IT QUICKLY.** At the first sign of pain, apply a cold compress (a small bag of ice cubes wrapped in a thin cloth) to the lower back for 15 to 20 minutes at a time, every 2 to 3 hours. Keep it cold for 24 to 48 hours. Cold reduces inflammation and helps prevent painful muscle spasms, says Andrew J. Cole, M.D.

The easiest approach is to use a gel pack, available at sporting goods and medical supply stores. The packs remain flexible even after they're chilled in the freezer. They mold themselves to the contours of your lower back, putting the cold right where you need it. In a pinch, you can even apply a bag of frozen vegetables. Wrap either one in a thin towel first to protect your skin.

■ **USE A HEATING PAD.** After applying cold for a day or two, switch to heat, advises John J. Triano, D.C., Ph.D. Apply a hot-water bottle or a heating pad to your lower back for 15 minutes at a time. Repeat the treatment every hour, and keep doing it as long as it seems to help. Heat relaxes muscles and helps prevent painful spasms. It also increases circulation and helps flush pain-causing toxins from around the nerve.

No matter how much better heat makes you feel, don't use it for more than 15 minutes at a time. "Applying heat for longer can result in rebound swelling, which will make the pain worse later," says Dr. Triano.

■ **TAKE ANTI-INFLAMMATORY MEDICA- TIONS.** When you first feel the pain of sciatica, take aspirin, ibuprofen (Motrin), naproxen (Aleve), or other nonsteroidal anti-inflammatory drugs (NSAIDs), Dr. Cole advises. They inhibit the body's production of prostaglandins, inflammatory chemicals that increase pain and swelling. Take the medications four times daily, following label instructions.

If aspirin or ibuprofen upset your stomach, it's fine to take acetaminophen (Tylenol). But keep in mind that it mainly works as a pain reliever. It has little effect on inflammation.

"I usually recommend naproxen," says Dr. Triano. "It's a good anti-inflammatory and is somewhat less likely than aspirin or ibuprofen to cause stomach upset."

■ **GO FOR A SWIM.** Or simply walk in water. The combination of warm water and gentle exercise will often loosen muscles and help relieve spasms and pain. Plus, water supports the body, which may relieve painful pressure on the back.

"Swimming and aquatic exercises are among the best rehabilitation tools available," says John G. Heller, M.D. It is especially effective for people who find other types of exercise initially too painful.

Most health clubs offer aquatics classes, he notes, and local arthritis associations often sponsor aquatics classes at community centers or YMCAs. The movements used in the classes are perfect for those with a history of back pain or sciatica, says Dr. Heller.

Swimming isn't recommended at the peak of an attack, but it's fine once the pain diminishes somewhat, Dr. Heller says. It's also a good preventive strategy for those who have had sciatica in the past.

■ **WALK IF IT'S COMFORTABLE.** Walking is one of the best exercises for relieving and preventing sciatica. It keeps muscles limber and improves circulation throughout the body, including the area of the damaged nerve.

If you're in the acute stage of sciatica and walking causes sharp, stabbing pains, don't do it, Dr. Triano says. "But if you've had the pain for more than a few days and it's mainly a dull, aching feeling, it's important to gently push through the discomfort with walking or other forms of gentle exercise."

■ **STRENGTHEN YOUR TRUNK MUSCLES.** Also called the pelvic girdle, these are the muscles that surround and support the spine. "The basic crunch is a good exercise for strengthening the muscles," says Dr. Cole.

Crunches are easy to do. Lie on your back with your knees bent at about a 90-degree angle and your feet flat on the floor, your arms at your sides. Using your upper abdominal muscles, raise your head and shoulders off of the floor. Your arms should be extended out in front. Then lower your shoulders to the floor in a slow, controlled motion. You don't want to raise your shoulders more than an inch or two, because that overstrains the muscle that links the lumbar spine to the legs and increases tension on the lower back, Dr. Cole says.

■ **GET A MASSAGE.** It won't reverse underlying nerve or disk damage, but it can reduce muscle spasms and increase flexibility. "Massage makes people feel better, and that can allow their rehabilitation to advance," says Dr. Cole.

■ **LET YOUR LEGS DO THE WORK.** Whether you currently have sciatica or have had it in the past, proper body mechanics—the ways you move every day—are essential. Bending from the waist, for example, is about the worst thing you can do. If you're doing anything more strenuous than picking up a sock, kneel or squat and use your leg muscles to push back up. Bending can trigger sciatica because it puts tremendous strain on the lower back, says Dr. Cole.

■ **HOLD THINGS CLOSE TO YOUR BODY.** Whether you're carrying a bag of groceries or a laundry basket, hold it as close to your body as possible, Dr. Cole advises. Holding weight close to your body takes some of the pressure off the lower spine.

■ **SUPPORT YOUR LOWER BACK.** Sciatica can take weeks or even months to improve. In the meantime, giving your back extra support—place a pillow or a rolled-up towel behind you when you're sitting—reduces pain and helps the injured area heal more quickly, says Dr. Triano.

Even better are pillows that inflate automatically with the turn of a valve. Available at sporting goods stores and stores that specialize in back care, they allow you to easily change the firmness every 15 to 20 minutes. "They're a superb way of inexpensively minimizing back pain," says Dr. Triano.

Just don't think of back supports as a substitute for exercise and strong supporting muscles of the back, says Dr. Heller. Such muscles derived through disciplined exercise become your internal back support.

■ **TAKE FREQUENT BREAKS.** Sitting is surprisingly hard on the lower back, especially when the sciatic nerve is inflamed and irritated. In fact, sitting without a back support can put about twice as much pressure on the spine as standing.

"If you have sciatica, your enemy is a prolonged, static posture," Dr. Triano says. "The elastic properties of your tissues are used up in about 20 minutes. After that, you're going to experience increased stress on the area."

If your job requires a lot of sitting, give your back a break and get up every 15 to 20 minutes, or whenever your back starts feeling tense or tired. Walk around for a few minutes. Stretch. Give your muscles a chance to unwind before sitting back down again. "Keep this in mind during lengthy car or plane trips, too," notes Dr. Heller.

■ **PUT A FOOT UP.** The back naturally has a slight curve, but when you're standing flat-footed, the curve is accentuated, which can aggravate a sensitive sciatic nerve. A more "relaxed" posture affords slightly more room for the nerves.

"One of the best things you can do when you're standing is to alternately prop one foot up and then the other," says Dr. Triano. Elevating one foot slightly increases the "free" space around the sciatic nerve, and shifting from one foot to the other on a regular basis helps maintain elasticity in the spi-

What the Doctor Does

Martha Howard, M.D., used this exercise when she had sciatica, and it kept her sister-in-law, who's in her seventies, pain-free for a decade.

Lie on your back on a bed—if you have a firm mattress—or on the floor. Bend your knees, and place your feet flat on the bed. Slowly extend your right leg, keeping your heel down, until it has reached its full length. Your heel should slide along the surface of the bed as you extend your leg. Do not lift or raise your leg throughout the exercise. You shouldn't feel a stretch or strain. Slowly bring your right leg back to the starting position and repeat the move with your left leg. Do 10 on each side, over time adding 2 at time to reach 30 on each side.

nal disks and surrounding tissues, he explains.

Whenever possible, rest your foot on a short stool or a step when standing. At the grocery store, rest one foot on the lower part of the shopping cart. On the street, use a curb or the base of a lamppost. Many people with sciatica find that elevating one foot even a few inches is often enough to temporarily eliminate the pain.

■ **STAY OUT OF THE CAR.** Apart from the fact that most car seats are notoriously hard on the lower back, cars vibrate at four to five cycles per second—a frequency that can damage disks, increase muscle inflammation or spasms, and generally increase strain on the sciatic nerve.

Until your back is better, spend as little time in the car as possible. Even when your pain is gone, it's a good idea to limit driving time to 2 hours daily.

■ **TRY STRETCHING AND FLEXIBILITY EXERCISES.** They are among the best ways to reduce the inflammation and muscle spasms that often accompany sciatica, says Dr. Triano.

Everyone responds differently to exercises. Some people do best with extension exercises, which include lying facedown, arching your back, and raising up on your elbows. Others require flexion movements—for example, lying on your back and bringing your knees to your chest. You'll have to experiment a bit to discover what works best for you.

"Stretching exercises encourage motion of the spine and associated joints, muscles, and ligaments, which can prevent adhesions or stiffness from scar tissue formation after an injury," says Dr. Heller. "If the exercises make you feel better, keep doing them. But they should never make pain worse or cause it to radiate down one or both legs. If they do cause pain, it's the wrong exercise for you and you should seek professional advice."

■ **GET PLENTY OF SLEEP.** It's hard to do when you're hurting, but studies have shown that the body undergoes much of its healing during sleep. If pain is keeping you awake, try elevating your knees with a small pillow: It takes some of the pressure off the nerve, says Dr. Triano. If you usually sleep on your side, curl up and put a pillow between your knees.

■ **IF YOU SMOKE, TRY TO QUIT.** Cigarette smoke weakens the spinal disks and slows recovery if you're experiencing sciatica. If you need surgery for sciatica, smoking increases the risk that the operation won't be successful. "Some surgeons won't operate unless patients quit smoking," says Dr. Cole.

PANEL OF ADVISORS

ANDREW J. COLE, M.D., IS A CLINICAL PROFESSOR IN THE DEPARTMENT OF PHYSICAL MEDICINE AND REHABILITATION AT THE UNIVERSITY OF WASHINGTON MEDICAL CENTER IN SEATTLE AND PRESIDENT AND MEDICAL DIRECTOR OF NORTHWEST SPINE AND SPORTS PHYSICIANS, PC, IN BELLEVUE, WASHINGTON.

JOHN G. HELLER, M.D., IS A PROFESSOR OF ORTHOPEDICS SURGERY AT EMORY UNIVERSITY SCHOOL OF MEDICINE IN ATLANTA.

MARTHA HOWARD, M.D., IS MEDICAL DIRECTOR OF WELLNESS ASSOCIATES OF CHICAGO, AN INTEGRATIVE MEDICINE CENTER.

JOHN J. TRIANO, D.C., PH.D., IS A PROFESSOR OF RESEARCH AT THE CANADIAN MEMORIAL CHIROPRACTIC COLLEGE AND ASSOCIATE PROFESSOR OF REHABILITATION SCIENCE AT MCMASTER UNIVERSITY IN ONTARIO, CANADA. HIS DOCTORATE IS IN SPINE BIOMECHANICS. HE SPECIALIZES IN PREVENTION, TREATMENT, AND REHABILITATION OF NECK AND BACK DISORDERS.

Seasonal Affective Disorder

12 Steps to a Brighter Outlook

Each autumn, as the days grow shorter, millions of people get the blues. They may experience mild to severe depression, weight gain, lethargy, a desire to sleep more, and an increased appetite or cravings for carbohydrates such as cakes and cookies. Almost magically in spring, their symptoms wane. They feel energized, sociable, and generally happy. Their malady: seasonal affective disorder, or SAD, a form of depression most likely to occur in winter.

For about 5 percent of people, the condition is severe enough to interfere with daily activities, work, and relationships, says Norman E. Rosenthal, M.D. Another 15 percent experience milder symptoms known as subsyndromal SAD (S-SAD).

Scientists have studied SAD as a psychological disorder since the 1980s, when Dr. Rosenthal, formerly of the National Institute of Mental Health, named the illness.

Researchers don't fully understand what causes SAD, only that it is connected to light received by the brain through the eyes. One theory is that light affects the hormone melatonin, which peaks in the brain at night and regulates your internal body clock. Another theory holds that light tinkers with the neurotransmitter serotonin, a mood-regulating chemical in the brain.

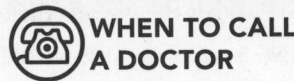

WHEN TO CALL A DOCTOR

Severe seasonal affective disorder can be helped by antidepressants such as selective serotonin reuptake inhibitors (SSRIs). See a doctor if your symptoms are getting in the way of your work or relationships, says Norman E. Rosenthal, M.D.

Also get help if you feel despair about the future or are suicidal, or if you have major sleep or eating changes, such as a weight gain of 15 or 20 pounds.

"It's a matter of degree and a matter of dysfunction, versus unpleasantness or inconvenience," Dr. Rosenthal says. If self-help strategies aren't effective, seek guidance as well.

Don't use light therapy without consulting your physician and your eye doctor, says Brenda Byrne, Ph.D. Some medications may make your eyes sensitive to light.

Because other conditions such as low thyroid functioning can mimic SAD, talk with your doctor before attempting to treat yourself, especially if you are severely depressed. Some of the suggestions below may complement treatment. If your symptoms are mild, try a few of these tips to dash the winter blues.

■ **BRING IN THE LIGHT.** Make your home shine, says Dr. Rosenthal. Add more lamps, brighten rooms with light-colored paint and carpets, raise window shades, and open draperies.

■ **DUPLICATE THE SUN.** Specially designed light fixtures, boxes, and visors offer full-spectrum lighting that replicate natural light without the harmful ultraviolet rays. Light therapy is a proven treatment for SAD. Typically, people with SAD benefit from sitting in front of a light box for 30 minutes to 2 hours daily, Dr. Rosenthal says.

A study of 96 Canadians with SAD found that light therapy was just as effective as Prozac, at improving mood. The light therapy brought relief after only 1 week, compared with Prozac which took twice as long. As a bonus, light therapy doesn't come with side effects such as agitation or difficulty sleeping.

■ **AWAKEN TO LIGHT.** If your symptoms are mild, put a bedroom light on a timer set to come on about an hour before you arise in the morning, says Dr. Rosenthal. "It helps people wake up in the morning, it helps them to feel better—even though it's just a regular bedside lamp—simply because the eyes are so very sensitive at that hour of the morning," he says. For

more severe SAD, purchase a specially designed dawn simulator.

■ **TAKE A WINDOW SEAT.** Sit by a window at work if you can. "Everybody wants a window seat," Dr. Rosenthal says. Even though the window's glass diminishes the sunlight's potency, you'll likely reap some mood-enhancing benefits.

■ **WALK OUTSIDE.** Go outdoors on a bright winter day, and you'll naturally soak up some of that feel-good light, says Dr. Rosenthal. Even on a cloudy day, you'll get more light than you would indoors. And it doesn't matter if you are bundled up. It's the light that is received through the eyes that helps to lift your mood. Aim for at least 30 minutes daily for an emotional and physical boost.

■ **GET FIT.** Whether you walk, jog, or cycle indoors or out, aerobic activity heightens mood-boosting brain chemicals that banish winter blues, says Dr. Rosenthal. For a one-two punch against SAD, combine exercise with light. For example, walk outside or set up a light box in front of your stationary cycle.

■ **MANAGE STRESS.** Don't set deadlines for winter if you have a choice. Similarly in winter, avoid long days of work that keep you out of the light. "Understand that winter is a time of year when you don't deal so well with stress," Dr. Rosenthal says.

■ **PREPARE FOR WINTER.** Anticipate those months when your overall energy may flag, says Brenda Byrne, Ph.D. Instead of waiting until the holiday season to shop for gifts or address greeting cards, for example, complete those tasks in the warmer months, when you're likely to feel more energetic.

■ **PENCIL IN A VACATION.** Then follow through. Even 3 or 4 days in a warm, sunny climate may pull you out of the doldrums, especially if your blues are mild. "Most people notice that within a few days, they really do feel better," says Dr. Byrne.

■ **SEEK WARMTH.** Some experts believe that temperature affects seasonal changes in behavior, says Dr. Byrne. "Lots of people with SAD also hate cold weather and tell me they can't get warm in winter, no matter how many layers of socks they put on," she says. People who dislike cold may simply avoid the outdoors in winter and get less sunlight, worsening their blues. Some possible strategies for staying warmer: Nudge the thermostat upward, wrap yourself in an electric blanket, or sip hot beverages.

■ **CURB CARBS.** "Many, many SAD patients claim to be carbohydrate addicts," says Dr. Rosenthal. But overdosing on carbohydrate-rich foods—comfort foods such as candy, cookies, cakes, potatoes, breads, and pastas—can lead to lethargy and weight gain. Substitute protein-dense meals, especially in the morning and afternoon. Instead of cereal at breakfast, try an omelet. Rather than a sandwich at lunch, opt for a chicken Caesar salad without the croutons.

What the Doctor Does

Martha Howard, M.D., bought a desk lamp called the Lights of America Sunlight Fluorescent Desk Lamp ($48.90, www.esplighting.com). "I turn it on every evening for about an hour while I check e-mails and work on my computer at my desk after work," she says. The special type of bulb in the lamp "extends" your daylight, fooling your body into thinking the day is longer.

■ **SUPPLEMENT YOUR DIET.** Reach for a daily multivitamin containing ample amounts of the Bs, such as vitamin B_6, thiamin, and folic acid, says Dr. Rosenthal. Studies show that the B vitamins, in particular, can enhance mood.

PANEL OF ADVISORS

BRENDA BYRNE, PH.D., IS A PSYCHOLOGIST WITH MARGOLIS BERMAN BYRNE HEALTH PSYCHOLOGY IN PHILADELPHIA AND THE FORMER DIRECTOR OF THE SEASONAL AFFECTIVE DISORDER PROGRAM OF THE LIGHT RESEARCH PROGRAM AT JEFFERSON MEDICAL COLLEGE OF THOMAS JEFFERSON UNIVERSITY IN PHILADELPHIA.

MARTHA HOWARD, M.D., IS MEDICAL DIRECTOR OF WELLNESS ASSOCIATES OF CHICAGO, AN INTEGRATIVE MEDICINE CENTER.

NORMAN E. ROSENTHAL, M.D., IS THE MEDICAL DIRECTOR OF CAPITAL CLINICAL RESEARCH ASSOCIATES IN THE NORTH BETHESDA–ROCKVILLE AREA AND HE MAINTAINS A PRIVATE PRACTICE, BOTH IN SUBURBAN MARYLAND. HE IS A FORMER SENIOR RESEARCHER AT THE NATIONAL INSTITUTE OF MENTAL HEALTH AND IS AUTHOR OF *WINTER BLUES: SEASONAL AFFECTIVE DISORDER* AND *THE EMOTIONAL REVOLUTION.*

Shingles

15 Tips to Combat the Pain

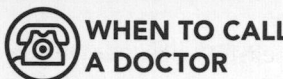
WHEN TO CALL A DOCTOR

If you have symptoms of shingles and notice a rash beginning to develop, it's important that you see a doctor as soon as possible, preferably within 72 hours. That's because the three antiviral drugs approved to treat shingles need to be started early in the course of the illness. When they're taken right away, these drugs have been proven to shorten the time of viral activity, help the rash to heal more quickly, and reduce the intensity and duration of shingles pain.

Also if your shingles pain is more than you can stand, see your doctor as soon as possible. This is no time for stoicism. Ignore your discomfort, and you could end up with irreversible nerve damage and years of pain, says Leon Robb, M.D.

It's a medical mystery. Shingles arises when the long-dormant chickenpox virus, known as herpes zoster, suddenly reawakens in nerve cells, making its way to the skin in a swath of burning pain, tingling, and numbness. On the skin's surface, it may cause a painful rash and blisters, generally on the chest or back, but sometimes on the face, arms, legs, even inside the mouth.

Scientists don't know why chickenpox leads, years later, to shingles in some people. Stress, illness, and a vulnerable immune system are thought to be contributing factors.

With the advent of the chickenpox vaccine for children, shingles will probably one day be just a footnote in medical history books. That offers little comfort to today's sufferers, many of whom are older adults. One in four people who have had chickenpox develop shingles.

As if the rash, blisters, and pain of a shingles outbreak weren't enough, in some people shingles pain may persist long after the rash disappears. This complication, called post-herpetic neuralgia, results from damaged nerve fibers. It can be exceedingly painful and difficult to treat. Around 40 percent of the people who get shingles develop post-herpetic neuralgia, which has been described as "the worst kind of pain imaginable."

It's important to see your doctor for this complicated condition.

Meanwhile, here's what you can do to make yourself as comfortable as possible.

AT THE OUTSET

Here is what the experts recommend for the beginning stages of shingles.

■ **REACH FOR PAIN RELIEF.** Jules Altman, M.D., favors Extra-Strength Tylenol.

■ **TAKE ST. JOHN'S WORT.** This herbal remedy may help to reduce nerve pain and has antiviral properties as well, says Sota Omoigui, M.D. He recommends taking 200 to 300 milligrams of St. John's wort two or three times daily until the pain is gone.

Note: Don't combine St. John's wort with any other medications. Lab studies found it boosts the power of a liver enzyme known as CYP3A4, which plays a role in dismantling more than half of all medicines.

■ **REACH FOR LARREA TRIDENTATA EXTRACT.** This traditional American Indian herb has antiviral properties and can be used for herpes simplex, says Cynthia Mervis Watson, M.D. She recommends taking 50 to 100 milligrams three times a day with food from the time of diagnosis until the shingles outbreak is gone.

■ **TRY LYSINE.** A number of studies show that the amino acid lysine can help inhibit the spread of the herpes virus. Not all studies on lysine point to that conclusion, however.

Trying lysine supplements at the onset of shingles can't hurt and might help, says Leon Robb, M.D.

Taking 1,000 milligrams of lysine three times a day with antioxidants can also reduce the severity of the virus, says Dr. Watson.

FOR SHINGLES BLISTERS

Once blisters appear, there are several ways you can get relief.

■ **DO NOTHING.** Leave the blisters alone unless your rash is really bad, says Dr. Robb. "You can retard healing if you irritate the skin by applying too many skin creams and ointments."

■ **MAKE A CALAMINE LINIMENT.** This recipe comes from James J. Nordlund, M.D. You may be able to get your local pharmacist to make it for you.

To calamine lotion add 20 percent isopropyl alcohol and ½ to 1 percent each of phenol and menthol. If the phenol is too strong or the menthol too cool, dilute the liniment with equal parts water.

"Use this as often as you want in the course of a day until the blisters are dried and scabbed over," says Dr. Nordlund. "Then stop using it."

■ **CONCOCT A CHLOROFORM-AND-ASPIRIN PASTE.** Mash two aspirin tablets into a powder. Add 2 tablespoons of chloroform and mix. Put the paste onto the affected skin with a clean cotton ball. You can apply the paste several times a day. You can also ask your pharmacist to make this mixture for you, Dr. Robb says.

The chloroform is said to dissolve soap residue, oil, and dead cells in the skin. That leaves the aspirin to soak into the skin folds and

---

Roll Up Your Sleeve

Just in case you're turning the page thinking you can't get shingles because you didn't have chickenpox, hold on. If you didn't have chickenpox as a child, you're at a greater risk for getting a more virulent adult form of it, which can lead to hepatitis, pneumonia, or heart failure. Fortunately, you can get protection with the chickenpox vaccine, called Varivax.

On the other hand, if you have had chickenpox, another vaccine called Zostavax can protect you from getting shingles. A federal panel of immunization experts suggests that everyone 60 and older receive the vaccine, which reduces the risk of a shingles episode by about 50 percent. If you do get sick, symptoms are 67 percent less severe, found a Centers for Disease Control and Prevention study.

Can't remember if you had chickenpox or not? A simple blood test can tell if you carry antibodies. If you have antibodies and you're younger than age 60, you don't need either vaccine. However if you're 60 or older and you have antibodies, you need the Zostavax vaccine. If you don't have antibodies and you're younger than age 60, you need the Varivax vaccine. If you're 60 or older and you don't have antibodies, you're an unusual case. Talk with your doctor about which vaccine is right for you.

---

desensitize the affected nerve endings. You should begin to feel better in 5 minutes. The relief can last for hours, even days. Skip this tip if you're allergic to aspirin.

■ **APPLY A WET DRESSING TO SEVERE ERUPTIONS.** Take a washcloth or towel, dip it in cold water, squeeze it out, and apply it to the affected area, says Dr. Nordlund. "The cooler it is, the better it feels," he says.

■ **STAY COOL.** Avoid anything that will make your blistered skin hotter. Heat will just macerate the skin, says Dr. Robb.

■ **SINK INTO A STARCH BATH.** If you have shingles on your head, skip to the next tip. But if the problem is below your neck, this can help. Just throw a handful of cornstarch or colloidal oatmeal, such as Aveeno, into your bathwater and settle in for a good soak, says Dr. Nordlund.

"People find this helpful, although the relief may not last long," he says. "I often have my patients do this 20 minutes before bed, then they take something for the pain to help them sleep."

■ **ZAP THE INFECTION WITH HYDROGEN PEROXIDE.** If the blisters become infected, try dabbing them with hydrogen peroxide. Don't dilute it. Straight out of the bottle is fine, says Dr. Robb.

■ **USE AN ANTIBIOTIC OINTMENT.** But be careful about which one you choose. Neomycin and Neosporin are notorious skin sensitizers, says Dr. Nordlund. Polysporin and erythromycin are better choices.

POSTBLISTER CARE

You may have some discomfort even after the blisters are gone. Here's what to do.

■ **TRY ZOSTRIX.** Zostrix is an over-the-counter remedy for shingles pain. Its active ingredient is capsaicin, found in hot peppers and used to make cayenne pepper. Scientists believe it works by blocking the production of a chemical needed to transmit pain impulses between nerve cells.

Using this topical ointment on blistering skin, however, is "like putting hot peppers on active shingles," says Dr. Altman. "The idea behind Zostrix is its counterirritant effect. It is for healed skin that has a pain sensation, not for an open, oozing infection."

■ **GET THE BENEFITS OF CAPSAICIN IN YOUR DIET.** Sprinkling cayenne pepper on your food may speed pain relief because it contains the same extract as the capsaicin in pain-relieving creams. Put it on eggs, soups, and casseroles, or use it in marinades and sauces.

■ **CHILL OUT WITH ICE.** If you still have pain after the blisters have healed, put ice in a plastic bag and stroke the skin vigorously, says Dr. Robb. "What we're trying to do here is confuse the nerves."

■ **SEEK EMOTIONAL HELP.** Sometimes, for some people, long-lasting shingles pain may point to some underlying emotional need that's not being met, says Dr. Altman. Is the pain diverting your attention away from some other problem? Or is the pain diverting much-needed attention to you? It's an issue to consider, he says, and one that you may want to discuss with your doctor.

PANEL OF ADVISORS

Shinsplints

11 Ways to Soothe Sore Legs

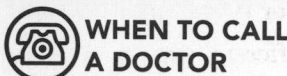

WHEN TO CALL A DOCTOR

Because some experts believe shinsplints may actually be stress fractures in an early stage, telling the difference between the two is sometimes tricky. Even so, shinsplints can become full-blown stress fractures with continued abuse, so seeing your doctor for an early diagnosis is crucial.

"With a stress fracture, you're going to have pinpoint pain, about the size of a dime or quarter," says trainer Marjorie Albohm. "If somebody asks you where it hurts, you'll be able to go right to it, put one or two fingers on it, and tell them exactly where it is. It'll be right on or around a bony area, and it's point-specific. A shinsplint will be an aching discomfort up and down the whole lower leg."

Shinsplints aren't hard to get. Faulty posture, poor shoes, fallen arches, insufficient warmups, poor running mechanics, poor walking mechanics, and overtraining can lead to the telltale shin pain.

Shinsplints are one of the most common and disabling conditions in aerobics. Long-distance runners have probably suffered with them since the first road was paved.

Most people know when they have shinsplints, but very few—experts included—know what they are. Most doctors prefer the terms *tendinitis*, or *periostitis*, though they can't say for certain which of those terms, if either, actually describes the condition.

Some say shinsplints are the start of a stress fracture. Others contend they are a muscle irritation. Still others think they are an irritation of the tendon that attaches muscle to the bone.

The symptoms of shinsplints are often confused with those of stress fracture. But shinsplints typically include pain in the shin of one or both legs, though there may or may not be a specific area of tenderness. Pain and aching will be felt in the front of the leg after activity, although it may occur during activity as the condition progresses.

The remedies here are designed to help keep that shinsplint condition from progressing to the point of stress fracture and to let you continue your active lifestyle without causing undue harm. Let pain be your guide. If anything recommended here causes increased discomfort, don't do it.

■ **TAKE A BREAK.** If walking or running is giving you shinsplints, cut back for 3 to 8 weeks to give the tissues time to heal. Keep in shape by cross-training with low-impact exercises such as cycling or swimming. When you're ready to walk or run again, go on a dirt path and limit it to 20 minutes at a moderate pace. Increase your distance or speed slightly each week. If you feel sore again, dial it back for a few days, and when you resume again take it even more slowly.

■ **START WITH THE GROUND.** Hard, unyielding surfaces can produce shinsplints in an instant. "Start by looking at the surface," says athletic trainer Marjorie Albohm. "If you're walking, running, dancing, playing basketball, or whatever on a surface that has no give, then you need to change that."

For people involved in aerobics, injuries are highest on concrete floors covered with carpet, while wood floors over air space are the least damaging. If you're doing aerobics on a nonresilient floor, make sure that the instructor teaches only low-impact aerobics or that high-quality foam mats are provided. For runners, choose grass or dirt before asphalt, and asphalt before concrete. Concrete, however, is the hardest on your legs and should be avoided.

Depending on where you live, you might have the best of both worlds—soft sidewalks. More than 140 cities in 28 states, including Washington, D.C., and Seattle, have installed sidewalks made from old car tires called Rub-

bersidewalks. This product was invented by a California-based company as an environmental measure, but the added benefit is decreased impact and a more forgiving landing should you take a spill.

■ **THEN MOVE TO THE SHOES.** If you can't change your surface, or if you find that's not the problem, look at different footwear. Choose a shoe with good arch support, shock absorption, and fit, says Albohm.

For people who participate in activities that cause a lot of forefoot impact such as aerobics, judge a shoe on its ability to absorb shock in that area. The best test is to try the shoes on in the store and jump up and down, both on the toes and flat-footed. The impact with the floor should be firm but not jarring.

For runners, the choice is a bit more difficult. Research has shown that about 58 percent of all runners with shinsplints also pronate excessively (meaning the foot rolls to the inside). Choosing a shoe for pronation control sometimes means less cushioning. If you're a pronator with shinsplints, motion-control shoes are probably what you need most. These shoes are rigid and durable, and they limit pronation.

■ **CHANGE SHOES OFTEN.** One way to get as much cushioning as possible in your shoes is to change them frequently. Runners should replace their shoes every 300 miles, says Gary M. Gordon, D.P.M. Less mileage means new shoes once a year. People who participate in aerobics, tennis, or basketball twice a week need new shoes two or three times a year, while those who participate up to four times a week need them every 2 months.

■ **PUT IT ON RICE.** As soon as you notice shinsplint pain, follow the rules of RICE: rest, ice, compression, and elevation for 20 to 30 minutes a day. The experts swear by it.

Keep your icing routine simple, Albohm says. Just prop the leg up, wrap it with an elastic bandage, and place the ice pack on it for 20 to 30 minutes.

■ **GO FOR CONTRAST.** A variation on the RICE treatment is the contrast method, which seems especially effective for pain on the inner leg. With this method, alternate 1 minute of ice with 1 minute of heat. Do this before any activity that can cause shinsplint pain, and continue it for at least 12 minutes.

■ **MASTER MASSAGE.** "For shinsplints in the front of the leg, you want to massage the area right near the edge of the shin—not directly on it," says masseur Rich Phaigh. "If

you work right on the bone, it just seems to make the inflammation worse."

To massage away shinsplint pain, sit on the floor with one knee bent and the foot flat on the ground. Start by lightly stroking both sides of the bone using the palms of your hands, gliding them back and forth from knee to ankle. Repeat this stroking motion several times. Then wrap your hands around the calf and, using the tips of your fingers, stroke deeply on each side of the bone from ankle to knee. Cover the area, using as much pressure as possible.

"What you want to do is restore length and relieve tightness in the tendons at the top and bottom of the shins," Phaigh says, noting that a good massage helps improve circulation in the area, too.

■ **CORRECT FAULTY FEET.** Flat feet or very high arches can sometimes cause shinsplints, Dr. Gordon says. "If you have flat feet, the muscle on the inside of your calf has to work harder and gets fatigued quicker," he says, "making the bone take more of a pounding."

If you're flat-footed, you may need additional shock-absorbing material or arch support in your shoes. Inserts are available at sporting goods stores, but it might be best to see a podiatrist before adding inserts on your own.

Pain on the outside of the lower leg is sometimes associated with very high arches, Dr. Gordon says. "Relieving pain requires a lot of stretching exercises, as well as strengthening the muscles and maybe adding orthotics."

Favorite Fixes

WHAT IT IS: Stretching helps keep the calf muscles limber.

WHY IT WORKS: It relieves the tightness across your shins.

HOW TO USE IT: "To stretch the calves, which can relieve tightness across the shins, I stand on a step or curb and hang my heels over the edge," says Maggie Spilner, a writer and editor in Easton, Pennsylvania. "It's very effective."

■ **STRETCH THOSE CALVES.** Stretching the Achilles tendon and the calf muscles is an excellent preventive measure for shinsplints, Albohm says. "If you're a woman wearing 2-inch heels every day, you're not stretching either of those at all."

Stretching helps, because shortened calf muscles tend to throw more weight and stress forward to the shins. Place your hands on a wall, extend one leg behind the other, and press the back heel slowly to the floor. Do this 20 times and repeat with the other leg.

■ **NOW TEND TO THE TENDONS.** Dr. Gordon offers this simple technique for stretching the Achilles tendon: Keep both feet flat on the ground about 6 inches apart. Then bend your ankles and knees forward while keeping your back straight. Go to the point of tightness and hold for 30 seconds. "You should feel it really stretching down in the lower part of the calf," he says. Repeat the exercise 10 times.

■ **STRENGTHEN YOUR MUSCLES.** To help keep your shinsplints from coming back, strengthen the muscles in the front of your lower leg, the anterior tibialis, with this simple exercise. Stand and lift your toes toward your shins 20 times. Work up to three sets. After that, to add resistance, place a 2- or 3-pound ankle weight across your toes.

PANEL OF ADVISORS

MARJORIE ALBOHM IS A CERTIFIED ATHLETIC TRAINER AND PRESIDENT OF THE NATIONAL ATHLETIC TRAINERS ASSOCIATION IN DALLAS. SHE SERVED ON THE MEDICAL STAFFS FOR THE 1980 WINTER AND 1996 SUMMER OLYMPICS AND THE 1987 PAN AMERICAN GAMES.

GARY M. GORDON, D.P.M., IS CHIEF OF PODIATRY AT THE UNIVERSITY OF PENNSYLVANIA SPORTS MEDICINE CENTER AND HAS A SPORTS MEDICINE PRACTICE IN GLENSIDE, PENNSYLVANIA.

RICH PHAIGH IS THE OWNER OF A THERAPEUTIC MASSAGE CLINIC IN EUGENE, OREGON. HE HAS TAUGHT MORE THAN 250 CLASSES IN ADVANCED THERAPEUTIC TECHNIQUES IN THE UNITED STATES AND ABROAD. HE HAS WORKED ON THE LIKES OF RUNNING STARS ALBERTO SALAZAR AND JOAN SAMUELSON.

Side Stitches

6 Ways to Avoid the Nuisance

A stitch or catch in the side—a sharp, temporary pain—is caused by a stretching of the ligaments that run downward from the diaphragm to hold up the liver. You breathe once for each two strides, and you breathe out when one foot, usually the right, strikes the ground. So your diaphragm goes up when the force of your foot strike causes your liver to go down. This stretches the ligament and makes it hurt, explains Gabe Mirkin, M.D.

This often happens to runners.

You also can get side stitches from walking, or even laughing. Here's how to handle them.

■ **STOP.** When the pain hits, stop whatever you are doing. You need to relax to calm your twitching muscle.

■ **SLOW DOWN AND WALK.** If you're running when you get a stitch, sometimes just slowing to a walk is enough to calm that jerking muscle, says Suki Munsell, Ph.D. When the twinge fades, speed up again.

■ **PRESS HERE.** Stop running and press your fingers deep into your liver to raise it up toward your diaphragm, says Dr. Mirkin. This releases the stretched ligaments. At the same time, purse your lips and blow out as hard as you can against tightly held lips.

This lowers your diaphragm. The pain will disappear and you will be able to resume running.

■ **BREATHE IN, BREATHE OUT.** Continue to massage your aching side and work to slow your breathing to a regular pace. Getting your breathing back to a steady rhythm will help stop the ache.

■ **MASSAGE YOUR DIAPHRAGM.** Like any muscle, the diaphragm needs to be warmed up before it exercises. So before you stretch your legs, give your diaphragm a breath massage and get it in working order. Sit on the floor and place one hand on your chest, the other on your belly. As you breathe, both hands should move up and down, indicating that you're using your full breathing capacity, including your diaphragm because a warmed diaphragm is less likely to stitch.

■ **STOP TO GO.** Any aerobic activity will slow or stop the digestive process while the blood rushes to help the muscles. That's why runners are told not to eat at least 2 hours before a race. It's also the reason runners sometimes get diarrhea if they drink a lot of water during a race.

Their advice? Be careful what and when you eat before you exercise. Eat plenty of fiber. Try to have a bowel movement before you begin any exercise if you are prone to side stitches.

PANEL OF ADVISORS

GABE MIRKIN, M.D., IS A BOARD-CERTIFIED PHYSICIAN IN SPORTS MEDICINE AND PRACTICES IN KENSINGTON, MARYLAND. HE IS AUTHOR OF A NUMBER OF BOOKS ON THE SUBJECT.

SUKI MUNSELL, PH.D., IS A REGISTERED MOVEMENT THERAPIST AND FOUNDING DIRECTOR OF THE DYNAMIC HEALTH AND FITNESS INSTITUTE IN MARIN COUNTY, CALIFORNIA. A FITNESS CONSULTANT, SHE HAS A DOCTORATE IN MOVEMENT EDUCATION AND BODY TRANSFORMATIONS.

Sinusitis

13 Infection Fighters

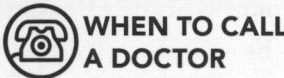

WHEN TO CALL A DOCTOR

If you've tried self-treatment for 3 to 4 days and still have sinus pain, pressure, and stuffiness, you need to see a doctor to help clear up the infection and drain your sinuses, advises Terence M. Davidson, M.D. "Otherwise, your sinuses could abscess into your eye, or worse, into your brain."

You may also have chronic sinusitis, which can be a recurrent or prolonged disorder lasting for months or even years. Depending on the cause, you may need to take a longer course of antibiotics than for acute sinusitis, or undergo a sinus drainage procedure or surgery to break up the blockage. A sinus specialist can perform x-rays or other tests to discover what's causing your congestion, be it bacteria, an obstruction such as polyps, allergies, untreated acute sinusitis, or a sensitivity to medications such as birth control pills or aspirin.

Sinuses are air-filled pockets that serve as small air-quality-control centers under your cheekbones, above your eyes and nose, and behind your eye sockets. It's their job to help warm, moisten, purify, and generally condition the air you breathe before it hits your lungs. When your sinuses are functioning properly, entering bacteria get trapped and filtered out by mucus and minute nasal hairs called cilia.

This little air-flow system may gum up, however, if something impedes the cilia, if a cold clogs the sinus openings, or if an allergen swells the sinus linings. Then air gets trapped, pressure builds, the mucus stagnates, and bacteria or other organisms can breed. Infection and inflammation of the sinuses can set in, a disorder called sinusitis.

When you try to sleep, it's as if you've sprung a slow leak. All night long, the drip, drip of nasal fluid trickles down your throat, sending you into coughing spasms.

Pressure and pain around the face, teeth, or eyes, and often a headache and a thick green or yellow nasal discharge, are the hallmarks of acute sinusitis. You may run a fever as well. Acute sinusitis is usually caused by viruses or bacteria and can last a month or longer.

If you get clogged up too many times, you may wind up with a permanent thickening of the sinus membranes and a chronic stuffy nose. Less common than acute sinusitis, chronic sinusitis is caused by allergies—especially to dust, mold, pollen, and certain fungi—or other conditions and typically lasts longer than 8 weeks.

Doctors generally prescribe antibiotics to clear the infection if it's bacterial. However, they often suggest you wait it out for a week. After 7 days, about three-quarters of sinus infections will improve without prescription medications, especially if the condition is mild,

with only moderate pain and a fever of less than 100°F. If symptoms are the same or worse, or if they initially improve but then get worse, it's a good sign that the infection is bacterial.

In the meantime, you can take a number of steps to feel better. Here's what the doctors say you can do to unstuff your sinuses, reduce pain and pressure, and get the air flowing freely.

■ **GET STEAM ON THE RUN.** If stuffiness hits during the day when you're at work or on the run, get a cup of hot coffee, tea, or soup, cup your hands over the top of the mug, and sniff, suggests Howard M. Druce, M.D. It won't work as well as a steam bath, but it will provide some relief.

■ **HUMIDIFY YOUR HOME.** Running a humidifier in your bedroom prevents your nasal and sinus passages from drying out, says Bruce W. Jafek, M.D. Just make sure you clean it once a week so that fungi don't invade your humidifier.

You can use either a cool-mist or a warm-mist humidifier. Dr. Jafek suggests starting with a cool-mist machine. Though the room won't heat up like it would with a warm-mist unit, cool-mist machines may be safer because they won't cause a burn if accidentally tipped, he says.

■ **TRY A STEAM SHOWER.** Put a few drops of eucalyptus oil on the floor of a hot, running shower. Inhale the steam. The humidity will help to keep the mucus flowing and your sinuses drained.

Note: This could be slippery, so be careful

Cures from the Kitchen

The way to find sinus relief may be through your stomach—eating foods that make your eyes water or nose run will help burst through your sinus blockage, says Howard M. Druce, M.D. Here's what he recommends.

GARLIC. This pungent herb contains the same chemical found in a drug that makes mucus less sticky, says Dr. Druce.

HORSERADISH. This pungent root contains a chemical similar to one found in decongestants, he says. The bottled variety works just fine.

CAJUN SPICE SEASONING. You probably can't go wrong if you order Cajun food. These spicy dishes are made with cayenne chile peppers, which contain capsaicin, a substance that can stimulate the nerve fibers and may act as a natural nasal decongestant. Other hot peppers contain this potent compound as well. Look for the smaller varieties. They're usually hotter and have more capsaicin than the larger types—or use ground red pepper (cayenne) or other ground chile powders in cooking.

551

getting into and out of the shower. Also, the room may become too hot for children.

■ **BATHE YOUR NOSTRILS DAILY.** To flush out stale nasal secretions, Dr. Jafek suggests using saline nasal sprays or drops, such as Breathe Right or Ayr. Or make your own solution by mixing 1 teaspoon of table salt with 2 cups of warm water and a pinch of baking soda. Pour the liquid into a squirt bottle or medicine dropper, tilt your head back, close one nostril with your thumb, and squirt the solution into the open nostril while sniffing. Then blow that nostril gently. Repeat on the other side. You can also use a mister to spray the solution into your nostrils, but keep your head in an upright position.

■ **MOISTURIZE.** People complain of postnasal drip, but it is not a disease, says Hueston King, M.D. Your nose provides nearly all of the moisture for your lungs and respiratory system. A healthy nose produces between 1 and 3 quarts of clear, watery mucus a day. But this moisturizing mucus decreases as we age. As it decreases, you notice the *other* type of nasal mucus more, the sticky nasal mucus that picks up contaminants and takes them to your throat where they are swallowed and destroyed by stomach acid. That mucus is what we call postnasal drip.

To replace the lost moisturizing mucus, try Ponaris Nasal Emollient. (It's so effective that it's stocked on the space shuttle for the astronauts.) It comes as nose drops, but it works much better as a spray, so pour it into a nasal spray bottle and use as needed, says Dr. King.

What the Doctor Does

From the time I was 6 years old, I had chronic sinus congestion, says Martha Howard, M.D. I got rid of it at age 66, using NeilMed Sinus Rinse. My whole sinus health has been better ever since!

To use the rinse, add it to water. Lean over a sink and squeeze the squishy, plastic bottle containing the rinse so the solution goes up your nose, and then blow your nose. That's it. It's easy to use and because it contains baking soda (along with the salt that's in most nasal rinses), it doesn't burn your nostrils.

I also use a product called Neti Wash Plus with Zinc, which also contains echinacea and goldenseal, two herbs with mild, natural antibiotic action. You can buy both of these products online and at drugstores.

■ **USE MEDICATED NASAL SPRAYS SPARINGLY.** Medicated nose sprays or drops, such as Afrin or Neo-Synephrine, are fine to use in a pinch, but frequent use of these products could actually prolong the condition or even make it worse, says Terence M. Davidson, M.D. It's what specialists call the "rebound effect."

Initially, the sprays shrink your nasal linings, explains Dr. Davidson. "But then the mucosa reacts by swelling even more than before, creating a vicious cycle of use. It can take weeks for the swelling to finally subside after you stop using the sprays."

■ **GET SOME OTC RELIEF.** Try over-the-counter decongestants such as Sudafed, pain relievers such as acetaminophen (Tylenol), and sinus-irrigating rinses (such as SinuCleanse) to feel better.

■ **APPLY PRESSURE.** Rubbing your sore sinuses brings a fresh blood supply to the area and soothing relief, suggests Dr. Jafek. Press your thumbs firmly on both sides of your nose and hold for 15 to 30 seconds. Repeat.

■ **USE HEAT.** Apply moist heat to tender sinuses, to ease sinus pain, Dr. Druce says. Place a warm washcloth over your eyes and cheekbones and leave it there until you feel the pain subside. It may take only a few minutes.

■ **EAT AN ANTI-INFLAMMATORY DIET.** The foods you eat play a tremendous part in your health, says Martha Howard, M.D. Avoid wheat and dairy products as much as possible. Instead, focus on fish, chicken, and fresh fruits and vegetables. As a bonus, eating this way keeps you from consuming processing chemicals, such as dyes and additives. This anti-inflammatory diet will help ease the systematic inflammation that is contributing to your sinus woes.

PANEL OF ADVISORS

TERENCE M. DAVIDSON, M.D., IS A PROFESSOR OF HEAD AND NECK SURGERY AND DIRECTOR OF THE NASAL DYSFUNCTION CLINIC AT THE UNIVERSITY OF CALIFORNIA, SAN DIEGO, MEDICAL CENTER.

HOWARD M. DRUCE, M.D., IS A CLINICAL PROFESSOR OF MEDICINE IN THE DIVISION OF ALLERGY AND IMMUNOLOGY AT THE UNIVERSITY OF MEDICINE AND DENTISTRY OF NEW JERSEY/NEW JERSEY MEDICAL SCHOOL IN NEWARK.

MARTHA HOWARD, M.D., IS MEDICAL DIRECTOR OF WELLNESS ASSOCIATES OF CHICAGO, AN INTEGRATIVE MEDICINE CENTER.

BRUCE W. JAFEK, M.D., IS A PROFESSOR IN THE DEPARTMENT OF OTOLARYNGOLOGY AT THE UNIVERSITY OF COLORADO SCHOOL OF MEDICINE IN DENVER. HE SERVED AS CHAIR OF THE DEPARTMENT FOR 22 YEARS BEFORE RETURNING TO CLINICAL PRACTICE AND TEACHING.

HUESTON KING, M.D., IS A CLINICAL PROFESSOR OF EAR, NOSE, AND THROAT AT THE UNIVERSITY OF FLORIDA MEDICAL SCHOOL IN GAINESVILLE. HE IS ALSO A RETIRED EAR, NOSE, AND THROAT SPECIALIST IN VENICE, FLORIDA.

Snoring

13 Tips for a Silent Night

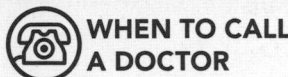
WHEN TO CALL A DOCTOR

Modern science is now proving what Shakespeare wrote long ago in *The Tempest:* "Thou dost snore distinctly. There's meaning in thy snores." In general, says Philip Smith, M.D., the louder your snore, the more likely it's related to a medical problem.

"If home remedies don't ease your snoring or if you have snoring *and* chronic stuffiness, or snoring *and* heartburn, see a doctor," says James Herdegen, M.D.

Snoring has long been the subject of jokes, cartoons, and sitcom episodes, but in a significant number of people, it is no laughing matter. Snoring can be a serious problem, disrupting normal sleeping patterns and disturbing partners as they try to sleep through the noise.

Snoring is extremely common, affecting the sleep habits and lives of 90 million American adults and their partners. Sixty-seven percent of married adults say their partners snore. One British survey found that if your spouse snores, by your 50th wedding anniversary, you'll have lost about 4 years' worth of sleep!

Besides just feeling sleepy all the time and the risk of nodding off during *Lost*, people who don't get enough sleep can develop memory and mood problems, and they're more likely to be involved in car accidents. (Researchers in New Zealand discovered that people who had fewer than 5 hours of sleep the previous night increased their chances of a car crash by a whopping 170 percent.)

Clinically, moderate snorers are those who snore every night but perhaps only when on their backs or only part of the night, says Philip Westbrook, M.D.

A wind ensemble located in the back of the throat orchestrates the sound made by a snorer. "The tissue in the upper airway in the back of the throat relaxes during sleep," says Philip Smith, M.D. "When you breathe in, it causes this tissue to vibrate. The effect is very similar to a wind instrument."

A physician should evaluate heavy snorers to make sure they don't have a serious sleeping disorder called sleep apnea. For light or occasional snoring, here are a number of ways to have a silent night.

■ **GO ON A DIET.** Lose weight, says Jacob Teitelbaum, M.D. If you are overweight, you probably have gained weight on inside of your neck as well. If your collar size is 17 or over, you may be obstructing your airway. It's like pinching a balloon.

"You don't have to be a 2-ton Tony to develop snoring. Just being a little overweight can bring on a problem," says Dr. Smith. But the more overweight you are, the more likely it is that your airway collapses while you sleep, causing snoring.

A reasonable goal: Lose 10 percent of your body weight.

■ **AVOID ALCOHOL.** Because alcohol relaxes the muscles in your throat, uvula, and palate, it makes snoring even worse. Don't drink for at least 3 hours before bedtime.

■ **STAY OFF YOUR BACK.** Sleeping in the supine position almost always makes snoring worse, says Dr. Westbrook.

Sew a pocket on the back of a T-shirt and place a tennis ball in the pocket. Use the T-shirt as a pajama top and sleep in the shirt. Rolling onto the hard ball will train you to stay off your back, says James Herdegen, M.D.

■ **PROP YOURSELF UP.** Try propping your head up with an extra pillow. This will open your airway more and alleviate the snoring.

■ **RAISE THE HEAD OF YOUR BED.** Elevating the bed can help minimize snoring. "Elevate the upper torso, not just the head," says Dr. Westbrook. "Put a couple of bricks under the legs at the head of your bed."

■ **TRY THIS PILLOW.** The FDA-approved Sona pillow ($69.99, www.sonapillow.com), developed by a Harvard-trained neurologist, is specially designed to tilt your head and open your airways. In one study conducted at Florida Hospital in Kissimmee, the pillow decreased or eliminated snoring in nearly every patient studied and reduced sleep interruptions from an average of 17 an hour to fewer than 5.

■ **DECONGEST YOUR NOSE.** If you have a cold, the snoring can get very loud, says Dr. Herdegen. Decongestants can help, such as antihistamines containing cetirizine hydrochloride (Zyrtec) or nasal sprays such as Afrin. They can shrink nasal mucosa and improve airflow to reduce snoring. However, if you use nasal sprays chronically, they can actually make you more stuffy, not less. Try them for 3 days, then give them a rest or see a doctor.

■ **HUMIDIFY YOUR ROOM.** Another way to unstuff your nose is to run a humidifier in your bedroom at night, says Dr. Herdegen. This will help encourage your sinuses to drain. Smearing some Vicks VapoRub on your chest at night will help open up your nasal passages, too, easing your snoring.

■ **GET HELP FOR HEARTBURN.** "Some people who snore actually have esophageal reflux; the acid can get up into your voice box

When Snoring Is Serious

One of the worst problems associated with snoring is a condition called sleep apnea, a potentially life-threatening disorder, in which breathing actually stops during sleep for at least 10 seconds and up to a minute, or even longer.

This can happen hundreds of times a night, contributing to high blood pressure, cardiovascular disease, memory problems, weight gain, impotency, and headaches. Sleep-deprived apnea patients have job-related problems and may be unsafe behind the wheel, according to the Washington, D.C.–based American Sleep Apnea Association.

Recent Yale University research shows that sleep apnea can double your risk of having a stroke. It also raises blood pressure and the risk of blood clots, the researchers say.

Sleep apnea afflicts more than 12 million Americans, especially overweight men older than 40. But women and children can have sleep apnea, too.

Symptoms of sleep apnea include loud snoring, that is, loud enough to be heard outside the room; snoring punctuated by periods of silence, gasping, or choking; and extreme tiredness during the day. If this sounds like you, see your doctor. It's usually treated with lifestyle modifications, such as exercise to lose weight, or in more severe cases, with a breathing mask that keeps airways open.

To find out the extent of your snoring, head to a local sleep clinic. For the address of a sleep clinic near you, contact the American Academy of Sleep Medicine, One Westbrook Corporate Center, Suite 920, Westchester, IL 60154, or visit the Web site at www.aasmnet.org.

If you're not sure just how loud or frequent your snoring is, tape record yourself at night, suggests James Herdegen, M.D.

and cause irritation and swelling," says Dr. Herdegen. If your snoring is caused by acid reflux, in addition to trying over-the-counter acid-suppressing medications such as omeprazole (Prilosec), try elevating the head of your bed as mentioned earlier. This will tip your body a bit so the acid can't reflux up as high at night.

■ **SUPPRESS YOUR COUGH.** If you're getting over a cold and have a postcold cough, it might be irritating your upper airway, causing swelling and aggravating your snoring, says Dr. Herdegen. Try taking an over-the-counter cough medication. Guaifenesin (Robitussin), for example, will ease your cough and also help loosen your nasal secretions.

■ **STRIP IT.** If you snore but you don't have underlying sinus problems or coughing, you might turn down the volume by wearing an over-the-counter nasal strip, such as Breathe

Right, says Dr. Herdegen. These adhesive strips pull open the nasal passages so they're less narrow, giving you better airflow.

■ **GET M.A.D.** A mandibular advancement device, also known as an oral appliance, is shaped like a nighttime mouth guard. It keeps the lower jaw pushed out, widening the airway and reducing noisy turbulence. Studies show that it is 90 percent effective at reducing snore noise. It costs $500 to $1,000 and lasts for at least 3 years. You can get fitted for one by your dentist.

For a less expensive option, you can buy an over-the-counter device called a snore guard, says Dr. Herdegen. You boil the device and then fit it into your mouth to create an impression of your teeth and dental structure. The goal is to bring your lower jaw forward a bit to make the back of your throat less crowded.

■ **LEARN TO DIDGERIDOO.** In a Swiss study of 25 sleep apnea patients, doctors asked half to practice the Aboriginal wind instrument for 25 minutes, 6 days a week. After 4 months, the people who played the didgeridoo reported fewer symptoms, such as daytime sleepiness, and their bed partners said they experienced a third less nighttime noise.

Turns out the didgeridoo requires a breathing technique that strengthens muscles in the upper airways. The researchers says you'd likely get similar results with other wind instruments, such as flute, oboe, or clarinet.

■ **CONSIDER A SPRAY.** If all else fails, you might want to give an anti-snoring spray a try, says Dr. Herdegen. These sprays lubricate the back of the throat thereby preventing tissues from sticking together and allowing air to pass through more easily.

PANEL OF ADVISORS

JAMES HERDEGEN, M.D., IS MEDICAL DIRECTOR OF THE SLEEP SCIENCE CENTER AT THE UNIVERSITY OF ILLINOIS IN CHICAGO.

PHILIP SMITH, M.D., IS A PROFESSOR OF MEDICINE AND A PHYSICIAN IN THE DIVISION OF PULMONARY AND CRITICAL CARE, WHO SPECIALIZES IN SLEEP DISORDERS, AT THE JOHNS HOPKINS UNIVERSITY SCHOOL OF MEDICINE IN BALTIMORE.

JACOB TEITELBAUM, M.D., IS A BOARD-CERTIFIED INTERNIST AND MEDICAL DIRECTOR OF THE FIBROMYALGIA AND FATIGUE CENTERS, WITH LOCATIONS THROUGHOUT THE COUNTRY.

PHILIP WESTBROOK, M.D., IS CHAIRMAN OF THE BOARD AND MEDICAL DIRECTOR OF ADVANCED BRAIN MONITORING, A COMPANY IN CARLSBAD, CALIFORNIA, WHICH DEVELOPS SOFTWARE AND TECHNOLOGY THAT CAN BE INTEGRATED INTO A PORTABLE DEVICE FOR RECORDING SNORING AND SLEEP APNEA. HE IS ALSO CHIEF MEDICAL OFFICER FOR VENTUS MEDICAL, INC., A COMPANY THAT HAS DEVELOPED A TREATMENT FOR SLEEP APNEA. HE WAS FOUNDER AND FORMER DIRECTOR OF THE SLEEP DISORDERS CENTERS AT THE MAYO CLINIC IN ROCHESTER, MINNESOTA, AND CEDARS-SINAI MEDICAL CENTER IN LOS ANGELES; PRESIDENT OF THE AMERICAN ACADEMY OF SLEEP MEDICINE; AND EDITOR OF THE JOURNAL *SLEEP MEDICINE REVIEWS*.

Sore Throat

14 Ways to Put Out the Fire

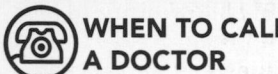
**WHEN TO CALL
A DOCTOR**

A strep throat is an extremely painful bacterial infection that may come on suddenly. Fortunately, says Hueston King, M.D., the vast majority of bacterial infections, including strep, generally respond quite well to one course of an appropriate antibiotic.

Because sore throats can have so many causes, some symptoms need to be evaluated by a doctor. These include:

■ Severe, prolonged, or recurrent sore throats

■ Difficulty breathing, swallowing, or opening the mouth

■ Joint pains, earache, or a lump in the neck

■ Rash or a fever above 101°F

■ Hoarseness lasting 2 weeks or longer

■ White patches on your throat (look with a flashlight)

■ Blood in saliva or phlegm

A burning, irritated throat can disrupt your sleep, interfere with your work, and make you feel generally miserable. Your raw throat may be an early warning sign of a cold, the flu, or some other viral or bacterial infection. Sometimes a sore throat is just a minor irritation caused by winter's low humidity or too much cheering at a football game.

Whatever the cause, here's how doctors say you can feel better fast.

■ **SUCK ON LOZENGES.** If your sore throat is caused by a viral infection, antibiotics won't help it. Most lozenges are only soothing, but medicated lozenges containing phenol, such as Cepastat, may do some good, says Hueston King, M.D. The phenol can kill surface germs, keeping the invaders in check until your body has a chance to build up its resistance. Phenol's mild anesthetic action numbs raw nerve endings so that your throat doesn't feel as scratchy. These lozenges come in various strengths, so follow package directions to find out how often you should use them.

■ **GARGLE!** If it hurts when you swallow, the sore area may be high enough in your throat that gargling will bathe and soothe it, says Dr. King. So gargle frequently with one of the solutions on the next page. But be aware that if you're hoarse or have a cough, the sore spot is farther down, and gargling won't help.

■ **Baking Soda.** Combine 2 teaspoons of baking soda with 16 ounces of warm water. Gargle and swish your mouth with this solution, says R. Thomas Glass, D.D.S., Ph.D. If you store the solution in a plastic bottle with a cap, it will last for several days.

Dr. Glass suggests buying the smallest box of baking soda and keeping the opened box in a ziplock bag to retain the baking soda's potency.

■ **Salt.** Gargling with saltwater is a time-tested remedy for a sore throat. Simply mix 1 teaspoon of salt into 8 ounces of water. Warm water is particularly soothing. But here's how to take it to the next level. Simply Gargle packets are individually wrapped liquid doses that contain a premixed amount of water, salt, vitamin C, and grapeseed extract. Break open the packet, gargle with the contents, and then spit it out. No cup, no fuss, no mess.

You can buy a 12-pack of them for around $7 at drugstores.

■ **GET UP A HEAD OF STEAM.** In the face of a worse-than-normal dry or sore throat, try inhaling steam from your bathroom tap, says Jason Surow, M.D. Run very hot water in the bathroom basin to build up steam. With the water running, lean over the sink, drape a towel over your head to capture some of the steam, and inhale deeply through your mouth

> ## What the Doctor Does
>
> Irwin Ziment, M.D., has heard of a home-made gargle for sore throat that consists of a mixture of horseradish, honey, and cloves in warm water. If you try it, use it carefully, he advises; otherwise, it could irritate your throat even further. There have been a few reports of toxicity with ingestion of clove oil, but cloves appear to be safe. In fact, they're widely used in commercial foods, beverages, and toothpastes.

and nose for 5 to 10 minutes. Repeat several times a day if necessary. Personal facial steamers, such as HoMedics and Conair, are also available in department and discount stores and drugstores.

■ **OPEN YOUR NOSE.** If part of the reason you're breathing through your mouth is because your nose is clogged, says Dr. Surow, open it with an over-the-counter medicated decongestant nasal spray or drops, such as Afrin or Neo-Synephrine. But you should limit its use to a day or two.

■ **INHALE SEA BREEZES.** If you can't actually go someplace humid, such as the seashore, get the same sort of salty atmosphere from a saline nasal spray or drops, available at any drugstore. When you inhale the mist, says Dr. Surow, the salt-based spray moistens your nose and drips down the back of your throat to help increase humidity there. Among the brands available are Ocean, NaSal, and Ayr.

To make your own saltwater rinse, Robert Rountree, M.D., recommends stirring about $1/4$ teaspoon of sea salt and $1/8$ teaspoon of baking soda into 4 ounces of warm water. To apply, lean forward over a sink, breathe through your mouth (to prevent the solution from coming out of your mouth and creating a very unpleasant choking sensation), and tilt your head to the left side. Pour the mixture into your right nostril. Tilt your head to the right to rinse the left nostril.

■ **INCREASE YOUR FLUID INTAKE.** Take in as much fluid as you can to hydrate your parched throat tissues, says Dr. Surow. Although it doesn't really matter *what* you drink, he says, here are a few things to avoid: Thick, milky drinks coat your throat and may produce mucus, making you cough and further irritating tissues. Orange juice may burn an already inflamed throat, and caffeinated beverages have a diuretic effect.

■ **TRY THIS TEA.** In one study, researchers gave 60 people with sore throats either a tea called Throat Coat, which contains marshmallow and licorice roots and slippery elm bark, or a placebo beverage four to six times

a day for about a week. The people who drank the herb tea reported only half as much pain as those who drank the placebo tea did. You can buy Throat Coat online and in health food stores.

Note: If you have allergies or high blood pressure, discuss it with your doctor before drinking the tea.

■ **CONSIDER THIS AFRICAN FLOWER.** *Pelargonium sidoides* is native to South Africa. A member of the geranium family, it has deep burgundy flowers and heart-shaped leaves. Nine studies show that pelargonium shortens the severity and duration of sore throats. The herb contains polyphenol compounds that stimulate the immune system and help it to wipe out viruses and bacteria.

Try Umcka ColdCare by Nature's Way. A 4-ounce bottle costs around $15 online and at health food stores. Be sure to follow the instructions on the label.

■ **TOSS YOUR TOOTHBRUSH.** Believe it or not, says Dr. Glass, your toothbrush may be perpetuating—or even causing—your sore throat. Bacteria collect on the bristles, and any injury to the gums during brushing injects these germs into your system.

"As soon as you start feeling ill, throw away your toothbrush. Often that's enough to stop the illness in its tracks," he says. "If you do get sick, replace your brush *again* when you start to feel better and when you feel completely well. That keeps you from reinfecting yourself."

Cures from the Kitchen

 Sore throat relief could be just a few ingredients away. Try the following recipe for relief.

Mix together 1 clove (antiseptic and fights infection) with ¼ teaspoon of powdered ginger (fights inflammation) and ⅛ teaspoon of cinnamon (reduces inflammation). Infuse the tea in 2 cups of boiling water. Stir in 4 teaspoons of raw honey (which is soothing and sweet). Sip the tea throughout the day until your throat feels better.

What the Doctor Does

Hueston King, M.D., takes 500 milligrams of vitamin C and 400 IU of vitamin E each day to protect himself from exposure to respiratory infections that can lead to sore throat.

Taking the combination of these vitamins when you have an infection is helpful for combating both viral and bacterial infections.

■ **MITIGATE THE MUCUS.** If you have thick mucus in addition to your sore throat, try taking guaifenesin (Mucinex), says Dr. Surow. This increases the water content of mucus and lets it flow without getting stuck in the throat.

■ **GET HELP FOR HEARTBURN.** Chronic sore throats may be caused by acid reflux, when acids leak out of the stomach into the throat, causing a chronic low-grade throat irritation, says Dr. Surow. Signs of this include heartburn, a bitter taste in the mouth, and a sore throat after eating or while lying down. As a first-line treatment, try an over-the-counter antacid such as Tums, Maalox, or Mylanta.

■ **ALLEVIATE ALLERGIES.** Another condition that can cause chronic low-grade throat inflammation is inhalant allergies, such as pollen, indoor molds, or dust mites, says Dr. Surow. To start, try taking an over-the-counter nonsedating allergy medication containing cetirizine hydrochloride, such as the antihistamine Zyrtec or Claritin.

■ **GIVE IT A REST.** If your throat is sore, it needs rest, says Dr. King. The throat is a muscular structure, and it tires just like any other muscle. Speak in a soft voice, mostly a monotone. But don't whisper, however, because it quickly leads to a stage whisper, which causes even more strain.

PANEL OF ADVISORS

R. THOMAS GLASS, D.D.S., PH.D., IS A PROFESSOR OF FORENSIC SCIENCES, PATHOLOGY, AND DENTAL MEDICINE AND AN ADJUNCT PROFESSOR OF MICROBIOLOGY AT OKLAHOMA STATE UNIVERSITY CENTER FOR HEALTH SCIENCES, IN TULSA. HE IS A PROFESSOR EMERITUS AT THE UNIVERSITY OF OKLAHOMA GRADUATE COLLEGE AND THE UNIVERSITY OF OKLAHOMA COLLEGES OF DENTISTRY AND MEDICINE, WHERE HE SERVED AS CHAIR OF THE DEPARTMENT OF ORAL AND MAXILLOFACIAL PATHOLOGY AND PROFESSOR OF PATHOLOGY.

HUESTON KING, M.D., IS A CLINICAL PROFESSOR OF EAR, NOSE, AND THROAT AT THE UNIVERSITY OF FLORIDA MEDICAL SCHOOL IN GAINESVILLE. HE IS ALSO A RETIRED EAR, NOSE, AND THROAT SPECIALIST IN VENICE, FLORIDA.

ROBERT ROUNTREE, M.D., IS A HOLISTIC PHYSICIAN IN BOULDER, COLORADO, AND COAUTHOR OF *IMMUNOTICS*.

JASON SUROW, M.D., IS AN EAR, NOSE, AND THROAT SPECIALIST AT ENT AND ALLERGY ASSOCIATES IN MAHWAH, NEW JERSEY.

IRWIN ZIMENT, M.D., IS PROFESSOR EMERITUS OF CLINICAL MEDICINE IN THE DEPARTMENT OF MEDICINE AT UCLA SCHOOL OF MEDICINE IN LOS ANGELES.

Splinters

7 Ways to Get Them Out

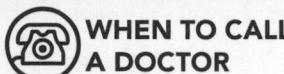

WHEN TO CALL A DOCTOR

Call a health professional if the splinter is very large or deeply embedded and can't be pulled out easily, says Dee Anna Glaser, M.D. Deep splinters may require a doctor to make a small incision to extract it. "But, unless the splinter is removed, it will almost always become infected," she says.

Speaking of infection, those with diabetes or compromised immunity should see a physician if they have a deeply embedded splinter, suggests Dr. Glaser. "These people are at a greater risk for more serious infection."

Yet another instance to make a doctor's visit is if the splinter is a piece of metal, not wood, and your last tetanus shot was more than 5 years ago, says Dr. Glaser.

In the well-known fable *Androcles and the Lion*, a tiny splinter brought the mighty lion to his knees. And if you've ever had a spiky splinter puncture your tender skin, you can relate.

Getting a splinter in the hand or foot—or worse, someplace even more sensitive—pains even the strongest of us. Unfortunately, removing those little suckers can often be just as troublesome.

"Splinters are small pieces of wood, glass, metal, or other matter that gets caught under your skin," says Dee Anna Glaser, M.D. "Even though they're often small, they tend to hurt. Whether they are buried deep or not, you need to remove them as soon as possible so they don't cause infection."

Here's what some of the pros recommend for painless removal—or at least somewhat painless—to keep that splinter from becoming a real thorn in your side.

■ **ENLIST SOME OUTSIDE HELP.** First, get a loved one to sterilize a tweezers by cleaning it with rubbing alcohol, or heating it with a lighter or hot match. "It's hard to cause yourself pain, so ask a husband, wife, or someone else who cares about you to lend you a gentle, helping hand," says Dr. Glaser.

Grab the protruding end of the splinter with the sterilized tweezers and gently pull it out in the direction it entered, says Dr. Glaser. If the splinter is embedded in the skin, sterilize a needle with rubbing alcohol, a lighter, or a match, then make a small hole in the skin over the end of the splinter. Then, lift the skin to expose the splinter, put the needle under the splinter until it can be grasped with the tweezers, and pull it out.

Last, have your helper check to make sure that the entire splinter is gone. If not, repeat the previous steps. "For really small splinters or If you don't get the entire splinter on the first try, use a magnifying glass for a closer look," says Dr. Glaser.

■ **CLEAN UP YOUR ACT.** After the whole splinter is out, clean the wound with hydrogen peroxide, allowing the bubbles to work on the area, says Joseph Bark, M.D.

Then apply a bandage, if needed, to keep the wound clean; otherwise, leave it open to the air, says Dr. Glaser. Either way, be on the lookout for signs of infection (redness, pus, increased pain, swelling, and even red streaking in that area). "Applying an antibiotic ointment once the area is cleaned will help the healing process," she says.

■ **TAKE PREVENTIVE MEASURES.** Dr. Glaser says that some splinters can be avoided with an ounce or two of prevention. She recommends the following.

■ Wear shoes outdoors at all times and whenever you walk on unfinished wood floors, wooden decks, or boardwalks.

■ Clean up all broken glass and metal shavings around the house immediately. Be careful when handling broken glass, and wear hard-soled shoes to protect your feet.

■ Wear work gloves when handling plants with thorns, sharp tips, and spines.

■ Be careful when applying friction to an object while performing tasks such as woodworking. "If you're not careful, a small portion of that wood can dislodge into your skin," says Dr. Glaser. "So again, wear gloves."

PANEL OF ADVISORS

JOSEPH BARK, M.D., IS A DERMATOLOGIST IN LEXINGTON, KENTUCKY, AND DIRECTOR OF SKIN SECRETS, A COMPREHENSIVE SKIN-CARE FACILITY.

DEE ANNA GLASER, M.D., IS A PROFESSOR IN THE DEPARTMENT OF DERMATOLOGY AT ST. LOUIS UNIVERSITY SCHOOL OF MEDICINE IN MISSOURI.

Sprains

17 Self-Care Strategies

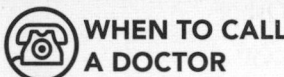 WHEN TO CALL A DOCTOR

All sprains are painful, and it's difficult even for doctors to tell right away if the injuries involve torn tissue, fractured bone, or other serious problems.

If there's a lot of swelling or bruising, or if the pain seems unusually severe, it's a good idea to get to an emergency room for x-rays, says Michael Osborne, M.D.

Sprains should start feeling better within a few weeks, Dr. Osborne adds. Even if the initial discomfort is mild, see your doctor if there isn't noticeable improvement within 2 to 4 weeks.

Ligaments are tough bands of tissue that wrap around your ankle and other joints, lending support and stability. They have a little bit of give, but only a little. If stretched beyond their usual limits, they can become damaged or inflamed—or, in other words, sprained.

"The usual time for a sprain to heal is about 6 weeks, but that's only if it's treated properly," says John M. McShane, M.D. "People tend to ignore sprains, which can result in chronic problems."

Many sprains can be treated at home without medical attention, Dr. McShane adds. Here's what you need to do.

■ **REST THE JOINT.** Sprains don't necessarily hurt a lot at first, and people may assume it's okay to keep doing the activity that got them into trouble in the first place. But pushing an injured joint too hard makes the damage worse.

"Minor sprains need a couple of days of rest," says Dr. McShane. You don't have to limit your daily movements altogether, but you will want to avoid vigorous activities that stress the injured area.

■ **ICE IT IMMEDIATELY.** Applying cold to a sprain deadens pain and reduces internal bleeding or the accumulation of fluids in the injured area. It's important to ice sprains immediately because swelling is hard to reverse once it's under way.

"Use ice cubes or crushed ice," Dr. McShane says. "Put the ice in a ziplock plastic bag, seal it, wrap it in a thin towel, and put it over the sore spot. Keep icing the area as long as it hurts, especially if there's any swelling."

If you don't have ice, open the freezer and take out a bag of frozen vegetables. A bag of peas or corn is pliable enough to mold around the joint and apply cold right where it's needed, says Michael Osborne, M.D.

■ **OR USE A GEL PACK.** Available at drugstores and sporting goods stores, gel packs stay flexible even when frozen and mold themselves to the contours of the joint. "Gel packs get colder than ice and can actually cause frostbite if they're put directly on the skin," Dr. McShane says. So when using a gel pack, make sure to put a cloth between it and the skin, and don't leave it on for more than 15 minutes at a time.

■ **WRAP THE JOINT.** Compressing the area with an elastic bandage helps prevent fluid from accumulating, which reduces swelling and pain. Wrapping a joint also restricts movement, which helps the injured ligaments heal.

Don't make the bandage so tight that it cuts off circulation, Dr. McShane adds. If the area beyond the sprain feels numb or cold, or if the bandage itself is uncomfortably tight, loosen it a bit.

"You should be able to slip a finger snugly under the bandage," Dr. McShane says.

■ **USE AN AIRCAST ON THE ANKLE.** Available at some drugstores and from mail-order catalogs, Aircasts can be pumped up with air to put even pressure on the ankle. "They help keep the swelling down and prevent the joint

from moving too much," says Dr. McShane.

Another option is an elastic "tube" bandage. Available at some drugstores and most medical supply stores, the tubes come in different sizes for different joints. They support healing by applying even pressure all the way around the joint, Dr. Osborne explains. Their one downside is that they can shift as you wear it, which may allow swelling in some areas.

■ **PUT GRAVITY ON YOUR SIDE.** For the first day or two after a sprain, elevate the area for as long as possible. If you've sprained your ankle, for example, put a few pillows underneath your calf. If you've sprained your wrist, keep your hand above chest level. Elevating the joint aids lymphatic drainage from the area and keeps swelling to a minimum, says Dr. Osborne.

■ **TAKE AN OVER-THE-COUNTER ANTI-INFLAMMATORY.** Aspirin, ibuprofen, and other nonsteroidal anti-inflammatory drugs (NSAIDs) inhibit the body's production of prostaglandins, inflammatory chemicals that cause swelling and delay healing time. They are often used as the first treatment for overuse injuries.

"Acetaminophen is used for pain relief, but it doesn't have any effect on swelling," says Dr. McShane. You'll get better results with aspirin, ibuprofen, or naproxen (Aleve). The drugs work equally well, but naproxen is more convenient because you to take it only twice a day.

One caveat: If the injury is severe, wait until the bleeding has stopped or the swelling has stabilized before taking NSAIDs, because they also inhibit blood clotting and may complicate recovery time.

■ **RELIEVE STIFFNESS WITH HEAT.** You don't want to treat a sprain with a heating pad or hot-water bottle in the first 48 to 72 hours after the injury, because heat increases circulation and may increase swelling. But after several days, when swelling has subsided, applying heat—or soaking the area in a whirlpool or hot bath—may help you feel more comfortable, says Dr. Osborne.

Heat also improves the flow of nutrients to the injured area while removing painful metabolic by-products.

■ **HOBBLE TO THE HEALTH FOOD STORE.** Pick up a tube of comfrey ointment. Comfrey is a fuzzy-leaved weed that grows in marshes. As far back as 400 B.C., it's been used to treat bruises and broken bones. In fact, its scientific name (*Symphytum officinale*) is derived from the Greek word *symphytum*, which means "to knit together." In the 1600s, herbalists used comfrey to heal wounds, sores, burns, and swelling.

Today, we know that comfrey is high in allantoin, which reduces inflammation and stimulates the growth of healthy tissue. In one study, researchers applied comfrey ointment to some people with sprained ankles and applied the traditional prescription anti-inflammatory lotion diclofenac gel to other people. After 1 week, the people who used the comfrey were better healed and reported 92

percent less pain. The people who used the prescription gel had only 84 percent less pain.

Good brands include Nature's Way and Herbalist & Alchemist. Follow the label directions. And use comfrey only in ointment form. The FDA warns that comfrey supplements can contribute to liver damage.

■ **START WITH GENTLE EXERCISES AS SOON AS POSSIBLE.** It's normal for ligaments to be somewhat tight after a sprain. To prevent stiffness and restore joint mobility, it's helpful to do range-of-motion exercises once you're through the initial, painful phase.

Moving the joint may be painful at first, but that's okay. In fact, it's beneficial to gently push the joint slightly farther than it wants to go, says Dr. McShane. "Ligaments actually heal better when they're slightly stressed," he explains.

If you're recovering from an ankle sprain, for example, use that foot to "sketch" the entire alphabet once or twice a day. Imagine that your big toe is the tip of a pen, he says. Using the ankle to move the foot, form each letter of the alphabet, from A to Z, in the air.

"That helps get the range of motion back, and it reduces swelling as well," says Dr. McShane.

■ **WEAR A BRACE.** If you have a history of ankle sprains, consider wearing a brace. Available at drugstores, braces support and protect the joint, which can speed healing and reduce the risk of additional sprains. Some people with sprain-prone ankles wear braces whenever they do "risky" activities, such as play tennis or basketball.

■ **GET THE RIGHT SHOES.** If you've sprained your ankle once, you may have a higher risk of future sprains. One way to prevent problems is to buy shoes designed for the activities you do most. "Don't wear running shoes for playing basketball or racquetball," says Dr. McShane. "They don't provide ankle stability, and they may actually create a tendency for the ankle to roll in or out."

■ **STRENGTHEN THE JOINT.** Once the sprain is better, it's worth taking the time to strengthen and condition the joint, which reduces stress on the ligaments. Ankle sprains are so common that you might want to focus on that area of the body—both for relieving stiffness and for preventing future problems. Your risk of ankle sprains increases with age, but these exercises can help you prevent them.

"The ankle may be weak after a sprain, so you'll want to start with range-of-motion exercises, then progress to strengthening exercises," says Dr. Osborne. Try these exercises, for example.

■ Put a few cans of soup or vegetables into a plastic grocery bag, slip your foot

through the handles, and lift your toes toward the ceiling. Hold the weight for about 3 seconds, then lower it.

■ Put your foot against a wall or another immovable object, and flex and relax the muscles. This type of isometric exercise improves bloodflow and exerts beneficial stress on the ligaments and other tissues.

■ Sit with your legs straight in front of you, and flex the top of your foot back toward your body. Hold for a moment, then relax.

■ Sit and loop a towel or an elastic cord around your foot, then flex the muscles in different directions against the resistance.

PANEL OF ADVISORS

JOHN M. MCSHANE, M.D., IS A CLINICAL ASSOCIATE PROFESSOR OF FAMILY MEDICINE AT JEFFERSON MEDICAL COLLEGE OF THOMAS JEFFERSON UNIVERSITY AND DIRECTOR OF SPORTS MEDICINE AT THOMAS JEFFERSON UNIVERSITY HOSPITAL, BOTH IN PHILADELPHIA.

MICHAEL OSBORNE, M.D., IS AN ASSISTANT PROFESSOR OF PHYSICAL MEDICINE AND REHABILITATION AT THE MAYO CLINIC IN ROCHESTER, MINNESOTA.

Stress

23 Tips to Ease Tension

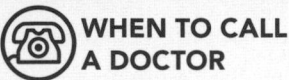

WHEN TO CALL A DOCTOR

Too much stress can directly threaten your health.

If your symptoms are new and have no obvious cause, especially if they interfere with your quality of life, see a doctor.

Any of the following stress-related symptoms may indicate that you should seek medical help promptly.

- Frequent headaches, jaw clenching, or pain
- Gritting or grinding teeth
- Stuttering or stammering
- Tremors, trembling of lips or hands
- Neck ache, back pain, or muscle spasms
- Light-headedness, faintness, or dizziness
- Ringing, buzzing, or "popping sounds"
- Frequent blushing or sweating
- Cold or sweaty hands and feet
- Dry mouth or problems swallowing

Stress. It really should be a four-letter word. Here in the 21st century, it's as pervasive as the everyday air that we breathe and is as contagious as the common cold.

Because stress is so difficult to avoid, why not make it work *for* you instead of against you? Stress is a force you can turn to your advantage. You don't have to run from it, and you *don't* have to go to a stress-management seminar to find out how to manage it. The following doctor-tested tips show you how to combat stress—and win. For relief when the world has you in a headlock, read on.

■ **GET A NEW ATTITUDE.** It's not what's out there that's the problem, it's how you *react* to it. How you react is determined by how you *perceive* a particular stress.

Changing the way you think—viewing a difficult assignment at work as a chance to improve your skills, for example—can change a life of stress and discomfort into a life filled with challenge and excitement.

■ **THINK POSITIVELY.** Thinking about a success or a past achievement is excellent when you're feeling uncertain—before a presentation, for example, or a meeting with your boss.

■ **TAKE A MENTAL VACATION.** "Taking a mini vacation in your mind is a very good way to relieve or manage stress," says Ronald Nathan, Ph.D.

"Imagine yourself lying in warm sand on a beach in the Bahamas, a gentle breeze coming off the ocean, the surf rolling in quietly in the background. It's *amazing* what this can do to relax you."

■ **USE AFFIRMATIONS.** Have a list of affirmations ready that you can start repeating when you feel stressed. They don't have to be complicated. Just chanting "I can handle this" to yourself or, "I know more about this than anyone here," will work. It pulls you away from the animal reflex to stress—the quick breathing, the cold hands—and toward the reasoned response, the intellect, the part of you that really *can* handle it.

The result? You calm down.

■ **COUNT TO 10.** Refusing to respond to a stress immediately can help defuse it, Dr. Nathan says. Making a *habit* of pausing and relaxing just for a few seconds before responding to the routine interruptions of your day can make a clear difference in the sense of stress you experience. When the phone rings, for example, breathe in deeply. Then as you breathe out, imagine you are as loose and limp as an old rag doll.

"One of the things pausing like this does is give you a feeling of control," Dr. Nathan says. "Feeling in control is generally less stressful than feeling out of control. Make a habit of using rapid relaxation during the pause before you answer the phone. Deliberately pausing can become an instant tranquilizer."

■ **LOOK AWAY.** "If you look through a window at a far-distant view for a moment, away from the problem that's producing the stress, the eyes relax. And if the eyes relax, the tendency is for you to do the same," Dr. Nathan says.

■ **GET UP AND LEAVE.** "Take a pot off the burner and it quits boiling," says Dr. Nathan. "Leaving the scene can also give you a fresh new perspective."

■ **TAKE SEVERAL DEEP BREATHS.** Belly breathing is what some people call it. It's an old and useful method for reducing temporary anxiety and nervousness.

The correct way to breathe? Abdominally—feeling your stomach expand as you inhale, collapse as you exhale. While there are many different breathing techniques to calm the mind, the simple "So Hum" meditation breathing is best for starters. Inhale deeply and say "soooooo," then slowly exhale with "hummmm." Pull your stomach in tight. Breathing slowly, fully, and calmly at the first signs of stress will change your attitude and life forever.

The basic idea is to stay calm. When you're experiencing stress, your pulse races and you start breathing very quickly. "If you can't fight and you can't flee, then relax and flow," says Dr. Nathan.

■ **GET A WORKOUT.** Exercise is one of nature's best tranquilizers. It burns off the by-products of stress and uses the fight-or-flight response much the way it was intended, says Dr. Nathan. And stretching after a workout is especially helpful for releasing tight jaw and shoulder muscles.

■ **MASSAGE YOUR TARGET MUSCLES.** Most of us have particular muscles that knot up under stress. It's sort of a vicious circle:

Stress produces adrenaline, which produces muscle tension, which produces more adrenaline, and so on. A good way to break the circle is to find out what your target muscles are—the ones that get tense under pressure, usually in the back of your neck and upper back—and massage them for a couple of minutes whenever you feel tense.

■ **PRESS ON YOUR TEMPLES.** This application of acupressure—the system that uses pressure points to relieve pain and treat a variety of ailments—works indirectly. Massaging nerves in your temples relaxes muscles elsewhere, chiefly in your neck.

■ **DROP YOUR JAW AND ROLL IT LEFT TO RIGHT.** People under pressure have a tendency to clench their teeth. Dropping the jaw and rolling it helps make those muscles relax, and if you relax the muscles, you reduce the sensation of tension.

■ **STRETCH YOUR CHEST TO ACHIEVE BETTER BREATHING.** The tense musculature of a person under stress can make breathing difficult, and impaired breathing can aggravate the anxiety you already feel. To relax your breathing, roll your shoulders up and back, then relax. The first time, inhale deeply as they go back and exhale as they relax. You may do this at the same time you are doing So Hum breathing. Repeat four or five more times, then inhale deeply again. Repeat the entire sequence four times.

■ **RELAX ALL OVER.** Easier said than done? Not if you know how. A technique called progressive relaxation can produce immediate and dramatic reductions in your sense of stress by reducing physical tension.

Starting at top or bottom, tense one set of muscles in your body at a time, hold for a few seconds, then let them relax. Work your way through all major body parts—feet, legs, chest and arms, head and neck—and then enjoy the sense of release it provides. Fifteen minutes of meditation can give the body the rest of 1 hour of sleep.

■ **TAKE A HOT SOAK.** Water is an enormous help when you're under stress, says G. Frank Lawlis, Ph.D. When we're tense and anxious, bloodflow to our extremities is reduced. Hot water restores circulation, convincing the body it's safe and that it is okay to relax. Add Epson salts or lemon juice for an even more relaxing experience, says Dr. Lawlis.

If you have no time for a bath, try placing warm washcloths on your feet, hands, and forehead. Cold water is a no-no; it *mimics* the stress response, driving blood away from the extremities, and the result is that tension increases.

An alternative at the workplace: Run hot water over your hands until you feel tension start to drain away.

■ **MOVE AROUND.** Regular exercise, of course, builds stamina that can help anyone battle stress. But even something as casual as a walk around the block can help you throw off some of the tension that a rough business meeting or a family squabble leaves you carrying around.

The Way to Inner Peace

Transcendental meditation, yoga, Zen meditation—they *all* work by inducing something called the relaxation response, a body state first identified and named by Herbert Benson, M.D.

"This phenomenon shuts off the distracting, stressful, anxiety-producing aspects of what is commonly called the fight-or-flight response," Dr. Benson writes in his book *Your Maximum Mind*.

In primitive situations, where dangers from wild animals might have been the order of the day, the fight-or-flight response was quite useful. In our own time, however, this response tends to make us more nervous, uncomfortable, and even unhealthy.

A person experiencing the relaxation response turns off all the hormones and behaviors that make him nervous. Basically any kind of meditation produces it, though most traditional forms require some degree of training and a good amount of self-discipline.

Dr. Benson suggests the following basic program for eliciting the response.

One, pick a focus word, phrase, or prayer ("peace," or "the Lord is my shepherd," for example) that is firmly rooted in your personal belief system. Two, sit quietly, close your eyes, and relax. And three, repeat your focus word each time you exhale. Continue this for 10 to 20 minutes.

Tips: Practice at least once a day, and don't worry about how you're doing. If you realize that you've been distracted by thoughts, this is normal and should be expected. Simply say, "Oh, well," and return to your focus.

■ **CHEW GUM.** Whenever you use the action of chewing, you flood the temporal lobe in the front of your brain with chemicals that help you de-stress, says Dr. Lawlis.

■ **STRESS EAT (THE RIGHT WAY).** Really, it's okay, as long as you eat the right foods. Chomping a few almonds, for example, helps relieve stress and anxiety, says Dr. Lawlis. So does eating strawberries and other fruits. "What we found in the research is that strawberries increase pain endorphins, especially when you eat the leaves along with the berry. And bananas contain tryptophan, which promotes muscle relaxation," he adds.

■ **LISTEN TO RELAXATION CDS OR MP3S.** Relaxation is the opposite of tension—the antidote for stress. And relaxation CDs can be very effective at easing tension. Options come in voice only, voice with music, or nature sounds—wind in the trees, surf on the sand, says Dr. Nathan. "All you need is a CD player or an iPod, and a headset to block out distractions and avoid disturbing others." (To listen to a free, 6-minute sample of Dr. Nathan's new relaxation program, visit www.relaxfastforfree.com.)

■ **TUNE IN THE MUSIC.** Of course, relaxation CDs and MP3s work, but they aren't your only option. The right music soothes as perhaps nothing else does. Music by itself is a very great stress reducer, says Dr. Lawlis.

■ **FIND THE RHYTHM.** Rhythmic movement stimulates neural chemicals in your system that help you relax, says Dr. Lawlis. Listening to music with repetitive drumming accomplishes a similar effect. "Something about rhythm trains the brain toward lower stress levels and balances the various parts of the brain that seem to be excited during a stress response," says Dr. Lawlis.

■ **STOP AND SMELL THE ROSES . . . OR ANY FLOWERS.** Breathing in pleasant aromas is an easy way to change your mental state, especially when combined with breathing techniques, says Dr. Lawlis. "When you smell scents like lavender, lilac, honeysuckle, or cedar, you change your brain chemistry," he explains.

There's some scientific evidence of this, but we know it on a basic level. "When we get in trouble and want to change the mental state of the person who's mad at us, we bring flowers, and we also send flowers to people in the hospital. Why? Probably to diminish their stress," he says.

You can buy essential oils at the health food store. But Dr. Lawlis recommends the real thing, fresh flowers.

PANEL OF ADVISORS

HERBERT BENSON, M.D., IS DIRECTOR EMERITUS AT THE BENSON-HENRY INSTITUTE FOR MIND BODY MEDICINE AT MASSACHUSETTS GENERAL HOSPITAL, AND ASSOCIATE PROFESSOR OF MEDICINE AT THE MIND/BODY MEDICAL INSTITUTE AT HARVARD MEDICAL SCHOOL.

G. FRANK LAWLIS, PH.D., IS A PSYCHOLOGIST, RESEARCHER, AND COFOUNDER OF THE LAWLIS AND PEAVEY CENTERS FOR PSYCHONEUROLOGICAL CHANGE IN LEWISVILLE, TEXAS. HE IS THE CHIEF CONTENT ADVISER FOR THE *DR. PHIL SHOW* AND AUTHOR OF *THE STRESS ANSWER*, *THE ADD ANSWER*, AND *THE IQ ANSWER*.

RONALD NATHAN, PH.D., IS A CLINICAL PROFESSOR AT ALBANY MEDICAL COLLEGE IN NEW YORK AND AUTHOR OF *THE FAST TECHNIQUE FOR STRESS RELIEF*.

Sunburn

24 Cooling Treatments

It's fun to play in the sun, but if you aren't careful, too much exposure to the sun's ultraviolet (UV) rays can cause a red, painful sunburn. While a mild sunburn may seem like a temporary inconvenience, a severe sunburn can cause serious symptoms, including swelling, blistering, fever, and dehydration. Although most people today know they should limit time in the sun and use sunscreen to prevent sunburn and some forms of skin cancer, 42 percent of people polled admitted to suffering at least one sunburn per year, according to a recent report by the Skin Cancer Foundation.

How long you can stay out in the sun before burning depends on your coloring. People with fair complexions, blue or green eyes, freckles, and light-colored hair get sunburned in the least amount of time.

But no matter your coloring, you may not realize you've stayed out too long until after you've come in from the sun, says Norman Levine, M.D. A sunburn leaves your skin cells damaged and inflamed. The pain may worsen in the next day or two, and the damaged skin may peel in about a week.

Prevention is key, but if you do get sunburned, stay comfortable

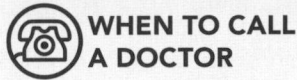

WHEN TO CALL A DOCTOR

A severe burn can take a lot out of you, says Rodney Basler, M.D. Consult a doctor if you experience nausea, chills, fever, faintness, extensive blistering, general weakness, patches of purple discoloration, or intense itching. If the burn seems to be spreading, you could have an infection compounding the problem.

while your body heals itself with the following expert advice and tips.

■ **APPLY SOOTHING COMPRESSES.** Following a burn, the skin is inflamed. Cool it down by applying ice water soaks, which can be soothing and may make the burn heal a little faster, says Dr. Levine. Add a few ice cubes to tap water, then dip a cloth into the liquid and lay it over the burn. Repeat every few minutes as the cloth warms. Apply several times a day for 10- to 15-minute stretches.

■ **SOOTH THE RED WITH WHITE.** If your sunburn is mild (no blisters), apply distilled white vinegar to the sunburned areas. "The acetic acid in the vinegar acts as a topical NSAID," says Audrey Kunin, M.D.

■ **SOAK THE PAIN AWAY.** If you've been sunbathing all day in a skimpy suit, you'll need allover cool comfort. Try soaking in a cool bath, says Dr. Levine. Add more water as needed to maintain a comfortably cool temperature. To soothe pain and itching, add baking soda or Aveeno colloidal oatmeal to your bathwater and soak for 15 to 20 minutes.

But go easy on soap. It can dry and irritate burned skin. If you must use soap, use only a mild brand and rinse it off very well. Do not soak in soapy water. Likewise, stay away from bubble baths.

■ **MOISTURIZE YOUR SKIN.** Soaks and compresses feel good and give temporary relief, says Rodney Basler, M.D. But they can make your skin feel drier than before if you don't apply moisturizer immediately afterward. Pat yourself dry, then smooth on some bath oil. Let it soak in for a minute, then apply a moisturizing cream or lotion, such as Eucerin. Some people like a topical cream called Wibi, which contains a little bit of cooling menthol, he adds.

■ **CHILL OUT.** For added relief, try chilling your moisturizer before applying it.

■ **SEEK HYDROCORTISONE RELIEF.** Soothe skin irritation and inflammation with a topical lotion, spray, or ointment containing 1 percent hydrocortisone, such as Cortaid or

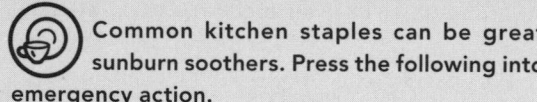

Cures from the Kitchen

Common kitchen staples can be great sunburn soothers. Press the following into emergency action.

CORNSTARCH. Add enough water to cornstarch to make a paste. Apply directly to the sunburn.

FAT-FREE MILK. Mix 1 cup fat-free milk with 4 cups water, then add a few ice cubes. Apply compresses for 15 to 20 minutes; repeat every 2 to 4 hours.

LETTUCE. Boil lettuce leaves in water. Strain, then let the liquid cool for several hours in the refrigerator. Dip cotton balls into the liquid and gently press or stroke onto irritated skin.

OATMEAL. Wrap dry oatmeal in cheesecloth or gauze. Run cool water through it. Discard the oatmeal and soak compresses in the liquid. Apply every 2 to 4 hours.

TEA BAGS. If your eyelids are burned, apply tea bags soaked in cool water to decrease swelling and help relieve pain. Tea has tannic acid, which seems to ease sunburn pain.

YOGURT. Apply yogurt to all sunburned areas. Rinse off in a cool shower, then gently pat skin dry.

Cortizone-10 (available at drugstores). Hydrocortisone has anti-inflammatory fighting ability, which means it will reduce redness and ease the pain of mild sunburns, says Coyle S. Connolly, D.O. "Use 2 or 3 times a day."

■ **SAY GOOD-BYE WITH ALOE.** "There is also evidence in medical literature that aloe vera may really help wound healing," says Dr. Basler. Simply break off a leaf and apply the juice. But test a small area first, he cautions, to make sure you're not allergic to aloe.

If you don't have an aloe plant handy, apply refrigerated (chilled) pure aloe vera gel (available in pump bottles at most drugstores), says Dr. Connolly. Apply as often as needed until the redness and pain subside. "The trick is using chilled not room temperature aloe vera gel," says Dr. Connolly.

■ **EAT RIGHT AND STAY HYDRATED.** Maintaining a balanced diet will provide the nutrients your skin needs to regenerate itself. Staying well hydrated by drinking lots of water will help counteract the drying effects of a sunburn.

■ **RAISE YOUR LEGS.** If your legs are burned and your feet are swollen, elevate your legs above heart level to help stop the swelling, says Dr. Basler.

■ **BE CAREFUL WITH BLISTERS.** If blisters develop, you have a pretty bad burn. If they bother you and they cover only a small area, you may carefully drain them, says Dr. Basler. But do not peel the top skin off—you'll have less discomfort and danger of infection if

What the Doctor Does

Rit Sun Guard is sun protection for your skin that you wash into your clothing. It is available at some supermarkets, drugstores, mass merchandisers, and online at www.dermadoctor. com. "This product increases the capability of fabric to stop ultraviolet (UV) rays from reaching the skin, and it's the relative equivalent of an SPF of 30," says Audrey Kunin, M.D.

Simply add it to the wash cycle, rinse, and dry your clothes as usual. One treatment of Rit Sun Guard stays in clothing for more than 20 washings, says Dr. Kunin.

"Your typical T-shirt has a UV protection factor of 5, but adding Rit Sun Guard to the wash cycle will increase that factor to 30," she says.

air does not come in contact with sensitive nerve endings.

To drain the fluid, first sterilize a needle by holding it over a flame. Then puncture the edge of the blister and press gently on the top to let the fluid come out. Do this three times in the first 24 hours, says Dr. Basler. Then leave the blisters alone.

■ **TAKE SOME ASPIRIN.** This old standby can help relieve the pain, itching, and swelling of a mild to moderate burn. "Take two tablets every 4 hours," says Dr. Basler. Acetaminophen and ibuprofen will work just as well; follow label instructions for dosages. If you know you got too much sun, try taking aspirin *before* the redness appears.

■ **DON'T MAKE THE SAME MISTAKE TWICE.** After you've been sunburned, it takes 3 to 6 months for your skin to return to

Are You Photosensitive?

We're not asking if you like to have your picture taken. The question is whether certain drugs increase your sensitivity to the sun and lead to a burnlike dermatitis.

Antibiotics, tranquilizers, and antifungal medications can cause reactions, says Rodney Basler, M.D. So can oral contraceptives, diuretics, drugs for diabetes, and even PABA-containing sunscreens. Always ask your doctor about potential side effects of any drugs you may be taking.

Even common foods can trigger a bad reaction. "Two young women I know tried to lighten their hair with lime juice," he says. "They didn't realize what a potent photosensitizer lime juice can be until they developed terrible dermatitis every place the juice had run down their faces and arms."

normal. When you get a sunburn and the top layer of skin peels off, the newly exposed skin is more sensitive than ever. This means you'll burn even faster than you did the first time, if you're not careful.

While the memory of your burn is still painfully fresh, brush up on your sun sense with these tips.

- Apply a sunscreen about 30 minutes before going out, even if it's overcast. (Harmful rays can penetrate cloud cover.) Don't forget to protect your lips, hands, ears, and the back of your neck, says Dr. Levine. Reapply as necessary after swimming or perspiring heavily.

- Pick a sunscreen with a sun protection factor (SPF) of at least 30, says Dr. Levine. Also look for the ingredients zinc oxide, titanium dioxide, or avoben-

zone in your sunscreen. These block both ultraviolet A and B rays.

- Take extra care between the hours of 10:00 a.m. and 3:00 p.m. (11:00 a.m. and 4:00 p.m., daylight saving time), when the sun is at its strongest.

- Wear protective clothing when not swimming. Hats, tightly woven fabrics, and long sleeves help keep the sun off your skin.

- Beware ice and snow. Don't let your guard down in winter. You can get a fierce burn from the sun's rays reflected off ice and snow.

- Take a sunshine supplement. Your skin makes vitamin D from ultraviolet rays, so diligently avoiding these rays may lead to a deficiency. "Vitamin D works to protect the body from cancer, and the trend away from sun exposure (to protect from both skin cancer and premature signs of aging) has led to a depletion in Vitamin D in many people," says Dr. Kunin.

■ Protect with pomegranate extract. This funny red fruit is rich in ellagic acid, which may help protect your skin against UVA- and UVB-induced cell damage, according to a 2008 study by the Department of Nutrition and Food Science at Texas A&M University. The reason may have something to do with the fruit's anti-inflammatory and antioxidant properties, the researchers speculate.

Other researchers from Japan found that pomegranate extract may slightly lessen pig-

mentation changes, such as freckles and stains, caused by UV rays.

PANEL OF ADVISORS

RODNEY BASLER, M.D., IS A DERMATOLOGIST AND ASSOCIATE PROFESSOR OF INTERNAL MEDICINE AT THE UNIVERSITY OF NEBRASKA COLLEGE OF MEDICINE IN LINCOLN.

COYLE S. CONNOLLY, D.O., IS A DERMATOLOGIST AND ASSISTANT CLINICAL PROFESSOR AT THE PHILADELPHIA COLLEGE OF OSTEOPATHIC MEDICINE AND PRESIDENT OF CONNOLLY DERMATOLOGY IN LINWOOD, NEW JERSEY.

AUDREY KUNIN, M.D., IS A COSMETIC DERMATOLOGIST IN KANSAS CITY, MISSOURI, THE FOUNDER OF THE DERMATOLOGY EDUCATIONAL WEB SITE WWW.DERMADOCTOR.COM, AND AUTHOR OF THE DERMADOCTOR SKINSTRUCTION MANUAL.

NORMAN LEVINE, M.D., IS A DERMATOLOGIST IN PRIVATE PRACTICE IN TUCSON, ARIZONA, AND A FORMER PROFESSOR OF MEDICINE IN THE DEPARTMENT OF DERMATOLOGY AT THE UNIVERSITY OF ARIZONA COLLEGE OF MEDICINE IN TUCSON.

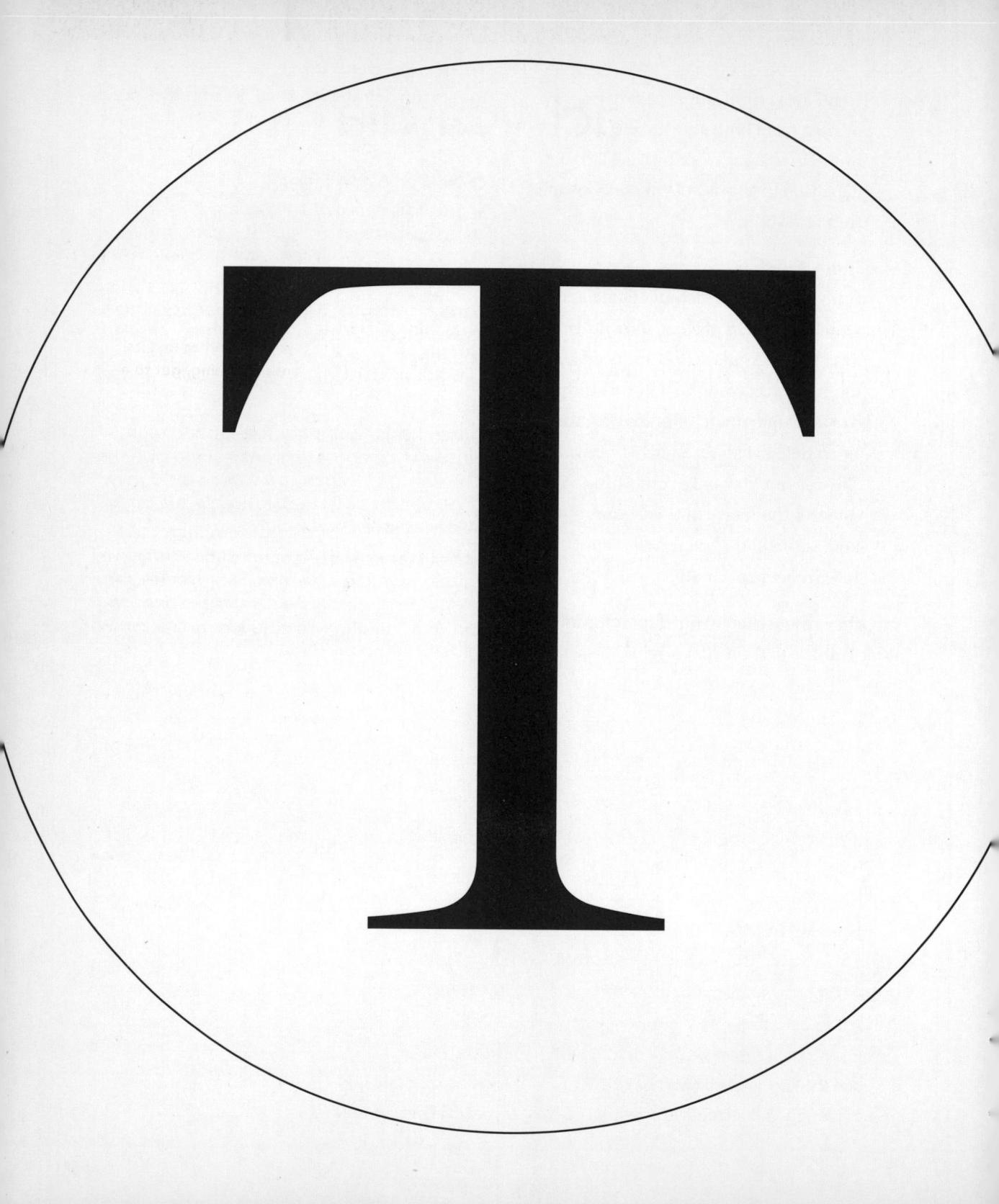

Tachycardia

13 Ways to Calm a Rapid Heartbeat

It comes on suddenly. Seventy-two beats a minute become 120 . . . 180 . . . 200 beats in only seconds. The rapid heartbeat makes it hard to breathe and causes nausea and heavy perspiring.

This is tachycardia—more specifically, paroxysmal atrial tachycardia—which means that your heart is racing, beating faster than 100 beats per minute. This occurs when your atria—the chambers in your heart that receive blood from the veins and pump it into the ventricles—get a little out of control. The atria are still keeping a steady rhythm, but the rhythm can be three times faster than normal.

Tachycardia is more common in women, but it also occurs in men. Even young people may experience this heart rhythm disturbance brought on by anxiety or exhaustion. Although tachycardia is generally not serious and doesn't signify heart disease, it may, however, cause serious or even life-threatening complications in people who already have heart disease. Symptoms vary but usually start and stop quickly.

Here's how to put the brakes on tachycardia.

■ **SLOW DOWN.** Think of that speeding heart as a flashing red light that says, "Stop what you're doing. Chill out. Rest." Rest, in fact, is your best mechanism for stopping an attack, says Dennis S. Miura, M.D., Ph.D. If you have trouble slowing down, try deep breathing techniques or use a home biofeedback system.

■ **TRY THE VAGAL MANEUVER.** How fast your heart beats and how strongly it contracts are regulated by sympathetic nerves and

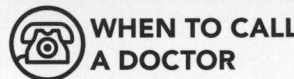

WHEN TO CALL A DOCTOR

If your heart has lost its sense of timing, get to a doctor—as soon as possible. "You should also notify your doctor if you have heart disease, shortness of breath, or trouble exercising," says Stephen R. Shorofsky, M.D., Ph.D. If you pass out or feel like you are going to pass out, call your doctor, he adds. This may indicate a more serious arrhythmia or condition.

"If your doctor has ruled out a serious condition, but you still have recurrent tachycardia symptoms that bother you physically or emotionally, seek an evaluation by an electrophysiologist," says Dennis S. Miura, M.D., Ph.D. "There are new drugs and new techniques that can help."

parasympathetic nerves (or vagal nerves). When your heart pounds, the sympathetic network is dominant. (That's the system that basically tells your body to speed up.) What you want to do is switch control to the mellower parasympathetic network. If you stimulate a vagal nerve, you initiate a chemical process that affects your heart in the same way that slamming on the brakes affects your car.

"Vagal maneuvers increase vagal tone, which tends to slow conduction from the top chambers of the heart to the bottom chambers," explains Stephen R. Shorofsky, M.D., Ph.D. "If the arrhythmia is using this pathway for a circuit, one blocked beat will terminate the circuit."

Doctors recommend these vagal maneuvers to break up supraventricular tachycardia (SVT), a common form of rapid heartbeat that arises from the upper chambers of the heart.

- Rub your eyeballs.

- Rub your neck where you feel your pulse. Have your doctor show you how and where.

- Hold your breath and bear down as hard as you can for as long as you can like you are having a bowel movement. This vagal maneuver is called a valsalva.

"Everybody has been constipated. And if you press down really hard, you get dizzy. The reason you get dizzy is because you slow your heart rate and your blood pressure disappears," says Dr. Miura.

■ **RELY ON THE DIVING REFLEX.** When sea mammals dive into the coldest regions of the water, their heart rates automatically slow. That's nature's way of preserving their brains and hearts. You can call on your own diving reflex by filling a basin with icy water and plunging your face into it for a second or two.

"Sometimes, that will interrupt the tachycardia," says Dr. Miura.

■ **CUT DOWN ON CAFFEINE.** Too much coffee, cola, tea, chocolate, diet pills, or stimulants in any form can put you at risk for tachycardia, says Dr. Miura. And skip the so-called energy drinks. Tachycardia is a commonly reported adverse effect from consuming caffeine in the quantities in most energy drinks, along with insomnia, nervousness, and headache, according to a study reported in the *Journal of the American Pharmacists Association.*

■ **GO EASY ON ALCOHOL.** Drinking alcohol—red wine, in particular—can trigger SVT. Try going without for several weeks and see if your symptoms improve.

■ **KICK THE BUTT.** Smoking is also associated with triggering tachycardia. If you don't smoke, don't start. And if you do smoke and have symptoms of tachycardia, consider it just one more reason to quit.

■ **GET YOUR FAIR SHARE OF MAGNESIUM.** In the muscle cells of the heart, magnesium helps balance the effects of calcium, which stimulates muscular contractions within the cell itself. Magnesium creates rhythmic contraction and relaxation, helping the enzymes in the cells pump calcium out, and making the heart less likely to get irritable. Magnesium can be found in such foods as soybeans, nuts, beans, and bran.

■ **KEEP POTASSIUM LEVELS UP.** Potassium is another mineral that helps slow heart action and reduce irritability of the muscle fibers. The mineral is found in fruits and vegetables, so getting enough shouldn't be difficult. But you can deplete it if your diet is high in sodium or if you use diuretics or overuse laxatives.

■ **GET MODERATE EXERCISE.** Getting in shape with moderate aerobic exercise tends to reset your resting heart rate at a lower level. Exercise also helps you get your aggressions out in a healthy way.

But check with your doctor before beginning a new exercise program. Some people may experience what's known as exercise-induced ventricular tachycardia, a more serious form of rapid heartbeat, says Dr. Miura.

PANEL OF ADVISORS

DENNIS S. MIURA, M.D., PH.D., IS AN ASSISTANT CLINICAL PROFESSOR OF MEDICINE AT THE ALBERT EINSTEIN COLLEGE OF MEDICINE OF YESHIVA UNIVERSITY AND DIRECTOR OF CARDIOLOGY AT THE BRONX-WESTCHESTER MEDICAL GROUP, BOTH IN BRONX, NEW YORK.

STEPHEN R. SHOROFSKY, M.D., PH.D., IS DIRECTOR OF THE ELECTROPHYSIOLOGY LABORATORY AT THE UNIVERSITY OF MARYLAND MEDICAL CENTER IN BALTIMORE, AND PROFESSOR OF MEDICINE AT THE UNIVERSITY OF MARYLAND SCHOOL OF MEDICINE.

Teething

9 Ways to Soothe the Pain

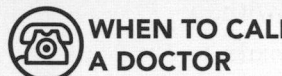

WHEN TO CALL A DOCTOR

It's normal for babies to develop low-grade fever while teething. But if the temperature is 100°F or higher, it means something else is going on in your baby's body. You should see your doctor.

Just one of the many miracles of life, an infant's teeth actually start developing months before birth. In fact, tooth buds begin appearing by the 7th week of pregnancy. By the time the baby is born, all 20 of the primary teeth that will sprout over the next $2\frac{1}{2}$ years are already present and accounted for in the jawbone.

Usually those first teeth start pushing 4 to 8 months after birth. Baby's gums become swollen and tender, and the little child becomes irritable and restless. Get ready—teething has begun.

An infant can react to this new sensation of teething in a variety of ways. Some babies will experience periods of irritability and pain and some will run low-grade fevers, always lower than 100°F, says Dorota Szczepaniak, M.D., FAAP. Teething infants enjoy chewing, but after the recent warning about possible toxic ingredients in plastic toys, doctors recommend natural methods to ease teething—all from ingredients readily available at home. Here is the current expert advice.

■ **COOL THOSE TEETH.** A wet washcloth placed in the freezer for 30 minutes makes a handy teething aid. "It's cold and crunchy, and infants enjoy it—just be sure to wash it after each use," says Dr. Szczepaniak. Avoid rubber teething rings filled with liquid because they can break and expose your baby to the chemical inside, she warns. And those recent warnings about chemicals in plastic make the rubber teething rings less desirable.

■ **DAB THE DROOL.** Drooling often occurs around the same time as teething, but new research suggests it is not caused by the teething. "Drooling has more to do with the child starting to make more saliva and not having yet learned how to swallow it," says Helen F. Neville, R.N. Wash the overflow off frequently with a warm washcloth to prevent a rash from developing on the baby's face.

If drool causes a rash on your baby's face, wipe gently—don't rub—with a soft cotton cloth. "You can also smooth petroleum jelly on the baby's chin before a nap or bedtime to protect the skin from further irritation," says Dr. Szczepaniak.

■ **MASSAGE THE GUMS.** Rub your baby's gums with a clean finger, gently but firmly. Or gently rub the gums with a small, cool spoon, says Dr. Szczepaniak.

Cures from the Kitchen

Instead of the typical teething ring, try giving your baby some frozen bananas in a product called Baby Safe Feeder. Designed to eliminate choking hazards for early eaters, the feeder looks similar to a pacifier with a small mesh bag (instead of a nipple) that can hold food for your baby to suck or chew. Most standard teething rings are flavorless, so just a little frozen fruit will give the baby an incentive to bite down and work those teeth through the gums.

■ **LISTEN TO GRANDMA.** Infants 6 months or older may get comfort from biting a hard teething cracker—a time-honored trick. Dr. Szczepaniak recommends using organic whole grain unsweetened biscuits with no salt added. You can also take a small slice of day-old bagel (with the crust) and let baby gnaw on it. Just make sure the chunk is big enough so it can't be swallowed and won't break into pieces, and it should not contain nuts, says Dr. Szczepaniak.

■ **OPT FOR A FRUIT POP.** Let your 6-month or older baby suck on an unsweetened fruit juice popsicle. "You can make popsicles yourself by freezing baby food fruits," says Dr. Szczepaniak.

■ **GAUZE THE GUMS.** If your baby hates the feel of a toothbrush, then wipe the teeth with gauze rather than a toothbrush, says Neville. When you do start brushing your infant's little teeth, make sure you use a child's soft toothbrush. And be gentle. Neville advises tasting the toothpaste. "For some sensitive kids, mint flavor is hot, peppery, and uncomfortable," she says. "So some parents find that changing the toothpaste makes the child more willing to get her teeth brushed."

■ **BAN THE BOTTLE.** Well, not completely. But once your baby is teething, make sure your child doesn't fall asleep with a bottle in her mouth. The milk or juice can pool in the mouth and start the process of tooth decay and plaque. But some kids really need those bottles, says

Neville. "Sucking is really important to them. If your child still needs a bottle, gradually dilute the milk with water. That way the child can suck on a bottle without damaging the teeth," she explains.

■ **CUDDLE AND COO.** "The children who are more sensitive are going to be in more pain, and the kids with a higher pain tolerance are going to float right through teething," says Neville. If your child is sensitive, he'll need more cuddling, holding, and soothing because of the pain.

■ **BE A CLOWN.** Sometimes a simple distraction can help your baby forget his pain temporarily, says Dr. Szczepaniak.

PANEL OF ADVISORS

HELEN F. NEVILLE, R.N., IS A SPECIALIST IN INBORN TEMPERAMENT AND FORMER INSTRUCTOR IN STRESS MANAGEMENT AT KAISER PERMANENTE HOSPITAL IN OAKLAND, CALIFORNIA. SHE IS AUTHOR OF *TEMPERAMENT TOOLS* AND *IS THIS A PHASE? CHILD DEVELOPMENT & PARENT STRATEGIES, BIRTH TO 6 YEARS.*

DOROTA SZCZEPANIAK, M.D., FAAP, IS ASSOCIATE DIRECTOR OF CLINICAL AFFAIRS AT THE SECTION OF GENERAL AND COMMUNITY PEDIATRICS, INDIANA UNIVERSITY SCHOOL OF MEDICINE, AND A GENERAL PEDIATRICIAN AT RILEY HOSPITAL FOR CHILDREN IN INDIANAPOLIS.

Temporomandibular Disorders

21 Ideas to Ease the Discomfort

Temporomandibular disorders, a group of diseases commonly known as TMD, are without a doubt among the most complex and controversial of all modern ailments.

While TMD is usually linked to problems with the muscles or joints (or a combination of the two), it sometimes involves related tissues, such as the ligaments or bone cartilage. Many experts believe that most cases have multiple causes. Trauma, stress, misaligned teeth, orthodontic treatment, and arthritis are just some of the factors associated with TMD. And still, other factors are yet to be discovered.

What is clearly known is that women appear to have TMD symptoms at about twice the rate of men. "Research suggests women's hormonal fluctuations during pregnancy and menopause may account for their higher incidence," says John C. Moon, D.D.S.

Fortunately in the majority of cases, TMD pain is temporary and can be relieved with simple measures. Here are a few that our experts recommend.

■ **ASSUME THE POSITION.** Your tongue's resting position should be on the top of your palate during the day, says Dr. Moon. This relieves tension in the jaw. If you can also maintain this position while you sleep, it might help curb teeth grinding.

■ **CHILL OUT.** Increase bloodflow to the area with an ice pack or bag of frozen peas wrapped in a towel. Cold packs are effective for relieving acute pain and reducing strain and swelling that go along with it, says Jerry F. Taintor, D.D.S. Apply to the

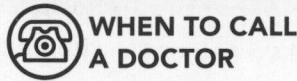

WHEN TO CALL A DOCTOR

The most common signs of temporomandibular disorders (TMD)—among them, facial and jaw joint pain or swelling; headaches; toothaches; aching neck, shoulders, or back; and a clicking, grating, or popping noise or pain when opening or closing your jaw—are usually nothing more than minor to moderate annoyances that will go away when the condition is treated. Few people develop significant long-term effects.

Some symptoms, however, are considered more serious and should be investigated by your doctor. Signs that your TMD is getting worse: You can't open your mouth or brush your teeth, or you are having sharp headaches.

affected area for 5 to 10 minutes or until it feels a little numb. Do not exceed 20 minutes. Repeat every 2 hours for up to 2 days or until the pain is relieved. Apply heat therapy, using a warm compress, for the same length of time.

■ **CUDDLE UP WITH A HEATING PAD OR HEAT PACK.** Heat can soothe muscles for recurrent or prolonged TMD. Apply a heating pad or pack several times a day, especially in the evening when symptoms often seem to worsen, says Dr. Taintor.

Basically, you want to use hot compresses for muscle aches around the jaw and temples, and use cold compresses for pain at the temporomandibular joint itself, says Andrew S. Kaplan, D.M.D.

■ **MASSAGE THE JAW.** You can also try gently stretching and massaging the jaw as long as the muscles don't cramp up. If you get the blood flowing in the area, you are likely to alleviate some of your symptoms, says Dr. Kaplan. This will help gradually increase your range of motion and strengthen the joint.

■ **TAKE AN ANTI-INFLAMMATORY.** Dr. Taintor suggests taking two ibuprofen tablets every 4 to 6 hours.

■ **CHECK YOUR BODY POSITION.** If you work at a desk, check your body position throughout the day. Make sure that you, and especially your chin, are not leaning over the desk. Your back should be supported. As a general guideline for sitting or standing, your cheekbones should be over your clavicles, and your ears should not be too far in front of your shoulders, he says.

If you have neck pain and headaches, attach an adjustable document holder to your computer monitor to minimize neck strain as you work. If you're on the phone all day, avoid tilting your head on your shoulder. Consider getting a headset, says Dr. Moon.

■ **SLEEP ON A WEDGE-SHAPED HEAD PILLOW.** A wedge pillow helps keep your neck and jaw in proper alignment because it positions you on an incline, says Dr. Moon. You can also tuck a pillow under your knees. Sleeping in this position—on your back throughout the entire night with your head, neck, shoulders, and upper back in alignment and less pressure on your lower back—can be very relaxing to your jaw joints and critical to overcoming TMD. But what if you generally sleep on your side? Try placing a beanbag on each side of your head to stop you from rolling into that position.

■ **LIMIT YOUR JAW MOVEMENT.** If you feel a yawn coming, try to restrict it by holding a fist under your chin, says Dr. Kaplan. Yawning can actually stress the jaw.

■ **DON'T CHEW GUM.** Repetitive chewing can stress the jaw and increase TMD symptoms, says Dr. Moon. Control other similar habits, such as biting your lips or fingernails, and use your pencil for writing, not chewing.

■ **STOP GRINDING YOUR TEETH.** Gnashing teeth, referred to by doctors as bruxism, is often associated with TMD and may be a

Seven Habits to Break

Overcoming temporomandibular disorders (TMD) is very much a matter of what you don't do, advises Andrew S. Kaplan, D.M.D. If any of these habits are yours—pay attention! These tips may be of help to you.

■ Don't sleep on your stomach with your head twisted to one side.

■ Don't lie on your back with your head propped up at a sharp angle for reading or watching television.

■ Don't cradle the telephone between your shoulder and chin.

■ Don't prop your chin on one or both of your hands for too long.

■ Don't carry a heavy shoulder bag with the strap on the same shoulder for an extended period.

■ Don't participate in situations, such as painting a ceiling or sitting in the front row during movies, that require looking up for long periods of time.

■ Don't grind or clench your teeth.

factor that exacerbates existing symptoms, says Dr. Kaplan.

■ **CREATE A RELAXING BEDTIME ROUTINE.** Going to sleep after a stressful day can lead to teeth grinding like nothing else. Don't go to sleep stressed. Wind down with quiet music, a gentle massage, or a few simple yoga stretches before you climb into bed, says Dr. Moon.

■ **USE A MOUTH GUARD.** Ask your dentist to fit you professionally with a mouth guard. These are far better than those sold in sporting goods stores and drugstores. A well-fitted mouth guard can help reduce nighttime grinding and clenching, says Dr. Moon.

If your symptoms seem worse in the morning, wear a mouth guard during the night. You may be grinding your teeth while you sleep. In some cases, bruxism can lead to poor sleep habits and aggravate symptoms.

■ **AVOID HARD, CRUNCHY FOOD.** Limit yourself to a soft diet to keep stress off the muscles and joints. Eat soft foods like pasta, fish, mashed potatoes, boiled chicken, and well-cooked vegetables. "Avoid hard-to-chew foods like steak, broiled chicken, salads (which require lots of lateral movement to chew), raw carrots, and celery," says Dr. Kaplan.

■ **CONSIDER ACUPRESSURE.** To find the point that will ease TMD cheek pain on the left side of your face, Albert Forgione, Ph.D., recommends the following: Place your left forearm on a table with your palm flat. Put the fingers of your right hand on your left forearm so your index finger is in the fold of your elbow and the rest of your fingers lay next to each other. Wiggle your left middle finger and feel the corresponding ligament move at the edge of your right index fingertip. Press moderately hard on this point for 15 seconds (the point will feel quite sensitive and will hurt if you have found the right spot). You may have to do this three times in a row, pausing briefly in between. Switch sides to relieve pain on the right side of your face.

Here's another one to try: Hegu is a point on the hand also known as large intestine 4. This point is considered to be the most powerful acupressure point in the body for head and face pain. Locate this point by placing the thumb of the opposite hand halfway between the index finger and the thumb on the hand that's on the same side as your face pain, then extend to the line of the first knuckle and push down. You can also apply ice wrapped in a small towel to easily stimulate the point with

both cold and pressure. Hold the ice in place for 20 minutes to provide several hours of relief from face pain or headache, says George E. Maloney, D.M.D., M.Ac.

PANEL OF ADVISORS

ALBERT FORGIONE, PH.D., IS A PAIN SPECIALIST AND DIRECTOR OF RESEARCH AT THE CRANIOFACIAL PAIN CENTER AT TUFTS UNIVERSITY SCHOOL OF DENTAL MEDICINE IN BOSTON.

ANDREW S. KAPLAN, D.M.D., IS A CLINICAL ASSOCIATE PROFESSOR OF DENTISTRY AT MOUNT SINAI SCHOOL OF MEDICINE OF NEW YORK UNIVERSITY AND A FORMER DIRECTOR OF THE TMJ AND FACIAL PAIN CLINIC AND ASSOCIATE ATTENDING DENTIST AT MOUNT SINAI HOSPITAL IN NEW YORK CITY.

GEORGE E. MALONEY, D.M.D., M.AC., IS AN ASSOCIATE PROFESSOR AT THE CRANIOFACIAL PAIN CENTER AT TUFTS UNIVERSITY SCHOOL OF DENTAL MEDICINE IN BOSTON.

JOHN C. MOON, D.D.S., IS A COSMETIC AND GENERAL DENTIST IN HALF MOON BAY, CALIFORNIA.

JERRY F. TAINTOR, D.D.S., IS A DENTIST IN PRIVATE PRACTICE IN MEMPHIS, TENNESSEE, THE FORMER CHAIR OF ENDODONTICS AT THE UNIVERSITY OF TENNESSEE COLLEGE OF DENTISTRY IN MEMPHIS, AND THE FORMER CHAIR OF ENDODONTICS AT THE UCLA SCHOOL OF DENTISTRY. HE IS AUTHOR OF *THE COMPLETE GUIDE TO BETTER DENTAL CARE.*

Tendinitis

10 Soothing Remedies

Like simple muscle soreness from overuse, tendinitis—inflammation in or around a tendon—can be painful. But where simple muscle soreness is temporary, tendinitis is tenacious. It's soreness that doesn't go away with a few hours of rest and an ice pack.

Tendon injuries are often related to problems with the underlying tendon prior to the injury, says Terry Malone, Ed.D. With each additional injury, tendon recovery becomes more limited and your risk of another injury increases. "We never really get back to normal after the first injury, which is why doctors often use the word *tendonosis* (a degenerative process) rather than *tendinitis* (an inflammatory process)," Dr. Malone explains.

The situation isn't hopeless. But if you continue to use the tendon in the same repetitive motion that triggered the problem in the first place, it's going to be very difficult to get better. This applies to everyone from world-class marathoners to window washers and typists.

Still, it's possible to lessen the effects of tendinitis and prevent intense flare-ups. The key is to unlock your mind and be free to change some of your old ways.

■ **GIVE IT A REST.** That's a hard thing for some people to do. But a runner with Achilles tendinitis, for example, can't realistically expect any improvement if he doesn't take at least a couple of days away from the pounding.

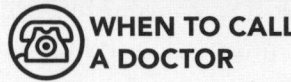

WHEN TO CALL A DOCTOR

If you only feel the pain of tendinitis during or after exercise, and if it isn't too bad, you may be thinking that you could run a race or swim laps with that same amount of pain—if you had to. Or maybe you already have.

In either case, you would be wise to realign your thinking. Avoid playing through pain unless your physician or physical therapist tells you otherwise.

If pain is severe and you continue to abuse the tendon, it may rupture. That could mean a long layoff, surgery, or even permanent disability.

In other words, exercising through tendon pain today could mean staying on the sidelines for the remainder of your tomorrows. To err on the safe side, back off if you're in pain, and see a physician if your pain is persistent.

Try reducing your mileage—or substituting non-weight-bearing activities such as swimming or upper-body training, as long as these don't aggravate the pain. Avoid walking or running uphill, because this increases the stretch on the tendon, irritating it and making it weaker, says Teresa Schuemann, P.T., S.C.S., A.T.C., C.S.C.S.

Regular calf stretches may help prevent Achilles tendinitis, says Michael J. Mueller, P.T., Ph.D.

When you return to walking, keep the foot in a neutral position by sticking to flat surfaces, and gradually increase your distance and intensity.

Of course, resting is easier said than done if the activity triggering your tendinitis is part of your job. If you have occupational tendinitis, it might not be a bad idea to save a day or two of vacation time for those flare-ups of tendinitis.

■ **BUT DON'T GIVE IT TOO LONG A REST.** Inactivity can worsen mild musculoskeletal pain because it prevents blood from flowing to that area. And if you stop working out and begin filling out, added weight will cause more stress on your musculoskeletal system.

Cut back on the intensity of your workouts, but not the frequency, says Willibald Nagler, M.D. If anything, you want to exercise more regularly to condition all your muscle groups and keep them from getting even stiffer.

You're better off with a little conditioning every day rather than heroic efforts once a week, says Dr. Nagler. Daily stretching, for instance, renders muscles more flexible, and in effect

gives them the same properties they had in younger years when they were more resilient.

■ **MAKE A CHANGE.** If your tendinitis is exercise induced, a new form of exercise may be just what your inflamed tendon needs. If you're a runner with tendon problems in the lower legs, for example, you can stay on the road if you're willing to hop on a bicycle, which will still give you a good upper-leg workout.

■ **HAVE A SOAK.** Taking a whirlpool bath or just soaking in warm bathwater is a good way to raise body temperature and increase bloodflow. Warming the tendon before stressful activity decreases the soreness associated with tendinitis.

■ **ICE IT.** In severe tendinitis flare-ups, limit or stop your activity and place cold packs on the injured area for 15 to 20 minutes, up to three or four times a day, to reduce inflammation and pain, says Dr. Mueller.

In general, ice is helpful after exercising for holding down both swelling and pain. People with heart disease, diabetes, or vascular problems, however, should be careful about using ice because the cold constricts blood vessels and could cause serious difficulties.

■ **WRAP IT UP.** Another alternative for reducing swelling is to wrap your pain in an elastic bandage. Just be careful not to wrap the inflamed area too tightly or to leave the area wrapped for so long that it becomes uncomfortable or interferes with circulation. (For more information about using an elastic bandage, see Sprains on page 564.)

■ **RAISE THE SQUEAKY WHEEL.** Elevating the affected area above heart level is also good for controlling swelling.

■ **GO OVER-THE-COUNTER.** Aspirin, ibuprofen, and naproxen (Aleve)—nonprescription nonsteroidal anti-inflammatory drugs—are effective temporary pain relievers for tendinitis. They also reduce inflammation and swelling, says Dr. Malone.

■ **WARM UP FIRST.** Warming up includes more than just temperature, says Dr. Malone. Always perform slow and controlled actions before higher speed actions. "We want to increase temperature but also stretch the muscle-tendon unit into the range of motion that is required for the activity," he explains. This minimizes the likelihood of injury and helps you stay safe during exercise. The idea is to increase temperature (often just general low-level exercises), then stretch, then move into the activities progressively.

"Interestingly, some recent data suggest significant stretching just before performance may actually decrease maximal levels of performance," says Dr. Malone.

But don't skip stretching altogether. Some studies indicate that people who are less flexible are more prone to develop tendinitis. So stretching should be a regular part of your routine.

■ **TAKE WORK BREAKS.** A simple way to at least temporarily relieve physical stress at work is to take frequent breaks and move,

What the Doctor Does

You feel a mild sting, a little pressure. You may wonder if you've wandered into a sci-fi movie; there's a big, ball-shaped device nestled next to your arm. But if you have an aching tennis elbow, you won't mind because a government-approved shock wave treatment could ease the pain.

In a study of 114 people whose tendinitis did not respond to other therapies, 64 percent of those treated with Sonocur Basic reported significantly less pain. During three 15- to 20-minute weekly sessions, the device sends out shock waves that stimulate bloodflow and the release of chemicals that start a healing process. This drug- and surgery-free therapy, widely used in Europe and Canada, is becoming more popular throughout the United States.

stretch, or at least change your position. Tendinitis can develop quite easily if you work in an awkward position, especially in the arms or wrists if you're working at a keyboard all day.

PANEL OF ADVISORS

TERRY MALONE, ED.D., IS A PROFESSOR OF PHYSICAL THERAPY AT THE UNIVERSITY OF KENTUCKY IN LEXINGTON.

MICHAEL J. MUELLER, P.T., PH.D., IS AN ASSOCIATE PROFESSOR OF PHYSICAL THERAPY AND DIRECTOR OF THE APPLIED BIOMECHANICS LABORATORY AT WASHINGTON UNIVERSITY SCHOOL OF MEDICINE IN ST. LOUIS.

WILLIBALD NAGLER, M.D., IS A PROFESSOR OF REHABILITATION MEDICINE AT NEW YORK WEILL CORNELL MEDICAL CENTER IN NEW YORK CITY.

TERESA SCHUEMANN, P.T., S.C.S., A.T.C., C.S.C.S., IS DIRECTOR OF THE PHYSICAL THERAPY AND SPORTS MEDICINE DEPARTMENT AND DIRECTOR OF THE SPORTS PHYSICAL THERAPY RESIDENCY PROGRAM AT SKYLINE HOSPITAL IN WHITE SALMON, WASHINGTON.

Tinnitus

19 Ways to Cope with the Din

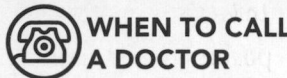

WHEN TO CALL A DOCTOR

Because tinnitus can be caused by so many things, including a tumor, Lyme disease, and other medical problems that are potentially serious, it's essential to see a doctor at the first sign of symptoms.

If you've started experiencing tinnitus and you're also taking prescription or over-the-counter medications, talk to your doctor or pharmacist. A number of drugs, including aspirin or antibiotics, can aggravate tinnitus in some people. Even drugs that help some people with tinnitus, such as antihistamines, may worsen it in others.

The noise of the modern world is bad enough, but people with tinnitus have the added burden of hearing sounds in their own heads. This irritating condition causes people to hear clicking, roaring, ringing, or buzzing sounds when no external sounds actually exist.

Doctors and audiologists think tinnitus is caused by damage to the microscopic hairs on auditory cells in the inner ear, which in turn causes portions of the brain to generate its own sound.

Persistent exposure to ear-splitting music or other loud sounds is the main cause of tinnitus. It has also been linked to hearing loss, circulatory problems, and middle-ear problems. Tinnitus is often accompanied by an intense sensitivity to sounds called *hyperacusis*.

Of the 50 million Americans who experience tinnitus, 12 million have it seriously enough to seek medical help for their condition. It can sometimes be eliminated by treating underlying medical problems, or it sometimes goes away on its own, but the main approach is to help people cope with the persistent noise—and to prevent it from getting worse. Here's what doctors advise.

■ **AVOID LOUD NOISES.** Table saws, power motors, and the ear-pounding volume of rock 'n' roll are just a few of the things that can damage auditory cells and make tinnitus worse.

"If you're 8 feet from someone and have to raise your voice to make yourself heard, the environmental noise is probably too loud and potentially damaging to the inner ear," says Douglas Mattox, M.D.

■ **PICK UP SOME EARPLUGS.** When you know you're going to be exposed to ear-splitting sounds—from a construction crew next door, for example—pick up some earplugs. Pharmacy earplugs work fine, but you'll do better with the type sold at music stores: They allow you to hear music or voices clearly, but at a greatly reduced volume.

Customized earplugs are available at audiology clinics or businesses that specialize in hearing aids.

■ **DON A SET OF EARMUFFS.** If you don't like the sensation of earplugs, drop by the hardware store and pick up a set of foam-filled safety muffs, which form a tight seal over the ears. "Ear muffs are the most effective sound defenders," says Dr. Mattox. You probably won't wear these out in public, to a Metallica concert, for example, but they may come in handy while running your table saw in the privacy of your basement.

■ **HUM AWAY NOISE.** One of the first lessons drummers learn is that humming for a few seconds during the loudest part of the song helps drown out the crashing sounds of cymbals. You can use the same technique whenever you're anticipating a loud noise—when you're walking past an idling bus, for example, or when you're using power tools at home.

Humming activates a muscle in the inner ear, which pulls tiny bones together and pre-

vents some sound waves from getting through. This helps protect you ears from prolonged exposure to loud noises.

■ **GIVE YOUR EARS A REST.** A single loud noise could potentially cause tinnitus, but persistent loud noises are more likely to be the problem. It's important to let the ears "rest" for about 16 hours after exposure to loud sounds. If you work in a noisy environment, wear earplugs to protect your hearing and keep your tinnitus from getting worse. And turn down the volume on the MP3 player and TV.

■ **ASK ABOUT A HEARING AID.** About 90 percent of those with severe tinnitus also have hearing loss. A hearing aid often helps both problems at the same time. One possible benefit of using a hearing aid to mask tinnitus is that you may experience several tinnitus-free hours after you take the hearing aid off (called residual inhibition).

■ **GET A WEARABLE SOUND GENERATOR.** Available from audiologists, a sound generator placed in the ear like a hearing aid fills the ear with a soft white noise. This white noise distracts the auditory pathways so your brain won't pay attention to the sounds of tinnitus.

■ **EAT LESS SALT.** Tinnitus is sometimes caused by Ménière's disease, a condition that results in excessive amounts of fluid in the ear, causing hearing loss, dizziness, fullness in the ear, and tinnitus. People with this condition should restrict their daily sodium intake to 2,000 milligrams by limiting the use of table salt, for example, and buying low-sodium soups, condiments, and other packaged foods.

■ **CUT BACK ON CAFFEINE.** If you drink a lot of coffee, tea, or cola, you might experience higher levels of tinnitus. Caffeine constricts blood vessels and temporarily raises blood pressure, which can make the sounds of tinnitus louder. Giving up caffeine isn't likely to eliminate the problem, but it might make a small difference in some people, says Dr. Mattox.

■ **DON'T SMOKE.** The nicotine in cigarettes and cigars has the same effect as caffeine: It constricts blood vessels and may make tinnitus sounds more noticeable.

■ **TRY "TINNITUS RETRAINING."** Studies have shown that when people subject themselves to a quiet sound—static or white noise from a sound generator that's just loud enough to mask the tinnitus sounds—the internal noise may diminish or even disappear.

Over a period of months, you'll find that the volume of sound needed to mask the tinnitus may get progressively lower.

■ **LEARN TO RELAX.** If you already have tinnitus, high levels of stress are likely to make the sounds seem louder. Everyone controls stress in different ways. Some people exercise. Others meditate, practice yoga, or retreat to the movies for the afternoon. You can buy audiotapes or CDs that explain how to relax. Or you can see a professional hypnotist or other therapists who will help you find ways to unwind on your own.

■ **LEARN TO DISTRACT YOURSELF.** It can be hard to ignore the sounds of tinnitus, but it's worth making the effort. The more you focus on the sounds, the more likely it is your brain will build additional neural pathways to make your listening more efficient. In other words, you may wind up hearing the annoying sounds even more, says Dr. Mattox.

"The most important thing is to keep the auditory system busy doing other things," Dr. Mattox says. "When you're working or doing other quiet activities, create a little ambient noise, like the sound of a small water fountain or an inexpensive noise generator."

An even easier solution is to turn on the radio. Just be sure to keep the volume low, Dr. Mattox advises. "You don't necessarily want sounds that you'll pay attention to or that you'll find distracting."

■ **GET MORE SHUT-EYE.** If tinnitus is keeping you up, try masking the noise with a white-noise machine, a fan, or soft music. If nighttime Zzzs still elude you, take a nap during the day. Contrary to conventional wisdom, research shows taking naps doesn't keep you from sleeping at night, says Sara Mednick, Ph.D. In fact, napping during the day lowers your risk of heart disease, and by association may reduce your risk of tinnitus. "Just limit you naps to $1\frac{1}{2}$ hours or less, and wake up at least 2 hours before bedtime."

■ **BREAK A SWEAT.** Daily aerobic exercise helps distract you from the noise and improves circulation. Better circulation may also help your cardiovascular health and reduce the incidence of vascular-related tinnitus.

■ **LISTEN TO THE SOUNDS OF NATURE.** A study in the *Journal of the American Academy of Audiology* found masking sounds with white noise or music reduced ringing in the ears better than no sound therapy at all. But when the researchers tested 10 digital white noise and custom sound formats to determine which sounds masked tinnitus the best, they found water and nature sounds significantly more effective in relieving tinnitus than the other eight digital sound formats.

■ **AVOID OVERDOSING ON ASPIRIN.** If you accidentally or intentionally pop large amounts of aspirin, you may hear warning bells. An overdose may affect your inner-ear cells and cause ringing in the ears. The higher the daily dose, the more likely you are to experience tinnitus. The symptom typically disappears when you stop taking aspirin. Many other medications carry the risk of tinnitus as a side effect. If you already have tinnitus, talk to your doctor before taking any new medication.

■ **STICK IT IN YOUR EAR.** Consider sticking it to your tinnitus with acupuncture. In a recent double-blind acupuncture and tinnitus study, researchers in Portugal asked acupuncturists to treat two groups of 76 tinnitus patients with acupuncture needles. But the acupuncturists didn't know what condition they were treating.

For the first group, the acupuncturists inserted the tiny needles in locations most likely to ease tinnitus. For the second group, the acupuncturists inserted needles in other points not likely to ease tinnitus. Although both groups reported some relief, people in the group that got the real treatments had a significantly greater reduction in tinnitus.

PANEL OF ADVISORS

DOUGLAS MATTOX, M.D., IS A PROFESSOR IN THE DEPARTMENT OF OTOLARYNGOLOGY–HEAD AND NECK SURGERY AT EMORY UNIVERSITY SCHOOL OF MEDICINE IN ATLANTA.

SARA MEDNICK, PH.D., IS AN ASSISTANT PROFESSOR AT THE UNIVERSITY OF CALIFORNIA, SAN DIEGO, A RESEARCH SCIENTIST AT THE SALK INSTITUTE FOR BIOLOGICAL STUDIES IN LA JOLLA, CALIFORNIA, AND AUTHOR OF *TAKE A NAP! CHANGE YOUR LIFE.*

Toothache

11 Tips for Pain Relief

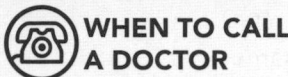

WHEN TO CALL A DOCTOR

A toothache can be a symptom of a wide range of problems. The pulp of your tooth or the gums around your throbbing cuspid could be infected. There could be decay in a molar. You may have a cracked bicuspid.

An injury, a piece of food caught between two teeth, or even a sinus problem may be at the root of your pain, says Jerry F. Taintor, D.D.S. The bottom line? If you have tooth pain, it's important to find out why. See a dentist whenever you have a toothache, even if the pain subsides. If you have an abscessed tooth, it may go into a state of dormancy and seem to be causing no problem, but don't be fooled, warns Dr. Taintor. "It's just waiting to come back with a vengeance." The next time, it might be much worse.

It's no wonder dentistry may have been one of the earliest medical specializations in ancient Egypt. Toothaches can be excruciatingly painful. The Egyptians used some bizarre methods to ward off tooth pain—for example placing a live mouse on the gums of a person with tooth pain. Mice have such good teeth, they reasoned, there should be some effect. By Roman times, things were only marginally better. One ancient scholar noted that a frog tied to the jaws would make teeth firmer, and that toothaches responded to eardrops made from boiling earthworms in olive oil.

The good news is, no rodents, amphibians, or worms need to be harmed to follow the advice we've gathered from *modern* dentists. Here's what they suggest for tooth pain.

■ **RINSE.** Take a mouthful of tepid water and rinse vigorously several times a day, says Jerry F. Taintor, D.D.S. If your toothache is caused by trapped food, a thorough rinse may dislodge the problem.

■ **LEAVE IT ALONE.** When your tooth hurts, it's tempting to keep checking to see exactly how much it hurts. But stop picking at it. "This means keeping things like toothpicks out of the cavity

Be Gentle to Tooth Sensitivity

If you can't even touch the tooth, that's an ache. But if the tooth is merely reacting to heat or cold, then it's a problem with sensitivity.

More than 40 million Americans have "dentinal hypersensitivity," and it begins when the dentin underneath the tooth enamel becomes exposed—usually at the gumline. Sensitivity can also occur from tiny cracks in the tooth, says John C. Moon, D.D.S.

Age, receding gums, surgery, and overzealous brushing with harsh toothpastes and hard brushes can expose dentin. Sometimes plaque attacks the tooth enamel and exposes the dentin.

If you're noticing sensitivity for the first time, it makes good sense to see your dentist to make sure you have no other problem. "Your dentist may recommend a prescription fluoride toothpaste (five times the fluoride strength of over-the-counter toothpastes) or a preparation containing amorphous calcium phosphate," says W. Brian Powley, D.D.S.

---

where one exists. Even keeping your tongue out of the area is helpful," says Dr. Taintor. You already have a problem; don't add to it!

■ **FLOSS GENTLY.** If swishing doesn't work, try to pry a small bit of food like a popcorn hull from between your teeth by flossing, says Dr. Taintor. Hold the floss firmly or use a floss threader that you can get from most pharmacies if you have trouble manipulating the floss with you fingers. Use an easy sawing motion.

Be gentle, but deliberate, says Dr. W. Brian Powley, D.D.S. Your gums are likely to be sore.

■ **RINSE WITH SALTY WATER.** After each meal and at bedtime, add ½ teaspoon of salt to an 8-ounce glass of tepid water, says Dr. Taintor. Hold each mouthful; roll it around your mouth. Spit.

■ **TRY A HAND MASSAGE.** Wrap a thin cloth around an ice cube and rub into the fleshy V-shaped area where the thumb and forefinger meet. Gently hold the ice on the area for 5 to 7 minutes. Amazingly, this technique can ease toothache pain. In one study, ice massage eased toothaches in 60 to 90 percent of the people who tried it. It works by sending rubbing impulses along the nerve pathways that the toothache pain would normally travel. Because the pathways can carry only one signal at a time, the rubbing impulse outweighs the pain.

■ **USE OIL OF CLOVES.** People have been using this remedy for many years. Drop a little directly onto the tooth, or dab a little on a cotton ball and pack it next to the problem tooth. Oil of cloves helps calm the inflamed nerves of the pulp of the tooth, explains John C. Moon, D.D.S.

■ **DON'T BITE.** If the toothache is caused by a bruise because you bit something hard, try not to use that area when you eat. If nothing is damaged, resting the tooth may ease the ache and allow it to heal on its own, says Dr. Moon.

■ **ICE IT.** Treat the problem as you would treat a bruise with ice. As with bruises, ice decreases the inflammation that is causing the pain, says Dr. Moon. Place ice in a small ziplock bag, seal it, wrap a thin cloth around it, and put it on the aching tooth or the adjacent cheek for 15-minute intervals at least three or four times a day.

■ **KEEP YOUR MOUTH SHUT.** If cold air moving past the tooth is a problem, just shut off the flow. But don't clench your teeth. Some toothaches happen because your bite isn't quite right. In this case, avoid shutting your mouth as much as possible until the dentist can take a look.

■ **SWALLOW ASPIRIN.** Don't believe that old-time remedy of placing an aspirin directly on the aching gum. This can cause an aspirin burn, says Dr. Taintor. On the other hand, you can take an aspirin every 4 to 6 hours for pain relief. Extra-strength Tylenol and ibuprofen will work just as well; the pain should start to subside in half an hour or so.

■ **NUMB THE PAIN.** For temporary relief, try a topical desensitizer. "Try over-the-counter benzocaine products such as Anbesol or Orajel," says Dr. Moon.

PANEL OF ADVISORS

JOHN C. MOON, D.D.S., IS A COSMETIC AND GENERAL DENTIST IN HALF MOON BAY, CALIFORNIA.

W. BRIAN POWLEY, D.D.S., IS A DENTIST IN PRIVATE PRACTICE IN PARADISE VALLEY, ARIZONA.

JERRY F. TAINTOR, D.D.S., IS A DENTIST IN PRIVATE PRACTICE IN MEMPHIS, TENNESSEE, THE FORMER CHAIR OF ENDODONTICS AT THE UNIVERSITY OF TENNESSEE COLLEGE OF DENTISTRY IN MEMPHIS, AND THE FORMER CHAIR OF ENDODONTICS AT THE UCLA SCHOOL OF DENTISTRY. HE IS AUTHOR OF *THE COMPLETE GUIDE TO BETTER DENTAL CARE.*

Tooth Stains

11 Brightening Ideas

Coffee, tea, colas, smoke, acidic juices, certain medications, and highly pigmented foods can take a dingy toll on pearly whites.

Not that teeth were ever meant to be totally white. The natural color of teeth is actually light yellow to light yellow-red. But as you age, your teeth tend to darken even more.

Over time, surface enamel cracks and erodes, exposing dentin, the less dense interior of the tooth, which absorbs food color. Stains also latch onto the plaque and tartar buildup on and between teeth, finding anchorage in crevices.

Many things can stain teeth, including antibiotics, quirks in individual metabolism, even a high fever.

The yellower your tooth stains, the easier it will be to remove them. Deep brown stains, such as those brought on by use of the antibiotic tetracycline during childhood when teeth are forming, can be very difficult to erase, says W. Brian Powley, D.D.S.

The good news is that many common stains—the coffee and cigarette variety—can often be washed away between professional cleanings. Here's how.

■ **BRUSH AFTER EVERY MEAL.** If you clean your teeth regularly and conscientiously, you have less chance of keeping stains on your teeth. "Brush in a circular motion (not back and forth)," says John C. Moon, D.D.S.

■ **CHECK YOUR PLAQUE QUOTIENT.** Rinse with a disclosing solution from your dentist to show where plaque remains on your teeth after brushing. Those spots are where your teeth will stain if you don't improve your brushing technique.

■ **RINSE OFTEN.** After every meal, rinse the food from your teeth, says Dr. Moon. If you can't get to a restroom, pick up your water glass, take a swig, then rinse and swallow at the table.

■ **SWITCH TO AN ELECTRIC TOOTHBRUSH.** Reluctant brushers do better with the electric version, and will clean their teeth more often than if they just used a manual toothbrush, says the Academy of General Dentistry. But when it comes to plaque removal, it depends more on the quality of your brushing than the type of toothbrush you're using.

■ **BE CHOOSY ABOUT YOUR MOUTH-WASH.** All mouthwash is fine for rinsing, but mouthwash that has an antibacterial action will reduce stain-catching plaque. And now you can find whitening mouthwash products made by Crest and Listerine that may help a little, says Dr. Moon.

■ **USE A WHITENING TOOTHPASTE OR TOOTH POLISH.** Dentists used to warn patients away from over-the-counter whitening products because they contained gritty abrasives that could erode the tooth enamel. But manufacturers have gotten better at using peroxide instead of abrasives to give you a slightly brighter after-brushing effect.

But don't expect miracles. Because peroxides in toothpastes or polishes stay on the tooth surface only for a brief period of time, they give just a bit of whitening and it doesn't last very long, says Dr. Moon. Even the lighteners you get at the dentist's office won't last

forever—there's no permanent solution, he explains. That's because after you get your teeth nice and white, you'll probably still be drinking tea, coffee, colas—the same things that stained your teeth in the first place.

■ **SIP THROUGH A STRAW.** To prevent staining, or restaining, after you've used a whitener, consider drinking beverages such as coffee, tea, and cola through a straw to avoid staining your teeth again. "You may not enjoy drinking a fine red wine this way, but overall you can limit your exposure," says Dr. Moon.

■ **SCRUB GENTLY.** Just as abrasive products could scrub away enamel, overly aggressive brushing can expose the deeper-hued dentin, which, ironically, could make your teeth look even dingier.

■ **TRY TOOTH STRIPS.** This product looks like packing tape, but it fits across your teeth. The strips keep peroxide on the teeth a little bit longer than a tooth polish, so they'll get them a bit whiter. They're simple, inexpensive, and safe, says Dr. Moon. Regular use can lighten your teeth 2 to 3 shades, compared with the 8 to 10 shades of lightening you can get from a dentist-directed home-bleaching program or in-office treatment.

■ **USE A BLEACH TRAY.** One of the most effective means of bleaching teeth is a home-bleaching program. Your dentist custom fits you with a mouth-guard-like tray that fits over your teeth. You fill it each night with a concentrated bleach solution and wear it for 1 to 2 hours per day, for 1 to 2 weeks, says Dr. Powley.

This option costs between $400 and $600. While more expensive, the results are dramatically more effective than you can obtain with over-the-counter products.

Some companies make over-the-counter bleaching kits that come with whitening gel and trays that fit onto your teeth. These one-size-fits-all trays don't conform specifically to the surfaces of your teeth and gums. Not only is the peroxide distributed unevenly over your tooth surfaces, but it also may irritate your gums. The reason professional bleaching methods work better is that they use a higher concentration of peroxide that penetrates the tiny tubules that run from the outside of your tooth into the dentin, where they oxidize the discoloration.

■ **DO IT ALL IN ONE VISIT.** If you're impatient because you have a wedding or special event coming up, a dentist can bleach your teeth in a 1- to 2-hour appointment by using a concentrated carbamide peroxide solution and a special light that "powers" the material into the dentin. The only downside is the cost, which can be $500 to $800.

But if you have sensitive teeth, be cautious with this method. "This method is like doing 1 or 2 weeks of treatments in 1 or 2 hours, which can worsen sensitivity," says Dr. Moon. If your teeth are already sensitive, Dr. Moon recommends using the slower, more conservative methods.

PANEL OF ADVISORS

JENNIFER JABLOW, D.D.S., IS IN PRACTICE AT PARK 56 DENTAL IN NEW YORK CITY.

JOHN C. MOON, D.D.S., IS A COSMETIC AND GENERAL DENTIST IN HALF MOON BAY, CALIFORNIA.

W. BRIAN POWLEY, D.D.S., IS A DENTIST IN PRIVATE PRACTICE IN PARADISE VALLEY, ARIZONA.

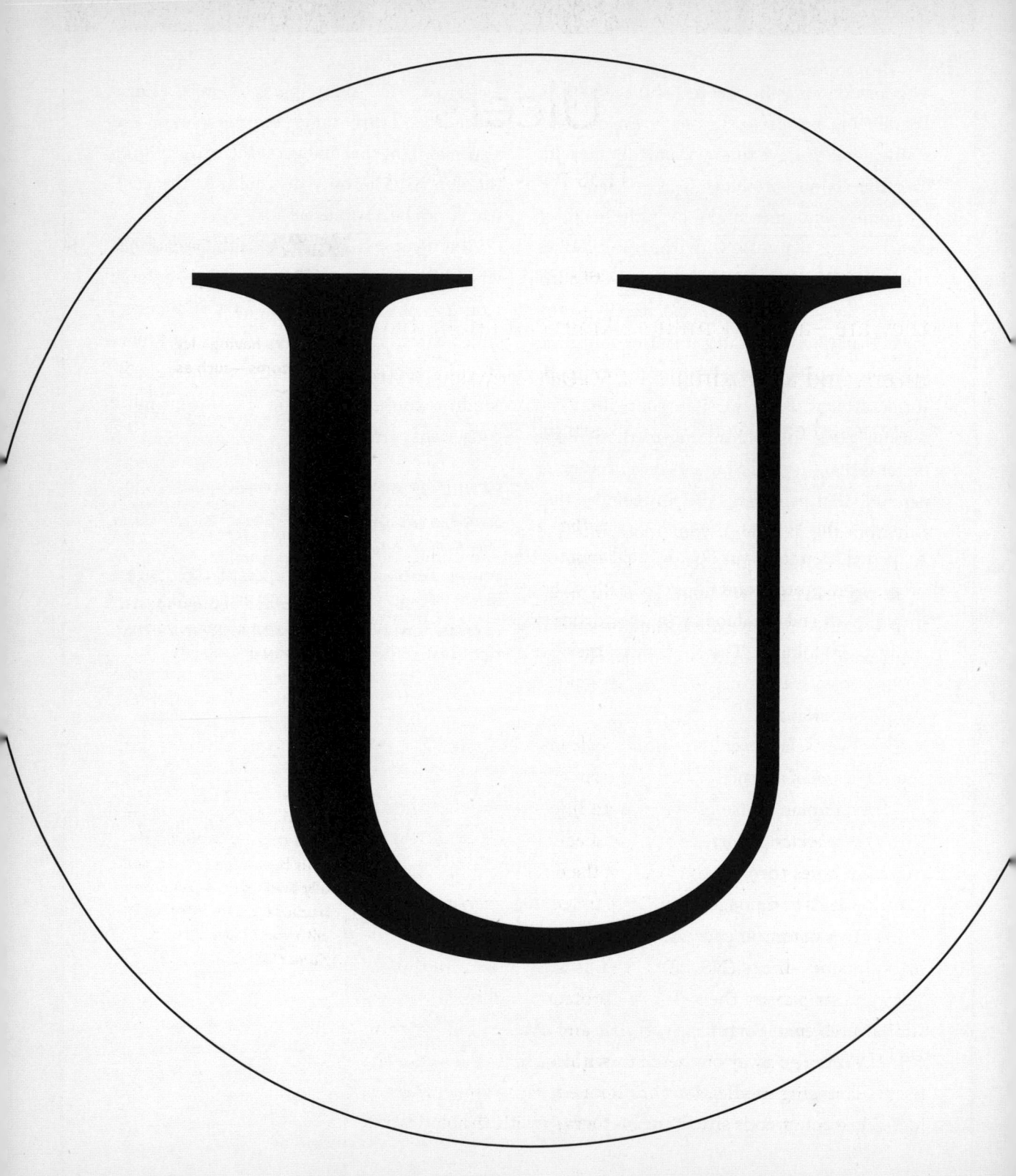

Ulcers

12 Tips for Quick Relief

The surprising thing about ulcers isn't how common they are—about 4 million American adults have ulcers, and approximately 350,000 new cases are diagnosed each year. What's surprising is that we don't get them more often.

Every time you eat, your stomach bathes foods in acids to continue digestion that was begun in the mouth. The same acids that break down protein and fat are actually strong enough to damage the stomach and the duodenum, the portion of the small intestine nearest the stomach. The only reason they don't is that the tissues are coated with a protective, spongelike mucous lining that resists the acidic onslaught.

Sometimes, however, the tissues break down and painful ulcers about the size of a pencil eraser may form.

One common cause of ulcers is an infection of the stomach with *Helicobacter pylori* (*H. pylori*), a corkscrew-shaped bacterium that bores through the lining of the duodenum or stomach, allowing acids to damage the delicate tissue underneath.

Another common cause is the overuse of nonsteroidal anti-inflammatory drugs (NSAIDs) such as aspirin and ibuprofen. They can strip away the stomach's protective lining and cause similar problems. Fortunately, gastric and duodenal ulcers from NSAIDs often go away on their own within 1 to 3 weeks once the tissue-damaging medications are stopped, says Samuel Meyers, M.D. He recommends simultaneous therapy with antibiotics and

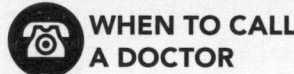

WHEN TO CALL A DOCTOR

If you're having ulcer symptoms—such as stomach pain, a "gnawing" feeling between meals or at night, a burning sensation beneath the breastbone, or black, tarlike stools—ask your doctor to test for the presence of the *Helicobacter pylori* bacterium. The infection can be detected with blood or breath tests. If you test positive, your doctor will probably put you on antibiotics for 1 to 2 weeks. In about 97 percent of cases, the ulcer never comes back.

It's common for people with ulcers to have "sewer breath" long before they have other symptoms. If your breath has an unusually foul odor, it could be because you're infected with the *H. pylori* bacterium. Call your doctor.

other medication to reduce stomach acidity.

"Ulcers due to *H. pylori* can recur sporadically unless the bacteria are eradicated," says Dr. Meyers. "This eradication lowers the recurrence rate to less than 3 percent. The pain in the meantime, however, can be intense."

To stop the pain, and to keep an ulcer from coming back, here's what doctors advise.

■ **GIVE UP ORANGE JUICE FOR A WHILE.** Doctors aren't sure why, but oranges—along with tomatoes and possibly grapefruit—may trigger the release of pain-causing chemical messengers, or neurotransmitters, in those with ulcers. If you think one of these foods might be contributing to your ulcer, try eliminating it from your diet for a few weeks. Then slowly add it back in and see if you notice a difference.

■ **DON'T FALL FOR THE MILK MYTH.** For a long time, doctors encouraged people with ulcers to drink milk. They thought milk's smooth texture would coat and soothe painful ulcers. Research has shown, however, that the protein and calcium in milk stimulate acid production and can make ulcers worse, says Dr. Meyers.

■ **SOOTHE WITH YOGURT.** Although milk can aggravate an ulcer, yogurt can actually soothe one. A review of studies suggests that while these friendly bacteria don't get rid of *H. pylori*, they may lower the levels of it in the stomach, and their antioxidant and anti-inflammatory properties may help heal the gastric mucosa.

The probiotics, or *friendly* bacteria, in yogurt, such as *Lactobacillus bulgaricus* and *L. acidophilus*, may be the therapeutic substance.

■ **GUARD WITH GARLIC.** Long known as a natural antibiotic, some alternative experts suspect that garlic may also inhibit the growth of *H. pylori*. In one laboratory study, the extract from the equivalent of two cloves of garlic was able to stop the growth of this ulcer-causing bacterium.

■ **ASK YOUR DOCTOR ABOUT LICORICE.** It's a traditional folk remedy for ulcers, and there's some evidence that it's effective. Licorice contains glycyrrhizic acid, a compound that is thought to soothe and strengthen the intestinal lining and help ulcers heal more quickly.

The average daily dose is 1.5 to 3 grams, says Dr. Meyers, but talk to your doctor before taking this amount because of the increased risk of high blood pressure. Licorice should not be used on a regular basis for a prolonged time—no longer than for 4 to 6 weeks.

■ **EAT MORE FREQUENTLY.** Even though the stomach's acid production increases during

Cures from the Kitchen

Folk healers have traditionally advised people to drink cabbage juice during ulcer flare-ups. It might be worth a try because cabbage contains an amino acid called glutamine, which is thought to speed intestinal healing.

Some alternative experts recommend juicing half a head of cabbage and drinking it once daily. Eating the same amount of raw cabbage will have similar effects—but don't bother with cooked cabbage, because heat cancels the beneficial effects.

and after meals, the presence of food in the stomach helps buffer the corrosive effects. Eating also increases bloodflow to the stomach, which helps protect it from digestive acids. Rather than having two or three large meals a day, eat five or six small meals daily.

■ **REDUCE THE STRESS IN YOUR LIFE.** For a long time, emotional stress was thought to be a leading cause of ulcers. Doctors now know that stress doesn't cause ulcers—but anxiety, tension, and a high-strung approach to life can increase the brain's perception of pain, says Dr. Meyers. If you already have an ulcer—or have had one in the past—it makes sense to include stress reduction in your overall treatment plan.

Everyone controls stress in different ways. Vigorous exercise—walking, running, or cycling, for example—is a great way to dispel tension at the end of hectic days. Others turn to more formal stress-reduction strategies, such as meditation, prayer, or deep breathing.

■ **QUIT SMOKING.** People who smoke are much more likely to get ulcers than those who don't smoke, Dr. Meyers says. Smoking slows the healing time of ulcers, increases the risk of relapses, and also may make the body more susceptible to infection-causing bacteria.

■ **DRINK ALCOHOL IN MODERATION.** Alcohol can erode the stomach's protective lining, resulting in inflammation and bleeding. It is even more likely to cause problems if you also smoke or take aspirin regularly, says Dr. Meyers.

What the Doctor Does

To stop the pain of ulcers, doctors recommend taking an antacid. During ulcer flare-ups, taking an antacid is the quickest way to relieve the pain, says Samuel Meyers, M.D.

Antacids contain calcium, aluminum, magnesium, or a combination. Aluminum causes constipation in some people, while magnesium can lead to diarrhea. "I advise people to evaluate their overall bowel habits, and choose an antacid based on that, as well as their overall calcium requirement," says Dr. Meyers.

For men, the daily alcohol limit should be two drinks; for women, the upper limit is one drink daily. If ulcers continue to cause problems, you may want to give up alcohol altogether.

■ **CUT BACK ON COFFEE.** Both regular and decaffeinated coffee increase levels of stomach acids. Coffee is unlikely to *cause* ulcers, but it can increase discomfort while an ulcer is healing, Dr. Meyers says.

■ **DRINK A LOT OF WATER.** Drink at least 2 quarts of water daily when ulcers are "active"—and have a full glass whenever you experience discomfort. "Drinking water helps dilute acid in the stomach," Dr. Meyers says. "Unlike milk, it doesn't stimulate the production of more acid."

PANEL OF ADVISORS

SAMUEL MEYERS, M.D., IS A GASTROENTEROLOGIST AND CLINICAL PROFESSOR OF MEDICINE AT THE MOUNT SINAI SCHOOL OF MEDICINE OF NEW YORK UNIVERSITY IN NEW YORK CITY.

Urinary Tract Infections
19 Germ-Fighting Strategies

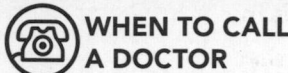

WHEN TO CALL A DOCTOR

Urinary tract infections respond very quickly to antibiotics, so call your doctor at the first sign of symptoms. It's especially important to make the call if you're having fever, chills, or nausea along with the usual sensations of burning or urgency. These are signs of a kidney infection, which can be serious without prompt treatment, says Larrian Gillespie, M.D.

Urinary tract infections are easy to treat, but that's hardly reassuring when you're rushing to the bathroom every 15 minutes to urinate—and experiencing burning, stinging pain.

Most urinary tract infections (UTIs) occur when bacteria from outside the body enter the urethra, the tube that carries urine from the bladder out of the body. Sex is a common cause of UTIs because intercourse can "massage" external bacteria into the urethra. UTIs are also common after menopause, when declines in estrogen make tissues in the vagina and urethra drier and, thus, more vulnerable to bacteria.

One in five women will get a UTI—in the urethra, bladder, or kidneys—at some point in her life. Some women get them over and over again. Men are much less likely to get UTIs because their extra inches of anatomy make it harder for bacteria to get inside.

Antibiotics are necessary to knock out urinary tract infections, says Larrian Gillespie, M.D. Once you start taking the drugs, the discomfort will usually disappear within a day or two. In the meantime, here are a few steps to make you more comfortable and help prevent the infection from coming back.

■ **DRINK A LOT OF WATER.** The more you drink, the more you urinate—and frequent urination helps flush harmful bacteria from the bladder, says Mary Jane Minkin, M.D. When you keep filling your bladder and flushing it out, you can reduce the number of bacteria and help improve your condition.

Water also dilutes the concentrated salts in urine, which can reduce discomfort when you have an infection. Try to drink at least 64 ounces of water each day.

■ **FIGHT BACTERIA WITH BAKING SODA.** At the first sign of symptoms, drink a solution made with ¼ teaspoon of baking soda mixed in 8 ounces of water. Continue this once a day until you can get a culture done at a doctor's office or clinic and can get on antibiotics. Baking soda makes the bladder environment more alkaline, which, thereby, reduces the ability of bacteria to multiply, says Dr. Gillespie.

■ **DILUTE THE BURN.** The concentrated salts in urine can cause stinging pain when you have a UTI. You can reduce discomfort by pouring body-temperature water over yourself while you urinate.

■ **RELAX WITH A HEATING PAD.** Applying heat to the abdomen is a great way to reduce cramps and painful pressure that sometimes accompany UTIs, says Dr. Gillespie. If you don't have a heating pad, a hot-water bottle or washcloth soaked in hot water works just as well.

■ **AVOID ORANGE JUICE FOR A FEW DAYS.** Along with strawberries, grapefruit, and pineapple, orange juice has a high acid content. When you have a UTI, it will increase the burn when you urinate, says Dr. Gillespie.

■ **DON'T DRINK COFFEE OR ALCOHOL.** When you have an infection, coffee and alcohol can make it painful to urinate, says Dr. Gillespie. Caffeine and alcohol also stim-

ulate the muscular walls of the bladder, which may increase urinary "urges" and cause additional discomfort.

■ **DRINK CRANBERRY JUICE.** Cranberry juice is a traditional remedy for preventing UTIs, and scientific research suggests it works. Cranberry juice is rich in proanthocyanidins, chemical compounds that appear to help prevent bacteria from sticking to cells in the urinary tract, says Beverly Kloeppel, M.D. If you can't find cranberry juice, look for cranberry juice concentrate that you can mix with water. You should avoid cranberry juice, however, if you have an overactive bladder, because it can irritate the bladder and make it more sensitive.

If you get frequent UTIs, the key is to drink tart cranberry juice, not sweet cranberry juice cocktail. Drink 8 ounces of unsweetened cranberry juice three times a day or take one 400 milligram capsule of cranberry concentrate twice daily for a few months to see if it makes a difference. "Long-term use of cranberry should be avoided if you have kidney stones," says Dr. Kloeppel.

"If you don't want to drink all the caloric cranberry juice, by all means get cranberry extract pills at the health food store. They do help," says Dr. Minkin.

While you're at it, add some blueberries to your breakfast cereal or morning smoothie—they're related to cranberries and contain the same active compounds, says Dr. Kloeppel.

■ **EAT MORE YOGURT.** The research isn't conclusive, but there's some evidence that the organisms in live-culture yogurt, *Lactobacillus acidophilus*, may help prevent unwanted bacteria from multiplying in the urinary tract and prevent UTIs, says Dr. Minkin.

Yogurt is especially helpful if you're taking antibiotics. While these drugs are very effective at killing harmful bacteria, antibiotics also kill "good" germs, which can lead to UTIs. Eating a cup of live-culture yogurt daily helps replenish beneficial bacteria while keeping the "bad" bugs away.

■ **WASH BEFORE SEX.** It's impossible to eliminate infection-causing bacteria from around the anus, but you can prevent them from gaining entry into the urinary tract by washing the genital area before having sex, says Dr. Minkin. This helps prevent the bacteria from being pushed up into the vaginal area and urethra.

■ **URINATE AFTER SEX.** It washes out bacteria that may have made it inside the urethra during intercourse, says Dr. Kloeppel.

■ **USE A LUBRICANT.** If you're experiencing vaginal dryness, it's important to use a water-based lubricant during sex. By decreasing friction, the extra lubrication lessens the possibility of inflammation in the external urethral area, which in turn makes it more difficult for bacteria to cause infection.

■ **CHANGE BIRTH CONTROL METHODS.** Studies have shown that women who use diaphragms and spermicides for birth control have a higher risk of UTIs, probably because use of these products irritates the urethral lining. If you get infections frequently, you may want to talk to your doctor about other forms of birth control.

■ **USE REGULAR TAMPONS.** Women tend to get more infections around the time of their periods. This is partly because the warmth and moisture of the blood provides a favorable environment for germs. In addition, supersize tampons can obstruct the bladder and prevent it from emptying completely. It's easier for bacteria to multiply when urine stays in the bladder for a long time, Dr. Gillespie says.

It's a good idea to use pads or regular-size tampons, says Dr. Gillespie. Change tampons every time you urinate, she adds.

■ **PRACTICE GOOD PERSONAL HYGIENE.** After using the bathroom, wiping from front to back helps ensure that anal bacteria doesn't get pushed forward toward the urethra, says Dr. Kloeppel.

■ **DON'T USE "FEMININE" PRODUCTS.** The chemicals in douches and deodorant sprays may irritate tender tissues in the urethra and vagina, making it easier for bacteria to thrive.

■ **SMELL THE AROMATHERAPY.** To speed healing of a UTI, add 20 drops each of eucalyptus and sandalwood essential oils, or juniper and thyme essential oils, to a hot bath. Soak in the tub for 10 minutes.

■ **HEAL WITH HERBS.** Capsules of uva ursi, also called bearberry, may help treat urinary tract infections, according to a report in the *Alternative Medicine Review*. These capsules are available in most health food stores. Follow the dosage recommendations on the label.

■ **GO HOT AND COLD.** Try contrasting sitz baths to increase circulation in the pelvis, suggests Tori Hudson, N.D. Soak in a shallow hot bath for 3 to 5 minutes, then sit in a basin of cold water for 30 seconds. "Repeat this sequence three times, finishing with cold water," says Dr. Hudson. "And if you don't have two tubs, you can alternate hot and cold compresses to the pelvic area." You can use this treatment once or twice a day, she says.

■ **RUB IT RIGHT WITH REFLEXOLOGY.** Reflexology is an ancient Chinese foot massage technique thought to restore the body's flow of energy (or qi). Certain reflex areas in the feet correspond to different parts of the body. For a UTI, the bladder point (near the heel, along the inside edge of the foot) and the kidney point (in the center of the foot) are most beneficial. You can work these points by pressing and rolling a tennis ball with the sole of each foot. Continue until any tenderness at the points subsides.

PANEL OF ADVISORS

LARRIAN GILLESPIE, M.D., IS A RETIRED ASSISTANT CLINICAL PROFESSOR OF UROLOGY AND UROGYNECOLOGY IN LOS ANGELES AND PRESIDENT OF HEALTHY LIFE PUBLICATIONS. SHE IS AUTHOR OF *YOU DON'T HAVE TO LIVE WITH CYSTITIS, THE MENOPAUSE DIET,* AND *THE GODDESS DIET.*

TORI HUDSON, N.D., IS A NATUROPATHIC PHYSICIAN, MEDICAL DIRECTOR OF A WOMAN'S TIME, P.C., A PROFESSOR AT NATIONAL COLLEGE OF NATUROPATHIC MEDICINE, PROGRAM DIRECTOR AT THE INSTITUTE OF WOMEN'S HEALTH AND INTEGRATIVE MEDICINE, AND ADJUNCT CLINICAL PROFESSOR AT BASTYR UNIVERSITY AND SOUTHWEST COLLEGE OF NATUROPATHIC MEDICINE.

BEVERLY KLOEPPEL, M.D., IS ASSOCIATE DIRECTOR OF STUDENT HEALTH AND COUNSELING AT THE UNIVERSITY OF NEW MEXICO IN ALBUQUERQUE.

MARY JANE MINKIN, M.D., IS A CLINICAL PROFESSOR AT YALE UNIVERSITY SCHOOL OF MEDICINE AND AN OBSTETRICIAN-GYNECOLOGIST IN NEW HAVEN, CONNECTICUT. SHE IS AUTHOR OF *A WOMAN'S GUIDE TO MENOPAUSE AND PERIMENOPAUSE* AND *A WOMAN'S GUIDE TO SEXUAL HEALTH.*

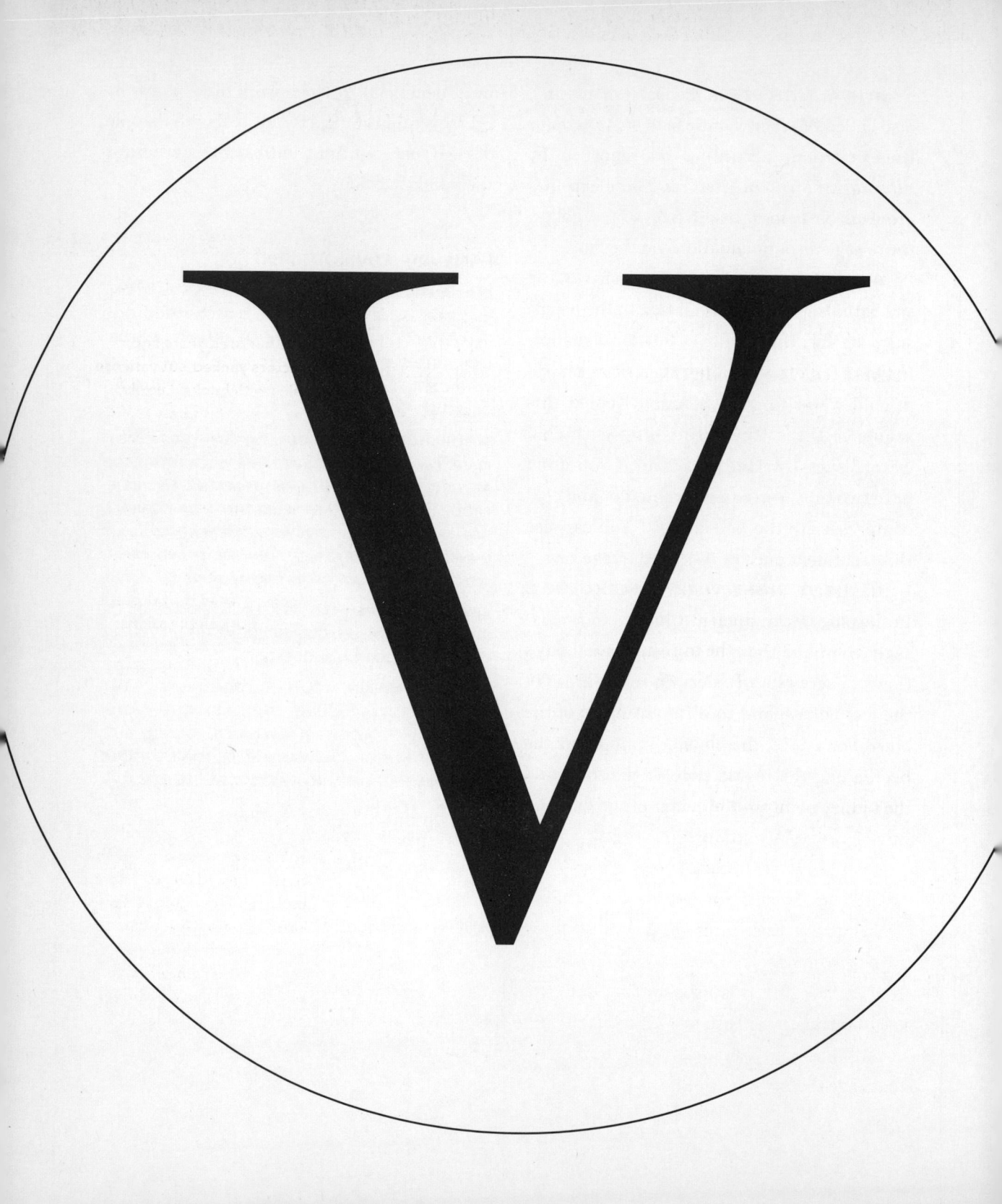

Varicose Veins

16 Helpers and Healers

Blue, swollen, lumpy-looking veins—and their cousins, the crimson "spider veins"—are only the most obvious signs of varicose vein disease. Veterans of this condition know all too well that these visible veins often come with achy, tired, listless legs.

Crossing the legs, wearing high heals, and standing on concrete floors have been blamed for causing varicose veins, but there's little medical evidence to support this, says Mark N. Isaacs, M.D. By far the most important factors are hormones and genetics. "When people ask me what they can do to prevent varicose veins, my best answer is, 'Get different parents the next time around,'" says Dr. Isaacs.

Although you can point to heredity and hormones, your age, occupation, weight, number of pregnancies, and even your shoes make the condition worse. Women are more likely to get varicose veins than men. In fact, according to a survey conducted by the American Society for Dermatologic Surgery, almost 300,000 vein-related procedures are done per year, and 86 percent of them are on women.

The condition is usually not life-threatening, so there's no reason to panic or rush to a doctor. If you have varicose veins, however, you—and your legs—will be better off knowing how to manage them.

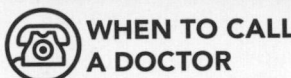

WHEN TO CALL A DOCTOR

One hundred years ago, doctors yanked out varicose veins with hooks. Luckily, the treatment today is much more humane—and helpful. Today, injection therapy is used with resounding success against even the wiliest varicose veins.

But when do varicose veins warrant a trip to the doctor? When they present two major complications: vein clotting and rupture.

Clots are usually visible as red lumps in the veins that don't decrease in size even when you put your legs up. The area around the clot will become very painful, sore, and tender.

Varicose veins around the ankle areas are more inclined to rupture and bleed. This is much more dangerous than clotting because you can lose blood very rapidly. If this happens, put pressure on it to slow the bleeding and get to your doctor.

Here's what our experts suggest.

■ **GET GRAVITY ON YOUR SIDE.** Varicose veins are weakened veins that lack the strength they once had to return blood to the heart. Veins in the legs are the most susceptible because they're farthest—and straight downhill—from the heart. Propping your legs up makes their job much easier. "Leg elevation uses gravity to help reduce pressure in the veins; unfortunately, it only works as long as your legs are elevated," says Dr. Isaacs.

■ **WEAR SUPPORT HOSE.** They help provide relief. These stockings, available in drugstores and department stores, resist the blood's tendency to pool in the small blood vessels closest to the skin. (Instead, the blood is pushed into the larger, deeper veins, where it is more easily pumped back up to the heart.)

■ **WEAR COMPRESSION STOCKINGS.** These special stockings, generally sold in medical supply stores rather than in drugstores, are to support hose what a .45 Magnum is to a BB gun. "They provide more pressure at the ankle, less pressure up at the thigh. This helps press the blood out of the veins and overcome the valves that don't work," says Tej M. Singh, M.D. Get measured for a good-quality stocking.

■ **WEAR SENSIBLE SHOES.** Avoid wearing heels higher than 1 inch. "High heels make you walk with your buttock muscles, but it is your calf muscles that decrease varicose veins," says Mitchel P. Goldman, M.D.

■ **WATCH YOUR WEIGHT.** Maintaining a healthy weight will eliminate excess pressure on your legs that cause veins to surface, says Robert Weiss, M.D. Losing weight may actually help prevent varicose and spider veins from developing in the first place, he adds.

■ **STAY AWAY FROM TIGHT-FITTING CLOTHING.** Restrictive clothing might actually trap blood, causing clots. Clothing around specific body parts, including the waist, legs, and groin area, can restrict circulation and lead to spider and varicose veins, says Dr. Weiss.

■ **BE SUSPICIOUS OF THE PILL.** Hormonal imbalances, which sometimes occur with birth control pills, can be the cause of spider veins. If your problem appeared after you started the Pill, there may be a connection.

■ **DON'T SMOKE.** A report from the landmark Framingham Heart Study noted a correlation between smoking and the incidence of varicose veins. The researchers conclude that smoking may be a risk factor for varicose veins.

■ **KEEP THOSE LEGS MOVING.** "Walking, cycling, and swimming all help keep up blood circulation in the legs and will reduce pressure and blood pooling," says Dr. Weiss. He also advises changing positions every 30 minutes while you're sitting to help bloodflow and keep veins healthy. Flex the muscles in your calves frequently at your desk, on long car trips, or on a plane to keep up circulation, he adds.

The leg muscles act as the pumps for the leg veins, so exercise that builds muscle tone in the calf and thigh muscles is very important, says Dr. Isaacs. Walking is the simplest leg exercise to build tone, he says.

In fact, the Framingham study found that sedentary adults were more likely to have varicose veins than those who were active.

■ **PROP WHILE YOU SLEEP.** "Sleep with two or three pillows under your lower legs so that your feet are higher than your heart," says Dr. Singh.

■ **FIND RELIEF WITH ORDINARY WATER.** Relief for varicose veins may be as close as your shower. While showering, alternate between applications of warm and cold water on your legs. Change temperatures at 1- to 3-minute intervals, and repeat the switch three times. The changing temperature gets your blood moving by expanding and contracting the blood vessels.

■ **BUT AVOID OVERHEATING.** Don't subject legs to excessive heat: Everyone enjoys a hot bath or relaxing in a hot tub on occasion, but it's important to keep it to a minimum, says Dr. Weiss. "The heat associated with baths and hot tubs will actually increase vein swelling and lead to blood pooling."

Cures from the Kitchen

Strangely enough, a high-fiber diet may be the key to preventing varicose veins. Straining to have a bowel movement puts pressure on the veins in your lower legs. Over time, this pressure promotes the development of varicose veins.

A high-fiber diet can stop this gradual development before it's too late. Fiber keeps waste moving freely through the system, so to speak, preventing straining and thus preventing varicose veins in the long run. Try to get around 25 grams a day from sources such as bran cereals, beans, and whole grains.

PANEL OF ADVISORS

MITCHEL P. GOLDMAN, M.D., IS MEDICAL DIRECTOR OF LA JOLLA SPA MD, IN LA JOLLA, CALIFORNIA, AND A VISITING CLINICAL PROFESSOR AT THE UNIVERSITY OF CALIFORNIA, SAN DIEGO SCHOOL OF MEDICINE.

MARK N. ISAACS, M.D., IS A PHLEBOLOGIST IN WALNUT CREEK, CALIFORNIA, WHO SPECIALIZES EXCLUSIVELY IN NONSURGICAL VEIN TREATMENT. HE IS ON THE TEACHING FACULTY OF THE AMERICAN COLLEGE OF PHLEBOLOGY AND THE EDITOR OF THE COLLEGE NEWSLETTER, *VEIN LINE*.

TEJ M. SINGH, M.D., IS AN ENDOVASCULAR SURGEON IN PALO ALTO, CALIFORNIA, AND CLINICAL DIRECTOR OF VASCULAR SURGERY AT EL CAMINO HOSPITAL IN MOUNTAIN VIEW, CALIFORNIA.

ROBERT WEISS, M.D., IS A DERMATOLOGIST IN HUNT VALLEY, MARYLAND, AN ASSOCIATE PROFESSOR OF DERMATOLOGY AT JOHNS HOPKINS IN BALTIMORE, THE PRESIDENT OF THE AMERICAN SOCIETY OF DERMATOLOGIC SURGERY, AND AUTHOR OF MANY MEDICAL TEXTBOOKS, INCLUDING *VEIN DIAGNOSIS & TREATMENT: A COMPREHENSIVE APPROACH*.

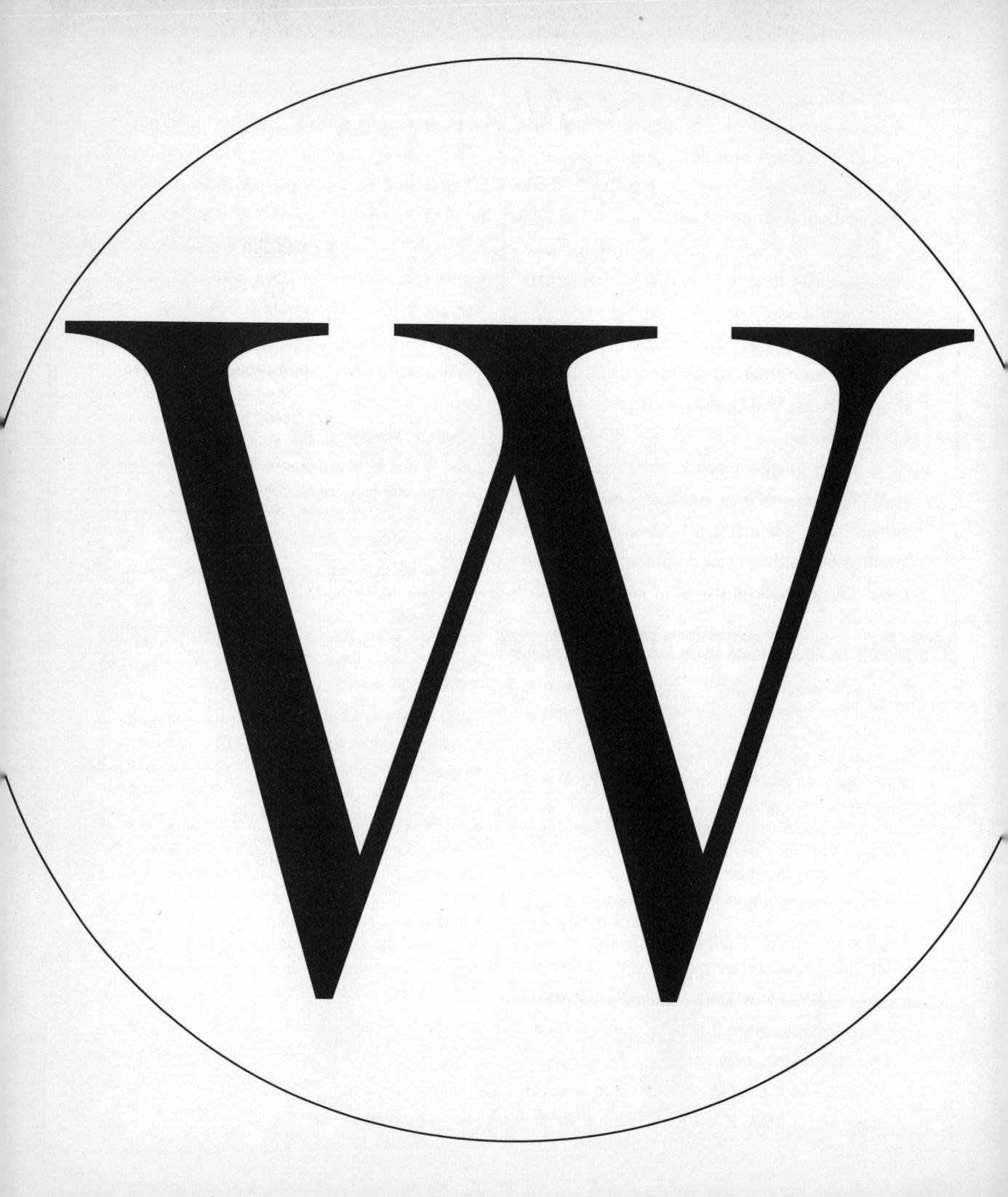

Warts

20 Healing Secrets

After acne, warts are the most common dermatological complaint that most people have.

At any one time, about 10 percent of people have a wart, says Robert Garry, Ph.D., and about 25 percent will get one sometime in their lives.

Warts are benign skin tumors that can occur singly or in packs on just about any part of the body. They come in several different varieties, each bearing its own special name, each caused by various strains of the papillomavirus. The virus masterfully tricks the body into providing it with free room and board in a sheltered "house"—the wart.

Unfortunately, standard medical treatments are often violent—burning, scraping, cutting, freezing, injecting, or zapping the wart with a laser. Many are also painful. Some even leave scars. The irony is, these techniques are not always effective. To add insult to injury, warts often reappear, no matter which treatment is used.

Knowing all this, you may want to try some home remedies before heading to the doctor's office. But be careful not to injure yourself with wart treatments. Give these simple techniques a try for several weeks before resorting to stronger measures.

Unless otherwise noted, the following are effective for both common warts and plantar warts (those found on the foot).

■ **LEAVE 'EM ALONE.** According to one estimate, 40 to 50 percent of all warts eventually disappear on their own—typically within 2 years. Children, in particular, often lose warts spontaneously.

Warts constantly shed infectious virus, though, cautions Marc A. Brenner, D.P.M. If left untreated, they may get larger or spread

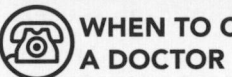
WHEN TO CALL A DOCTOR

If you have the slightest doubt about what you're dealing with, see a doctor. It could be a corn, callus, mole, or rarely skin cancer. "Note that warts may look different if found on the top of the foot (fleshy) versus the bottom of the foot (flat and roughened)," says Glenn Gastwirth, D.P.M.

In general, warts are pale, skin-colored growths with a rough surface, even borders, and blackened surface capillaries. Normal skin lines do not cross a wart's surface. And contrary to popular opinion, warts are very shallow growths—they don't have "roots" or "runners" that go down to the bone.

to other areas. So if your warts start multiplying, take action.

■ **CALL IN THE A-TEAM.** Dr. Garry has had great success applying vitamin A directly to warts. Simply break open a capsule containing 25,000 IU of natural vitamin A from fish oil or fish-liver oil, squeeze some of the liquid onto the wart, and rub it in. Apply once a day. He emphasizes that the vitamin should be applied to the skin only. Taken orally in large doses, vitamin A can be toxic.

Different warts respond differently to this treatment. Juvenile warts can disappear in a month, others in 2 to 4 months, but plantar warts might take 2 to 5 months longer, he says.

Dr. Garry recalls one woman who had

Cures from the Kitchen

When all is said and done, you never know just what will cure any particular wart. The remedy that so neatly dispatched one little growth might leave another completely unscathed. So perhaps your most powerful weapon in the war of the warts is an open mind. That's why you shouldn't overlook the healing potential of so-called folk cures, treatments that have never undergone formal scientific scrutiny but have worked just fine for many people. Here are a few that some folks swear by.

■ Apply clove oil or the milky juice of unripe figs directly to the wart.

■ Soak lemon slices in apple cider with a little salt. Let stand 2 weeks. Then rub the lemon slices on the wart.

■ Rub the wart with a piece of chalk or a raw potato.

■ Tape the inner side of a banana skin to a plantar wart.

more than 200 warts on her hand. By persisting with the vitamin A therapy for 7 to 8 months, she was able to get rid of all but one stubborn wart under her fingernail.

■ **PRACTICE GOOD FOOT HYGIENE.** Warts can be contagious. So keep your feet clean, avoid walking barefoot, and wear socks with your shoes, preferably socks that draw moisture away from the skin, says Glenn Gastwirth, D.P.M. "And avoid picking at warts with your fingers," he adds.

■ **STAY DRY.** Warts thrive on moisture, so keeping your feet very dry may help eliminate plantar warts. Dry your feet with a blow-drier, says Dr. Brenner. "Many people with plantar warts have hyperhidrosis (sweaty feet). If you control the sweating, you may be able to control the warts," he adds. "You can try an antiperspirant for feet, such as Lavilin."

To banish a plantar wart without chemicals, change your socks at least three times a day, says Dr. Brenner. At the same time, apply a medicated foot powder such as Zeasorb-AF frequently—10 times a day if necessary.

■ **OPT FOR A NONPRESCRIPTION PRODUCT.** Probably the most popular commercial wart remedies are the over-the-counter (OTC) salicylic acid preparations. Salicylic acid is believed to work against warts by softening and dissolving them. These products come in liquid, gel, pad, and ointment form.

Liquid products like Compound W are effective on small warts. One good thing about Compound W is that it contains a little oil,

How to Avoid a Wart

Warts are caused by a virus. Someone with a wart sheds the virus onto a moist surface (in a locker room, bathroom, or nail salon) and you pick it up the same way you do any viral infection. If you're susceptible to the virus and you have a cut or crack in the skin for it to take hold, you'll get a wart. It's that simple. Even so, there are a few things that you can do to lessen your chances.

Keep your shoes on. The wart virus thrives in a very moist environment, says Suzanne M. Levine, D.P.M., P.C., so always wear sandals around swimming pools, health clubs, and locker rooms to avoid foot contact with the virus. By not going barefoot, you also avoid getting the minute cracks or cuts in your feet the virus needs to enter.

Change shoes frequently. Because the wart virus breeds in moist places, you should change your shoes frequently and allow shoes to dry out between wearings, says Dr. Levine.

Clean up. "At a health club or gym, you might even want to clean the shower out first with a product like Lysol," says Dr. Levine. "Even just household bleach works to kill viruses and bacteria."

Look but don't touch. "Warts spread easily," says Marc A. Brenner, D.P.M. "So if you have one on the bottom of your foot, for instance, try not to touch it with your hand. If you have even a small cut on your finger, you risk getting a wart there."

Pamper your cuticles. If the wart virus enters a cut or can opening around your cuticle, it can cause a particularly nasty type of wart. Called periungual warts, they're very difficult to treat, says Dr. Levine. "If you do get a cut in the cuticle, put on a topical antibiotic cream (such as bacitracin) and cover it with a bandage until it heals."

Keep your feet dry. Making sure your feet are dry, including between the toes, will help prevent infections from fungi, bacteria, and viruses, says Dr. Levine. If you visit a nail salon, make sure it has a clean environment (sterilized instruments, scrubbed wash basin).

Play it cool. "My own feeling is that people seem to be more susceptible to warts when they're under stress and eating poorly," says Dr. Levine. "And the warts seem to spread more then." So try to take it easy.

which makes it less irritating to the skin than some other salicylic acid products, says Suzanne M. Levine, D.P.M., P.C.

Dr. Brenner advises, however, that the liquid and gel products, which typically contain only about 17 percent salicylic acid, may not be strong enough to work on plantar warts, which have thick calluses covering them.

Follow these three rules for dealing with any over-the-counter product, says Dr. Gastwirth. "First, be certain that it *is* a wart you're treating (see "When to Call a Doctor" on page 619).

Woo Woo for Warts?

As difficult as it is to cure warts with medicine, wouldn't it be great if you could just wish your warts away? It turns out there is real scientific evidence that you can psych out your warts with a little help from self-hypnosis. According to a recent scientific review of studies, psychotherapeutic treatment with and without hypnosis is an effective way to reduce or eliminate viral warts. This method involves using guided imagery and hypnotic suggestions to boost your immune system.

In one study, psychotherapists hypnotized 17 people who had warts on both sides of their bodies for a series of five sessions and told them that their warts would disappear only from one side. Another 7 people were not hypnotized and were instructed to abstain from using any wart remedies. Three months later, more than half of the hypnotized group had lost at least 75 percent of the warts on the suggested side. The people who hadn't been hypnotized still had their warts.

Imagine your warts away. The power of suggestion alone—without hypnosis—may be equally effective at wasting warts, the researchers say. To try it at home, imagine that your warts are shrinking, that you can feel the tingling as your warts dissolve and your skin becomes clear. Do this for 5 minutes every day.

Be a believer. The power of suggestion is a well-known phenomenon among doctors. In fact, believing in the cure is the power behind the placebo effect. Strong belief in a cure may also explain the continued popularity of such offbeat, old-fashioned folk remedies as rubbing the wart with a penny and then burying the penny under the porch.

To try this at home, simply believe that your warts will go away just as they did for those in the hypnosis study. You are getting very sleepy . . .

Second, follow all of the package instructions to the letter. And third, if the wart does not respond within a reasonable amount of time—say, a week or two—see a doctor." If you have diabetes, a circulatory or cardiovascular problem, or an active skin infection, then do not use a caustic compound on your feet, says Dr. Gastwirth.

Be cautious or avoid freezing sprays, says Coyle S. Connolly, D.O. "When used improperly, these products may cause skin injury."

■ **DO IT WITH DUCT TAPE.** Covering warts with duct tape zaps warts better than cryotherapy (freezing), according to a study published in the *Archives of Pediatrics and Adolescent Medicine*. In the study, the duct tape method eliminated 85 percent of the warts after 2 months, compared with 60 percent with the freezing method.

To use duct tape with over-the-counter preparations, follow this procedure, says Dr. Connolly:

- Bathe the area in warm water for at least 10 minutes to soften the thick callus overlying the wart.

- Scuff the area in a gentle yet vigorous manner with an emery board or file. This makes it easier for the salicylic acid to penetrate the callus.

- Apply a salicylic acid liquid once during the day and once at night.

- Cut a piece of duct tape to size (slightly larger than the wart) and leave it on overnight.

- Repeat this sequence of duct tape use for 10 nights, skip 10 nights, then apply for 10 more nights, all the while using the acid application during the day. Remember, warts are stubborn and may take weeks of treatment.

■ **PAD THE WART.** Compound W Pads work fairly well for plantar warts and can also be effective on hand warts, although it's harder to keep the patch in place on the hand.

"The main drawback to pads," says Dr. Levine, "is that people often use too large a piece, which exposes the surrounding skin to serious irritation. And they put on a new pad every day. Pretty soon they have an ulcer around the wart that's far worse than the wart they started with. The best course of action is to follow the directions on the label."

To ensure a good fit, cut out a little cardboard template in exactly the shape and dimensions of your wart. Then use that template to precut a supply of patches from the adhesive plaster. Lightly coat the normal skin surrounding the wart with petroleum jelly to prevent any medication from touching your skin.

■ **GO WITH AN OINTMENT.** Rounding out the salicylic acid arsenal is 60 percent ointment. For best results, says Dr. Levine, soak the wart area in lukewarm water for about 10 minutes before applying ointment to allow for greater penetration. Dry well, then apply a drop of the ointment to the wart. Cover with a bandage. If you're dealing with a plantar wart, do this at bedtime so that you won't have to walk around on the wart and rub off the ointment. In the morning, soak the area again and lightly pumice off any softened skin.

PANEL OF ADVISORS

MARC A. BRENNER, D.P.M., IS FOUNDER AND DIRECTOR OF THE INSTITUTE OF DIABETIC FOOT RESEARCH IN GLENDALE, NEW YORK. HE IS PAST PRESIDENT OF THE AMERICAN SOCIETY OF PODIATRIC DERMATOLOGY AND AUTHOR AND EDITOR OF VARIOUS BOOKS.

COYLE S. CONNOLLY, D.O., IS A DERMATOLOGIST AND ASSISTANT CLINICAL PROFESSOR AT THE PHILADELPHIA COLLEGE OF OSTEOPATHIC MEDICINE AND PRESIDENT OF CONNOLLY DERMATOLOGY IN LINWOOD, NEW JERSEY.

ROBERT GARRY, PH.D., IS A PROFESSOR OF MICROBIOLOGY AND IMMUNOLOGY AT TULANE UNIVERSITY SCHOOL OF MEDICINE IN NEW ORLEANS.

GLENN GASTWIRTH, D.P.M., IS EXECUTIVE DIRECTOR OF THE AMERICAN PODIATRIC MEDICAL ASSOCIATION.

SUZANNE M. LEVINE, D.P.M., P.C., IS A PODIATRIC SURGEON AND CLINICAL PODIATRIST AT NEW YORK HOSPITAL–CORNELL MEDICAL CENTER. SHE IS AUTHOR OF *YOUR FEET DON'T HAVE TO HURT.*

Weight Problems

34 Ways to Win the Battle of the Bulge

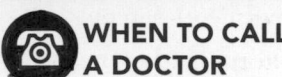

WHEN TO CALL A DOCTOR

It's a good idea to talk with your doctor if you think you may need to lose weight. Doing so is especially important if you have reached or are near menopause, or if you have risk factors for developing a chronic disease associated with overweight and obesity, such as a smoking habit, a sedentary lifestyle, high blood sugar, or abnormal blood fats. Weight loss during menopause may increase the rate at which bone density is lost. Tell your doctor about your efforts to lose weight—you may need supplemental calcium.

On any given day, about half the women and a third of the men in America are trying to shed pounds. That's 106 million dieters!

Meal planning, portion control, strength training, aerobics—that all sounds like so much work! But if your goal is healthy weight loss, you'll agree later that it was all worth it. Ready to give it a try? The following expert advice and support is sure to motivate you and keep all that effort working for you efficiently and effectively.

The following pages show how to use your mind, mouth, and muscles to control your weight.

USE YOUR MIND

Many weight-loss efforts fail from our improper mind-set, says Gary Foster, Ph.D., who views the process of cutting pounds from a psychologist's perspective. Here's how to use your mind to lose your girth.

■ **RESIST THE HARD SELL.** Regardless of all the get-thin-quick pitches you see stapled to telephone poles and hear on the radio, the best way to lose weight and keep it off is to make permanent changes to your eating and exercise habits, says Marsha D. Marcus, Ph.D.

Easy answers to a difficult task like losing weight and keeping it off are certainly appealing. But if a weight-loss pitch sounds too good to be true—no matter how convincing—then it is.

■ **CHOOSE GOALS WISELY.** Despite the inspiring advertisements of skinny people holding up the huge clothes they used to

wear, the best goal for weight loss is to lose *10 percent of your body weight*, Dr. Foster says.

It's hard to think small in our bigger-is-better culture. In one of Dr. Foster's studies, a group of obese women reported how successful they would consider different amounts of weight loss. They called a 25 percent weight loss one they wouldn't be happy with, and a 17 percent weight loss one they could not view as successful in any way. Such unreasonable expectations can seriously undermine motivation and the ability to maintain long-term weight loss, Dr. Foster says.

People who set themselves up by shooting for too high a goal, like losing 100 pounds, do one of two things. Many engage in super-human behaviors, eating even less, exercising even more, which leads to eventual perceived failure because nobody can continue living that way long term. Others just give up from the get-go and say, "To heck with it if this is the best I can do."

Instead, Dr. Foster recommends figuring out how much 10 percent of your body weight is and shooting for that. For example, if you weigh 150 pounds, you'd strive to lose 15 pounds. For most people, it will take about 6 months to achieve this initial goal, says Dr. Foster.

■ **REMEMBER THAT A LITTLE GOES A LONG WAY.** Once you've figured out how much total weight to lose, at first plan on losing ½ to 1 pound a week, advises Joanne Larsen, R.D. "When we go on a very low calorie diet or get way too much exercise and lose more than 2 pounds per week, our body goes into starvation mode. When our body's in starvation mode, it burns fewer calories," she says, and it resists your efforts to lose more weight.

■ **LOWER STRESS.** One of the major factors in weight gain is stress. When you're under stress your body will accumulate fat, and it doesn't stop until you train it to do something else, says G. Frank Lawlis, Ph.D. Find positive ways to deal with your stress. For example, take a yoga class, take a bath, or listen to soothing music. But avoid self-medicating with food, says Dr. Lawlis.

A high-stress work environment can make you want to grab a high-calorie fast-food snack or processed convenience food, especially in the late afternoon and early evening, say researchers at Monell Chemical Senses Center in Philadelphia.

Instead, have some healthier snacks on hand, like celery with peanut butter.

■ **CURB YOUR CRAVINGS.** Emotional eating is a major issue because we learn it from the day we're born. "As babies we cry and we get milk," says Dr. Lawlis. "When we fuss, we get food." Rather than forbid the foods you love, find healthier foods that have the same sensory properties. For example, if you crave crunchy-salty foods when you're angry, satisfy your craving with dry popcorn or lightly salted carrots before you dive into the corn chips and fried chicken.

You're also likely to crave more calories

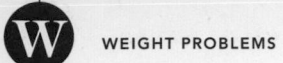

from fatty foods the week before your menstrual period, according to a recent study at New York State Psychiatric Institute and Department of Psychiatry. So carefully plan your meals ahead of time.

■ **THINK YOURSELF THIN.** If you think of yourself as always being overweight or obese, you always will be, says Dr. Lawlis. So to change your body, you first have to change your body image. "You're not going to be your teenage self again with an 18-inch waist, but a realistic self-image is really important to maintain," says Dr. Lawlis.

■ **ENJOY YOUR SUCCESS.** Once they've shed 20 pounds or so, many clients tell Dr. Foster that they sleep better, can climb stairs more easily, and have more energy to play with their grandkids.

Take time to notice and celebrate these successes. Then, go out and treat yourself to a new dress or a manicure.

■ **GO A WHILE AND REST.** Once you've reached your goal of losing 10 percent of your body weight, your next goal should be to simply maintain that weight for a while.

"Try to stay at that weight for at least another 6 to 8 months or a longer period of time than it took to lose that initial amount. Really get a sense of what it is to live in your skin at that weight," Dr. Foster says. If the time is right and you're ready and willing for even more weight-loss effort, *then* start peeling off another reasonable amount.

"You'll be in a much better position to know what's required to lose weight after you've maintained the loss. If I'm not banging my head against the wall just to maintain my weight, then the prospect of losing more weight is a little more appealing," he says.

■ **MAKE CHANGES YOU CAN LIVE WITH.** Even if you can totally cut out fast food, greasy movie-theater popcorn, and other tempting foods while you're losing weight, you'll need to learn that you can enjoy all foods, including those, in moderation for the rest of your life.

"I think that for people with weight problems, it's a question of a lifetime of self-management. That's not to say that one has to *diet* over one's lifetime. We have to say yes to ourselves and enjoy our food, but we also have to learn to say no," Dr. Marcus says.

■ **BECOME MORE AWARE OF YOUR EATING BEHAVIOR.** In order to *change* your eating behavior, you first have to *understand* that behavior. It's a two-step process, says Dr. Marcus. First, start paying attention to what, when, where, and with whom you're eating, how you feel, and what kind of activities you're doing throughout the day. Next, think about what triggers the eating. If you are hungry, then, of course, eating is the appropriate response. But many things other than hunger stimulate eating. Triggers could be the sight or smell of a certain food, boredom, or stress, says Dr. Marcus.

■ **MAKE A GOOD REFLECTION.** Hang a full-length mirror in your home, Larsen sug-

How Much Is Too Much?

Most health professionals use a tool called the body mass index (BMI) to determine if someone falls into either the "overweight" or the "obesity" category. The BMI measures body weight relative to height, which usually correlates to the your of body fat. People who have a BMI of 30 or higher are classified as obese—meaning, in most cases, at least 30 pounds overweight. This category includes a person who is 5 feet 4 inches and weighs 1/4, or a 5-foot 10-inch person who tips the scales at 209 pounds.

People with a BMI of 25 to 30 are considered overweight, because they weigh more than the standard for their height. The excess weight can come from muscle, bone, or body water as well as fat. This means that certain individuals, such as a bodybuilder or a person with a large frame, can be overweight but not overly fat. BMI values below 25 and down to 18.5 are considered normal or healthy weight.

You can calculate your own BMI by dividing your weight in pounds by your height in inches squared, then multiplying by 703. Or go to the Web site of the National Heart, Lung, and Blood Institute and use the automatic BMI calculator available there. You will also find tables that have the BMI already calculated.

Another key tool to determine overweight is waist circumference, which is an obvious indicator of abdominal fat. You can determine your waist circumference by standing and placing a measuring tape snugly around your waist. Health risks rise as waist measurement increases, especially if it's greater than 35 for women or 40 for men.

gests. Many overweight people prefer mirrors that show only their face, and they don't see the full image that everyone else sees.

You can find full-length mirrors in department stores for less than $20. Take a good look in it regularly.

■ **WEIGH YOURSELF DAILY.** If you use the scale wisely, you'll know when you gain 5 pounds. You can then reduce your eating and bump up your exercise, says Larsen. "It is easier to catch a small weight gain than chase a larger one."

USE YOUR MOUTH

Sure, it's easy to say that the secret to weight loss is to eat fewer calories than you burn. Sadly, because of our fast-paced, sedentary lifestyle, eating well isn't that simple in daily life.

■ **EAT AT LEAST THREE MEALS A DAY TO FUEL YOUR ACTIVITIES.** At the very least, start the day with a good breakfast. "If you skip meals, you will be too hungry and may binge on whatever food you can eat fast, quickly consuming more calories than you need. It takes 20 minutes for a message to get from your stomach to your brain that you are full," says Larsen.

■ **DITCH THE DIET FOODS.** Sure, you can buy reduced-fat versions of foods, but cooking from scratch will let you determine how much fat and salt your meal contains. "Cooking from scratch saves money, too, because processed and prepared foods are more expensive," says Larsen.

■ **FORGET THE "BAD FOODS" LISTS.** The minute someone tells us not to eat something, we're sunk—sooner or later we're going to indulge, and while we're at it we'll probably overindulge to make up for feeling deprived. The problem isn't just eating "bad" foods, it's eating larger portions than we need, says Larsen. Cut down the portions of all food, and eat more whole grains, fruits, vegetables, and dairy, she says.

■ **FIGURE OUT WHAT YOU NEED.** An estimate of how many calories you should consume each day to lose weight safely is 10 calories per pound of body weight per day. If you weigh 180 pounds, try to keep it at 1,800 calories per day.

Your individual needs may differ from this, however, depending in part on your body composition and activity level. Gender and genetics have a strong impact on how your body uses and stores food. For example, women's hormones tend to encourage fat storage. A dietitian can help you figure out a more precise calorie number, Larsen says. To find a dietitian, ask at your local hospital, or

visit the Web site of the American Dietetic Association, at www.dietitian.com and click on Find a Dietitian. For a do-it-yourself calorie count, click on the Web site's Healthy Body Calculator.

■ **EAT A BALANCED DIET.** A high-protein and low-carbohydrate diet, which bumps up the meat and cuts out the bread, pasta, and fruit, have been very popular.

Though people might lose weight while enjoying steak, eggs, and beef jerky, it's partly from fluid loss as their bodies turn food into energy, and partly because they're eating fewer calories. Using so much protein as fuel can leave you fatigued and constipated, and it puts more demands on your kidneys as they filter excess protein, posing special risks to those with diabetes, says Mary Friesz, R.D., Ph.D.

A diet that's ultralow in fat isn't good either. In reasonable amounts, the fat in your food makes you feel full and makes you want to stop eating. For example, when you choose fat-free ice cream, you may wind up eating more because it's less satisfying—and getting more calories than if you'd eaten a bit of regular ice cream. In the end, it's the calories that count, Dr. Friesz says.

The balanced diet that experts recommend for weight loss or weight maintenance is simple. Each day, try to get about *half* of your calories from carbohydrates. Good sources of carbohydrates include fruits, vegetables, whole grain breads, pasta, rice, and milk. Try to include at least five servings of veggies and two fruits a day rather than filling up on bread and pasta, says Dr. Friesz. And go for whole grains and legumes over refined flour and simple sugars.

About a *quarter* of your calories should come from protein. Good sources include lean cuts of beef, chicken breast, fish, and beans. If you're a vegetarian, have rice during the same day as beans to ensure that you receive complete proteins.

The last *quarter* of your calories should come from fats and oils. The best are olive and canola oils. These are the healthiest for your heart, but they're still high in calories, so don't go overboard with them.

■ **KEEP TRACK OF YOUR CALORIES.** Larsen suggests using a food diary, whenever possible, to record what you've eaten each day, how many calories the foods contain, along with the other details of your eating behavior.

"Keeping food records is the only way to know whether you're on track or not. Here's a comparison," she says. Imagine that you write checks and put money in your checking account, but you don't write down the amount of the check, and you never balance your checking account. You'd have no idea where you're at financially. It's the same thing with losing weight.

■ **EAT FREQUENTLY.** Instead of eating all your food in two or three sittings, eat four to six smaller meals throughout the day, says Dr. Friesz. When you eat smaller, more frequent meals each day as opposed to a couple of belly busters, your body is more likely to use the calories instead of packing them away as fat, she says. You'll also ensure that you aren't starving when you pull up to the table, which increases your chances of wolfing down more than you need.

Just make sure that the total calories in your small meals don't exceed the amount of calories you should be consuming each day.

■ **BE CREATIVE AT THE RESTAURANT.** You know when you eat out that the waiter is likely to drop a calorie bomb onto your table that can devastate your hips for months to come. "If you're full when you leave the table, you ate too much. That's your body's way of saying, 'There's too much here for me to digest at one time,'" Dr. Friesz says. You need to stop before that, when you still have room for food but don't have that hunger feeling. Instead of eating until you hurt:

- Split an entrée with your spouse or friend.

- Order a child-size entrée.

- Ask the waitress to box up half the meal, and take it home to enjoy later.

- Ask for the pasta separately. Side servings of pasta are usually about 1½ cups, but bottom servings can be twice that amount.

- Get butter, sour cream, and other toppings on the side, and add just enough for flavoring. If you get a stuffed baked potato, for example, and can still taste it, you're doing well.

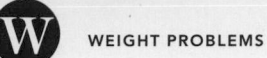

■ **STRIVE FOR 25.** Eating at least 25 grams of fiber each day is especially important if you're trying to lose weight. Foods rich in fiber tend to be nutritious, filling, lower-calorie choices, Larsen says.

You can accumulate a total of 25 grams of fiber in a day by having a cup of bran flakes for breakfast, toasting a whole wheat English muffin for your morning break, tossing ½ cup of chickpeas into your lunch salad, snacking on a large apple, and stir-frying ½ cup of broccoli for dinner.

■ **GUZZLE—DON'T GOBBLE.** Drink eight 8-ounce glasses of water each day. Keeping some water in your stomach most of the time can help fool it into thinking it's full, Larsen says.

USE YOUR MUSCLES

More important than what you eat is how you move. If you go on a really low-calorie diet and don't exercise, you risk losing muscle, says Rob Huizenga, M.D.

"Diet is vastly over-relied on and overused and is really not the way to go for health, looks, or optimal body composition," says Dr. Huizenga, who formed his opinions based on his work with professional athletes, women athletes, and people attempting to lose weight on the TV show *The Biggest Loser*.

"You need to lose fat, not weight, and you've got to get healthy by exercising to lose fat," says Dr. Huizenga.

Here's how to wield the power of exercise to your advantage.

■ **GO FOR A BLEND.** The best exercise program combines aerobic exercise, strength training, and stretching. Aerobic exercise that is continuous, such as cycling, walking, and swimming, strengthens your heart and is best for reducing your risk of many chronic diseases. "Stop-start" activities, such as racquetball, are not as beneficial.

Strength training involving calisthenics or weight lifting makes your muscles stronger and helps maintain muscle mass. This becomes more important as we get older, because our muscle mass starts diminishing in our early twenties. If you don't use your muscles, they decline in size. Muscle tissue burns more calories, so the more muscle mass you have, the more calories you expend just by standing still. The daily difference isn't large, but it's huge over time.

■ **DON'T GO FOR ALL-OR-NOTHING.** Initially, plan to exercise for 20 minutes for a minimum of 3 days a week. Build up to 30 to 40 minutes at a time. The more days you exercise, the better, but 3 days is a good starting point if you haven't been exercising.

If your size or fitness level prevents you from working out for 20 minutes a day, start with just 15 minutes and gradually work your way up. Don't put off exercising if time is an issue. Even exercising for 10 to 15 minutes intermittently through the day helps strengthen your heart. And just a few minutes of exercise done regularly will eventually make it easier to go for longer periods.

■ **FIND EXERCISES YOU ENJOY.** List all the activities you might enjoy, then alternate among them whenever you wish. Adding variety may make it easier to stick with your program.

■ **BE ABLE TO SPEAK.** While you're doing aerobic exercise, exert yourself at a moderate intensity level. You should be able to carry on a conversation punctuated by moderately heavy but not comfortable breathing.

■ **PLAY THESE NUMBERS IN THE WEIGHT ROOM.** Adults get the greatest gains in muscle strength and muscle endurance by using weights that they can comfortably lift for a set of 8 to 12 repetitions. If you can't lift a weight 8 times, decrease the weight. If you can easily lift it 12 times, bump up the weight a few pounds.

Ideally, you should lift weights three times a week. If you can hit the gym or exercise at home that often, you need to do each set of repetitions only once. If you lift weights 2 days a week, do two or three sets of each exercise.

■ **SEEK HELP.** It's a good idea to talk to a qualified trainer to ensure that you're choosing the right exercises to safely work all the major muscles in your body. If you don't belong to a gym, hire a personal trainer for a few sessions to get you started. Look for someone who is certified by the National Strength and Conditioning Association (NSCA) as a certified strength and conditioning specialist or certified personal trainer.

■ **MAKE EXERCISE A PRIORITY.** If you're not accustomed to exercising regularly, schedule it in advance as an appointment on your calendar or electronic planner, Dr. Friesz suggests. Otherwise, you'll forget or find an excuse not to do it. After 3 months, it should become a habit, she says.

PANEL OF ADVISORS

GARY FOSTER, PH.D., IS CLINICAL DIRECTOR OF THE WEIGHT AND EATING DISORDERS PROGRAM AT THE UNIVERSITY OF PENNSYLVANIA IN PHILADELPHIA.

MARY FRIESZ, R.D., PH.D., IS A NUTRITION AND WELLNESS CONSULTANT AND A CERTIFIED DIABETES EDUCATOR IN BOCA RATON, FLORIDA, AND AUTHOR OF *FOOD, FUN N' FITNESS: DESIGNING HEALTHY LIFESTYLES FOR OUR CHILDREN* AND *WHAT IS NORMAL EATING: UNDERSTANDING EATING IN TODAY'S SOCIETY.*

ROB HUIZENGA, M.D., IS AN ASSOCIATE PROFESSOR OF MEDICINE AT THE UNIVERSITY OF CALIFORNIA IN LOS ANGELES, THE DOCTOR BEHIND THE HIT TV SHOW *THE BIGGEST LOSER,* AND AUTHOR OF *WHERE DID ALL THE FAT GO?: THE WOW PRESCRIPTION TO REACH YOUR IDEAL WEIGHT—AND STAY THERE!*

JOANNE LARSEN, R.D., HAS WORKED IN HEALTH CARE FACILITIES, TAUGHT AT THE UNIVERSITY LEVEL, AND DESIGNED NUTRITION SOFTWARE. SHE CREATED ASK THE DIETITIAN AT WWW.DIETITIAN.COM AND DESIGNED AND EDITED THE AMERICAN DIETETIC ASSOCIATION'S ONLINE DIET MANUAL.

G. FRANK LAWLIS, PH.D., IS A PSYCHOLOGIST, RESEARCHER, AND COFOUNDER OF THE LAWLIS AND PEAVEY CENTERS FOR PSYCHONEUROLOGICAL CHANGE IN LEWISVILLE, TEXAS. HE IS THE CHIEF CONTENT ADVISER FOR THE *DR. PHIL SHOW* AND AUTHOR OF *THE STRESS ANSWER, THE ADD ANSWER,* AND *THE IQ ANSWER.*

MARSHA D. MARCUS, PH.D., IS A PROFESSOR OF PSYCHIATRY AND PSYCHOLOGY AND CHIEF OF THE BEHAVIORAL MEDICINE AND EATING DISORDERS PROGRAM IN THE DEPARTMENT OF PSYCHIATRY AT THE UNIVERSITY OF PITTSBURGH SCHOOL OF MEDICINE.

Wrinkles

17 Age-Defying Secrets

Doctors often recommend active skin care treatment for wrinkles. Active skin care creams contain one or more of six ingredients that do more than just moisturize the skin. They also help reduce wrinkles, make skin look brighter and more youthful, and stimulate fibroblasts (connective tissue cells that make collagen), which helps reduce fine lines and blotches.

Using an "active agent" helps hydrate the skin, says Audrey Kunin, M.D. If your skin still feels dry even after using the active cream with a sunscreen, add a moisturizer, she says.

The ingredients to look for in some product samples are vitamin C (found in many topical creams), GHK copper peptides (Neutrogena Visibly Firm), glycolic acid (Total Skin Care Glycolic Gel), N6 furfuryladenine (Kinerase cream or lotion), alpha lipoic acid (Z. Bigatti Re-Storation Deep Repair Facial Serum), and tretinoin, a vitamin A derivative (RoC Retinol ActifPur Anti-Wrinkle Treatment).

The quality of many fine wines and single-malt scotches improves dramatically with age. Unfortunately, our skin doesn't. Rather, it loses moisture, elasticity, and resiliency as we age, causing it to wrinkle.

Skin undergoes two types of aging, says Coyle S. Connolly, D.O. The first, intrinsic aging, is genetically programmed. You can't do much about that without the help of a dermatologist. The second—extrinsic aging, or photoaging—is the result of damage primarily from too much sun.

You can fight photoaging every step of the way by making smart choices. Here's what the experts advise to keep wrinkles—those reminders of how much mileage you have on your odometer—from taking too much of a toll on your skin.

- **SLEEP ON YOUR BACK.** Sleeping on one side or the other or on your belly with your face mashed into the pillow causes wrinkles, says Dr. Connolly. Some stomach sleepers develop a diagonal crease on their foreheads, running above their eyebrows. Sleeping on your back may eliminate this problem.

- **HOLD YOUR HEAD UP.** Don't let leaning on your hands become a habit. The constant pressure may lead to wrinkling, says Dr. Connolly.

- **WEAR SUNGLASSES.** One real problem area for wrinkles is around the eyes. These wrinkles, called crow's-feet, often result from squinting. One way to avoid them or lessen their severity is to wear sunglasses whenever you go outside. A pair of UV-coated glasses can also protect your eyes from a type of melanoma that can form at the back of the eye, says Audrey Kunin, M.D.

■ **RELAX YOUR FACIAL MUSCLES.** Excessive frowning or smiling, or any other much-repeated facial expression, deepens wrinkles.

For the same reason, experts advise *against* facial exercises. Facial exercises build facial muscles just like biceps curls build biceps, says Dr. Kunin. Normal, everyday repeated movements cause enough wrinkles. Smiling causes crow's-feet, frowns result in deep crevices between your brows, and lifting your brows in surprise leaves you with lines across your forehead.

■ **QUIT SMOKING.** Smoking makes your skin age faster, says Dr. Connolly. And for several reasons. It robs your complexion of oxygen and important nutrients and damages the collagen fibers that keep your skin firm and elastic. Constantly pursing your lips to inhale and squinting your eyes to avoid the smoke contribute even more premature wrinkles. But it's not only your facial skin that suffers from a tobacco habit. A recent study at the University of Michigan suggests smoking is linked to skin aging, even in the upper inner arms.

■ **BE SUN SMART.** Most wrinkles are the result of too much sun. Today's tan leads to tomorrow's wrinkles, whether it's achieved indoors or outside. "Obviously, excessive exposure to sunlight is going to increase your chances of developing wrinkles," says Dr. Kunin. Wear your sunscreen, preferably with a sun protection factor (SPF) of 30 and with

both ultraviolet (UV) A and B protection (also known as broad-spectrum). Dr. Kunin recommends titanium oxide or zinc oxide.

Dr. Connolly couldn't agree more: "I cannot overemphasize the need to use sunscreen every day. That means on cloudy days and in winter months, not just in summer." Apply sunscreen first thing in the morning whenever you're going to go outside, even on cloudy days. If you have dry skin, look for a sunscreen that contains a moisturizer. The moisturizer in the sunscreen plumps the skin and helps prevent overdrying, says Dr. Connolly.

■ **WASH IN SUNBLOCK.** Rit Sun Guard is sun protection for your skin that you wash into your clothing. "This product increases the capability of fabric to prevent UV rays from reaching the skin and is the relative equivalent of an SPF 30 rating for sunscreen," says Dr. Kunin.

Simply add it to the wash cycle, rinse, and dry your clothes as usual. One treatment of Rit Sun Guard is good for more than 20 washings, says Dr. Kunin. "Normally, clothing has an SPF of 4, making it worthless when it comes to screening out the longer UVA rays. While these rays may not cause a sunburn like UVB, they are more likely to cause skin damage that leads to wrinkles and skin cancer down the road," she says.

■ **BAN TANNING BEDS.** Twenty minutes of tanning-bed use is equivalent to an entire day at the beach without sunscreen. Avoid them like the plague to keep from damaging

your skin, suggests Dr. Kunin. "If you want to look tan, use a self-tanner lotion and perhaps a bronzer with your makeup foundation," she says.

■ **WEAR A HAT.** Whether you're heading to the beach or spending extended time in the midday sun, put on a hat with a 4-inch-wide brim to keep the sun off your face and neck, says Dr. Kunin.

But steer clear of straw hats that are unlined and loosely woven. They allow the sun's rays to penetrate directly through the hat. Also keep in mind that baseball caps don't protect your ears, the back of your neck, or even most of your face from full-bore sun.

Choose a hat with an extra-long bill and sun-protective cloth inside, says Dr. Kunin. "It gives you the extra protection you need to limit your chances of developing wrinkles."

■ **STAY OUT OF THE MIDDAY SUN.** That's 10:00 a.m. to 4:00 p.m. during spring, summer, and fall, or 10:00 a.m. to 2:00 p.m. during winter. These peak hours are when the ultraviolet radiation is the strongest.

■ **BE A SHADY PERSON.** Wrinkles are caused by excessive sun exposure, so periodically retreat to a shady spot on sunny days. At the beach or in your backyard, sit under a large umbrella. While on hikes or on the water, if it's not too hot out, wear tightly woven clothing. It helps keep UV rays off your skin.

■ **USE MOISTURIZER.** If you have dry skin, daily use of a moisturizer can plump up your skin and temporarily hide smaller wrinkles that form on the skin surface, says Dr. Connolly. "It's not a long-term solution for wrinkles, but it will give your skin a healthier look."

■ **GIVE ME A "C."** Apply a topical vitamin C cream or ointment on a daily basis. You'll notice a marked improvement in your skin's overall quality, says Dr. Connolly. "Vitamin C creams help build collagen and gobble up free radicals, which if left unchecked will cause your skin to age or wrinkle," he says. Vitamin C creams and ointments are available over-the-counter in many drugstores.

■ **RELY ON RETINOL.** Apply retinol creams at night to fill out lines. Retinol creams are weaker and gentler than prescription Retin-A, says Dr. Connolly. They may be a little drying, so use them every other night if redness or excessive dryness occurs, he adds.

■ **SLOUGH OFF THE CELLS.** Alpha hydroxy acids (AHAs), found in plants and fruits, are available in creams, lotions, and gels. They act by defoliating dead skin cells on the surface to uncover the younger cells underneath. And they fill in the areas that cause wrinkles. Glycolic acid is the most common AHA, and there are fragrance-free versions of AHAs for sensitive skin around the eyes.

If your skin is too sensitive for AHAs, you might try beta hydroxy acids (BHAs), such as salicylic acid. It's available in moisturizers and cleaners, and it exfoliates the skin like an AHA but with less irritation.

■ **DINE ON FISH AND FLAX.** Two dietary adjustments can help to maintain proper skin moisture. Eat fish such as salmon, trout, sardines, and tuna, which are rich in omega-3 fatty acids, at least twice a week to help replenish moisture to dry skin. Flax oil, which also is loaded with omega-3s, can be mixed into fruit juice or drizzled on salad and vegetables. It is perishable, so it must be refrigerated.

■ **PUT ON SOME PAPAYA.** Try using a papaya peel twice a month. The same protein-eating enzymes that make this tropical fruit a good digestive agent can also break down your outer layer of skin. Grind 2 tablespoons of washed and peeled papaya in a food processor, and add 1 tablespoon of dry oatmeal (the oatmeal helps remove debris from the skin). Pat this mixture onto clean skin and let it set for 10 minutes. Then remove it with a wet washcloth, wiping in an outward, circular motion.

PANEL OF ADVISORS

COYLE S. CONNOLLY, D.O., IS A DERMATOLOGIST AND ASSISTANT CLINICAL PROFESSOR AT THE PHILADELPHIA COLLEGE OF OSTEOPATHIC MEDICINE AND PRESIDENT OF CONNOLLY DERMATOLOGY IN LINWOOD, NEW JERSEY.

AUDREY KUNIN, M.D., IS A COSMETIC DERMATOLOGIST IN KANSAS CITY, MISSOURI, THE FOUNDER OF THE DERMATOLOGY EDUCATIONAL WEB SITE WWW. DERMADOCTOR.COM, AND AUTHOR OF *THE DERMA-DOCTOR SKINSTRUCTION MANUAL.*

First Aid for Medical Emergencies

WHEN LIGHTNING STRIKES

In most major disasters, it's common practice for emergency personnel to temporarily bypass those show no signs of life and tend to the wounded instead. But according to Robin Peavler, M.D., a lightning strike is a different animal.

"Say that you're at a sporting event and lightning strikes a section of metal bleachers," Dr. Peavler says. "Contrary to what you might think, you treat those who aren't breathing first. A lightning strike stuns the diaphragm, and often a little mouth-to-mouth resuscitation is all that's needed to bring the person back."

As this book has shown, you can treat any number of minor injuries and illnesses on your own, often using remedies you already have on hand. A medical emergency, however, ups the ante. In this case, the care you provide while you wait for emergency medical personnel to arrive can make all the difference in the outcome. Doing as much advance preparation as possible can help you stay calm and act confidently no matter what the circumstances.

In fact, one of the best things you can do to prepare for a medical emergency—and our team of experts is in universal agreement on this—is take a community first-aid course. Nothing beats hands-on training for learning the necessary skills. Your local hospital or American Red Cross chapter can provide information about classes available in your area.

With the strategies here, you'll be able to navigate the most common medical emergencies in a pinch. Just bear in mind that you're dealing with a genuine emergency, requiring urgent medical attention. You should call 9-1-1 or have someone call for you while you're administering care. Your task is to stabilize the illness or injury and then monitor the situation until EMTs or hospital personnel can take over.

WOUNDS

Even the toughest among us tend to get squeamish at the sight of blood, which is usually the biggest problem with any sort of flesh wound. The person might get woozy and pass out, which would complicate matters even more, says Robin Peavler, M.D. That's why Dr. Peavler's first piece of advice for treating a wound is to keep the person relaxed. Encourage him to stay calm by taking a few deep breaths. If he's standing and he becomes light-headed, ask him to sit down.

To treat the wound itself, follow these tips.

■ **APPLY PRESSURE.** Using a clean, dry cloth, apply firm pressure directly over the wound for 10 minutes, advises Mark Levine, M.D. This should help stop the bleeding. "Don't use so much pressure that it hurts you or the person," Dr. Levine says. "And be sure to keep it on for the full 10 minutes. People tend to check the wound every 30 seconds or so, which doesn't really help stop the bleeding."

■ **CHECK THE WOUND.** After 10 minutes, remove the cloth and check the wound. "If it's still spurting blood, cover it up and call for help," Dr. Peavler says. This time, he adds, try leaving the cloth in place for 30 minutes.

■ **CLEAN THE WOUND.** If the wound has stopped bleeding, your next step is to flush it with clean water, Dr. Levine says. If any debris remain that you can easily remove, do so with a pair of tweezers that you've sterilized with alcohol.

■ **HEAD TO THE HOSPITAL.** If you're unsure whether the wound is severe enough to require medical care, it's best to err on the side of caution, Dr. Peavler says. In general, any wound that is more than ¼-inch deep, has jagged edges, or has muscle or fat protruding from it will need stitches to heal properly. "Another area of concern is tingling or numbness away from the site of the cut," Dr. Levine says. "For example, if person says he can't feel his fingers after getting a cut on his arm, he definitely needs medical attention."

■ **DON'T USE A TOURNIQUET.** Many people assume, incorrectly, that a more serious wound calls for a tourniquet. The reality is that a tourniquet can damage surrounding tissue by cutting off bloodflow, Dr. Peavler notes. "I'd use a tourniquet only if I were dealing with a severed limb," he says. In such a situation, you'd wrap a clean cloth—even a T-shirt or handkerchief will do—close to the wound and twist it tightly. A first aid course will provide more guidance here.

BROKEN BONES

Broken bones account for nearly 7 million doctor or hospital visits every year, which means the odds are good that you'll encounter one at some point. But a break isn't always obvious. Hip fractures are common among the elderly, for example, but they frequently go undetected. If an elderly person takes a tumble, look at her hips and legs. "If the hips are sideways and the legs are different lengths, then it's a broken hip," Dr. Peavler says. In that case, you should call for help immediately.

Any broken bone requires prompt medical attention. Here's what to do while you wait for help.

■ **APPLY ICE.** For a less severe break, a bag of ice can do wonders to ease the pain and swelling. Leave the ice on the break for as long as it feels comfortable.

■ **ASSESS WHETHER TO MOVE THE PERSON.** The conventional wisdom is to not attempt to move someone who's suffered a broken bone. In reality, it's more of a judgment call, Dr. Peavler says. If the person has a broken arm, for example, but is okay otherwise, then he or she probably can tolerate being driven to the hospital. A broken leg, hip, back, or neck is an altogether different story; in this case, the person should be immobilized while you wait for help.

■ **MAKE A BRACE.** A broken bone in an arm or leg can cause tremendous pain if allowed to shift around. You can prevent this from happening by fashioning a splint for the limb. "Even a rolled-up magazine can work in a pinch," Dr. Peavler says. You can tie the splint in place above and below the break with strips of cloth.

UNCONSCIOUSNESS

Watching someone faint or lose consciousness can be especially scary, because unless the person has a known medical condition, you can't be sure what caused the episode in the first place. This is a situation in which medical attention is absolutely necessary, even if the person comes to after a few minutes. You can help by doing the following.

■ **IF POSSIBLE, GET THE PERSON INTO THE PROPER POSITION.** The objective here is to keep blood flowing to the brain. This means putting the person flat on her back, with her feet slightly elevated on a pillow or rolled-up towel, Dr. Peavler says. Of course, you should do this only if you witness the person's collapse and you're reasonably confident that he or she doesn't have any broken bones. Otherwise, you could do more harm than good.

■ **CHECK THE VITALS.** Make sure the person is breathing and has a pulse. You can do this by listening and watching for signs of respiration, and by feeling the carotid artery on either side of the neck. (Try finding your own now, using the index and middle fingers of either hand to press gently on the side of your neck.) This is where training in rescue breathing and CPR can come in handy.

■ **CONSIDER THE POSSIBILITY OF HEART ATTACK OR STROKE.** If the person has a known history of heart trouble, this could be to blame for the current medical crisis. Ask yourself, has the person been complaining of other symptoms? The classic symptom of a heart attack is prolonged pain or tightness in the chest (lasting 5 to 10 minutes), accompanied by shortness of breath and sweating, Dr. Peavler notes. Tingling pain on one side of the body may foretell a stroke.

Be sure to inform the EMTs or emergency-room personnel of any other symptoms leading up to the person's collapse, as well as any underlying medical problems. But don't be surprised if the cause of the collapse turns out to be something else entirely. "The symptoms of heart attack or stroke can be very difficult to interpret," says Stephen Schenkel, M.D. "Unfortunately, heart attacks don't read text-books."

■ **WATCH FOR VOMITING.** If the person begins to vomit while lying on his or her back, it can obstruct his or her airways and lead to choking. In this situation, "very carefully roll the person's body as a single unit onto one side," Dr. Peavler says. "Then clean out the mouth and check that the person is still breathing."

BREATHING TROUBLE

For someone who is having difficulty breathing, a "watch and wait" approach is best. Call for help, and then stay with the person to monitor his or her condition. Here, too, a bit of fact-finding can help the EMTs target a response once they arrive on the scene. You can start by looking for clues in the person's health history.

■ **IN AN INFANT OR TODDLER, CONSIDER CROUP AS A CAUSE.** Common in children under age 5, croup is characterized by a harsh cough that's reminiscent of a seal barking. "The sound freaks out parents, but it usually isn't that big of a deal," Dr. Peavler says. "Some-times the parents will be getting ready to take the child to the hospital, and as soon as they hit the cool air outdoors, the cough subsides." Running a humidifier or holding the child upright can help as well. If the cough doesn't clear in a few days, though, it's time to see a doctor.

■ **PAY ATTENTION FOR INSECT STINGS.** Getting stung by a bee or wasp is painful for anyone. For some, though, a sting can trigger what's known as anaphylactic shock, in which the immune system overreacts by flooding the body with antibodies. This hyper-response can lead to difficulty breathing and severe swelling, among a number of other frightening symptoms.

If the person has been stung and is known to be allergic to stings, ask whether he or she has an EpiPen. This device delivers a small shot of epinephrine that can prevent full-blown anaphylaxis. In the absence of an EpiPen, an antihistamine such as Benadryl can be an effective substitute.

If anaphylaxis has an upside, it's that the first episode may not be quite so severe, as the body is still trying to figure out how to react to the sting, Dr. Schenkel says. It doesn't always play out this way, he adds, but it's a possibility. If the person complains of other symptoms besides difficulty breathing, such as tingling in the ears or an all-over sick feeling, he or she should see an allergist once the current medical crisis passes. The next time, the reaction could be much worse.

■ **ASK ABOUT ASTHMA.** Adult-onset asthma is becoming more common, and the first episode can be especially frightening to someone who hasn't experienced it before. If the person doesn't have a history of asthma, he or she should see a doctor for proper diagnosis and treatment—usually consisting of an inhaler or another medication.

POISONING

Poisoning is more common among children than adults. But a child may be too sick or too frightened to tell you what's wrong. Look for symptoms such as an unusual odor coming from the child's mouth, redness or irritation around the mouth, vomiting, and confusion or sleepiness. That said, if you have any reason to suspect poisoning, don't second-guess yourself in the absence of symptoms. This is a situation where you'd rather be safe than sorry.

■ **CALL FOR HELP.** Before you do anything else, grab the phone and dial 1-800-222-1222, which is the national toll-free hotline for the American Association of Poison Control Centers. "Your call will automatically be routed to the center in your area," Dr. Schenkel says. "The centers are staffed by trained professionals who are very good at walking you through what to do."

■ **READ THE LABEL.** If you spot an open or empty bottle, the label may provide instructions for what to do in case of ingestion. Read this information carefully.

■ **REMOVE THE POISON.** If you're able, remove any remaining poison from the mouth, taking care not to push any of it into the child's throat. If the substance is on the child's skin or in his or her eyes, flush it away with cool water. Taking the child outside into fresh air may help, too.

■ **BUT DO *NOT* INDUCE VOMITING.** As Dr. Peavler explains, some poisons—such as gasoline and wood finishes—can cause more damage coming up than they did going down. That's why you should never induce vomiting. Along the same line, don't give the child ipecac syrup, which is an emetic (or vomit inducer).

CHOKING

You may have heard of something called the universal sign for choking: arms crossed over the chest, hands clutched to the throat. Of course, someone who's choking may not think to use the sign. That's why you should watch for other warning signs, such as an inability to talk, cough, or breathe—all indicators of an obstructed airway—or a blue tinge to the lips or face.

By far the best technique for clearing an obstructed airway is the Heimlich maneuver. But it needs to be done properly to ensure both your safety and the safety of the person whom you're trying to help. Here's what you need to know.

■ **GO FIVE-AND-FIVE.** Most experts recommend alternating the Heimlich maneuver with back blows. To perform the back blows, stand behind the person and strike him or her between the shoulder blades with the heel of your hand. Repeat five times, and then follow up with five Heimlich. Continue the five-and-five sequence until you dislodge the food or object from the airway.

■ **USE PROPER TECHNIQUE.** For the Heimlich maneuver to be effective, you need to do it the right way. The person should bend forward slightly, with you still standing behind. Make a fist with one hand and position it just above the person's navel. Place your other hand on top of your fist, then push in and up. "Pushing up slightly forces the air outward," Dr. Peavler explains.

Incidentally, you can perform the Heimlich on yourself, if there's no one around to help you. Just lean against a countertop, table, or another hard surface with your fist on your abdomen as above. By pressing against the surface, you thrust your fist in and upward.

■ **CHANGE YOUR STRATEGY, IF NECESSARY.** If the person should go unconscious while you're administering back blows and Heimlichs, carefully lower him or her to the floor. Then continue trying to dislodge the food or object by switching to chest compressions, just as for CPR. (If you enroll in a CPR course, you'll learn how to handle choking emergencies as well.)

"A person who goes unconscious tends to relax, which may make it easier to remove the obstruction from the airway," Dr. Peavler says. Look inside the person's mouth for the food or object; if you see it, try to hook it with your finger, taking care not to push it into the throat.

PANEL OF ADVISORS

MARK LEVINE, M.D., IS AN EMERGENCY ROOM PHYSICIAN AT BARNES-JEWISH HOSPITAL IN ST. LOUIS, MISSOURI.

ROBIN PEAVLER, M.D., IS A BOARD-CERTIFIED EMERGENCY PHYSICIAN AT EPHRAIM MCDOWELL REGIONAL HOSPITAL IN DANVILLE, KENTUCKY.

STEPHEN SCHENKEL, M.D., IS CHIEF OF EMERGENCY MEDICINE AT MERCY MEDICAL CENTER IN BALTIMORE.

A Home Remedy First-Aid Kit

A first aid kit filled with bandages, ointment, tweezers, and other necessities is just what you want to have on hand to tend to minor medical emergencies. (For more details on assembling your own first-aid kit, visit the Ready America Web site at www.ready. gov). But a more unconventional kit—consisting of household items like cayenne powder and apple cider vinegar—can be helpful in certain situations.

With guidance from Gayle Eversole, Ph.D., N.D., founder and director of the Creating Health Institute and The Oake Centre for natural health education in Moscow, we've put together a "home remedy" first-aid kit that's meant as a complement to your conventional kit. Here's what you'll want inside.

■ **CAYENNE POWDER.** Just a little cayenne powder mixed with hot water can help stop bleeding, soothe ulcers, fight colds and flu, and clear chest congestion. Dr. Eversole recommends 35,000 heat unit, non-irradiated cayenne powder.

■ **LAVENDER OR TEA TREE OIL.** Both of these oils have antiviral, antibacterial, and antifungal properties. You can use either one to soothe scrapes and burns, as well as reduce the stinging and swelling of bug bites. Just apply the undiluted oil directly to the skin.

■ **APPLE CIDER VINEGAR.** You can mix a teaspoon in a glass of water to soothe an upset stomach; make a 50/50 solution with water and spray on sunburned skin; or soak a bandage in the same solution and wrap around a sprained ankle.

■ **PEPPERMINT TEA.** A cup of tea can ease a headache, soothe an upset stomach, and reduce tension. Diluted, it can even soothe a baby's colic.

■ **GINGER.** It's known as a stomach soother, and rightfully so. Ginger is great for just about any gastrointestinal symptoms, including motion sickness and morning sickness during pregnancy. Make a tea by steeping a tablespoon of ground fresh ginger in hot water for 10 minutes, then straining.

■ **CAROB POWDER.** A tablespoon of this powder can quell diarrhea symptoms. Just add a dash of cinnamon and mix it into water or milk.

■ **MILD LIQUID SOAP.** You want a mild, natural, nonantibacterial soap on hand for cleaning cuts and scrapes. Dr. Eversole recommends Dr. Bronner's Baby Mild Liquid Soap (www.drbronner.com).

Home Remedies for Dogs and Cats

Anyone who has ever brought home a cuddly puppy or a rambunctious kitten knows the joy of pet ownership. And their numbers are rising. According to the 2007 edition of the American Veterinary Medical Association's *U.S. Pet Ownership and Demographics Sourcebook*, there are 82 million pet cats in America and 72 million pet dogs.

Unfortunately, loyalty and playfulness aren't the only things pets bring into the home. Along with the fun may come a variety of unpleasant surprises: skunk odor and fleas, to name just two. The good news is that a host of old-fashioned home remedies and safe new products can protect you and your pet from many common problems. Here's what the experts recommend.

SKUNK STINK SOLUTIONS

Skunks are nocturnal, so chances are your pet's encounter with one of the brazen, odoriferous black-and-white critters will occur at night, when pet stores and dog-grooming parlors are closed. Even though there are a variety of commercial products that make skunk odor disappear, there are also several homemade remedies that you can use right away. For best results, try them outside (if weather permits).

■ **START WITH THE FACE.** Dogs usually get sprayed in the face, which is why certified dog trainer Steve Brooks starts by washing out his dog's eyes with a saline solution. "This will prevent irritation and help keep your dog calm," he says.

■ **GET READY TO RUMBLE.** Before you go toe-to-toe with this nasty stench, you'll want to take some precautions to keep it off yourself, says Brooks. If you're handling a dog, gather some old towels, an apron, a smock, and rubber gloves, and put them on before the bathing begins.

■ **USE THEM ALL AT ONCE.** If you're a dog owner, you have no doubt heard a grocery list of ways to deal with "skunk stink." Tomato juice? Check. Vinegar-and-water douche? Check. Even mouthwash and dishwashing liquid make it onto many people's lists.

The reality, explains Brooks, is that they *all* work well. "There's a reason everybody talks about all these different remedies, and that's because they're all effective," he says.

Of course, skunk stench is a powerful opponent, so no matter what you use, it's going to take several rinses to get it all out. That's why Brooks takes the novel approach of rinsing with all of them—or at least as many as he has handy. "I think that the tomato juice works best, so I'll start there and rub the dog down well," he says. "Then I rinse that off and follow with vinegar. Then I'll use tomato juice again, and try mouthwash or dishwashing liquid the next time. But I apply tomato juice for every other step."

■ **FOLLOW UP.** Even after rinsing your dog four or five times, Brooks recommends repeating the routine the next day. "There's no

sugar-coating it," he says. "It takes persistence to get rid of that smell."

■ **TRY A HOMEMADE SOLUTION.** Another stink stopper that can be whipped up from items you might have on hand comes from Jean Hofve, D.V.M. She recommends mixing 1 quart of 3 percent hydrogen peroxide, 1 teaspoon of dishwashing liquid, and a $\frac{1}{4}$ cup of baking soda. "Wear eye protection when you mix these together because when you add the baking soda, it will fizz," she says. "Sponge it on the dog immediately while the mix bubbles. Really drench the most skunky areas. Lather it up, leave it on for a few minutes, and rinse thoroughly."

■ **GO WITH A COMMERCIAL PREPARATION.** If your dog gets skunked a lot, you might want to look into commercially available products for de-stinking. Ann Hohenhaus, D.V.M., recommends a product called Skunk-Off. "This works great, and, as an aside, it also works well to help remove the smell from anal glands," she says.

■ **SECURE THE PERIMETER.** Once you finally get that awful smell to go away, the best way to stop the problem is to make your yard a skunk-free zone. There are several strategies to take, explains Brooks. First, don't leave out any food or trash. Second, try placing rags soaked with ammonia or sprinkled with human hair around your yard. "For some reason, these things seem to scare away rodents," he says.

Finally, if you have a skunk trapped under a porch or house, Brooks recommends leaving an escape hatch for the skunk. "Go to the end of the porch opposite it's exit route, and place a radio playing loud music there," he says. "This should scare it out."

FREEDOM FROM FLEAS

Fleas are as prolific as they are resilient. Consider the facts. In 9 months, the time it takes to make one human baby, two fleas can generate *millions* of descendants. Adult fleas live 1 to 2 months on pets; they can survive the most frigid winters; and immature fleas can go 6 to 12 months without eating. But they're more than a simple nuisance: Fleas can cause anemia in pets and transmit disease and parasites.

Given all this, it's no surprise that people have long been working on the perfect flea fighter. Unfortunately, several of the most commonly known flea remedies don't work, and some of them can be downright dangerous to your pets. "There are several urban myths regarding oral flea repellants, including Brewer's yeast, garlic, and apple cider vinegar," says Cori Gross, D.V.M. "The general consensus among veterinarians is that these remedies don't work very well. Garlic can be toxic in high doses, leading to a life-threatening anemia, and vinegar can lead to gastrointestinal upset."

The other thing to be wary of are flea collars. "Flea collars do not work," says Dr. Gross. "They just make the fleas jump away from the collar, down to the animal's rump!" Luckily, there are plenty of simple successful flea-fighting strategies.

■ **GROOM YOUR PET FREQUENTLY.** Rather than relying on gimmicks, the best approach is to brush your pet often, using a flea comb that traps the insects and keeps them from jumping off. "As you comb, pull fleas off the pet, dip the comb into hot soapy water, and slide the fleas off into the water," says Dr. Gross. Another approach, says Brooks, is to brush your pet as it stands on a white sheet, or shine a flashlight on the pet's coat so you can easily see any fleas.

■ **KEEP BATH TIME SIMPLE.** Bathing your pet is another way to control fleas, but contrary to what you may think, you don't need fancy shampoos and rinses. "Giving your pet a bath will drown fleas, but frequent bathing or harsh soaps can damage the skin," says Dr. Hofve. "Mild shampoo is just as effective and less toxic than those designed to kill fleas."

The key, says Brooks, is to soak the dog in the water long enough to take care of all the fleas. Ten minutes ought to do the trick.

■ **RELY ON AVON.** To keep fleas from coming back, several experts recommend Avon's Skin-So-Soft bath oil. Long used by women as a luxuriating bath soak, it also seems to make fleas flee from your dog. Just spray it on once a week.

■ **DON'T GIVE FIDO'S PRODUCTS TO FLUFFY.** Whatever product you decide to use to rid your pets of fleas, just be very careful that they don't end up in the wrong paws. "Never, ever use a product made for dogs on a cat," says Dr. Hofve. "Ingredients that are safe for dogs can be fatal to cats."

■ **CLEAN OUT THE HOUSE.** If you found some fleas, they're not confined to your pets—your house is going to need a good cleaning, too. Our experts recommend sprinkling the floor with borax, letting it set for a few hours, and then vacuuming it up.

■ **SUPERCHARGE YOUR VACUUM.** If the fleas somehow make it through this gauntlet in one piece, Dr. Hofve has a surefire way to stop them in their tracks. "To keep them from hatching or escaping, discard the bag immediately, or use a flea spray in the vacuum bag or container," she says.

■ **DEBUG THE BEDDING.** Your pet's bedding is another likely hiding spot, so be sure to wash it all in hot, soapy water to get rid of any fleas that may be shacked up there, says Dr. Gross.

■ **GET THEM AT NIGHT.** Even after all of this, the craftiest of fleas may still find a good hiding spot in your house. Brooks has a solution for rooting them out. He recommends waiting until night, and then placing a candle in the middle of a pan of water. "The fleas will be attracted to the light and will get trapped in the water," he says. "You can also use a fluorescent light in the middle of a piece of fly paper if you're worried about the fire hazard from the candle."

■ **TAKE CARE OF THE YARD.** If your pets have fleas, they had to pick them up somewhere, and your yard is a likely spot. One strategy that Dr. Hofve employs to control fleas in your yard is to sprinkle a safe, natural pesticide known as "diatomaceous earth" under bushes, decks, and other shady areas where animals hang out. "These measures will help control flea populations outdoors—and minimize the number of critters hitching a ride in on your dog," she says.

■ **KEEP CATS INSIDE.** Dr. Hofve's final flea-fighting strategy is also the easiest. "Just keep your cat indoors," she says. "It's safer—for many reasons!"

TICK TALK

Ticks suck blood from warm-blooded creatures. They can spread Rocky Mountain spotted fever, Lyme disease, and ehrlichiosis. The good news is that ticks are easier to control than fleas.

■ **GROOM THEM AWAY.** After your dog comes in from the fields or woods, go over him with a fine-toothed flea comb, says Richard Pitcairn, D.V.M., Ph.D. This helps catch ticks that haven't attached themselves yet. Concentrate on the neck and head, and in and around the ears. Ticks love to burrow in these areas because they are warm and protected.

■ **PULL THEM OUT.** If you should find a tick already attached, clean your hands, the area around the site of the bite, and a pair of tweezers with disinfectant. Use your fingers if you wear latex gloves. Grab the tick as close to your pet's skin as possible, then pull gradually and slightly twist. If you pull slowly, you will get the head out, too. But if you don't, it's not a major concern. Leaving the head embedded may cause a minor inflammation, but it clears up rapidly, Dr. Pitcairn says. Be sure to wash your hands thoroughly after removing a tick.

TAME UNWELCOME MATS

Anyone who has furry friends knows that hair mats happen, and the best way to avoid them is with regular and frequent brushing. Even then, some will develop. When your pet gets tangles, here's what you need to know.

■ **BRUSH SLOWLY.** The main thing you want to do is prevent any pain to your pet. So Dr. Gross recommends brushing at the mat gently and slowly, starting at the base of the hair and working your way out.

■ **SHAVE, DON'T CUT.** If that won't work, take a pair of clippers and shave out the mat, says Dr. Gross. "Never attempt to cut the hair out with scissors," she says. "Mats pull up on the skin, so its easy to cut the skin while trying to cut out the mat."

■ **BUY A BETTER BRUSH.** For preventing future mats, Dr. Hofve recommends getting the right kind of brush. "Many brushes tend to skim over the surface of the fur and don't get to the dead hair underneath," she says. "A wire-toothed slicker brush, metal comb, or a product like the Furminator will make the job easier."

■ **ADD SOME OMEGA-3S.** A pet food supplemented with omega-3 fatty acids will keep the skin and coat healthy, says Dr. Hofve. Several pet foods are supplemented with omega-3 fatty acids. Just be sure to check the label.

■ **RELY ON YOUR GROOMER.** If all else fails, it's best to head to the groomer or veterinarian to remove mats rather than risk hurting your pet. "Worst case, your vet may need to sedate the pet to deal with a major disaster," says Dr. Hofve. "A mild sedative will reduce both the time and the stress of mat removal—which is especially important for cats and many small dogs."

STICKER SOLUTIONS

Most of the time, prickly stickers that get caught in your pet's fur are just an annoyance. They're a hassle to remove, and if you leave them in, they can mat fur. But sometimes they're more hazardous. Foxtails, for instance, can literally burrow their way into ears and through skin and body openings, causing severe infections, Dr. Pitcairn says. That's why removing stickers is essential.

■ **COMB OR BRUSH THEM OUT.** Use a metal comb with wide teeth to pull stickers out of fur before matting begins. Hold the comb against the skin to make the grooming easier.

■ **USE YOUR FINGERS.** If there are only a few stickers or if they are in the ears or between the toes, use your fingers to pull them out. (If this job is bothersome, just think, at least they're not ticks!) If the sticker is too deep in the ear for you to reach, however, don't try to remove it. You may push it right through the eardrum, Dr. Pitcairn warns. Instead, put some vegetable or mineral oil in the ear to soften the sticker and take your pet to the veterinarian as soon as possible.

EVICT EAR MITES

Pets with ear mites scratch their ears frequently, especially if the ear is touched. If you look down the ear canal, you'll see dark, dry debris, like coffee grounds. In most animals the infestation will clear up even without treatment. "If it doesn't, then it may indicate a low level of health in the animal," says Dr. Pitcairn.

Ear mites can be confused with excessively waxy and irritated ears, a whole different thing from ear mites. "Waxy ears will have a lot of moist, brown, and oily substance—excessive ear wax—instead of the dry 'coffee-ground' look," says Dr. Pitcairn.

Although prescription medication is a common method of attack, Dr. Pitcairn recommends these natural remedies.

■ **TRY THE HERB MITE HELPER.** Mix ½ ounce of almond oil and 400 IU of vitamin E in a dropper bottle, Dr. Pitcairn says. Once a day for 3 days put a warmed dropperful or two in each ear and massage the ear well. Let your pet shake its head, then clean out the opening with cotton swabs (don't stick the swab into the ear canal). The oily mixture smothers the mites and helps healing.

■ **SEND YELLOW DOCK TO THE RESCUE.** After 3 days of almond oil treatments, let your pet's ears rest for 3 more days. Then try this approach to inhibit or kill the mites. In 1 pint of boiling water add 1 slightly rounded teaspoon of the herb yellow dock. Remove from the heat, cover tightly, and steep for 30 minutes. Strain, and let cool until the liquid is warm but not hot. Once a day for 3 days, put a warmed dropperful or two in each ear and massage the ear well. Let your pet shake its head, then clean out the opening with cotton swabs (don't stick the swab into the ear canal). Refrigerate the mixture between uses. Let your pet's ears rest for 10 days. Then do another round of 3-day yellow dock treatment.

DEAL WITH DIGESTIVE PROBLEMS

Anyone who has come home from work to find a doggy "accident" on the floor knows how hard they take it, and how embarrassed they are about it. But oftentimes, they just can't help it. Just like people, dogs get sick from time to time. And when we're not there, they have nowhere else to go.

An unexpected accident should also be taken quite seriously, as it could be an indication that your dog is ill, says Susan Nelson, D.V.M. Still, as long as the pet is acting normally and there is no blood in the stool, she says that it's okay to try a few at-home remedies to ease your dog's troubled tummy.

■ **GO WITH SOMETHING BLAND.** Dr. Hohenhaus says that the tried-and-true approach to getting your dog's digestive system back on track is a bland meal. "Feeding a bland diet of boiled chicken and white rice for a day or two and gradually reintroducing the pet's regular diet may resolve the problem," she says. Also, make sure your dog has plenty of water, as diarrhea can be very dehydrating.

■ **TRY SOME YOGURT.** Sometimes taking antibiotics for another reason can leave your dog feeling queasy. In this instance, Dr. Hohenhaus says that a tablespoon of plain yogurt added to your dog's food each day might be the answer. "The healthy bacteria in the yogurt help replenish the normal intestinal bacteria killed by the antibiotic. The bacteria are essential for digestive health," she says.

■ **GIVE PUMPKIN A SHOT FOR CONSTIPATION.** Sometimes your dog's problem isn't keeping it in, but getting it out. And though nobody is quite sure why, canned pumpkin seems to work great for getting your dog's system working again. Brooks uses 1 tablespoon for small dogs and 2 tablespoons for larger dogs.

HELP ACHING HIPS

Dogs are no different than the rest of us—their bones and joints start to ache as they get older. And few things are sadder than seeing your faithful companion struggling to get up to be at your side. Fortunately, there are several easy things you can do at home to ease his pain. Here's what can help.

■ **GIVE GLUCOSAMINE A TRY.** As soon as your pet reaches middle age or shows any sign of stiffness, Dr. Gross says it's time to try oral glucosamine. And if your pet is obese, start incorporating this supplement into its regimen—obese pets have a greater risk of developing arthritis at a younger age. "The dose is 250 milligrams per day for a cat or small dog and 500 milligrams per 25 pounds for large dogs," says Dr. Gross. "For the first 6 weeks, give it twice daily, and then decrease to once daily."

■ **PUT YOUR DOG ON A DIET.** Just like you, the best thing for your dog's health is to lose excess pounds. "The extra weight puts pressure on the joints, causing them to age faster," says Dr. Gross. So make sure you're giving your dog the right amount of food, or try a special weight-loss formula. Most dog food brands have their special version.

■ **BUY THE RIGHT BED.** Beds that are too soft will cause problems for your dog's joints. "Dogs need decent support, or it's harder for them to get up. This is one reason why I don't have a waterbed anymore!" says Dr. Hofve. "For older animals, a heated bed—one made specifically for pets—may be helpful during cold weather."

PANEL OF ADVISORS

STEVE BROOKS IS A CERTIFIED DOG TRAINER AND FOUNDER OF STEVEBROOKSK9U IN LOS ANGELES.

CORI GROSS, D.V.M., IS A FIELD VETERINARIAN FOR VETERINARY PET INSURANCE AND A PRACTICING VETERINARIAN NEAR SEATTLE.

JEAN HOFVE, D.V.M., IS THE FORMER EDITOR IN CHIEF OF THE *JOURNAL OF THE AMERICAN HOLISTIC VETERINARY MEDICAL ASSOCIATION* AND CURRENT PRESIDENT OF THE ROCKY MOUNTAIN HOLISTIC VETERINARY MEDICAL ASSOCIATION.

ANN HOHENHAUS, D.V.M., IS A STAFF VETERINARIAN AT THE ANIMAL MEDICAL CENTER IN NEW YORK CITY.

SUSAN NELSON, D.V.M., IS AN ASSISTANT PROFESSOR OF CLINICAL SCIENCES AT KANSAS STATE UNIVERSITY COLLEGE OF VETERINARY MEDICINE IN MANHATTAN.

RICHARD PITCAIRN, D.V.M., PH.D., IS ON THE STAFF OF THE ANIMAL NATURAL HEALTH CENTER IN EUGENE, OREGON, AND AUTHOR OF *DR. PITCAIRN'S COMPLETE GUIDE TO NATURAL HEALTH FOR DOGS AND CATS.*

Index

Underscored page references indicate boxed text.

Wounds. *See also* Bites, scratches, and stings;
    Cuts and scrapes
    first-aid care for, 633
    promoting healing of, 529–31
Wrinkles, 628–31
Wrist pain. *See* Carpal tunnel syndrome
Wrists
    preventing muscle pain in, 428–29
    strengthening, 472
Wrist splints, for carpal tunnel syndrome, 116

Y

Yawning
    for earache, 232
    temporomandibular disorders and, 586
Yeast infections. *See* Vaginal and yeast infections
    chafing from, 118
    dandruff from, 166
Yellow dock, for ear mites in pets, 645
Yellow jacket stings, 61
Yoga
    preventing neck pain from, 449
    for treating
        chronic back pain, 47
        constipation, 149
        eyestrain, 246
        fatigue, 252
        insomnia, 369
        premenstrual syndrome, 491
        restless legs syndrome, 518
Yogurt
    lactose intolerance and, 392
    for preventing
        canker sores, 111
        urinary tract infections, 607–8

for treating
    bad breath, 49
    diarrhea in pets, 645–46
    irritable bowel syndrome, 374–75
    sunburn, 574
    ulcers, 604

Z

Zinc, for treating
    burnout, 93
    cuts and scrapes, 162
    diabetes, 195
    foot odor, 275
    genital herpes, 285
    prostate problems, 497
    wounds, 530
Zinc lozenges
    for preventing flu, 265
    for treating
        colds, 129
        coughs, 153
Zinc oxide, for treating
    chapped lips, 127
    hives, 343
Zinc solution, for cold sores, 137
Zostavax vaccine, for preventing shingles, 542
Zostrix, for shingles pain, 543
Zovirax, for treating
    cold sores, 136
    genital herpes, 283, 284